C. A. Yankah ■ Y. Weng ■ R. Hetzer ■ (Eds.)

Aortic Root Surgery

C. A. Yankah   Y. Weng   R. Hetzer
(Eds.)

Aortic Root Surgery

The Biological Solution

With 271 Figures in 434 Separate Illustrations,
Most in Color, and 108 Tables

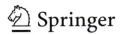

CHARLES A. YANKAH, MD, PhD
Professor of Surgery

YUGUO WENG, MD
Professor of Surgery

ROLAND HETZER, MD, PhD
Chairman,
Professor of Surgery

Deutsches Herzzentrum Berlin
& Charité Medical University Berlin
Augustenburger Platz 1
13353 Berlin, Germany

ISBN 978-3-7985-1868-1 Springer-Verlag Berlin Heidelberg New York

Bibliographic information published by Die Deutsche Nationalbibliothek
Die Deutsche Bibliothek lists this publication in the Deutsche Nationalbibliografie;
detailed bibliographic data is available in the Internet at http://dnb.d-nb.de.

This work is subject to copyright. All rights are reserved, whether the whole or part of the material is concerned, specifically the rights of translation, reprinting, reuse of illustrations, recitation, broadcasting, reproduction on microfilm or in any other way, and storage in data banks. Duplication of this publication or parts thereof is permitted only under the provisions of the German Copyright Law of September 9, 1965, in its current version, and permission for use must always be obtained from Steinkopff Verlag. Violations are liable for prosecution under the German Copyright Law.

Springer Medizin
  Springer-Verlag GmbH, a member of Springer Science+Business Media

springer.de

© Springer-Verlag Berlin Heidelberg 2010
  Printed in Germany

The use of general descriptive names, registered names, trademarks, etc. in this publication does not imply, even in the absence of a specific statement, that such names are exempt from the relevant protective laws and regulations and therefore free for general use.

Product liability: The publishers cannot guarantee the accuracy of any information about the application of operative techniques and medications contained in this book. In every individual case the user must check such information by consulting the relevant literature.

Medical Editor: Dr. Annette Gasser   Production: Klemens Schwind
Cover Design: WMX Design GmbH, Heidelberg
Typesetting: K+V Fotosatz GmbH, Beerfelden

SPIN 80044028   85/7231-5 4 3 – Printed on acid-free paper

To our families and loved ones,
whose unrelenting understanding of the
demands of our surgical and scientific lives
made this book possible

■ Preface

The surgical results of bioprosthetic aortic valve replacement in the 1960s and 1970s were not very satisfactory. The search for the ideal substitute for the diseased aortic valve led Donald Ross to develop the concept of the aortic allograft in 1962 and the pulmonary autograft in 1967 for subcoronary implantation, and later, in 1972, as a full root for replacing the aortic root in the infected aortic valve with a root abscess. The aortic allograft and pulmonary autograft surgical procedures were revolutionary in the history of cardiac valve surgery in the last millennium because they compete well with the bioprosthesis, are nonthrombogenic (thus, requiring no postoperative anticoagulation), are resistant to infection, restore the anatomic units of the aortic or pulmonary outflow tract, and offer unimpeded blood flow and excellent hemodynamics, giving patients a better prognosis and quality of life.

Surgery for congenital, degenerative, and inflammatory aortic valve and root diseases has now reached a high level of maturity; yet an ideal valve for valve replacement is not available. Therefore, surgeons are focusing their skills and their clinical and scientific knowledge on optimizing the technical artistry of valve-sparing procedures. In his honored guest address titled *Cardiac Valve Surgery – the "French correction"* delivered at the 63rd annual meeting of the American Association for Thoracic Surgery, April 25–27, 1983, Professor Alain Carpentier cautiously concluded on the basis of his experience with the first 95 cases of aortic valve repair and root remodeling between 1971 and 1982 that "it is too early to recommend these techniques. However they are a valuable alternative to valve replacement in children" (J Thorac Cardiovasc Surg (1983) 86:323–337). The ensuing 38 years have witnessed the advancement of his techniques of nonthrombogenic aortic valve repair and annuloplasty by Duran, Yacoub, David, and Elkins to become a realistic surgical procedure for selected groups of patients. David furthermore stressed the importance of the aortic sinotubular junction as a stabilizing factor for leaflet coaptation in the aortic root remodeling procedure.

Still the well-known dilemmas remain: on the one hand, the unpredictable durability of aortic valve repair and root remodeling procedures and of biological substitutes but, on the other hand, the need for anticoagulation in mechanical valves that otherwise guarantee long-term functioning. The choice of procedure is determined by the patient's age, metabolic and bleeding disorders, bleeding preconditions and such important issues as the desire to bear children in young women. Our approach has been problem-oriented and is largely based on 23 years' experience of 7000 patients with aortic valve and root diseases at the Deutsches Herzzentrum Berlin.

It is for the busy practitioner that the Berlin Heart Valve Symposium held November 27–30, 2008, was organized, and we are grateful to be able to complement our experience with that from other institutions in chapters for this third symposium volume on *Aortic Root Surgery – The Biologic Solution* by internationally renowned experts in this field.

This volume focuses on current surgical approaches to and evolving trends in aortic valve repair and root remodeling techniques and replacement, the Ross operation, advances in minimally invasive transfemoral and transapical aortic valve replacement, ablation techniques for atrial fibrillation, tissue engineering of heart valves, multimodality imaging, and anticoagulation. The Ross operation has earned an important place in the pediatric and adolescent age group, because of the potential of the pulmonary autograft to grow, whereas the use of aortic allograft has been limited to the reconstruction of the right ventricular outflow tract (RVOT) and to the treatment of complicated active infective endocarditis. Besides cellular allografts and decellularized allografts (SynerGraft, CryoLife Inc. Atlanta, GA, USA), several biological xenografts such as the Contegra bovine jugular vein conduit (Medtronic, Inc., Minneapolis, MN, USA) and the AutoTissue (AutoTissue, Berlin) have been used to reconstruct the RVOT after Ross operation, but none could last for the lifespan of the patient without potential drawbacks. The chapter on tissue engineering discusses the state-of-the-art of decellularized allograft tissue for repopulation of autologous cells to form biocompatible tissue and, therefore, enhance durability in younger age groups. The spectacular innovative minimally invasive transcatheter aortic valve replacement technology with the Edwards Sapien, CoreValve, and Sadra Lotus valves which was pioneered by Cribier, Grube, Webb, Mohr, and Walther is an option that may offer hope to patients who have few or no treatment alternatives because of high operative risks.

We trust that our efforts have resulted in a volume that will provide a highly authoritative reference source for the family practitioner, internist, pediatrician, cardiologist, and cardiovascular nurse and surgeon treating patients with aortic root disease.

Berlin, August 2009
CHARLES A. YANKAH, MD, PhD
YUGUO WENG, MD
ROLAND HETZER, MD, PhD

Contents

Imaging of the aortic root

Perioperative imaging for assessing aortic
and mitral valve diseases and surgical procedures ... 3
M. Kukucka

Innovations in aortic valve surgery

The aortic root 13
C. A. Yankah, M. Pasic, E. Ivanitskaia-Kühn,
J. Kempfert, T. Walther, F. W. Mohr, R. Hetzer

Percutaneous transluminal aortic valve replacement:
The CoreValve prosthesis 22
U. Gerckens, L. Büllesfeld, G. Latsios, R. Müller,
B. Sauren, S. Iversen, E. Grube

Transapical aortic valve implantation
– a truly minimally invasive option
for high-risk patients 32
J. Kempfert, F. W. Mohr, T. Walther

From minimally invasive
to percutaneous aortic valve replacement 46
L. Conradi, H. Treede, H. Reichenspurner

Sutureless equine aortic valve replacement 57
S. Martens

The Ross operation: Aortic valve and root replacement with pulmonary autograft

Pulmonary autograft or aortic allograft for surgical treatment of active infective aortic valve endocarditis: a review of the literature 67
C. A. YANKAH

The Ross operation:
two decades of clinical experience 74
J. F. M. BECHTEL, H.-H. SIEVERS, T. HANKE, U. STIERLE,
A. J. J. J. C. BOGERS, W. HEMMER, J. O. BÖHM, J. G. REIN,
C. A. BOTHA, R. LANGE, J. HÖRER, A. MORITZ, T. WAHLERS,
U. F. W. FRANKE, M. BREUER, K. FERRARI-KÜHNE,
R. HETZER, M. HÜBLER, G. ZIEMER, A. W. GORSKI,
J. J. M. TAKKENBERG, M. MISFELD
on behalf of the German-Dutch Ross Registry

Aortic valve repair and valve sparing root procedures

The bicuspid aortic valve 89
J. F. M. BECHTEL, M. MISFELD, C. SCHMIDTKE,
H.-H. SIEVERS

From dynamic anatomy to conservative
aortic valve surgery: the tale of the ring 102
E. LANSAC, I. DI CENTA

Yacoub/David techniques for aortic root operation:
success and failures 133
J. F. M. BECHTEL, H. H. SIEVERS, T. HANKE, E. I. CHARITOS,
C. SCHMIDTKE, E. G. KRAATZ, U. STIERLE, M. MISFELD

Aortic annuloplasty 144
W. F. NORTHRUP III, S. D. ROLLINS

Correction of aortic valve incompetence
combined with ascending aortic aneurysm
by relocation of the aortic valve plane
through a short-length aortic graft replacement 178
R. HETZER, N. SOLOWJOWA, M. KUKUCKA,
C. KNOSALLA, R. RÖTTGEN

Using BioGlue to achieve hemostasis
in aortic root surgery 185
S. A. LeMaire, J. S. Coselli

Endocarditis

Challenges in the surgical management
of infective endocarditis 195
C.-A. Mestres, J. M. Miró

Clinical results of the Shelhigh® stentless bioprosthesis
in patients with active infective endocarditis:
8-year single center experience 210
M. Musci, Y. Weng, H. Siniawski, S. Kosky, M. Pasic,
M. Hübler, A. Amiri, J. Stein, R. Meyer, R. Hetzer

Double valve endocarditis and evolving
paraannular abscess formation 223
H. Siniawski, M. Dandel, H. B. Lehmkuhl,
C. A. Yankah, R. Hetzer

Aortic root abscess:
reconstruction of the left ventricular outflow tract
and allograft aortic valve and root replacement 243
C. A. Yankah, M. Pasic, H. Siniawski, Y. Weng,
R. Hetzer

Implantation techniques of freehand subcoronary
aortic valve and root replacement with a cryopreserved
allograft for aortic root abscess 274
C. A. Yankah, M. Pasic, Y. Weng, R. Hetzer

Surgery for atrial fibrillation

Cryoablation for the treatment of atrial fibrillation
in patients undergoing minimally invasive mitral valve
surgery – Technique and recent results 291
J. Passage, M. A. Borger, J. Seeburger, A. Rastan,
T. Walther, N. Doll, F. W. Mohr

Minimally invasive endoscopic ablation on the beating
heart in patients with lone atrial fibrillation   302
U. ROSENDAHL, J. ENNKER

Hemodynamic evaluation of the bioprosthetic aortic valves

Evaluation of bioprosthetic valve performance as a
function of geometric orifice area and space efficiency
– a reliable alternative to effective orifice area   313
J. SAUTER

Long-term results of biological valves

Stentless bioprostheses

Stented and stentless aortic bioprostheses:
competitive or complimentary?   341
W. R. E. JAMIESON

Edwards Prima Plus Stentless Bioprosthesis:
long-term clinical and hemodynamic results   346
A. FABBRI, A. D'ONOFRIO, S. AURIEMMA, G. D. CRESCE,
C. PICCIN, A. FAVARO, P. MAGAGNA

The Cryo-Life O'Brian stentless valve: 1991–2008   356
U. HVASS, T. JOUDINAUD

Medtronic stentless Freestyle®
porcine aortic valve replacement   366
J. ENNKER, A. ALBERT, I. FLORATH

The ATS 3f Aortic Bioprosthesis   386
J. L. COX

The Vascutek Elan stentless porcine prosthesis –
the Glasgow experience   396
G. A. BERG, P. SONECKI, R. B. S. BERG, K. J. D. MACARTHUR

Sorin pericardial valves – Operative technique
and early results of biological valves   406
S. BEHOLZ, S. MEYER, N. VON WASIELEWSKI,
W. F. KONERTZ

Stented bioprostheses

The changing role of pericardial tissue
in biological valve surgery: 22 years' experience
with the Sorin Mitroflow stented pericardial valve ...   417
C. A. YANKAH, M. PASIC, J. STEIN, C. DETSCHADES,
H. SINIAWSKI, R. HETZER

20 years' durability of Carpentier-Edwards Perimount
stented pericardial aortic valve   441
E. BERGOËND, M. R. AUPART, A. MIRZA, Y. A. MEURISSE,
A. L. SIRINELLI, P. H. NEVILLE, M. A. MARCHAND

Twenty-year experience with the St. Jude Medical
Biocor bioprosthesis in the aortic position   452
W. EICHINGER

20-Year durability of bioprostheses
in the aortic position   463
W. R. E. JAMIESON

Clinical results including hemodynamic performance
of the Medtronic Mosaic porcine bioprosthesis
up to ten years   470
F.-C. RIESS, R. BADER, E. CRAMER, L. HANSEN,
B. KLEIJNEN, G. WAHL, J. WALLRATH, S. WINKEL,
N. BLEESE

Aortic root replacement
with the BioValsalva prosthesis   487
D. PACINI, R. DI BARTOLOMEO

Valve replacement in renal dialysis patients:
bioprostheses versus mechanical prostheses   498
W. R. E. JAMIESON, V. CHAN

Replacement of bioprostheses
after structural valve deterioration   503
C. A. YANKAH, M. PASIC, H. SINIAWSKI, J. STEIN,
C. DETSCHADES, A. UNBEHAUN, N. SOLOWJOWA,
S. BUZ, Y. WENG, R. HETZER

Predictors of patient's outcome

Predicted outcomes after aortic valve replacement
in octogenarians with aortic stenosis 523
C. Piper, D. Hering, G. Kleikamp, R. Körfer,
D. Horstkotte

Predicted patient outcome after bioprosthetic AVR
and the Ross operation 530
J. J. M. Takkenberg, M. W. A. van Geldorp

Anticoagulation

Anticoagulation and self-management of INR:
mid-term results 541
H. Körtke, J. Gummert

Tissue engineering

Biomatrix-polymer hybrid material
for heart valve tissue engineering 551
C. Stamm, N. Grabow, G. Steinhoff

Standards for the in vitro fabrication of heart valves
using human umbilical cord cells 564
C. Lüders-Theuerkauf, R. Hetzer

Tissue engineering with a decellularized valve matrix   574
W. Konertz, S. Holinski, S. Dushe, A. Weymann,
W. Erdbrügger, S. Posner, M. Stein-Konertz,
P. Dohmen

Regularatory issues on tissue valves

Human tissues for cardiovascular surgery:
regulatory requirements   581
D. M. FRONK, J. D. FERROS

Concluding remarks   588
– Acknowledgments   590
C. A. YANKAH

Atlas of biological valves   591
C. A. YANKAH

Subject index   599

Authors

MATTHIAS BECHTEL, MD, PhD
Universitätsklinikum
Schleswig-Holstein
Campus Lübeck
Klinik für Chirurgie
Ratzeburger Allee 160
23538 Lübeck
Germany

SVEN BEHOLZ, MD, PhD
Cardiovascular Surgery
Charité –
University Medicine Berlin
Charité Place 1
10117 Berlin
Germany

GEOFFREY A. BERG, ChM FRCS
Glasgow Heart and Lung Centre
Golden Jubilee National Hospital
Beardmore Street, Clydebank
West Dunbartonshire G81 4HX
Scotland

ERIC BERGOËND, MD, PhD
Professor of Surgery
Service de chirurgie cardiaque
Hôpital Trousseau
C.H.R.U. de Tours
37000 Tours cedex 9
France

LENARD CONRADI, MD
Universitäres Herzzentrum
Klinik und Poliklinik
für Herz- und Gefäßchirurgie
Martinistrasse 52
20246 Hamburg
Germany

J. S. COSELLI, MD
Professor of Surgery
The Texas Heart Institute
at St. Luke's Episcopal Hospital
and the Division of
Cardiothoracic Surgery
Michael E. DeBakey
Department of Surgery
Baylor College of Medicine
One Baylor Plaza, BCM 390
Houston, Texas 77030
USA

JAMES L. COX, MD
Professor of Surgery
Medical Director
ATS Medical, Inc.
3905 Annapolis Lane, Suite 105
Minneapolis MN 55447
USA

MICHAEL A. BORGER, MD, PhD
Professor of Surgery
Herzzentrum Leipzig
Struempellstrasse 39
04289 Leipzig
Germany

WALTER EICHINGER, MD, PhD
Professor of Surgery
Städtisches Klinikum München
Klinik für Herzchirurgie
im Klinikum München-
Bogenhausen
Englschalkinger Str. 77
81925 München
Germany

JÜRGEN ENNKER, MD, PhD
Professor of Surgery
Klinik für Herz-, Thorax-
und Gefäßchirurgie
Mediclin Herzzentrum
Lahr/Baden
Hohberweg 2
77933 Lahr
Germany

ALESSANDRO FABBRI, MD, PhD
Professor of Surgery
Division of Cardiac Surgery
San Bortolo Vicenza Hospital
Viale Rodolfi 37
36100 Vicenza
Italy

EBERHARD GRUBE, MD, PhD
Chief, Professor of Medicine
Medizinische Klinik
Kardiologie – Angiologie
HELIOS Klinikum Siegburg
Ringstrasse 49
53721 Siegburg
Germany

J. GUMMERT, MD, PhD
Chairman, Professor of Surgery
Herz- und Diabeteszentrum NRW
Klinik für Thorax- und Kardiovaskularchirurgie
Georgstrasse 11
32545 Bad Oeynhausen
Germany

DAVID M. FRONK, PhD
Vice President
Regulatory Affairs and Quality Assurance CryoLife, Inc.
CryoLife, Inc.
1655 Roberts Blvd., NW
Kennesaw, GA 30144
USA

ROLAND HETZER, MD, PhD
Chairman
Professor of Surgery
Deutsches Herzzentrum Berlin
Augustenburger Platz 1
13353 Berlin
Germany

ULRIK HVASS, MD, PhD
Professor of Surgery
Assistance hôpitaux
publique de Paris
Groupe Hospitalier
Bichat Claude Bernard
46, rue Henri-Huchard
75877 Paris Cedex 18
France

W. R. ERIC JAMIESON, MD
Professor of Surgery
3500 Jim Pattison Pavilion
Vancouver General Hospital
899 West 12th Avenue
Vancouver
Canada V5Z1M9

JÖRG KEMPFERT, MD
Universität Leipzig
Herzzentrum
Klinik für Herzchirurgie
Strümpellstrasse 39
04289 Leipzig
Germany

WOLFGANG F. KONERTZ,
MD, PhD
Chairman
Cardiovascular Surgery
Charité –
University Medicine Berlin
Charité Place 1
10117 Berlin
Germany

HEINRICH KÖRTKE, MD, PhD
Herz- und Diabeteszentrum
NRW
Klinik für Thorax- und
Kardiovaskularchirurgie
Georgstrasse 11
32545 Bad Oeynhausen
Germany

MARIAN KUKUCKA, MD
Deutsches Herzzentrum Berlin
Institut für Anästhesiologie
Augustenburger Platz 1
13353 Berlin
Germany

EMMANUEL LANSAC, MD, PhD
Professor of Surgery
Service de chirurgie
cardiovasculaire
Hôpital Foch
40 Rue Worth
92150 Suresnes
France

SCOTT A. LEMAIRE, MD
Professor of Surgery
The Texas Heart Institute
at St. Luke's Episcopal Hospital
and the Division
of Cardiothoracic Surgery
Michael E. DeBakey
Department of Surgery
Baylor College of Medicine
One Baylor Plaza, BCM 390
Houston, Texas 77030
USA

CORA LÜDERS-THEUERKAUF,
PhD
Deutsches Herzzentrum Berlin
Labor für Tissue Engineering
Augustenburger Platz 1
13353 Berlin
Germany

SVEN MARTENS, MD, PhD
Professor of Surgery
Klinik für Thorax-, Herz-
und Thorakale Gefäßchirurgie
Universitätsklinikum Frankfurt
Theodor Stern Kai 7
60590 Frankfurt
Germany

CARLOS-A. MESTRES,
MD, PhD, FETCS
Consultant,
Infectious Diseases Service
Associate Professor of Medicine
Hospital Clinic Universitari
Helios-Villarroel Building
Villarroel, 170
08036-Barcelona
Spain

FRIEDRICH-WILHELM MOHR,
MD, PhD
Chairman, Professor of Surgery
Universität Leipzig
Herzzentrum
Klinik für Herzchirurgie
Strümpellstrasse 39
04289 Leipzig
Germany

MICHELE MUSCI, MD
Deutsches Herzzentrum Berlin
Abt. für Herz-, Thorax-
und Gefäßchirurgie
Augustenburger Platz 1
13353 Berlin
Germany

WILLIAM F. NORTHRUP III, MD
Vice President
Medical Relations and Education
CryoLife, Inc.
1655 Roberts Blvd. NW
Kennesaw, GA 30144
USA

DAVIDE PACINI, MD
Cardiac Surgery Department
University of Bologna
Policlinico S. Orsola-Malpighi
Via Massarenti 9
40138 Bologna
Italy

JÜRGEN PASSAGE, MD
Universität Leipzig
Herzzentrum
Klinik für Herzchirurgie
Strümpellstrasse 39
04289 Leipzig
Germany

CORNELIA PIPER,
MD, PhD, FESC
Herz- und Diabeteszentrum
NRW
Klinik für Kardiologie
Georgstrasse 11
32545 Bad Oeynhausen
Germany

FRIEDRICH-CHRISTIAN RIESS,
MD, PhD
Chefarzt der Abteilung
für Herzchirurgie
Albertinen-Krankenhaus
Süntelstrasse 11a
22457 Hamburg
Germany

ULRICH ROSENDAHL, MD
Klinik für Herz-, Thorax-
und Gefäßchirurgie
Mediclin Herzzentrum
Lahr/Baden
Hohberweg 2
77933 Lahr
Germany

JOE SAUTER, MS, PE
SORIN GROUP
CarboMedics, Inc.
14401 W. 65th Way
Arvada, CO 80004-3599
USA

HANS-H. SIEVERS, MD, PhD
Chairman, Professor of Surgery
Universitätsklinikum
Schleswig-Holstein
Campus Lübeck
Klinik für Chirurgie
Ratzeburger Allee 160
23538 Lübeck
Germany

HENRYK SINIAWSKI, MD, PhD
Deutsches Herzzentrum Berlin
Charité Medical University
Berlin
Augustenburger Platz 1
13353 Berlin
Germany

CHRISTOF STAMM, MD, PhD
Deutsches Herzzentrum Berlin
Augustenburger Platz 1
13353 Berlin
Germany

J.J.M. TAKKENBERG, MD, PhD
Dept of Cardio-Thoracic
Surgery, Bd563
Erasmus MC
PO Box 2040
3000CA Rotterdam
The Netherlands

THOMAS WALTHER, MD, PhD
Professor of Surgery
Universität Leipzig
Herzzentrum
Klinik für Herzchirurgie
Strümpellstrasse 39
04289 Leipzig
Germany

CHARLES A. YANKAH, MD, PhD
Professor of Surgery
Deutsches Herzzentrum Berlin
& Charité Medical University
Berlin
Consultant Cardiothoracic
& Vascular Surgeon
Augustenburger Platz 1
13353 Berlin
Germany

Imaging of the aortic root

Perioperative imaging for assessing aortic and mitral valve diseases and surgical procedures

M. Kukucka

During the past decade, the use of echocardiography in the perioperative period and, in particular, of intraoperative transesophageal echocardiography (iTEE) has expanded rapidly [1]. The performance, interpretation, and clinical application of echocardiography in the perioperative environment are complex and require appropriate knowledge, technical skills, and complete familiarity with operative concerns.

History

In the latter half of the 1970s, it became apparent that the techniques for measuring cardiac output and various pressures were not fully adequate to assess rapid changes in ventricular compliance and ventricular performance which occurred during cardiac surgery.

To solve this problem, a great deal of research was required to obtain information on ventricular dimensions and volumes. At about this time, transthoracic echocardiography became recognized as an effective method for assessing left ventricular dimensions and performance. In 1978, employment of epicardial echocardiography using a commercially available M-mode transthoracic probe was evaluated to monitor left ventricular function in patients undergoing cardiac surgery. This technique was useful but quite cumbersome and suffered from a number of inherent problems (difficulty with probe position, interruption of the surgical procedure, etc.).

The first publication concerning usage of TEE was by Frazin et al. in 1976 [2]. His group used TEE in patients with COPD to make echocardiographic imaging possible but was not enthusiastic about this approach because patients found it very difficult to swallow the probe. Further development was associated with cardiac anesthesia and cardiac surgery. Yasu Oka and colleagues [3] described the use of TEE for the intraoperative monitoring of left ventricular function using M-mode echocardiography. The next improvement was reached with the application of phased array technology, which made two-dimensional echocardiography possible [4].

Application in cardiac surgery

TEE is used during cardiac surgery, where it has been instrumental in advancing valvular reconstruction, congenital heart repair, and minimally invasive techniques. Although the use of TEE in a "rescue" role (to diagnose the cause of life-threatening hypotension during surgery) is accepted, the routine use of TEE in all patients undergoing cardiac surgery remains somewhat controversial. More recent clinical opinion is that iTEE may provide new information regarding cardiac pathology in approximately 10% to 40% of patients undergoing cardiac surgery and that this new information may prompt alterations in surgical management in approximately 4% to 15% of such patients [5, 6]. In our institution, we use iTEE in about 80% of cases, and always if there are unclear hemodynamic disturbances or unexpected pharmacological support becomes necessary.

Indications for iTEE

Intraoperative echocardiography has both diagnostic and monitoring functions that are useful in many types of cardiac surgery procedures (Table 1).

Why iTEE before cardiopulmonary bypass?

It is axiomatic that all elective patients undergoing cardiac surgery have a full diagnostic workup and a definite surgical plan before arriving in the OR. Despite this, there may be findings on the echocardiogram prior to

Table 1. Indications for iTEE

- Mitral disease
- Aortic disease
- Tricuspid disease
- Prosthetic function
- Revascularization
- Surgery on aorta
- Transplantation/assist devices
- Congenital heart surgery
- Monitoring

cardiopulmonary bypass (CPB) that alter management by refining the preoperative diagnosis and surgical procedure. Such changes are more common in mitral valve (MV) than aortic valve (AV) operations [7]. Even in patients in whom no major change in plan occurs, the pre-CPB echocardiogram provides an updated understanding of the specific valvular anatomy and the mechanism of dysfunction, which help to refine the surgical technique. These changes result from the improvement in resolution of TEE over preoperative transthoracic echocardiography (TTE) and from changes in hemodynamic conditions or ischemia between the time of preoperative testing and the time of surgery.

iTEE in patients undergoing mitral valve surgery

To assess the mechanism of mitral regurgitation, we use the segmental approach to the mitral valve (Fig. 1). Clearly determination of leaflet and segment pathology helps the surgeon to choose the appropriate surgical technique. Carpentier's functional classification (Table 2) assists in distinguishing between normal, excessive, and restrictive leaflet motion. It is also

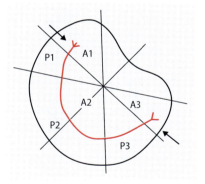

Fig. 1. Segmental approach for MV assessment. Posterior leaflet is divided into three scallops (P1–3) and anterior leaflet has three zones (A1–3). The lines show imaging possibilities in standard TEE views. Upper arrow marks anterolateral commissure, lower arrow posteromedial commissure

Table 2. Carpentier's functional classification of MV disease

Type I *Normal leaflet motion*	Type II *Excessive leaflet motion*	Type III *Restrictive leaflet motion*
▪ Annular dilatation ▪ Leaflet perforation ▪ Leaflet cleft	▪ Chordal rupture ▪ Chordal elongation ▪ Papillary muscle rupture ▪ Papillary muscle elongation	▪ Commissure fusion or thickening ▪ Chordal shortening ▪ Regional wall motion abnormalities ▪ Left ventricular aneurysm

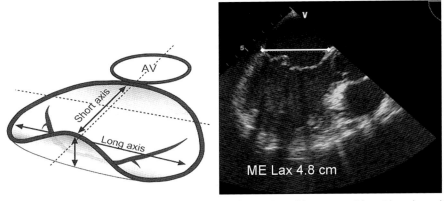

Fig. 2. Mitral valve annulus. Dilatation appears in short axis and is measured in midesophageal long axis view. In this case severe dilatation to 4.8 cm

necessary to answer the question of whether there is organic (leaflet defect) or functional (without leaflet defect) pathology of the MV. Pathoanatomical assessment of the annulus (dilation, calcification) (Fig. 2) completes the complex set of answers required to make the decision on MV reparability.

For quantification of MV regurgitation (MVR) in the OR, we use vena contracta measurements and calculation of regurgitant orifice and regurgitant volume using the proximal isovelocity surface area (PISA) method. Vena contracta is identified as the proximal width of a regurgitant jet. These two methods are relatively independent of loading, and the PISA method also allows exact quantification of regurgitant volume.

It is well known that MVR depends on different loading conditions and afterload. Induction of general anesthesia decreases the systemic vascular resistance and reveals the relative hypovolemia. Gisbert et al. [8] compared MV regurgitation severity preoperatively, under general anesthesia, and following afterload increase. They concluded that severity of organic and functional MVR decreases from baseline with general anesthesia and increases with phenylephrine in the OR (Fig. 3). Shiran et al. [9] studied a similar question in patients with ischemic MVR. They adjusted preload using fluids (PCWP > 15 mmHg) and afterload using phenylephrine (SP of ≥160 mmHg) and concluded that loading stress test can be useful to avoid underestimation of MVR severity. MVR may also be underestimated preoperatively, especially when studied after aggressive vasodilator and diuretic therapy.

Pre-CPB echocardiography is completed with the assessment of other valve disease (functional tricuspid regurgitation) and quantification of left and right ventricular function to provide comparable information for the post-CPB study.

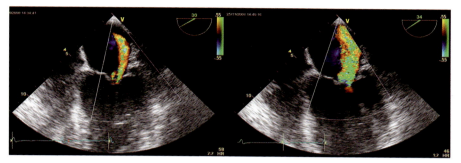

Fig. 3. Left: Mitral valve regurgitation after induction of general anesthesia (BP 90/60 mmHg). Right: Mitral valve regurgitation after bolus of norepinephrine and BP 130/85 mmHg

In the post-CPB study the following need to be investigated:
- Severity and mechanism of residual regurgitation
- Detection of systolic anterior motion of anterior mitral leaflet and left ventricular outflow obstruction
- Quantification of mitral opening area
- Identification of new regional wall motion abnormality
- Assessment of global left and right ventricular function.

iTEE evaluation during transapical aortic valve replacement

iTEE is usually used in patient selection and monitoring during the use of new, innovative surgical techniques. Conventional surgical aortic valve replacement is a standard procedure that has been performed for more than five decades with excellent short- and long-term outcomes. With an increasing life expectancy more elderly patients are being diagnosed with aortic stenosis. Beside advanced age, additional perioperative risk factors may be present such as low ejection fraction, pulmonary hypertension, respiratory dysfunction, and renal failure or peripheral arterial occlusive disease. Such comorbidities are associated with an increased perioperative morbidity and mortality. Thus, despite the good results of valve surgery, there may well be a role for less invasive transcatheter aortic valve implantation.

Preprocedure iTEE should include complete evaluation with imaging of the valve and aortic root. Geometric measurements of the aortic valve annulus in the midesophageal long axis view (Fig. 4) guide the intraoperative decision on prosthesis size. Also, the evaluation of coexisting valvular lesions and assessment of left ventricular function are essential. In patients with depressed LV function the primary decision for cardiopulmonary bypass will be discussed. Postprocedure iTEE assesses the global and regional

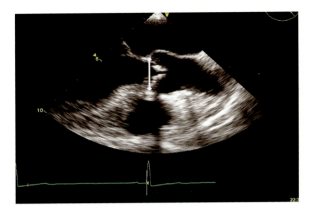

Fig. 4. Measurement of aortic valve annulus in midesophageal long axis view

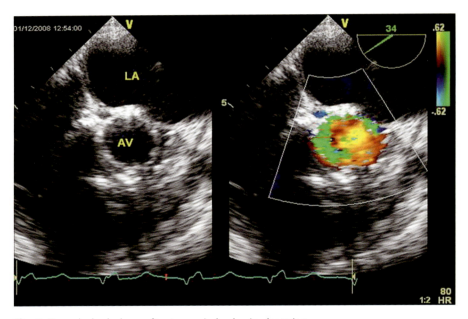

Fig. 5. Paravalvular leakage after transapical valve implantation

LV function, the location and degree of aortic regurgitation and the patency of coronary arteries and rules out such complications as hemopericardium and aortic dissection. If significant aortic regurgitation is found, the difference between paravalvular (Fig. 5) and valvular (Fig. 6) regurgitation should be recognized and the decision made for second balloon dilatation or valve-in-valve implantation. In our experience, it should be taken into account that there may be unusual and numerous regurgitant jets, so

Perioperative imaging for assessing aortic and mitral valve diseases and surgical procedures   9

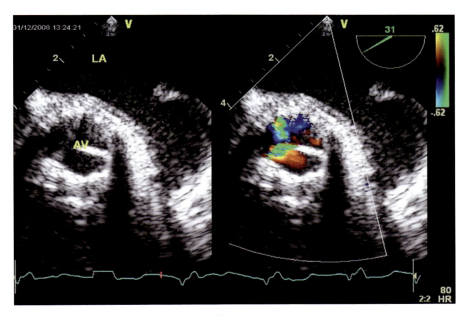

Fig. 6. Valvular leakage after second valve dilatation

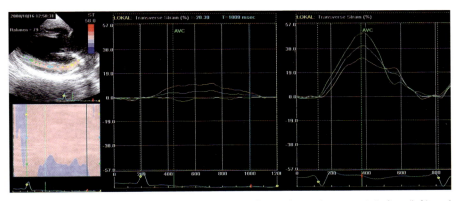

Fig. 7. Radial strain of anterior wall (basal, midpapillar and apical segment) before (left) and after (right) valve implantation shows essential improvement of systolic function

that complete probe rotation with short/long axis view imaging of the AV is necessary to detect the jets. In addition to conventional qualitative methods for the assessment of regional myocardial function, we also quantify radial and longitudinal deformation using strain calculation (Fig. 7) to identify the immediate functional changes.

The future

In the near future, the possibility of real-time single-beat 3D echocardiography will enable not only better anatomical imaging but also the exact quantification of such parameters as end-diastolic and end-systolic volumes and regional and global deformation (strain).

Conclusion

Intraoperative TEE during valve surgery is advantageous to refine the preoperative diagnosis and the surgical mission, to check the results of the surgical procedure, to make the decision for a second CPB run, to optimize the surgical outcome, to monitor the cardiac function, and to guide pharmacological therapy. The intraoperative assessment of valve disease severity is possible using dynamic quantitative echocardiography.

References

1. Shanewise JS, Cheung AT, Aronson S et al (1999) ASE/SCA guidelines for performing a comprehensive intraoperative multiplane transesophageal echocardiography examination: recommendations of the American Society of Echocardiography Council for Intraoperative Echocardiography and the Society of Cardiovascular Anesthesiologists Task Force for Certification in Perioperative Transesophageal Echocardiography. Anesth Analg 89:870–884
2. Frazin L, Talano JV, Stephanides L et al (1976) Esophageal echocardiography. Circulation 54:102–108
3. Matsumoto M, Oka Y, Strom J et al (1980) Application of transesophageal echocardiography to continuous intraoperative monitoring of left ventricular performance. Am J Cardiol 46:95–105
4. Souquet J, Hanrath P, Zitelli L et al (1982) Transesophageal phased array for imaging the heart. IEEE Trans Biomed Eng 29:707–712
5. Minhaj M, Patel K, Muzic D et al (2007) The effect of routine intraoperative transesophageal echocardiography on surgical management. J Cardiothorac Vasc Anesth 21:800–804
6. Click RL, Abel MD, Schaff HV (2000) Intraoperative transesophageal echocardiography: 5-year prospective review of impact on surgical management. Mayo Clin Proc 75:241–247
7. Sheikh KH, de Bruijn NP, Rankin JS et al (1990) The utility of transesophageal echocardiography and Doppler color flow imaging in patients undergoing cardiac valve surgery. J Am Coll Cardiol 15:363–372
8. Gisbert A, Souliere V, Denault AY et al (2006) Dynamic quantitative echocardiographic evaluation of mitral regurgitation in the operating department. J Am Soc Echocardiogr 19:140–146
9. Shiran A, Merdler A, Ismir E et al (2007) Intraoperative transesophageal echocardiography using a quantitative dynamic loading test for the evaluation of ischemic mitral regurgitation. J Am Soc Echocardiogr 20:690–697

Innovations in aortic valve surgery

The aortic root

C. A. Yankah, M. Pasic, E. Ivanitskaia-Kühn,
J. Kempfert, T. Walther, F. W. Mohr, R. Hetzer

Introduction

The shape of the aortic valve leaflet was first described by Philiston [1] in the 4th century BC as semilunar, and in 1513 Leonardo da Vinci [3] depicted in a drawing the geometry of the orifice of an opened and closed aortic valve as triangular and with three adjacent hemispherical forms, respectively (Figs. 1–3). Valsalva described the aortic sinuses in 1740 and suggested that the coronary artery filling takes place in the sinuses during diastole [4]. Recent echocardiographic and computed tomographic descriptions of the aortic valve and root diseases [5–7] and their relationship to the coronary artery origins have documented the importance of imaging the aortic root and the impact on the technical artistry of aortic root replacement, valve-sparing surgery, and minimally invasive transcatheter aortic valve replacement (Figs. 4–7) [8–12]. In fact, 2.9% of adults older than 65 years have calcific aortic stenosis [7].

The mechanism of aortic valvotomy for a calcified aortic stenosis and the transcatheter placement of the aortic valve prosthesis are best understood with knowledge of all anatomic units of the aortic root and its neighboring structures [13].

The anatomic units of the aortic root

The topographic anatomy of the aortic valve leaflets (cusps), the interleaflet triangle, and the sinuses of Valsalva are designated by their relationship to the coronary arteries.

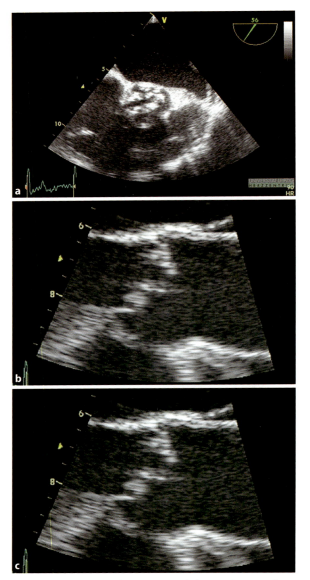

Fig. 1. Echocardiographic imaging of the aortic root: short and long axis view. **a** Short axis view: severe AS: AVA 0.5 cm^2; **b** long axis view: aortic valve annulus $\varnothing$ 24 mm; **c** mild mitral regurgitation, moderate tricuspid regurgitation

The aortic root | 15

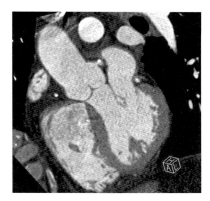

Fig. 2. Cardiac computed tomographic view of the aortic root: end-systolic phase. The anatomic relationship between the aortic annulus and the coronary artery are shown

Fig. 3. a The aortic valve in systole. **b** Opened leaflets in a triangular configuration. **c** The aortic valve in diastole in a configuration of three adjacent hemispheric form

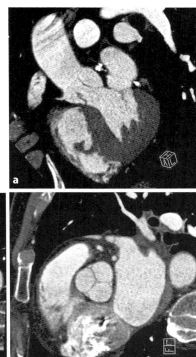

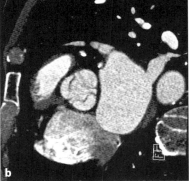

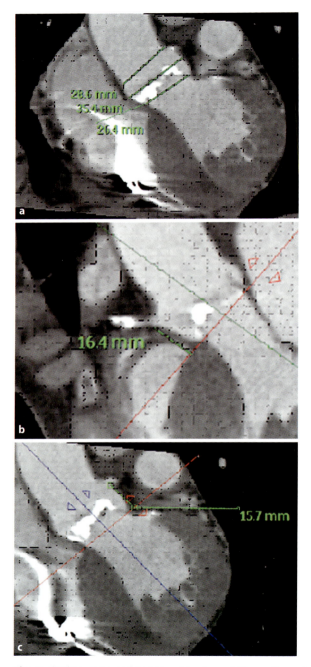

Fig. 4. Cardiac computed tomographic view of the aortic root. **a** Annulus 26 mm, **b** distance to left main coronary artery: 16 mm, **c** distance to RCA 16 mm

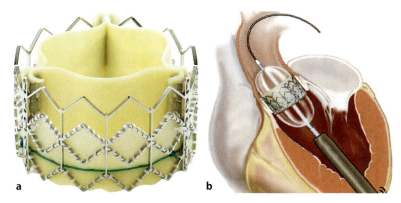

Fig. 5. a The Edwards Sapien transcatheter self-expandable pericardial valve. **b** Transapical implantation of the Edwards Sapien self-expandable sutureless pericardial valve in the aortic root

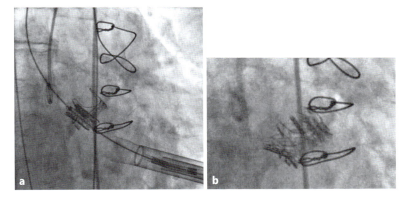

Fig. 6. Transapical valve-in-valve implantation of Edwards Sapien valve in a bioprosthesis after structural valve deterioration. **a** Introduction of the unexpanded Edwards Sapien valve into the bioprosthesis after balloon dilatation. **b** Implanted self-expandable Edwards Sapien valve in the bioprosthesis

The aortic annulus

The aortic annulus is the site where the ventricular musculature changes to that of the fibroelastic wall, the ventricular arterial junction to which the semilunar trileaflet aortic valve is attached. It represents the hemodynamic site between the left ventricle and the aorta.

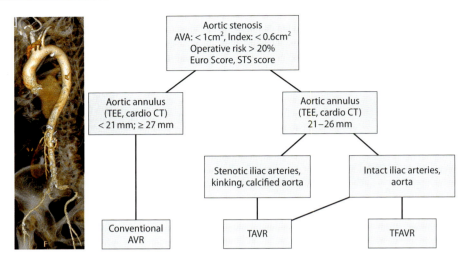

Fig. 7. Synopsis of a symptomatic aortic stenosis for transcatheter aortic valve replacement (*AVA* aortic valve area, *STS* Society of Thoracic Surgeons, *TEE* transesophageal echocardiography, *CT* computed tomography, *AVR* aortic valve replacement, *TAVR* transapical aortic valve replacement, *TFAVR* transfemoral aortic valve replacement)

The semilunar leaflets

The noncoronary leaflet (NCL) is described as the posterior leaflet. The left coronary leaflet (LCL) is described as the anterolateral leaflet, and the right coronary leaflet (RCL) as the anteromedial leaflet. The RCL is lower than the LCL and the NCL, while the RCL and the LCL originate from the myocardium (Figs. 3 and 4).

The aortic sinuses of Valsalva

Distal to the leaflet attachments are the sinuses of Valsalva (Fig. 2). The left and the right coronary sinuses (LCS, RCS) of Valsalva give rise to the LCA and RCA. The LCS is described as the anterolateral sinus and the RCL as the anteromedial sinus (Fig. 4). The noncoronary sinus (NCS) is the posterior sinus. The base of the NCS is a fibroelastic tissue which continues to the aortic mitral septum. At the base of the LCS and RCS, a crescent ventricular musculature is incorporated as part of the ventricular arterial segment.

The commissures

The highest point of the trileaflet aortic valve attachment is the commissure which is anchored within the sinuses of Valsalva in a crown-like fashion to form a cylindrical aortic root. The right or the posterior commissure is located between the noncoronary and the left coronary sinuses, and is located directly above the mid-point of the anterior mitral leaflet of the mitral valve. The left posterior commissure is located between the left and the right coronary sinuses. The anterior commissure is located between the right and the noncoronary sinuses in the region of the membranous septum.

Interleaflet triangle (the trigonum)

The triangular space below two commissures is the interleaflet triangle, which is a less dense connective tissue that is pliable and flexible. The right or the posterior interleaflet triangle is located between the noncoronary and the left coronary sinuses, and is located directly above the midpoint of the anterior mitral leaflet of the mitral valve. The left posterior interleaflet triangle is located between the left and the right coronary sinuses. The anterior interleaflet triangle is located between the right and the noncoronary sinuses in the region of the membranous septum.

The sinotubular junction

The sinotubular junction is the highest point of the sinuses of Valsalva and is located distal to the commissures and the cylindrical aortic root. It is the site at which the sinuses of Valsalva and the cylindrical aortic root change in diameter to form the ascending aorta (Figs. 2 and 4).

The coronary arteries

The right and the left coronary arteries originate from the anteromedial and anterolateral sinuses of Valsalva, respectively. Impingement of the coronary artery during an aortic root procedure may carry a high operative risk. Therefore, topographic evaluation of the distances between each coronary artery and the aortic annulus is important when planning aortic root procedures. The relationship of the coronary arteries to the prosthesis in the supraannular position are an important determining factor for unimpeded coronary blood flow during aortic root replacement and reimplantation of the coronary arteries, the Bentall-deBono procedure, valve replacement with a high-profile prosthesis and transcatheter aortic valve replacement with the Edwards Sapien and CoreValve (Fig. 5) [8–12, 14–17].

Comments

Currently, the aortic root is an area of innovative surgery. The recent development of transapical and percutaneous sutureless aortic valve replacement is an example of history repeating itself. The first clinical rapid sutureless fixation of a mechanical valve in the aortic position was introduced by Magovern and Cromie in 1962 [17, 18]. There are two first-generation transcatheter biological aortic valve replacements, the Edwards Sapien and the CoreValve for transapical and transfemoral approaches, being used in multiple centers in Europe, while two other devices, the Sadra Lotus and the Direct Flow Medical, are undergoing safety and efficacy testing [8–12, 19]. The latter devices are repositionable and retrievable in the aortic root and have smaller sheath diameters. Detailed knowledge of the anatomic units of the aortic root and its neighboring structures is necessary for the technical artistry of minimally invasive transcatheter aortic valve replacement.

Acknowledgment. The authors are grateful to Anne M. Gale, ELS, for editorial assistance, Julia Stein, MSc, for statistical assistance, Astrid Benhennour for bibliographic support, and Carla Weber for providing the graphics.

References

1. Leboucq G (1944) Une anatomie antique du Coeur human. Philiston de Locroi et le timee' de Plation. Rev Grecques 57:7
2. Sarton G (1952) A history of science. I Ancient science through the golden age of Greece. Harvard University Press, Cambridge, Massachusetts
3. Leonardo da Vinci (1977) Anatomical drawings from the Royal collections. The Royal Academy of Arts, London, p 35A
4. Valsalva AM (1740) Arteria magnae sinus. In: Morgagni JB (ed) Opera, pp 1–129
5. Siniawski H, Lehmkuhl H, Weng Y, Pasic M, Yankah C, Hoffman M, Behnke I, Hetzer R (2003) Stentless aortic valves as an alternative to homografts for valve replacement in active infective endocarditis complicated by ring abscess. Ann Thorac Surg 75:803–808
6. American College of Cardiology; American Heart Association Task Force on Practice Guidelines (Writing Committee to revise the 1998 guidelines for the management of patients with valvular heart disease); Society of Cardiovascular Anesthesiologists, Bonow RO, Carabello BA, Chatterjee K, de Leon AC Jr, Faxon DP, Freed MD et al (2006) ACC/AHA 2006 guidelines for the management of patients with valvular heart disease. Circulation 114:e84–e231
7. Otto CM, Lind BK, Kitzman DW, Gersh BJ, Siscovick DS (1999) Association of aortic valve sclerosis with cardiovascular mortality and morbidity in the elderly. N Engl J Med 341:142–147

8. Walther T, Simon P, Dewey T, Wimmer-Greinecker G, Falk V, Kasimir MT, Doss M, Borger M, Schuler G, Glogar D, Fehske W, Wolner E, Mohr F, Mack M (2007) Transapical minimally invasive aortic valve implantation. Multicenter experience. Circulation 116(Suppl I):I240–I245
9. Walther T, Dewey T, Borger M, Kempfert J, Linke A, Becht R, Falk V, Schuler G, Mohr F, Mack M (2008) Human minimally invasive off-pump valve-in-valve implantation: Step by step. Ann Thorac Surg 85:1072–1073
10. Grube E, Schuler G, Blumenthal L et al (2007) Percutaneous aortic valve replacement for severe aortic stenosis in high risk patients using the second- and current third-generation self-expanding CoreValve prosthesis: device success and 30-day clinical outcome. J Am Coll Cardiol 50:69–76
11. Webb JG, Chandavimol M, Thompson CR et al (2006) Percutaneous aortic valve implantation retrograde from the femoral artery. Circulation 113:842–850
12. Lieberman EB, Bashore TM et al (1995) Balloon aortic valvuloplasty in adults. Failure of procedure to improve long-term survival. J Amer Coll Cardiol 26:1522–1528
13. Bentall H, De Bono A (1968) A technique for complete replacement of the ascending aorta. Thorax 23:338–339
14. Petrou M, Wong K, Albertucci M, Brecker SJ, Yacoub MH (1994) Evaluation of unstented aortic homografts for the treatment of prosthetic aortic valve endocarditis. Circulation 90(Part 2):II-198–204
15. Yankah AC, Pasic M, Klose H, Siniawski H, Weng Y, Hetzer R (2005) Homograft reconstruction of the aortic root for endocarditis with periannular abscess: a 17-year study. Eur J Cardiothorac Surg 28:69–75
16. Yankah AC, Sievers HH, Buersch JH, Radtcke W, Lange PE, Heintzen PH, Bernhard A (1984) Orthotopic transplantation of aortic valve allograft. Early hemodynamic results. Thorac Cardiovasc Surgeon 32:92–95
17. Mogovern GJ, Kent EM, Cromie HW (1962) Sutureless artificial heart valves. Circulation 27:2784–2788
18. Zlotnick AY, Shiran A, Lewis BS, Aravot D (2008) A perfectly functioning Magovern-Cromie sutureless prosthetic aortic valve 42 years after implantation. Circulation 117:e1–e2
19. Walther T, Dewey T, Borger M, Kempfert J, Linke A, Becht R, Falk V, Schuler G, Mohr F, Mack M (2009) Transapical aortic valve implantation: Step by step. Ann Thorac Surg 87:276–283

Percutaneous transluminal aortic valve replacement: The CoreValve prosthesis

U. Gerckens, L. Büllesfeld, G. Latsios, R. Müller,
B. Sauren, S. Iversen, E. Grube

History of percutaneous aortic valve replacement

Open heart surgery with mechanical or porcine bioprosthetic valve replacement is the current gold-standard therapeutic approach for the vast majority of patients with severe aortic valve disease, offering symptomatic relief and improving long-term survival. However, the etiology of aortic stenosis in the Western population is primarily degenerative, and patients are typically elderly with multiple co-morbid conditions which increase surgical risk [1–3]. In high-risk patients with baseline features such as left ventricular failure, concomitant coronary artery disease, prior bypass graft surgery, chronic obstructive pulmonary disease and/or advanced age, expected operative mortality ranges from 10% to even 50% in high-risk patients subgroups [1]. Moreover, surgery is often not performed in high-risk patients. In the Euro Heart Survey, up to 33% of patients in NYHA functional class III/IV with a single diseased valve were declined for surgery or were never considered as surgical candidates, due to an expected short life expectancy and associated comorbid conditions [4]. Alternative techniques for treatment of high-risk patients are therefore needed.

Percutaneous treatment of aortic valve disease with implantation of a stent-based valve prosthesis has been evaluated in animal models over the past decade [5–10]. In 2002, Cribier et al. [11] performed the first human implantation of a balloon-expandable aortic valve prosthesis (Percutaneous Valve Therapy, PVT) in a patient with aortic valve stenosis considered inoperable due to severe comorbidities. Initial reports with this new percutaneous valve have been promising, though the optimal device and procedural technique are still evolving, and the restriction of PVT candidates to end-stage inoperable patients has clouded interpretation of the feasibility and safety of this procedure [12, 13].

A self-expanding aortic valve prosthesis intended for retrograde delivery across the aortic valve has been developed (CoreValve Irvine, CA, USA), to facilitate treatment of aortic stenosis. Following evaluation in animal models, this device was subsequently successfully implanted in a human being [14], and since 2004 its use was expanded in clinical use [15, 16]. In 2007 its use received a CE certification.

Patient population

Patients with severe native aortic valve stenosis are eligible for CoreValve implantation if they meet the following inclusion criteria:
- a native aortic valve stenosis with an aortic valve area < 1 cm^2
- aortic valve annulus diameter ≥ 20 mm and ≤ 27 mm, measured by means of echocardiography or CT
- diameter of the ascending aorta 3 cm above the annulus of ≤ 43 mm;
- high risk for surgery due to concomitant comorbid conditions, assessed and agreed to by both a cardiologist and a cardiothoracic surgeon.

The baseline risk of the patient population is estimated by the logistic EuroSCORE or STS score [1].

The patient selection procedure is given in Table 1.

General exclusion criteria include hypersensitivity or contraindication to any study medication; sepsis or active endocarditis; excessive femoral, iliac or aortic atherosclerosis, calcification, or tortuosity; aortic aneurysm; bleeding diathesis or coagulopathy.

Preinterventional morphological patient screening is carried out by means of transthoracic as well as transesophageal echocardiography, computerized multislice cardiac tomographic angiography (CTA), and an invasive cardiac evaluation with coronary arteriography and left ventriculography.

Device description and procedure

The CoreValve aortic valve prosthesis consists of a trileaflet bioprosthetic valve made originally of bovine and now of porcine pericardial tissue, which is mounted and sutured in a self-expanding nitinol frame (Fig. 1). The prosthetic frame is manufactured by laser cutting of a nitinol metal tube to a total length of 50 mm. The lower portion of the prosthesis has high radial force to expand and keep open the calcified leaflets and avoid recoil; the middle portion carries the valve and is constrained to avoid the coronary arteries; and the upper portion is flared to fixate the stent in the ascending aorta and provide longitudinal stability.

In total, three generation devices have been produced and used, with the differences being mainly the diameter of the upper segment and especially the diameter of the delivery sheath.

The third generation device was characterized by a broader upper segment for more secure fixation in the ascending aorta, which also allowed inclusion of patients with an ascending aorta diameter up to 43 mm. The first and second generation devices are constrained within a delivery

Table 1. Patient selection criteria for suitability for the CoreValve prosthesis according to the various diagnostic methods. (3rd generation 18 French device)

Anatomy	Non-invasive		Angiography			Selection criteria		
	Echo	CT/MRI	LV gram	AO gram	Coronary angiogram	AO & runoffs	Preferred	Borderline	Not acceptable
■ Atrial or ventricular thrombus	X						Not present		Present
■ Mitral regurgitation	X						≤Grade 1	Grade 2	>Grade 2
■ LV ejection fraction	X		X				>50%	30 to 50%	<20%
■ LV hypertrophy (wall thickness)	X						Normal to mild (0.6 to 1.3 cm)	Moderate (1.4 to 1.6 cm)	Severe (≥1.7 cm)
■ Sub-aortic stenosis	X	X					Not present		Present
■ Annulus (width)	X	X					20 to 23 mm—26 mm device 24 to 27 mm—29 mm device		<20 mm or >27 mm
■ Annulus-to-aorta (angle)		X	X	X			<30°	30 to 45°	>45°
■ AO root (width)		X	X	X			≥30 mm	27 to 29 mm	<27 mm (if sinus ≤15 mm)
■ Sinuses of valsalva (height)		X	X	X	X		≥15 mm	10 to 14 mm	<10 mm
■ Coronary ostia position (take-off)					X		High	Mid-sinus level	Low
■ Coronary disease						X	None	Mid or distal stenosis <70%	Proximal stenosis ≥70%

Table 1 (continued)

Anatomy	Non-invasive Echo	Non-invasive CT/MRI	Angiography LV gram	Angiography AO gram	Coronary angiogram	AO & runoffs	Selection criteria Preferred	Selection criteria Borderline	Selection criteria Not acceptable
■ Ascend aorta (width)		X	X	X			≤40 mm–26 mm device ≤43 mm–29 mm device		>43 mm
■ AO arch angulation		X		X		X	Large-radius turn		High angulation or sharp bend
■ Aorta & run-off vessels (disease)		X				X	None	Mild	Moderate to severe
■ Iliac & femoral vessels (diameter)		X				X	≥7 mm	Non-diabetic ≥6 mm	<6 mm

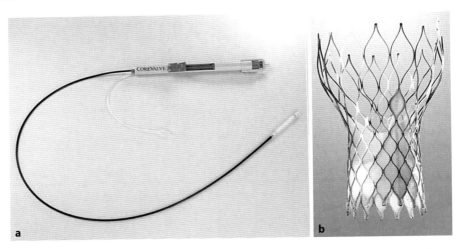

Fig. 1. The 18 French delivery catheter (**a**) and the 3rd generation CoreValve prosthesis (**b**)

sheath of 25 and 21 French diameter, respectively, with the smaller second generation device allowing access through smaller diameter vascular beds. However, most of the time this necessitated the use of surgical cut-down of the common iliac, the femoral or even the subclavian artery.

Improvement in the size of the prosthesis, in the form of a smaller (18 French) sheath necessary for the procedure, resulted in two major advantages: the device can be implanted even in patients with smaller peripheral arteries (common femoral artery >7 mm or even 6 mm in nondiabetic, noncalcified vessels). However, the main improvement of the introduction of the 18 French delivered CoreValve prosthesis is the implantation through a 18 French sheath, and at the end of the procedure the access site is sutured down by means of four prepositioned Prostar sutures (Prostar XL system), a well-known and long-practiced interventional technique [17]. This way, nowadays the procedure is purely interventional.

During the procedure the patient is mildly sedated but otherwise alert and not intubated. We do not use any more trans-esophageal echo or extracorporeal percutaneous femoro-femoral bypass or any other form of assist device, as requested per protocol for implantation of the first and second generation devices.

The procedure briefly is as follows: a pacemaker lead is placed in the right ventricular apex. Through initially a 9 French and eventually an 18 French sheath, a 0.035 super stiff guidewire is placed in the left ventricle, through a pigtail catheter. This guidewire has a short flexible atraumatic tip, which is bent by hand to form a loop which accommodates the left ventricle size. Over it, a balloon valvuloplasty is performed prior to device placement. Immediately afterwards, the CoreValve prosthesis passes the valve and is positioned. The advancement of the prosthesis through the 18

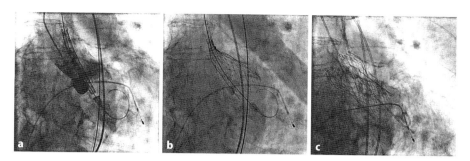

Fig. 2. Implantation of the CoreValve prosthesis at the native aortic valve anatomic position. Positioning by means of fluoroscopy and small contrast injections (**a, b**) and final angiographic result, with no aortic regurgitation (**c**)

French sheath, the peripheral vessels, the aortic arch and finally though the valve is accomplished using the push-and-pull technique over the super stiff guidewire. Accurate placement of the prosthesis is achieved by fluoroscopy and injection of small amounts of contrast through a pigtail catheter positioned in the aortic root (Fig. 2).

Aortography is performed at baseline and after valve placement to assess paravalvular regurgitation. Angiography is also performed after valve deployment to ensure coronary and/or bypass graft patency. Presence of a dicrotic notch as well as height of the DBP (diastolic blood pressure) and LVEDP (left ventricular end diastolic pressure) before and after the implantation are excellent hemodynamic markers, reflecting the presence and severity of possible paravalvular regurgitation. However, even in cases with moderate regurgitation, there are options available for further 'tuning' of the valve. In case of underexpansion, a further post dilatation of the already implanted valve can be carried out safely and efficiently, reducing effectively the regurgitation. Pulling of the CoreValve prosthesis in case of deep implantation is also feasible, by means of snare pulling. Noteworthy is the fact that all these manipulations can be carried out interventionally, avoiding the need of a cardiothoracic surgeon and the associated risks of turning the procedure into an open heart surgery.

As stated already, the 18 French femoral artery access site is sealed by means of four prepositioned Prostar XL sutures, tied together with a so-called sliding fisherman's knot (Fig. 3).

After the procedure, all patients are transferred to the intensive care unit for continuous monitoring. The temporary pacemaker cable remains for 24 to 48 hours, after which is either removed or substituted by a permanent pacemaker, if required by the patient's condition.

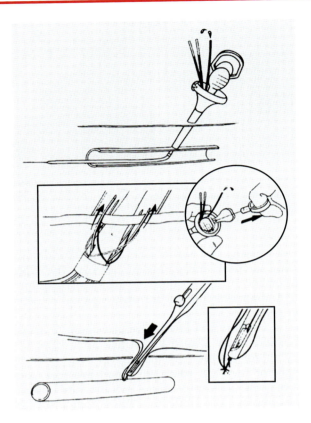

Fig. 3. Prostar XL device and its mode of employment

Medication

All patients receive acetylsalicylic acid (100 mg/d) before the procedure and lifelong afterwards. Also, all patients receive clopidogrel (300 mg loading dose) 75 mg/d for 6 months. During the intervention, patients receive weight adjusted heparin, with a target ACT of 250–300 s.

Outcomes following implantation

The follow-up consists of clinical questioning and transthoracic echocardiography, postprocedure, at hospital discharge, and at 15 and 30 days after device implantation. As part of the ongoing registry kept on all implantations, follow-up is also performed at 90 and 180 days.

Table 2. Procedural and 30-day outcomes following implantation of the 18 F CoreValve prosthesis. (European CoreValve registry)

	18F EE registry until April 2008 [18]	18F EE registry until August 2008 [19]
Patients	n = 646	n = 1243
30 day *all cause* mortality	52 (8.0%)	83 (6.7%)
Cardiac mortality	38 (5.9%)	48 (3.9%)
Pacemaker	60 (9.3%)	151 (12.2%)
Stroke	12 (1.9%)	17 (1.4%)
Valve dysfunction or valve migration	(0.0%)	(0.0%)

The data from the European multicenter evaluation registry inside the one year time frame that the 18 French CoreValve device is implanted under CE mark approval have already been published for 646 patients [18] Later data on an larger number of 1243 patients were also presented [19]. Table 2 shows cumulative data on the procedural and 30-day outcomes of these morbid, high-risk patients.

The immediate results are more than encouraging. All patients had a post-procedural invasive aortic valve gradient of 0–10 mmHg, and only 3% patient had an aortic regurgitation of more than 2+. As for their functional status, 80% of patients NYHA class III/IV symptoms before the procedure, of those almost everybody improved to class I/II.

Other conclusions that can be drawn by these data are as follows. First, the mortality rate of the procedure on these high-risk, very sick patients (mean logistic EuroSCORE was 23.1%) is quite acceptable. Even more importantly, the mortality rate, as well the rate of all complications, continues to decline over time. Of notice is that the implantation of a pacemaker (in 9.3%–12.2% of patients) is higher compared to the patients treated with conventional open heart surgical aortic valve replacement (6.0%–6.5%) [20, 21], since the nitinol frame CoreValve prosthesis applies constant pressure to the left ventricle outflow tract.

Stroke incidence, which was unacceptably high during the initial 25F and 21F studies, has declined to 1.9%–1.4% in the recent registry data [18, 19]. This is due to the smaller sheath size of 18 French, the shorter procedural time and the smoother passage of the prosthesis through the aortic arch. It is our belief that almost all cases of stroke are attributed to the valvuloplasty, during which fragmented calcified particles are freed by the aortic valve in the systemic circulation, and not to the prosthesis per se.

Also, none of the implanted devices showed any sign of malfunction or distal migration during the follow-up.

Conclusions

There is certainly a large need in cardiology for the development of an effective, interventional method for the treatment of degenerative calcified aortic valve stenosis. This need is not only necessitated by the large number of the patients who are considered inoperable for traditional open heart surgery, but also by the troublesome and potentially complicated course of thoracotomy, extracorporeal circulation, prolonged mechanical ventilation, etc.

After the initial safety and efficacy trials, the ongoing European Core-Valve registry demonstrates a high rate of procedural success and a low 30-day mortality in a large cohort of high-risk patients undergoing transcatheter aortic valve implantation with the CoreValve prosthesis. Long-term results and improvement in design and techniques will clarify many of the questions pending. Also, a randomized trial between percutaneous and surgical aortic valve replacement is already under way to further shed light.

To date, the percutaneous aortic valve replacement is one of the latest innovations in invasive cardiology, offering a new therapeutic option to many patients who until now are not being treated adequately.

References

1. Roques F, Nashef SA, Michel P, Gauducheau E, de Vincentiis C, Baudet E, Cortina J, David M, Faichney A, Gabrielle F, Gams E, Harjula A, Jones MT, Pintor PP, Salamon R, Thulin L (1999) Risk factors and outcome in European cardiac surgery: analysis of the EuroSCORE multinational database of 19030 patients. Eur J Cardiothorac Surg 15(6):816–822
2. Culliford AT, Galloway AC, Colvin SB, et al (1991) Aortic valve replacement for aortic stenosis in persons aged 80 years and over. Am J Cardiol 67:1256–1260
3. Kvidal P, Bergström R, Hörte L-G, Stahle E (2000) Observed and relative survival after aortic valve replacement. J Am Coll Cardiol 35:747–756
4. Iung B, Baron G, Butchart EG, Delahaye F, Gohlke-Barwolf C, Levang OW, Tornos P, Vanoverschelde JL, Vermeer F, Boersma E, Ravaud P, Vahanian A (2003) A prospective survey of patients with valvular heart disease in Europe: The Euro Heart Survey on Valvular Heart Disease. Eur Heart J 24(13):1231–1243
5. Andersen HR, Knudsen LL, Hasemkam JM (1992) Transluminal implantation of artificial heart valves: description of a new expandable aortic valve and initial results with implantation by catheter techniques in closed chest pigs. Eur Heart J 13:704–708
6. Bonhoeffer P, Boudjemline Y, Saliba Z, Hausse AO, Aggoun Y, Bonnet D, Sidi D, Kachaner J (2000) Transcatheter implantation of a bovine valve in pulmonary position: a lamb study. Circulation 102:813–816
7. Boudjemline Y, Bonhoeffer P (2000) Steps toward percutaneous aortic valve replacement. Circulation 105:775–776

8. Boudjemline Y, Bonhoeffer P (2002) Percutaneous implantation of a valve in the descending aorta in lambs. Eur Heart J 23:1045–1049
9. Sochman J, Peregrin JH, Pavnick D, Timmermans H, Rosch J (2000) Percutaneous transcatheter aortic disc valve prosthesis implantation: a feasibility study. Cardiovasc Intervent Radiol 23:384–388
10. Cribier A, Eltchaninoff H, Borenstein N (2001) Transcatheter implantation of balloon expandable prosthetic heart valves: early results in an animal model. Circulation 104:II552 (abstract)
11. Cribier A, Eltchaninoff H, Bash A, Borenstein N, Tron C, Bauer F, Derumeaux G, Anselme F, Laborde F, Leon MB (2002) Percutaneous transcatheter implantation of an aortic valve prosthesis for calcific aortic stenosis. Circulation 106(24): 3006–3008
12. Cribier A, Eltchaninoff H, Tron C, Bauer F, Agatiello C, Sebagh L, Bash A, Nusimovici D, Litzler PY, Bessou JP, Leon MB (2004) Early experience with percutaneous transcatheter implantation of heart valve prosthesis for the treatment of end-stage inoperable patients with calcific aortic stenosis. JACC 43(4):698–703
13. Bauer F, Eltchaninoff H, Tron C, Lesault PF, Agatiello C, Nercolini D, Derumeaux G, Cribier A (2004) Acute improvement in global and regional left ventricular systolic function after percutaneous heart valve implantation in patients with symptomatic aortic stenosis. Circulation 110(11):1473–1476
14. Grube E, Laborde JC, Zickmann B, Gerckens U, Felderhoff T, Sauren B, Bootsveld A, Buellesfeld L, Iversen S (2005) First report on a human percutaneous transluminal implantation of a self-expanding aortic valve prosthesis for interventional treatment of aortic valve stenosis. Catheter Cardiovasc Interv 66(4):465–469
15. Grube E, Laborde JC, Gerckens U, Felderhoff T, Sauren B, Buellesfeld L, Mueller R, Menichelli M, Schmidt T, Zickmann B, Iversen S, Stone GW (2006) Percutaneous implantation of the CoreValve self-expanding valve prosthesis in high-risk patients with aortic valve disease: the Siegburg first-in-man study. Circulation 114(15):1616–1624
16. Grube E, Schuler G, Buellesfeld L, Gerckens U, Linke A, Wenaweser P, Sauren B, Mohr FW, Walther T, Zickmann B, Iversen S, Felderhoff T, Cartier R, Bonan R (2007) Percutaneous aortic valve replacement for severe aortic stenosis in high-risk patients using the second- and current third-generation self-expanding CoreValve prosthesis: device success and 30-day clinical outcome. J Am Coll Cardiol 50(1):69–76. Epub 2007 Jun 6
17. Haas PC, Krajcer Z, Diethrich EB (1999) Closure of large percutaneous access sites using the Prostar XL Percutaneous Vascular Surgery device. J Endovasc Surg 6(2):168–170
18. Piazza N, Grube E, Gerckens U, den Heijer P, Linke A, Luha O, Ramondo A Ussia G, Wenaweser P, Windecker S, Laborde JC, de Jaegere P, Serruys P (2008) Procedural and 30-day outcomes following transcatheter aortic valve implantation using the third generation (18 Fr) CoreValve ReValving System: results from the multicentre, expanded evaluation registry 1-year following CE mark approval. EuroInterv 4:242–249
19. Grube E, Gerckens U (2008) Retrograde transfemoral aortic valve replacement – from early device prototypes to a routine cath lab procedure. Data on CoreValve registry presented at TCT, Washington, 12th–17th October 2008
20. Dawkins S, Hobson AR, Kalra PR, Tang AT, Monro JL, Dawkins KD (2008) Permanent pacemaker implantation after isolated aortic valve replacement: incidence, indications, and predictors. The Annals of thoracic surgery 85(1):108–112
21. Koplan BA, Stevenson WG, Epstein LM, Aranki SF, Maisel WH (2003) Development and validation of a simple risk score to predict the need for permanent pacing after cardiac valve surgery. Journal of the American College of Cardiology 41(5):795–801

Transapical aortic valve implantation –

a truly minimally invasive option for high-risk patients

J. Kempfert, F. W. Mohr, T. Walther

Introduction

Over the past few decades, conventional aortic valve replacement has evolved to a highly standardized procedure resulting in excellent clinical outcome. Today, isolated conventional aortic valve replacement (AVR) in low-risk patients is associated with a 30-day mortality of only 2–3% [1, 2].

Aortic valve stenosis, usually caused by degenerative disease, is the most frequent acquired heart valve lesion and predominantly affects elderly patients. Naturally these elderly patients often present with significant comorbidities resulting in an increased operative risk profile. Even in presence of an increased risk profile, aortic valve replacement can be performed in elderly patients with an acceptable clinical outcome leading to a significant improvement in the individual's quality of life [3]. According to the literature 30-day mortality after conventional aortic valve replacement in octogenarians is around 5–10% [4, 5], which is acceptable when taking into account the grave prognosis of elderly patients suffering from severe symptomatic aortic stenosis with mortality rates of up to 50% within the next year without surgical intervention [6].

To decrease the invasiveness of conventional aortic valve replacement several minimally invasive techniques using a limited surgical access (i.e., upper partial sternotomy) have been introduced recently to further improve clinical outcome [7].

The concept of transcatheter aortic valve implantation

Given these excellent results associated with conventional aortic valve replacement even in octogenarians, why would we need transcatheter aortic valve implantations? According to the data of the European Heart Survey one-third of all elderly patients suffering from severe symptomatic aortic stenosis were never referred to a cardiac surgeon because the referring cardiologists believed the surgical risk to be unacceptably high [8]. This is not true for the majority of elderly (octogenarian) patients who today are good candidates for conventional AVR, but there are certainly some patients with an excessive risk profile. So even with the minimally invasive technique for conventional AVR (i.e., partial upper sternotomy) the procedure still requires (partial) sternotomy, cardioplegic arrest and cardiopulmonary bypass. In contrast, when using a transcatheter technique it is feasible to implant an aortic valve prosthesis and avoid sternotomy, cardioplegic arrest, and probably most importantly even cardiopulmonary bypass. Theoretically, all these factors together should result in less surgical trauma, less cardiac impairment, and less inflammatory response leading to improved patient outcome. On the other hand, there may be an inherent additional risk with these new procedures when comparing them to the highly standardized conventional techniques. In addition long-term durability of the transcatheter valves is unknown despite promising in vitro tests and low transvalvular gradients. Therefore, transcatheter aortic valve implantation at present is exclusively targeting very high-risk patients suffering from severe symptomatic aortic stenosis.

▌ Transcatheter aortic valve prostheses

Presently, two systems are commercially available and have obtained CE mark approval recently. The first device is the CoreValve^{TM} system which is predominantly designed for transfemoral access. The valve is made from porcine pericardium and is mounted within a self-expandable nitinol stent 50 mm in length. The prosthesis is deployed within the aortic annulus extending above the level of the coronary ostia with a wide mesh allowing for unabated coronary flow. In contrast, the Edwards SAPIEN^{TM} (Fig. 1) valve is made from bovine pericardium including some anticalcification treatment (ThermaFix^{TM}) and is much shorter in height (14–16 mm). The SAPIEN^{TM} valve mimics the design of a conventional bioprosthesis and has

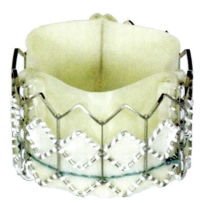

Fig. 1. Edwards SAPIEN^{TM} transcatheter heart valve

to be implanted in a strictly subcoronary position. The valve within a steel stent is anchored within the aortic annulus by active ballooning of the valve stent. The SAPIEN^{TM} system is at present the only commercially available device for transapical aortic valve implantation (TA-AVI) but can also be deployed using the retrograde transfemoral approach (TF-AVI).

Patient selection

Risk assessment

According to the literature, advanced age alone is not sufficient to deem a patient at high-risk for AVR [4]. Today several different scoring systems are used for risk assessment. The logistic EuroSCORE and the STS score are most frequently used in everyday clinical practice. The clinical practitioner when assessing the true risk for an individual patient needs to be aware of the known limitations of the current scoring systems. The logistic EuroSCORE tends to overestimate and the STS score to underestimate the actual risk for mortality in these complex patients [9]. Thus, careful clinical assessment is also crucial.

At present, we should restrain from including younger low-risk patients and strictly adhere to established inclusion criteria and to the recently published guidelines [10]. A suitable criteria for high risk is age >75 and a logistic EuroSCORE >20% and/or a STS score >10%. Beside age and risk scores, there are several clinical scenarios where a transcatheter approach might be beneficial:
- patients with patent bypass grafts,
- patients presenting with porcelain aorta,
- patients suffering from end-stage liver failure,
- history of chest radiation or mediastinitis.

Anatomical considerations

The SAPIEN^{TM} valve used for TA-AVI is currently available in two sizes: 23 mm and 26 mm (a larger 29 mm valve is under development). To safely anchor the prosthesis inside the aortic annulus, moderate oversizing of 2–3 mm should be performed. Thus, the cut-off diameter of the aortic annulus for the larger 26 mm valve is 24 mm. In addition to the diameter the pattern of calcification of the aortic valve should be assessed preoperatively. A concentric distribution of the calcium is more suitable for transcatheter AVI than eccentric calcification which may result in paravalvular leak or coronary obstruction. Assessment of the valve should be made by TEE preoperatively and the diameter of the annulus should be measured repeatedly in a strictly perpendicular long axis view (the largest diameter mea-

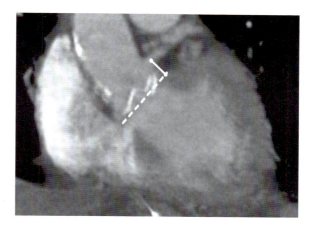

Fig. 2. Cardiac-CT demonstrating the diameter of the aortic annulus and the distance of the left coronary ostia to the aortic annulus

sured counts). In addition to TEE, a cardiac CT (Fig. 2) is of help to measure the distance between the coronary ostia and the level of the aortic annulus and thus provides an impression of where to position the prosthesis.

Transapical or transfemoral AVI?

To date, there is no scientific evidence proving the superiority of one of these approaches. The transfemoral (TF-AVI) access allows for a completely closed chest procedure without the need for intubation. On the other hand, the transapical technique (TA-AVI) offers several advantages:
- the short distance between left ventricular apex and aortic annulus allows for excellent steerability of the devices;
- the antegrade route eases crossing of the calcified stenotic valve, and
- avoids manipulation of the device around the aortic arch (stroke risk!);
- there is almost no limitation in the size of the delivery sheaths.

In clinical practice, both options should be carefully evaluated and then selected according to the individual patient characteristics. Severe peripheral vascular disease is a clear indication for the transapical approach.

TA-AVI – setup

The OR

The most important difference in transcatheter AVI compared to conventional techniques is the (almost) closed chest situation not allowing for direct vision of the working field. Therefore, optimal imaging is of utmost importance to ensure precise positioning of the prosthesis – the key step in any transcatheter AVI. The most suitable environment is a fully equipped hybrid-OR combining high quality fluoroscopy/angiography, transesophageal echo (2D and 3D/X-plane), cardiopulmonary bypass (on standby), and standard cardiac surgical equipment allowing for bailout to all conventional surgical techniques. If there is no such a hybrid-OR available, an "upgraded" cath-lab (by adding TEE, CPB and surgical equipment) is advantageous to ensure optimal imaging quality compared to a standard surgical theater with a mobile C-arm (inferior imaging quality).

The team approach

Despite the fact that some groups advocate TF-AVI as pure cath-lab procedures without the need for surgical participation and others argue that TA-AVI is strictly a surgical technique, we strongly believe in the concept of a true team approach. The specialized expertise of anesthetists (TEE, hemodynamic management), cardiologists (fluoroscopy, wire handling), and surgeons (surgical access, CBP, surgical bailout) should be combined to achieve optimal patient safety and outcome irrelevant of political borders.

TA-AVI – the procedure step by step

Anesthesia

Usually TA-AVI is performed under general anesthesia using a fast-track protocol resulting in relatively short ventilation times (approximately 80 min). In patients with severely decreased lung function, an awake procedure using thoracic epidural anesthesia only is feasible and has been successfully performed. The drawback of procedures without intubation is the lack of TEE imaging, which is crucial for sizing and valve function assessment.

The "safety net"

The patient is positioned supine with slightly elevated left chest. Prior to skin incision, a percutaneous arterial 6 French sheath is inserted into the femoral artery followed by a percutaneous wire in the femoral vein. The wire is advanced under TEE or fluoroscopic guidance to the right atrium. The 6 French arterial sheath is needed for aortic root angiography during the implantation process later. The percutaneous femoral vascular access acts as a "safety net" (Fig. 3) providing a bailout option. Using the Seldinger technique, the "safety net" facilitates percutaneous femoral-femoral cardiopulmonary bypass within minutes if required [11].

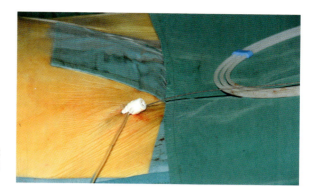

Fig. 3. Femoral "safety net": percutaneous venous wire and arterial 6F sheath

▌ Sizing and valve preparation

After repeat measurements of the aortic annulus by TEE (strictly perpendicular long axis view), the size of the transcatheter valve is selected to ensure adequate oversizing of at least 2 mm. The valve is then prepared and crimped on a balloon delivery catheter under sterile conditions in the operating room by a technician just prior to implantation. Attention in needed to double check the correct orientation of the valve on the delivery catheter for antegrade transapical or retrograde transfemoral implantation.

▌ Surgical access to the left ventricular apex

After obtaining femoral access, heparin is given at a dose of approximately 100 IU/kg aiming at an activated clotting time of 300 s.

For transapical access, an incision of 5–7 cm in length is placed 2 fingers submammary in the midclavicular line in the fifth or possibly sixth intercostal space (Fig. 4a). The left anterolateral minithoracotomy should result in straight access to the left ventricular apex. After opening the pericardium longitudinally, four pericardial stay sutures are placed to expose the apex and to allow for bilateral lung ventilation. An epicardial bipolar pacing wire is placed and tested. Two apical purse-string sutures (Prolene 2–0, large (MH) needle with 5 interrupted Teflon pledgets) are placed lateral to the LAD with sufficiently deep bites (approximately 3–5 mm, not penetrating completely) in the myocardium (Fig. 4b).

▌ Positioning of the fluoroscopic system

A strictly perpendicular angle to the aortic root is crucial for exact positioning of the prosthesis. Usually this is achieved by an angulation of LAO $\sim 10°$ and cranial $\sim 10°$. Further adjustment is carried out once the prosthesis is at the level of the aortic annulus and after the first aortic root angiography.

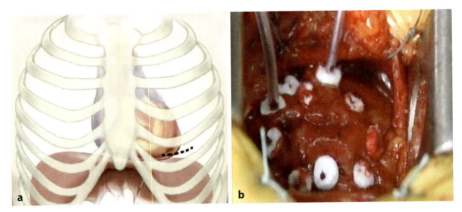

Fig. 4. a Transapical access and **b** left ventricular apex with purse-string sutures

▌ Hemodynamic management

Prior to valvuloplasty and valve implantation a systolic pressure above 120 mmHg (mean 80 mmHg) and sufficient volume preload is mandatory to ensure adequate coronary perfusion. After rapid ventricular pacing with 180–200 beats per minute to decrease left ventricular output temporarily during valvuloplasty and valve deployment, low-dose vasopressor support may be temporarily required. Good coordination of all specific procedural steps between cardiologist, anesthetist, and cardiac surgeon is crucial.

▌ Valvuloplasty and valve deployment

After apical puncture (orientation of the needle towards the right shoulder) a soft guidewire is inserted antegradely across the stenotic aortic valve, followed by a soft tip 14 F (30 cm long) sheath. With the help of a right Judkins catheter, a super stiff guidewire (Amplatz super stiff, 260 cm) is positioned across the aortic arch and into the descending aorta, all with minimal manipulation in the aortic arch. A 20 mm valvuloplasty balloon (filled with 1:4 diluted contrast agent) is placed in the aortic annulus and the tip of the 14F sheath retrieved into the left ventricle. Balloon valvuloplasty is performed during rapid ventricular pacing (RVP) when there is cessation of left ventricular ejection (Fig. 5).

After valvuloplasty, the balloon catheter is retrieved together with the 14 F sheath and the 26 F transapical delivery sheath is inserted bluntly (∼ 5 cm on the external indicators) over the stiff wire and the introducer retrieved (Fig. 6). The system is deaired, the valve introduced into the annulus, and the pusher retrieved. Valve positioning is performed under angiographic guidance aiming at implanting one third (maximum one

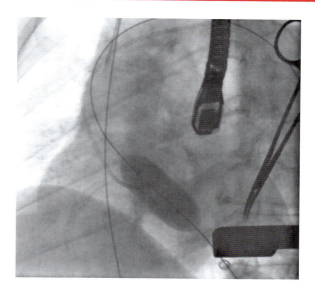

Fig. 5. Balloon valvuloplasty

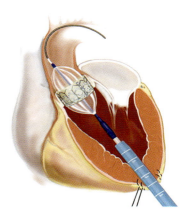

Fig. 6. Schematic TA-AVI

half) of the stent above and the other two thirds (minimum one half) below the level of the aortic annulus (Fig. 7). Once in a good position, online fluoroscopic imaging should be performed until valve implantation. Slight axial movement should be counteracted. An extra episode of RVP may be required to confirm optimal positioning.

A second episode of RVP is used for valve implantation (Fig. 8). Then the balloon is retrieved and regular cardiac function usually recovers. Valve function is assessed using TEE and angiographic control (Fig. 9). The wire is retrieved in case of good valve function without need for repeat balloon dilatation; the latter should be decided on an individual basis keeping patient-related factors in mind.

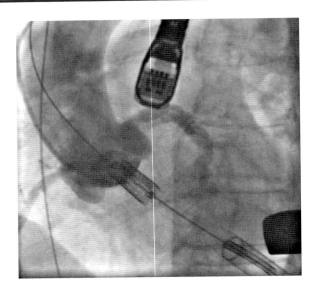

Fig. 7. Positioning of the SAPIEN™ prosthesis

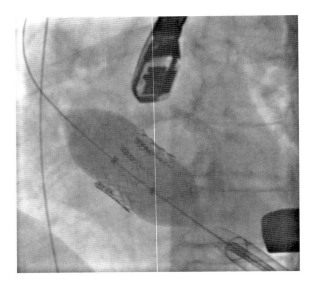

Fig. 8. Transapical valve implantation by balloon dilatation

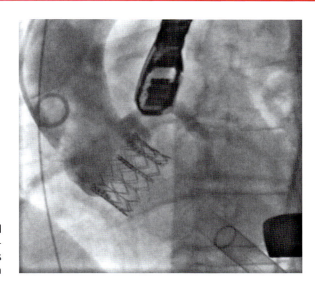

Fig. 9. Angiographic control after valve implantation showing patent coronary arteries and good aortic valve function

At the end of the procedure, the apical sheath is retrieved, the apical ventricular puncture site closed with the purse-string sutures, protamine administered, and the pericardium is slightly closed. A pleural chest drain is inserted, the incision controlled for bleeding, local anesthetic inserted and the chest wall closed in a routine fashion. The patient can usually be extubated early in the postanesthetic care unit and will be transferred to intermediate care afterwards.

How to achieve optimal outcome

"Anything can happen at any time" of the procedure. The mentioned "safety net" should be used in every patient to ensure CPB support within minutes, if required by hemodynamic deterioration.

Optimal imaging is of major importance during valve implantation. High quality fluoroscopic visualization of the aortic root will allow for exact positioning and placement of a transcatheter aortic valve. A modern hybrid operating theater will be the optimal surrounding for successful implementation of a joint transcatheter program.

Given a relatively new complex procedure aiming at very high-risk patients, complications will occur sooner or later. Therefore the whole team should be prepared to take appropriate action immediately, if required. Typical events are as follows:
- Hemodynamic deterioration after RVP or during valve positioning: consider early CPB support if inotropes are not sufficient.

- Apical tear or bleeding: consider additional pledget reinforced U-stitches. In case of major bleeding use CPB to unload the left ventricle.
- Suboptimal angle to the aortic root: re-assess the surgical access site. Try an intercostal space lower (or higher) more laterally (or medially) to obtain an axial approach inline with the aortic root.
- To avoid coronary obstruction, use preoperative cardiac CT assessment to measure the distance between the coronary ostia and the level of the aortic annulus. Try to aim at a very low position of the valve prosthesis to safely stay strictly subcoronary.
- In case of coronary obstruction, consider percutaneous interventions (left main or right ostia stenting) versus conversion to a surgical CABG procedure (beating heart) after hemodynamic stabilization with CPB.
- Severe paravalvular or central leak is rare. In case of moderate paravalvular leak consider reballooning.
- Central leak will increase after re-ballooning. In case of a moderate to severe central leak, the implantation of a second transcatheter valve prosthesis (valve-in-a-valve) is the only option.

The team approach is most important to safely implement a new technique even in high-risk patients. Optimal coordination during implantation is important, especially during critical steps of the procedure. Preoperative training is important and potential bailout strategies should be discussed by the team. Current strengths of the TA approach are the avoidance of the femoral arteries as well as a very low stroke risk due to minimal manipulations in the aortic arch. Therefore, this approach should be chosen in all patients with questionable or borderline femoral access vessels and in those with severe calcifications of the aorta. As peripheral vascular disease is a major risk factor in elderly patients, this has to be kept in mind whenever comparing transapical to transfemoral results at any later stage.

Postoperative care

After successful valve implantation the patients can usually be extubated within the first hour on ICU or PACU. Total AV blocks are not uncommon (up to 10%) and may occur with some delay. Therefore, patients should be kept on a monitor (or telemetric surveillance) for at least 5 d. Indication for permanent pacemaker implantation should be handled liberally.

Full anticoagulation is not required in case of stable sinus rhythm. Low dose aspirin and prophylactic low molecular heparin are sufficient.

Current results

After initial pioneering in the field of transcatheter valve therapy, transapical (TA) and transfemoral (TF) aortic valve implantation (AVI) have evolved to an almost routine procedure in specialized centers.

Table 1. Summary of published results with TA- and TF-AVI

Author	Approach	Valve	Design	n	logES	30-d mortality	Stroke	
Cribier	TF	SA	SC	27	~27	22.2	3.7	JACC (2006) 47:1214
Grube	TF	CV	SC	25	11	20	12	Circ (2006) 114:1616
Lichtenstein	TA	SA	SC	7	35	14	–	Circ (2006) 114:591
Grube	TF	CV	MC	86	21.5	12	10	JACC (2007) 50:69
Webb	TF	SA	SC	50	28	12	4	Circ (2007) 116:755
Walther	TA	SA	SC	30	27	10	–	EJCTS (2007) 31:9
Walther	TA	SA	MC	59	27	13.6	3.4	Circ (2007) 116:I–240
Walther	TA	SA	SC	50	27.6	8	–	EJCTS (2008) 33:983
Grube	TF	CV	MC	646	23.1	8	0.6	EuroInterv (2008) 4:242
Svensson	TA	SA	MC	40	35.5	17.5	–	Ann T Surg (2008) 86:46

TF transfemoral, *TA* transapical, *SA* SAPIEN™ prosthesis, *CV* CoreValve™ prosthesis, *SC* single center trial, *MC* multicenter trial, *n* patients included, *log ES* logistic EuroSCORE (%), *30-d mortality* all cause mortality within 30 days, *stroke* postprocedural new strokes (%)

Given the limitations of the current risk scoring systems available, results from different groups are difficult to compare on a scientific basis. There are no prospectively randomized clinical trials available at present. Table 1 gives an overview on the published results with TA- and TF-AVI. In the more recent series, results from experienced centers are good with 30-day mortality rates below 10%. When judging these results, we always have to take into account the high-risk profile of the patients included with a predicted (even though overestimated) risk for 30-day mortality of 20–30% by logistic EuroSCORE.

As demonstrated in Table 1, superiority of the transapical or the transfemoral approach is still unproven. A randomized, multicenter trial comparing TF-AVI, TA-AVI, and conventional aortic valve replacement would be warranted in order to identify optimal treatment strategies for high-risk patients suffering from severe symptomatic aortic valve stenosis.

At present TA-AVI offers a truly minimally invasive approach facilitating off-pump aortic valve implantation with good results even in high-risk patients with peripheral artery disease. Due to the antegrade approach minimal manipulation at the aortic arch is needed resulting in an extremely low stroke rate and the short distance from the apex to the aortic annulus allows for exact positioning of the prosthesis. In conclusion, TA-AVI is an elegant and safe option to treat high-risk patients by a transcatheter valve specialist team.

References

1. Aupart MR, Mirza A, Meurisse YA, Sirinelli AL, Neville PH, Marchand MA (2006) Perimount pericardial bioprosthesis for aortic calcified stenosis: 18-year experience with 1133 patients. J Heart Valve Dis 15:768–775; discussion 775–766
2. Brown ML, Pellikka PA, Schaff HV, Scott CG, Mullany CJ, Sundt TM, Dearani JA, Daly RC, Orszulak TA (2008) The benefits of early valve replacement in asymptomatic patients with severe aortic stenosis. J Thorac Cardiovasc Surg 135:308–315
3. Huber CH, Goeber V, Berdat P, Carrel T, Eckstein F (2007) Benefits of cardiac surgery in octogenarians – a postoperative quality of life assessment. Eur J Cardiothorac Surg 31:1099–1105
4. Filsoufi F, Rahmanian PB, Castillo JG, Chikwe J, Silvay G, Adams DH (2008) Excellent early and late outcomes of aortic valve replacement in people aged 80 and older. J Am Geriatr Soc 56:255–261
5. Melby SJ, Zierer A, Kaiser SP, Guthrie TJ, Keune JD, Schuessler RB, Pasque MK, Lawton JS, Moazami N, Moon MR, Damiano RJ, Jr. (2007) Aortic valve replacement in octogenarians: risk factors for early and late mortality. Ann Thorac Surg 83:1651-1656; discussion 1656–1657
6. Varadarajan P, Kapoor N, Bansal RC, Pai RG (2006) Clinical profile and natural history of 453 nonsurgically managed patients with severe aortic stenosis. Ann Thorac Surg 82:2111–2115

7. Murtuza B, Pepper JR, Stanbridge RD, Jones C, Rao C, Darzi A, Athanasiou T (2008) Minimal access aortic valve replacement: is it worth it? Ann Thorac Surg 85:1121–1131
8. Iung B, Cachier A, Baron G, Messika-Zeitoun D, Delahaye F, Tornos P, Gohlke-Barwolf C, Boersma E, Ravaud P, Vahanian A (2005) Decision-making in elderly patients with severe aortic stenosis: why are so many denied surgery? Eur Heart J 26:2714–2720
9. Dewey TM, Brown D, Ryan WH, Herbert MA, Prince SL, Mack MJ (2008) Reliability of risk algorithms in predicting early and late operative outcomes in high-risk patients undergoing aortic valve replacement. J Thorac Cardiovasc Surg 135:180–187
10. Vahanian A, Alfieri O, Al-Attar N, Antunes M, Bax J, Cormier B, Cribier A, De Jaegere P, Fournial G, Kappetein AP, Kovac J, Ludgate S, Maisano F, Moat N, Mohr F, Nataf P, Pierard L, Pomar JL, Schofer J, Tornos P, Tuzcu M, van Hout B, Von Segesser LK, Walther T (2008) Transcatheter valve implantation for patients with aortic stenosis: a position statement from the European Association of Cardio-Thoracic Surgery (EACTS) and the European Society of Cardiology (ESC), in collaboration with the European Association of Percutaneous Cardiovascular Interventions (EAPCI). Eur Heart J 29:1463–1470
11. Kempfert J, Walther T, Borger MA, Lehmann S, Blumenstein J, Fassl J, Schuler G, Mohr FW (2008) Minimally invasive off-pump aortic valve implantation: the surgical safety net. Ann Thorac Surg 86:1665–1668

From minimally invasive to percutaneous aortic valve replacement

L. Conradi, H. Treede, H. Reichenspurner

Introduction

The incidence of valvular heart disease (VHD) has steadily increased over the past few decades in western communities and is expected to continuously do so in the face of an aging population. The majority of valvular lesions in Europe and North America are of an acquired origin and occur in the fifth to eighth decade of life. Calcified aortic valve stenosis (AS) and degenerative mitral valve regurgitation (MR) are the two most frequent forms of acquired VHD and account for over 70% of cases in Europe [1]. In Germany, about 98 000 cardiac surgical procedures are performed annually. In 2008, 33 400 cases included valve procedures with 12 300 patients receiving isolated aortic valve replacement (AVR). Mortality rates have been stable around 3 to 4% for single AVR in spite of the ever increasing average patient age and associated comorbidities. The choice of prosthesis in the aortic position has shifted with the majority of diseased valves being replaced by a bioprosthesis today [2]. In contrast to coronary surgery where the decline in the number of operations has been accompanied by a rising procedural volume of percutaneous coronary interventions (PCI) since the late 1990s, valve surgery is still expanding.

Since the beginning of heart valve surgery in the early 1960s, repair or replacement of heart valves has become routine clinical practice. Improved heart valve prostheses and modern repair strategies have led to excellent results with low perioperative morbidity and mortality rates, and good long-term outcome, setting a high standard for new treatment options. However, the number of elderly patients, many of whom present with multiple comorbidities, is increasing. The share of octogenarians among the surgical candidates has tripled in the past 10 years, nearing 10% of all cases in Germany today. This development has triggered the introduction of less invasive surgical valve procedures to reduce operative trauma and to accelerate postoperative recovery. Traditionally, valvular heart surgery was performed through a full median sternotomy, employing cardiopulmonary bypass. Beginning in the early 1990s, minimally invasive techniques were developed, many of which have become standard care today with the same good results concerning perioperative morbidity and mortality and postoperative valve function along with faster patient recovery. More recently, the cardiovascular community has witnessed the advent of new interventional transcatheter valve procedures which hold the promise of an even less invasive treatment option.

Indications

Indications for aortic valve replacement (AVR) were determined by a joint task force of the American College of Cardiology (ACC) and the American Heart Association (AHA) in 1998 and were updated in 2008 [3]. In summary, AVR is indicated in all symptomatic patients with severe AS and in patients with asymptomatic severe AS undergoing cardiac surgery for other reasons. Many cardiac surgery centers have made it their practice to perform AVR along with concomitant cardiac surgery in cases of moderate AS, since the disease is known to progress over time [4]. There remains some controversy as to the treatment of asymptomatic patients with severe AS who have no other indication for surgery. The presence of a low gradient AS along with depressed left ventricular function may indicate excessive afterload (afterload mismatch) to be the cause of LV dysfunction and patients will usually benefit from surgery, especially if a substantial myocardial contractile reserve can be documented [5]. In asymptomatic patients with severe AS and normal left ventricular contractility, exercise testing may help determine treatment strategies.

Techniques of minimally invasive aortic valve surgery

The conventional approach to perform aortic valve surgery via full median sternotomy and cardiopulmonary bypass with cardioplegic arrest implies a profound interference with physiological body functions. Therefore, cardiac surgeons, spurred by the successes of laparoscopic procedures in general surgery in the early 1990s, attempted to minimize surgical trauma in heart valve surgery as well. Delos Cosgrove at the Cleveland Clinic and Lawrence Cohn at Brigham and Women's Hospital were the first to describe their experience with a nonsternotomy approach for aortic valve surgery [6, 7]. Initially they proposed a right parasternal incision and resection of the third and fourth costal cartilages to gain access to the proximal ascending aorta. Transsternal modes of access were also explored. Finally, these incisions were abandoned because of postoperative complications such as chest wall instability and lung herniation or because the price of sacrificing both internal mammary arteries using the transverse sternotomy approach seemed too high. In conclusion, the partial upper sternotomy approach eventually became the strategy of choice. Its routine clinical application was first described by Gundry and coworkers in 1998 [8] and has been adopted by most surgical units performing minimally invasive valve procedures today.

Our approach to minimally invasive aortic valve surgery at the University Heart Center Hamburg consists of a 5 to 6 cm skin incision beginning approximately 5 cm below the jugulum downwards. Dissection of subcutaneous tissue is followed by identification of the third or fourth right intercostal space. After partial upper median sternotomy using an oscillating saw, the dissection is continued into the third or fourth intercostal space, depending on the patient's individual anatomy. Care must be taken to strictly adhere to the sternal midline to avoid fracture of the sternal halves, even more so since only small sternal retractors will fit the incision, thus, distributing forces over a limited area of the sternal edges. The right internal mammary can usually be spared, the pleura remains intact in most cases. We use conventional aortic cannulae as employed for routine cardiac surgery, and small vacuum-assisted venous drainage cannulae to cannulate the ascending aorta and the right atrium directly via the incision. Some groups prefer to introduce the venous cannula via an additional incision below the processus xiphoideus or through an intercostal incision to minimize tubing in the operative field or to be able to retract the right atrium caudally for optimal visualization. When direct access is impossible, femoral cannulation can serve as an alternative. We use a continuous insufflation of CO_2 into the operative field in order to prevent the formation of gaseous emboli and to aide deairing towards the end of the operation. The following steps of the procedure are performed in a standard fashion. After crossclamping, antegrade cardioplegia is delivered via the aortic root or directly into the coronary ostia. A vent can be placed via the right upper pulmonary vein or alternatively in the pulmonary artery, depending on the surgeon's preference.

After replacement or repair of the aortic valve, the aortotomy is closed and the heart is deaired via the needle vent in the aortic root before and after release of the crossclamp by applying continuous suction (Fig. 1). Routine use of intraoperative transesophageal echocardiography is mandatory in order to control the filling state of the heart, for immediate control of the surgical result and to guide the deairing process.

Results after minimally invasive aortic valve surgery

During the last 10 years, many groups including our own [9] have conducted studies comparing outcomes after conventional versus minimally invasive aortic valve surgery. We presented the results of our experience at

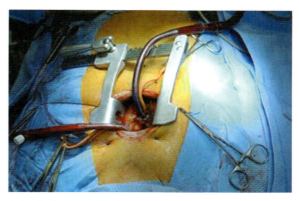

Fig. 1. Intraoperative setting for minimally-invasive AVR via partial upper sternotomy with regular cannulation. © University Heart Center Hamburg

the University Heart Center Hamburg at the 2007 annual meeting of the German Society of Thoracic and Cardiovascular Surgery in Hamburg [10]. Analyzing the results after 438 cases of isolated AVR, we found perioperative mortality to be 3% in the group receiving conventional isolated AVR. In the minimally invasive group, mortality was 0%. Although surgery and cross-clamp times were slightly shorter in the conventional group, patients receiving minimally invasive AVR had a lower rate of postoperative wound complications (1.5 vs. 2.7%) and a shorter duration of intensive care unit and overall hospital stay (55 ± 32 vs. 65 ± 67 h and 8.2 vs. 8.6 d respectively).

Most of the existing studies are of an observational and retrospective nature. There are, however, a few randomized studies. In 2002, Bonacchi and coworkers from Florence, Italy, published their results of 80 consecutive elective cases randomized either to a conventional sternotomy or a partial upper sternotomy group [11]. They found a significant reduction in postoperative blood loss, resulting in lower transfusion requirements in the ministernotomy group. Furthermore, partial sternotomy patients experienced a significantly improved recovery of respiratory function resulting in shorter mechanical ventilation, had a shorter duration of intensive care unit and overall hospital stay, and required significantly lower doses of analgetic medication postoperatively. Dogan and coworkers also reported significantly less blood loss and a better cosmetic result. In terms of safety and reliability both approaches were deemed similar [12]. Recently, Moustafa and coworkers from Mansoura, Egypt, affirmed these earlier results. Their findings included a cosmetic advantage, lower transfusion requirements due to less blood loss, greater sternal stability and earlier extubation and hospital discharge [13] for patients receiving minimally invasive AVR.

Most of the numerous other studies on this topic report similar findings, indicating that a minimally invasive approach to AVR is safe and not inferior to the conventional procedure. Advantages have been demonstrated concerning blood loss and faster postoperative recovery. However, concerning endpoints such as mortality, rates of perioperative myocardial infarction or cerebrovascular events, results remain controversial. Since the central part of the operation using a suture-based technique for implantation of modern, biological or mechanical valve prostheses has remained unchanged, the same excellent long-term results that have been observed after conventional AVR can be anticipated. The advantages of minimally invasive over conventional AVR have been recognized by the American Heart Association and have been included in the recommendations of the most recent Scientific Statement on percutaneous and minimally invasive valve procedures [14].

Percutaneous aortic valve replacement

While AVR via a partial upper sternotomy may offer some advantages in terms of reduced invasiveness, the need for extracorporeal circulation remains and excludes a substantial patient population from surgical treatment [15]. However, conservative management of AS is afflicted with a dismal prognosis [16]. Therefore, even less invasive, beating heart procedures have been developed. The implantation of a catheter-mounted valve prosthesis was first accomplished in an animal model in 1992 [17]. In 2002, Alain Cribier from Rouen, France, successfully implanted an interventional aortic valve prosthesis in a dramatic 'last resort' case of decompensated AS in a 57-year-old man who had been declined as a candidate for surgical AVR by several cardiac surgeons [18]. Since then, multiple improvements have been accomplished in terms of design and access for percutaneous AVR (pAVR). The initially chosen transvenous, antegrade, and transseptal route has been widely abandoned due to the complexity of the procedure. Today, there are two principle procedures for pAVR: a transfemoral, retrograde approach via puncture or cutdown of the femoral artery [19] or a transapical approach via a small left anterolateral thoracotomy [20]. Both types of procedures should be performed in a specially equipped hybrid operating room, providing the implanting personnel with adequate equipment should emergency conversion to surgery with cardiopulmonary bypass become necessary. Modern imaging techniques are essential to guide the implantation process. The combination of transesophageal echocardiography, fluoroscopy, and aortic angiography guarantees optimal conditions for pAVR.

For the transfemoral approach, local anesthesia may suffice, although we and most other groups currently prefer general anesthesia. There are at present two devices on the market and in clinical practice carrying CE mark approval, i.e., the balloon-expandable Sapien (Edwards Lifesciences,

Irvine, CA) and the self-expanding CoreValve (CoreValve Inc., Irvine, CA) prosthesis. Both are of a constructed, pericardial design and are mounted on compressible stents placed on delivery catheters until final positioning. The Edwards Sapien valve is crimped on a balloon catheter which allows for expansion of the valve and deployment in the aortic annulus after initial conventional balloon aortic valvuloplasty. Ventricular rapid pacing is used to minimize transvalvular flow at the time of implantation and, thus, ensure secure seating within the annulus. The CoreValve stent consists of a self-expanding nitinol mesh frame which allows for compression at low temperatures and resumes its original form when released at body temperature. The wide mesh covers the coronary ostia but allows for unimpeded coronary flow. Rapid ventricular pacing is not necessary during implantation of this type of valve.

Direct access to the left ventricular apex via a left anterolateral thoracotomy and subsequent transapical access to the aortic root represents a second alternative deployment route for transcatheter-based AVR without the need for cardiopulmonary bypass. After thoracotomy and opening of the apical pericardium the left ventricular apex is identified, Teflon-felt reinforced purse-string sutures are placed and the apex is directly punctured allowing for insertion of an introducer sheath in Seldinger's technique. Similar to the transfemoral approach, balloon valvuloplasty under rapid ventricular pacing prior to valve deployment may be necessary depending on the type of prosthesis used. After successful valve implantation, the guide wires and introducer sheath are removed and the access site in the ventricular apex is closed using the purse-string sutures.

Currently, there are several other systems for pAVR under development or in early clinical application. One of these, the Direct Flow Valve (Direct Flow Medical Inc., Santa Rosa, CA) is a stentless device made of bovine pericardial tissue encased in a conformable, polyester fabric cuff and designed for transfemoral implantation (Fig. 2). Two inflatable and deflatable ring balloons are used for subcoronary seating. After balloon valvuloplasty under rapid pacing, the catheter (with the valve enclosed in a jacket) is advanced to the aortic annulus and the ventricular and aortic rings are

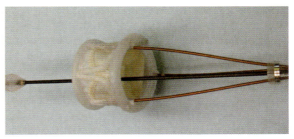

Fig. 2. Expanded direct flow aortic valve prosthesis attached to positioning/fill lumens. Reprinted with permission from [21]

successively inflated using a mix of saline and contrast agent. Because the rings between which the valve leaflets are suspended can be deflated, repositioning or even complete retrieval of the prosthesis is possible until definite device deployment. After correct positioning has been confirmed by transesophageal echocardiography, fluoroscopy, and aortography, the saline-contrast mix is replaced with a solidifying polymer. To date, the Direct Flow valve is the only repositionable and retrievable device in clinical application. The first implantation in humans was performed by our group in late 2007 and throughout 2008 at the University Heart Center Hamburg with promising preliminary results [21]. In a group of 15 patients with a mean logistic EuroSCORE of 24% and a median 30-day risk of mortality of 20% as predicted by the Society of Thoracic Surgeons Score procedural success was achieved in 12 patients (80%). Eleven patients were discharged with a permanent implant, surgical conversion became necessary in one patient on day two after valve intervention, due to incorrect sizing. The procedure resulted in a significant increase in aortic valve area (median 1.64 vs. 0.60 cm^2, p=0.0033) and a concomitant reduction in the mean pressure gradient (median 14.0 vs. 54.0 mmHg, p=0.0033) as well as marked hemodynamic and clinical improvement. At 30 days, one cardiac death and one major stroke were observed.

Results after percutaneous aortic valve replacement

At present, the results after pAVR in most studies are single center experiences with an observational character. Two of the most commonly used devices are the Edwards Sapien valve and the CoreValve system which have recently received CE mark approval. In most trials using these devices, pAVR procedures are performed in a high-risk patient population with reported logistic EuroSCORE ranging from 20 to 30%. Inhospital mortality rates are stated to be 10 to 20% with an incidence of periprocedural cerebrovascular events of 4 to 12% [22]. Freedom from structural valve deterioration has been documented in different studies for up to 4 years [23]. Concern has been expressed regarding issues like paravalvular regurgitation, coronary obstruction, the inability of most systems to recapture malpositioned valves, the incidence of atheromatous embolization and of course long-term durability of the new valve prostheses. Many of these issues will be addressed in future trials such as the currently ongoing North American PARTNER Trial (Placement of AoRTic TraNscathetER Valve Trial) which is randomizing high-risk patients to transfemoral or transapical pAVR using the Edwards Sapien valve or to standard of care (surgical AVR or medical therapy). Results can be expected in 2014.

Conclusions

Since the beginning of heart valve surgery in the early 1960s, replacement or repair of heart valves has developed to become routine clinical practice. The incidence of VHD has steadily increased over the past few decades in western communities and is expected to continuously do so in the face of an aging population. Conventional surgical AVR, most commonly for calcified AS yields excellent short- and long-term results which are documented in an extensive body of data on the subject, setting the gold standard for any aortic valve intervention. Even in high-risk patients outcomes are favorable and the operative risk is substantially lower than predictable by the usual risk stratification tools [24]. Indications for valve procedures are set down in well-approved guidelines of supernational institutions of the cardiovascular community and procedures are performed following standardized protocols. Beginning in the 1990s, minimally invasive aortic valve procedures were developed minimizing surgical trauma and resulting in decreased blood loss and faster patient recovery as documented in prospective randomized trials. Thus, the minimally invasive approach to aortic valve disease has become the standard of care at specialized centers such as our own. While AVR via a partial upper sternotomy offers some advantages in terms of reduced invasiveness, the need for extracorporeal circulation remains and excludes a substantial patient population from surgical treatment [15]. Therefore, interventional transcatheter-based beating heart procedures have been developed.

Since Alain Cribier reported the first in-man implantation in 2002, pAVR has seen a tremendous upsurge. Numerous different devices are available today and in clinical use by clinicians all over the world. Preliminary results of the second and third generation devices are encouraging and further improvements concerning deliverability and safety can be anticipated in the foreseeable future. However, results of pAVR always have to be matched with the superior outcomes of surgical AVR. Extensive data is available on the safety and long-term durability of surgical AVR. At present, most clinicians involved agree that pAVR should be restricted to patients deemed inoperable due to comorbidities. For all others, surgical AVR remains the gold standard. In view of the good results of conventional aortic valve surgery in otherwise healthy octogenarians, age alone should not determine treatment strategies. In their own interest, the protagonists of pAVR should adhere to strict trial protocols and refrain from merely following patients' requests for catheter-based and supposedly less harmful treatment. The current results do not justify the inclusion of patients for interventional treatment other than those with an unacceptable operative risk. At the University Heart Center Hamburg, we have established a close collaboration between cardiologists and cardiac surgeons to determine the optimal treatment strategy for each patient. If the risk of surgical AVR is deemed too high by both cardiologist and surgeon unanimously, interven-

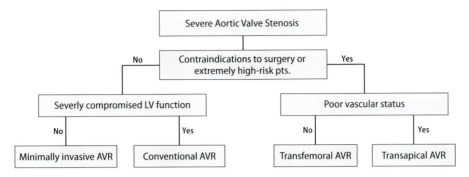

Fig. 3. Decision making at UHC Hamburg to determine the adequate treatment strategy for patients with aortic valve stenosis. © University Heart Center Hamburg

tional treatment via a transfemoral access is an option. In cases of severe peripheral vascular disease, a transapical approach can then be considered. All other patients presenting with severe aortic valve disease will undergo surgery using a minimally invasive approach whenever possible (Fig. 3).

In spite of the current limitations in the clinical applicability of pAVR due to technical deficiencies and unknown long-term performance of the current generation of devices, we are convinced that catheter-based valve techniques will gain increasing weight in the future. The role cardiac surgeons are going to play has yet to be determined. The renowned US cardiac surgeon and member of the Society of Thoracic Surgeons Board of Directors Michael Mack stated in a recent review article: "(...) just as in the dawn of the age of PCI, we have the choice; we can rest on our laurels, stand by our outcomes, and disparage the new treatments being invented. Alternatively, we can learn from the past, embrace change, gain the skill sets needed to participate and thrive, and be part of the process rather than be unengaged bystanders" [25].

References

1. Iung B, Baron G, Butchart EG, Delahaye F, Gohlke-Bärwolf C, Levang OW, Tornos P, Vanoverschelde JL, Vermeer F, Boersma E, Ravaud P, Vahanian A (2003) A prospective survey of patients with valvular heart disease in Europe: the Euro Heart Survey on Valvular Heart Disease. Eur Heart J 24:1231–1243
2. Leistungsstatistik DGTHG 2007
3. Bonow RO, Carabello BA, Chatterjee K et al (2008) 2008 focused update incorporated into the ACC/AHA 2006 guidelines for the management of patients with valvular heart disease: a report of the American College of Cardiology/American Heart Association Task Force on Practice Guidelines (Writing Committee to revise the 1998 guidelines for the management of patients with valvular heart disease).

Endorsed for the Society of Cardiovascular Anesthesiologist, Society for Cardiovascular Angiography and Interventions, and Society of Thoracic Surgeons. J Am Coll Cardiol 52:c1–142

4. Rosenhek R, Binder T, Porenta G et al (2000) Predictors of outcome in severe, asymptomatic aortic stenosis. N Engl J Med 343:611
5. Monin JL, Quere JP, Monchi M, Petit H, Baleynaud S, Chauvel C, Pop C, Ohlmann P, Lelguen C, Dehant P, Tribouilloy C, Gueret P (2003) Low-gradient aortic stenosis, operative risk stratification and predictors for long-term outcome: a multicenter study using dobutamine stress hemodynamics. Circulation 108:319–324
6. Cosgrove DM 3rd, Sabik JF (1996) Minimally invasive approach for aortic valve operations. Ann Thorac Surg 62:596
7. Cohn LH, Adams DH, Couper GS et al (1997) Minimally invasive cardiac valve surgery improves patient satisfaction while reducing costs of cardiac valve replacement and repair. Ann Surg 226:421
8. Gundry SR, Shattuck OH, Razzouk AJ, del Rio MJ, Sardari FF, Bailey LL (1998) Facile minimally invasive cardiac surgery via ministernotomy. Ann Thorac Surg 65:1100–1004
9. Detter C, Deuse T, Boehm DH, Reichenspurner H, Reichart B (2002) Midterm results and quality of life after minimally invasive vs. conventional aortic valve replacement. J Thorac Cardiovasc Surg 50:337–341
10. Reiter B, Beinke A, Wipper SH, Schönebeck J, Sprathoff N, Treede H, Boehm DH, Detter C, Reichenspurner H (2007) Minimal invasive aortic valve surgery: The development of a single center from the beginning until now. Thorac Cardiovasc Surg 55:S1
11. Bonacchi M, Prifti E, Giunti G, Frati G, Sani G (2002) Does Ministernotomy improve postoperative out come in aortic valve operations? A prospective randomized study. Ann Thorac Surg 73:460–466
12. Dogan S, Dzemali O, Wimmer-Greinecker G et al (2003) Minimally invasive versus conventional aortic valve replacement: a prospective randomized trial. J Heart Valve Dis 12:76–80
13. Moustafa MA, Abdelsamad AA, Zakaria G, Omarah MM (2007) Minimal vs. median sternotomy for aortic valve replacement. Asian Cardiovasc Thorac Ann 15:472–475
14. Rosengart TK, Feldman T, Borger MA, Vassiliades TA, Gillinov AM, Hoercher KJ, Vahanian A, Bonow RO, O'Neill W (2008) Percutaneous and minimally invasive valve procedures. A scientific statement from the American Heart Association Council on Cardiovascular Surgery and Anesthesia, Council on Clinical Cardiology, Functional Genomics and Translational Biology Interdisciplinary Working Group, and Quality of Care and Outcomes Research Interdisciplinary Working Group. Circulation 117:1750–1767
15. Nkomo VT, Gardin JM, Skelton TN, Gottdiener JS, Scott CG, Enriquez-Sarano M (2006) Burden of valvular heart diseases: a population-base study. Lancet 368:1005–1011
16. Lund O, Nielsen TT, Emmertsen K, Flo C, Rasmussen B, Jensen FT, Pilegaard HK, Kristensen LH, Hansen OK (1996) Mortality and worsening of prognostic profile during waiting time for valve replacement in aortic stenosis. Thorac Cardiovasc Surg 44:289–295
17. Andersen HR, Knudsen LL, Hasenkam JM (1992) Transluminal implantation of artificial heart valves. Description of a new expandable aortic valve and initial results with implantation by catheter technique in closed chest pigs. Eur Heart J 13:704–708
18. Cribier A, Eltchaninoff H, Bash A, Borenstein N, Tron C, Bauer F, Derumeaux G, Anselme F, Laborde F, Leon MB (2002) Percutaneous Transcatheter Implantation

of an Aortic Valve Prosthesis for Calcific Aortic Stenosis: First Human Case Description. Circulation 106:3006–3008
19. Webb JG, Chandavimol M, Thompson CR, Ricci DR, Carere RG, Munt BI, Buller CE, Pasupati S, Lichtenstein S (2006) Percutaneous aortic valve implantation retrograde from the femoral artery. Circulation 113:842–850
20. Walther T, Simon P, Dewey T, Wimmer-Greinecker G, Volkmar F, Kasimir M et al (2007) Transapical minimally invasive aortic valve implantation. Circulation 116:I240–I245
21. Schofer J, Schlüter M, Treede H, Franzen O, Tübler T, Pascotta A, Low RI, Bolling SF, Meinertz T, Reichenspurner H (2008) Retrograde transarterial implantation of a nonmetallic aortic valve prosthesis in high surgical-risk patients with severe aortic stenosis: A first-in-man feasibility and safety study. Circ Cardiovasc Intervent 1:126–133
22. Walther T, Chu MWA, Mohr FW (2008) Transcatheter aortic valve implantation: time to expand? Curr Opin Cardiol 23:111–116
23. Cribier A, Eltchaninoff H, Tron C (2006) Percutaneous implantation of aortic valve prosthesis in patients with calcific aortic stenosis: technical advances, clinical results and future strategies. J Invasive Cardiol 19:88–96
24. Collart F, Feier H, Kerbaul F, Mouly-Bandini A, Riberi A, Mesana TG, Metras D (2005) Valvular surgery in octogenarians: operative risks factors, evaluation of Euroscore and long term results. Eur J Cardiothorac Surg 27:276–280
25. Mack M (2008) Fool me once, shame on me. Fool me twice, shame on you. A perspective on the emerging world of percutaneous heart valve therapy. J Thorac Cardiovasc Surg 136:816–819

Sutureless equine aortic valve replacement

S. Martens

Introduction

Aortic valve replacement with mechanical or biological heart valves is the treatment of choice for aortic valve stenosis. With increasing patient co-morbidity and age, there is a trend towards biological valve implants avoiding long-term anticoagulation. In order to improve the hemodynamic and clinical outcome of patients after aortic valve replacement, stentless valves were introduced in the early 1990s. These valves were designed to result in lower transvalvular gradients.

The implantation technique of stentless valves is more demanding and time consuming, with consecutive prolongation of the aortic cross-clamp and cardiopulmonary bypass times. Cox and coworkers published their in vitro data on the newly designed 3f aortic bioprosthesis, a stentless bioprosthesis which consists of a tubular structure assembled from three equal sections of equine pericardial tissue [1]. Our group presented clinical and hemodynamic data on 24 patients operated between January and August 2002. While hemodynamic data were equivalent to other commercially available stentless valves, the implantation still required a cross-clamp time of 74 min [2].

In order to facilitate the surgical implantation, the 3f prosthesis was modified by addition of a self-expanding nitinol external frame, allowing for sutureless implant (Fig. 1): The ATS 3f Enable™ (ATS Medical, Minneapolis, MN, USA). The nitinol frame contributes to the fixation of the device in the deployed location through outward radial forces inherent in the material. To minimize the potential of paravavular leakage or migration, an oversized polyester flange was incorporated at the inflow aspect of the prosthesis. A total of 32 of these valves were implanted at our institution between July 2007 and November 2008. Because this patient cohort should profit from reduced implant times, we did not exclude patients at increased risk for perioperative morbidity and mortality from this trial; thus, also combined procedures with CABG and mitral tricuspid valve surgery were performed.

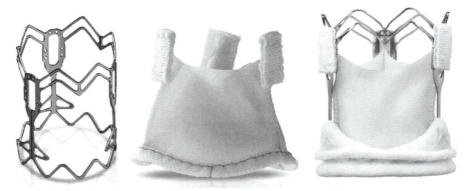

Fig. 1. The external self-expanding nitinol frame combined with the equine biologic 3f valve (Model 1000), resulting in a sutureless aortic valve prosthesis (ATS 3f Enable™)

Operative technique

In stand-alone procedures for aortic valve replacement, access to the mediastinal structures was obtained through partial upper sternotomy ending at the fourth (left) intercostal space.

Patients undergoing combined procedures with CABG received a complete sternotomy and preparation of the mammary artery and saphenous vein grafts, respectively. Cardiopulmonary bypass was instituted after cannulation of the ascending aorta or the right subclavian artery in patients at increased risk for cerebrovascular events. The right atrium was cannulated for venous drainage. For drainage of the left ventricle, a vent was introduced through the right upper pulmonary vein or the pulmonary artery, respectively. If complete sternotomy had been performed, the cardioplegic solution was applied through a retrograde catheter inserted in the coronary sinus. Patients operated on through partial sternotomy received antegrade cardioplegia through a needle vent in the ascending aorta, repeat application was performed using selective coronary ostial catheters. After aortic cross clamping, access to the aortic valve was obtained through transverse aortotomy, which was performed 2 cm above the sinotubular junction (Fig. 2). The aortic valve was inspected; the presence of a bicuspid valve was regarded as exclusion criteria according to the protocol. Attention was also paid to possible abnormalities of the coronary ostia or mismatch between the annulus and the sinotubular junction, respectively.

Excision of the aortic valve and debridement of the annulus was performed; afterwards we accurately sized the aortic annulus with especially designed sizers (Fig. 3). Because fixation of the valve in place is obtained through outward radial forces of the nitinol frame, care has to be taken for exact sizing. Paravalvular leakage might occur if the implant chosen is too

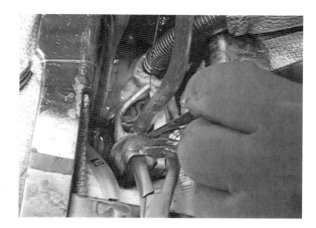

Fig. 2. The aortotomy is performed 2 cm above the sinotubular junction

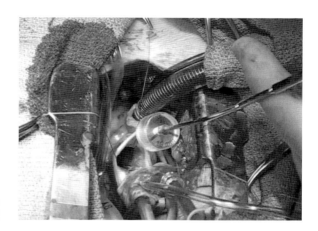

Fig. 3. Sizing is carefully performed as described in the text

small for the annulus. In case of oversizing, complete deployment of the valve might become impossible. The prosthesis requires rinsing in saline solution three times for 2 minutes each time. The time required for the rinsing process should be used for placement of a guiding suture (2/0 polyethylene) in the acoronary sinus, at the level of the deepest point of the annulus.

After the rinsing process is completed, the valve is placed in chilled physiological saline to make it pliable (Fig. 4). It is carefully folded under water to avoid damage of the frame. The valve is inserted in a specially designed deployment tool. The guiding suture is now attached to the superior portion of the polyester flange, in a position corresponding to the placement in the acoronary sinus. The valve is now inserted and deployed with special care taken to avoid rotation. Before the deployment is completed, through rinsing with warm saline solution, the positioning of the valve has

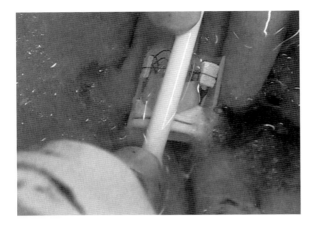

Fig. 4. Plication of the valve in chilled saline solution

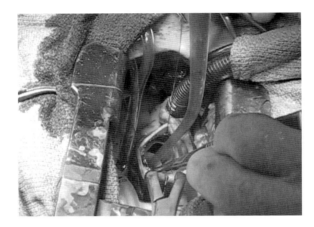

Fig. 5. The ATS 3f Enable™ valve after correct placement

to be meticulously inspected and, if necessary, corrected. If malpositioning occurs after complete deployment of the valve, rinsing with chilled saline enhances repositioning. The guiding suture is then tied down. In 9 patients of our series, we removed it without having observed postoperative displacement of the valve. The aortotomy is then closed in the regular fashion (Fig. 5).

Correct positioning of the valve prosthesis without paravalvular leakage was assessed intraoperatively by transesophageal echocardiography. Transthoracic echocardiography examinations were carried out at discharge, at 6 months, and at 12 months after surgery. Again, special attention was placed on the absence of valvular or paravalvular regurgitation, transvalvular gradients, and effective orifice area.

Clinical experience

From July 2007 through November 2008, 34 elective patients, who presented for isolated aortic valve replacement or combined procedures, were included in the study in our institution as a part of a multicenter trial. Mean age was 78±3 years, mean logistic EuroSCORE was 14; thus, our patients represented a high-risk cohort of cardiosurgical patients. Patients with acute infective endocarditis were excluded from this study.

Concomitant procedures were mitral valve and tricuspid valve repair (n=1), CABG (n=10), and subvalvular myectomy (n=5). Prosthetic valve sizes were 19 mm (n=1), 21 mm (n=9), 23 mm (n=9), 25 mm (n=13), and 27 mm (n=2). Two cases were abandoned intraoperatively due to misalignment of the valve (which was a 25 mm size in both cases). Although we felt that the reason for failure might have been oversizing, we converted to standard procedures with a 23 mm, commercially available bioprosthetic stented valve to avoid excess bypass time due to another pump run.

After initial deployment of the valve, exact positioning was time consuming, especially in the first cases of our series. Implantation of the valve required 9±5 min. Cardiopulmonary bypass and aortic cross-clamp time were 99±31 and 67±23 min, respectively. With increasing implant experience, procedural times were reduced.

No paravalvular leakage was detected in the operating room or at discharge. In one patient, mild paravalvular leakage was identified at the 6-month follow-up. However, 12 months after surgery it could not be detected any more. The transvalvular gradient at discharge was 10±6 mmHg (mean) and 18±9 mmHg (peak). The effective orifice area at discharge was determined to be 2.2±0.8 cm^2. Early mortality (<90 d) was 12.5% (4 patients); no valve-related mortality occurred.

Comments

The idea of a sutureless valve is not new: Magovern presented clinical results with a ball-cage-type prosthetic heart valve in the early 1960s [3]. However, the incidence of disabling thromboembolism (42%) and poppet failure (21%) was high with these early models [4]. First clinical experiences with a bioprosthetic valve designed for sutureless implant were published more than 40 years later by Wendt and coworkers [6]. To facilitate implantation, the 3f aortic bioprosthesis was modified with the addition of a self-expanding nitinol external frame that imparts flexibility. In their experience, three out of six patients presented with paravalvular leakage at follow-up; one of them underwent successful reoperation after 8 months.

The design of the valve implanted in this initial series was different regarding the polyester flange. The inferior aspect of the flange was enlarged in the current model, thus, allowing for broader coaptation with the annulus. In addition, up to three stay sutures were placed in the annulus in the initial series, possibly causing distortion of the valve. In our series of 32 implants, only one stay suture was tied down, while 9 implants did not receive a stay suture at all. Mild paravalvular leakage occurred in only one patient of our series after 6 months, which could not be detect any more after 12 months.

Percutaneous transfemoral aortic valve implantation found entrance into clinical practice. With transapical aortic valve implantation, a more surgical approach was developed [5]. One of the advantages is a significantly reduced stroke rate as compared to the transfemoral approach. With both techniques, the calcified aortic valve is just pressed into the aortic wall, without decalcification of the annulus. The rate of paravalvular leakage will always remain an important issue with this technology.

Implantation of a sutureless aortic valve prosthesis after resection of the native aortic valve, allowing for reduced CPB and aortic cross-clamp time, might be an alternative treatment option for patients at increased risk for morbidity and mortality after cardiac surgery. The transaortic approach adds the advantage of allowing for concomitant procedures as CABG or mitral/tricuspid valve surgery, as long as flexible implants are being used in the latter.

We have shown that sutureless valve implantation is possible and safe with the equine ATS 3f Enable™ valve. Exact positioning of the valve prosthesis is still time consuming, but with increasing experience, further reduction of aortic cross-clamp and CPB time seems possible. Hemodynamic features of the valve are promising. Despite encouraging short-term results with this new valve, we need data documenting long-term performance.

References

1. Cox JL, Ad N, Myers K, Gharib M, Quijano RC (2005) Tubular heart valves: a new tissue prosthesis design – preclinical evaluation of the 3f aortic bioprosthesis. J Thorac Cardiovasc Surg 130(2):520–527
2. Doss M, Martens S, Wood JP, Miskovic A, Christodoulou T, Wimmer-Greinecker G, Moritz A (2005) Aortic leaflet replacement with the new 3F stentless aortic bioprosthesis. Ann Thorac Surg 79:682–685
3. Magovern GJ, Cromie HW (1963) Sutureless prosthetic heart valves. J Thorac Cardiovasc Surg 46:726–736

4. Scott SM, Sethi GK, Flye MW, Takaro T (1976) The sutureless aortic valve prosthesis: experience with and technical considerations for replacement of the early model. Ann Surg 184(2):174–178
5. Walther T, Simon P, Dewey T, Wimmer-Greinecker G, Falk V, Kasimir MT et al (2007) Transapical minimally invasive aortic valve implantation: multicenter experience. Circulation 116(11 Suppl):I240–I245
6. Wendt D, Thielmann M, Buck T, Janosi RA, Bossert T, Pizanis N, Kamler M, Jakob H (2008) First clinical experiences and 1-year follow-up with the sutureless 3F-Enable aortic valve prosthesis. Eur J Cardiothorac Surg 33:542–547

The Ross operation: Aortic valve and root replacement with pulmonary autograft

Pulmonary autograft or aortic allograft for surgical treatment of active infective aortic valve endocarditis: a review of the literature

C. A. Yankah

The search for the ideal substitute for the diseased aortic valve led Donald Ross to develop the concept of the aortic allograft and pulmonary autograft for subcoronary implantation in the 1960s and in the early 1970s as a full root to replace aortic roots with abscesses [1–5]. Allograft aortic valve replacement was pioneered by two surgeons, Mr. Donald Ross himself in London and Sir Brian Barratt-Boyes in Auckland, New Zealand, independently of each other in 1962 [1, 6].

During the last century, the aortic allograft and pulmonary autograft surgical procedures revolutionized the history of cardiac valve surgery. They compete well with bioprostheses, being non-thrombogenic and, thus, requiring no postoperative anticoagulation. They are also resistant to infection and restore the anatomy of the aortic or pulmonary outflow tract, which ensures unimpeded blood flow and excellent hemodynamics, thus, offering patients a better prognosis of survival with good quality of life. Initial results were unsatisfactory due to technical problems of implantation and early tissue failure of the allograft valves due to lack of proper decontamination and preservation techniques.

Over time, the pulmonary autograft (Ross operation) has proven to be the preferred device for valve replacement in young patients in whom growth of the valve replacement is anticipated. It is a challenging double-valve procedure consisting of subcoronary aortic valve or aortic root replacement which requires surgical skill and experience to achieve good results. The operation technique has gained popularity and acceptance among today's pediatric surgeons.

Both the pulmonary autograft and aortic allograft have gained popularity in the management of acute endocarditis with root abscesses because of their resistance to infection. Aortic allograft is absolutely indicated for aortic root abscess with aortic ventricular dehiscence and drug addicts [10]. Their superiority over prosthetic valves has been demonstrated in many reports [7–13].

Results

The pulmonary autograft in the aortic position

The operative mortality rate for patients with endocarditis is reported to be 5–12% and the rate of reinfection is estimated to be 0–3% at 5 years [11, 12].

In patients with noninfected aortic root, hospital mortality is 0.6–3.9%. In the series of Elkins et al., in which most of the patients underwent root replacement, survival at 16 years was 82%, actuarial freedom from autograft reoperation and tissue failure was 80% and 74%, respectively, and for freedom from autograft endocarditis it was 95%. In children, actuarial freedom from autograft failure at 16 years was 83% and survival was 84%. The 16-year freedom from allograft reoperation was 82% [14]. Actuarial freedom from reoperation for the subcoronary implantation technique at 8 years in the series studied by Schmidtke et al. was 95% [11, 15].

The overall operative mortality reported from the German-Dutch Ross Registry in this volume was 1.4%; however, the rate of postoperative endocarditis for a pulmonary autograft in the aortic position and an aortic allograft in the pulmonary circulation was 14% and 21%, respectively [11].

Long-term results over 20 years are available only from the series of patients operated on by Ross himself. Of 225 survivors operated on by Ross, reoperation was performed in 17 (7.5%) patients due to technical failures and in 7 (3%) due to tissue failure during the 20 years of follow-up. There were 7 (3%) valve-related deaths and 8 (3.5%) other nonvalve-related deaths. The actuarial freedom from valve failure or reoperation on the aortic allograft in the pulmonary circulation was 81% and freedom from valve-related death was 97% (Table 2) [16].

Table 1. Surgical results of active infective native and prosthetic valve endocarditis according to type of valve replacement. A review of the literature

Source	Years	30-day mortality (%) Allo/PA	30-day mortality (%) Prosthesis	Reinfection/PL (%) Allo/PA	Reinfection/PL (%) Prothesis
Knosalla et al. [22]	11	8.5	23.5	3.2	27.1
Petrou et al. [17]	11	8.3	na	4.5	na
Haydock et al. [8]	15	17	20.7	na	na
Yankah et al. [10]	17	9.3	na	4.3	na
d'Udeckem et al. [23]	8	na	13	na	11.4
Niwaya et al. [12]	13	17	20	3	12.5
Niwaya et al. [12]	13	12	na	3	na

PA pulmonary autograft, *PL* paravalvular leak, *na* not available

Table 2. Long-term results of pulmonary autograft (the Ross operation) and allograft replacement of the aortic valve and root. A review of the literature*

	PA		Aortic allograft	
	Elkins et al.	Lund et al.	O'Brien et al.	Yankah et al.
Follow-up (years)	16	10/20	20	17
No. of patients	487	618	1022	203
Mean age at op. (years)	24	51	49	53
Hospital mortality (%)	3.9	5	3	2.3
Free of SVD (%)	74	62/18	na	na
Free of reoperation	80	81/35	50	72
Free of graft infection	95	93/89	89	90
Patient survival	82	67/35	40	64

* Elkins et al. [14], Lund et al. [7], O'Brien et al. [18], Yankah et al. [10].
PA pulmonary autograft

Aortic allograft in the aortic position

The operative mortality of allograft patients with active infective endocarditis was estimated to be 4–14% [10, 17]. Survival at 10 years and 15 years was 87% and 70%, respectively. The incidence of early reinfection was 1–4% and was associated with perivalvular leak and pseudoaneurysm formation [10, 17]. Freedom from recurrent infection and reoperation for all causes at 10 years and 15 years was 97% and 80%, respectively [17]. The reoperative hospital death rate after replacement of reinfected allograft ranged from 4 to 9.3% [9, 10, 17].

The 15- and 20-year survival of allograft patients with sterile aortic roots in our series was 65% and 58%, respectively. Late death was 5.6%. The estimated freedom from reoperation for all causes was 76% and 50% at 15 and 20 years, respectively. Actuarial freedom from structural deterioration at 15 years was 47% in patients under 20 years of age and 81% in patients between 41 and 60 years [18]. Freedom from explantation of undersized and matched allografts at 15 years was 48% and 77%, respectively [19].

Aortic root replacement

Patient survival was 71% for patients with a root replacement at 15 and 20 years. Freedom from structural valve deterioration (SVD) of 82.9% and 56% at 17 and 25 years, respectively, was documented [7, 10].

Freehand subcoronary aortic valve replacement

The survival rate of patients with subcoronary implantation was 45%, 33%, and 23% at 15, 20, and 25 years. Freedom from SVD was 63.5% and 15% at 17 and 25 years, respectively. Patients with undersized allograft and tailored aortic root who underwent freehand AVR had 48% and 13% freedom from reoperation at 10 and 15 years, respectively [7, 10].

Comments

Understanding of the use of pulmonary autografts and aortic and pulmonary allografts, from the bench to clinical practice, is probably universal for surgeons, especially those of the younger generation, homograft bankers, and scientists.

The surgeon has the medical and ethical responsibility to use a pulmonary autograft and aortic and pulmonary allograft valves to treat patient with aortic and pulmonary valvular disease. What we have accepted as critically important to pulmonary autograft and allograft recipients is the implanting surgeon's skill and scientific and clinical knowledge as well as quality control, which determine the outcome of the patient.

Lerich put it simply and effectively: "The great problem of surgery is a problem of knowledge." Allan Callow in Boston complemented this by saying that better science, which means better data, is making better medicine possible. Proof of the durability of viable allografts came from the longer follow-up series of Lund and O'Brien [18].

To provide perspective and to emphasize the state of the art, a brief review of current clinical practice is warranted. It is now recognized that the clinical results and durability of aortic and pulmonary allografts depend not only on tissue viability, recipient and donor age, and immune response, but also on valve sizing and the implantation technique.

A full root replacement is associated with a low incidence of valve dysfunction and of early reoperation. Aortic root tailoring or reduction annuloplasty of a large aortic annulus during freehand subcoronary aortic valve replacement appears to carry a high risk of valve failure and early reoperation. Patients with undersized allograft and tailored aortic root who underwent freehand AVR had freedom from reoperation of 48% and 13% at 10 and 15 years, respectively [7, 10]. In the learning phase of autograft, allograft root and freehand subcoronary aortic valve implantation, the rate of reoperation for technical, nonstructural valve failure will obviously be relatively high [7, 18]. The technical errors are associated with a geometric mismatch between the anatomic units of the aortic root, resulting in paravalvular leak, central leak, cusp rupture, leaflet prolapse or distortion, commissural displacement or progressive aortic root dilatation (annuloectasia, Marfan's syndrome).

Aortic annulus reinforcement with teflon or glutaraldehyde-fixed equine pericardial strips after aortic root replacement was suggested by Ross and others to prevent progressive annular dilatation of the pulmonary autograft and in patients with annuloectasia undergoing allograft root replacement [20, 21]. While others prefer the aortic root replacement technique for the Ross operation, Sievers has demonstrated that the freehand subcoronary implantation technique requires no aortic annulus reinforcement because the implantation technique itself provides protection against postoperative root dilatation and ensuing valve incompetence [11, 15]. It is, therefore, a fact that the implantation techniques of the pulmonary autograft constitute the technical artistry of the Ross operation.

The operative mortality rate of allograft patients with active infective endocarditis was estimated to be 4–14% compared to 5–12% for the Ross operation [10, 17]. Reoperative hospital death rate after replacement of reinfected allografts in our series was 9.3% and is comparable to that of other reports [17]. Recurrent endocarditis was the most common cause of death in allograft patients. The incidence of early reinfection was 1–4% as compared to 0–3% in autograft patients [10, 11, 12, 17]. Actuarial freedom from reinfection in allograft patients at 10 and 15 years was 81–97% and 72%, respectively [10, 17]. Survival at 10 and 15 years in endocarditis patients with allografts was found to be 82% and 70.4%, respectively [10, 17]. Survival of allograft patients at 15 and 20 years was 64.8% and 58%, respectively, in our series. In other series, survival of allograft patients at 15, 20, and 25 years was 48%, 35%, and 26% [7]. There was a significant difference in survival among patients with different allograft implantation techniques. Others reported long-term survival of 71% for patients with root replacement at 15 years; for patients with subcoronary implantation, it was 45%, 33%, and 23% at 15, 20, and 25 years, respectively [7, 10, 18]. Survival of autograft patients with root technique at 16 years was 82%, while in children it was 84% [21].

In O'Brien's follow-up of patients with allograft aortic valves, the estimated freedom from reoperation for all causes was 76% and 50% at 15 and 20 years, respectively. Structural deterioration at 15 years was 47% in patients under 20 years of age and 81% in patients between 41 and 60 years [18]. In other series, the actuarial freedom from allograft explantation at 15 years was 48% for undersized and 77% for matched valves [19]. Patients aged 53 years who were undergoing allograft aortic root replacement have shown freedom from reoperation for structural valve deterioration (SVD) of 82.9% and 56% at 17 and 20 years, respectively, as compared to 82% for autograft in patients aged 24 years at 16 years [7, 10, 21].

In conclusion, the pulmonary autograft in the aortic position (the Ross operation) should be considered the valve of choice for surgical treatment of active infective endocarditis in children and adolescents, although long-term data are not yet available. Allograft replacement of the aortic valve can be performed with good results but the risk of early degeneration limits its use in children, except in rescue operations.

Acknowledgment. The author is grateful to Anne M. Gale, ELS, for editorial assistance.

References

1. Ross DN (1962) Homograft replacement of the aortic valve. Lancet 2:487
2. Gonzalez-Lavin L, Graft D, Ross DN (1997) Indications and surgical technique of aortic valve replacement with the autologous pulmonary valve. In: Yankah AC, Yacoub MH, Hetzer R (eds) Cardiac valve allografts II: science and practice. Darmstadt: Steinkopff, pp 173–180
3. Gerosa G, McKay R, Ross DN (1991) Replacement of the aortic valve or root with a pulmonary autograft in children. Ann Thorac Surg 51:424–429
4. Somerville J, Ross D (1982) Homograft replacement of aortic root with reimplantation of coronary arteries. Results after one to five years. Br Heart J 47:473–482
5. Donaldson RM, Ross DN (1984) Homograft aortic root replacement for complicated prosthetic valve endocarditis. Circulation 70(Suppl I):I-178–I-181
6. Barratt-Boyes BG (1964) Homograft aortic valve replacement in aortic incompetence and stenosis. Thorax 19:131–135
7. Lund O, Chandrasekaran V, Grocott-Mason R, Elwidaa H, Mazhar R, Khaghani A et al (1999) Primary aortic valve replacement with allografts over twenty-five years: valve-related and procedure-related determinants of outcome. J Thorac Cardiovasc Surg 117:77–91
8. Haydock D, Barratt-Boyes B, Macedo T, Kirklin JW, Blackstone E (1992) Aortic valve replacement for active infectious endocarditis in 108 patients. A comparison of freehand allograft valves with mechanical prostheses and bioprostheses. J Thorac Cardiovasc Surg 103:130–139
9. Miller DC (1990) Predictors of outcome in patients with prosthetic valve endocarditis (PVE) and potential advantages of homograft aortic root replacement for prosthetic ascending aortic valve-graft infections. J Card Surg 5:53–62
10. Yankah AC, Pasic M, Klose H, Siniawski H, Weng Y, Hetzer R (2005) Homograft reconstruction of the aortic root for endocarditis with periannular abscess: a 17-year study. Eur J Cardiothorac Surg 28:69–75
11. Schmidtke C, Dahmen G, Sievers HH (2007) Subcoronary Ross procedure in patients with active endocarditis. Ann Thorac Surg 83(1):36–39
12. Niwaya K, Knott-Craig CJ, Santangelo K, Lane MM, Chandrasekaran K, Elkins RC (1999) Advantage of autograft and homograft valve replacement for complex aortic valve endocarditis. Ann Thorac Surg 67(6):1603–1608
13. Takkenberg JJ, Klieverik LM, Schoof PH, van Suylen RJ, van Herwerden LA, Zondervan PE, Roos-Hesselink JW, Eijkemans MJC, Yacoub MH, Bogers AJ (2009) The Ross procedure: A systematic review and meta-analysis. Circulation 119(2):222-228
14. Elkins RC, Thompson DM, Lane MM, Elkins CC, Peyton MD (2008) Ross operation: 16-year experience. J Thorac Cardiovasc Surg 136(3):623–630, 630.e1–e5
15. Sievers HH, Hanke T, Stierle U, Bechtel MF, Graf B, Robinson DR, Ross DN (2006) A critical reappraisal of the Ross operation: renaissance of the subcoronary implantation technique? Circulation 114(1 Suppl):I504–I511
16. Matsuki O, Okita Y, Almeida RS, McGoldrick JP, Hooper TL, Robles A, Ross DN (1988) Two decades' experience with aortic valve replacement with pulmonary autograft. J Thorac Cardiovasc Surg 95:705–711

17. Petrou M, Wong K, Albertucci M, Brecker SJ, Yacoub MH (1994) Evaluation of unstented aortic homografts for the treatment of prosthetic aortic valve endocarditis. Circulation 90(Part 2):II-198–II-204
18. O'Brien MF, Harrocks S, Stafford EG, Gardner MA, Pohlner PG, Tesar PJ et al (2001) The homograft aortic valve: a 29-year, 99.3% follow up of 1022 valve replacements. J Heart Valve Dis 10:334–344
19. Yankah AC, Klose H, Musci M, Siniawski H, Hetzer R (2001) Geometric mismatch between homograft (allograft) and native aortic root: a 14-year clinical experience. Eur J Cardio-thorac Surg 20:835–841
20. Carpentier A (1983) Cardiac valve surgery – The "French correction". J Thorac Cardiovasc Surg 86:323–337
21. Elkins RC (1996) Pulmonary autografts in patients with aortic annulus dysplasia. Ann Thorac Surg 61:1141–1145
22. Knosalla C, Weng Y, Yankah AC, Siniawski H, Hofmeister J, Hammerschmidt R, Loebe M, Hetzer R (2000) Homograft versus prosthetic valve for surgical treatment of aortic valve endocarditis with periannular abscess. Eur Heart J 21:490–497
23. d'Udekem Y, David TE, Feindel CM, Armstrong S, Sun Z (1997) Long-term results of surgery for active infective endocarditis. Eur J Cardiothorac Surg 11:46–52

The Ross operation: two decades of clinical experience

J. F. M. Bechtel, H.-H. Sievers, T. Hanke, U. Stierle,
A. J. J. J. C. Bogers, W. Hemmer, J. O. Böhm, J. G. Rein, C. A. Botha,
R. Lange, J. Hörer, A. Moritz, T. Wahlers, U. F. W. Franke,
M. Breuer, K. Ferrari-Kühne, R. Hetzer, M. Hübler, G. Ziemer,
A. W. Gorski, J. J. M. Takkenberg, M. Misfeld
on behalf of the German-Dutch Ross Registry

Until today, no perfect valve substitute has been developed. Some essential requirements for a perfect valve substitute are proposed in Table 1. Regarding the aortic valve, the Ross procedure (pulmonary autograft operation) is closer to this ideal than any other substitute in many ways. For this reason, it was enthusiastically adopted by many surgeons after it became widely known in the late 1980s and was technically simplified by Stelzer and Elkins [27] (total root replacment, Fig. 1). In recent years, however, several groups report high reoperation rates and a worrysome tendency for the development of neoaortic regurgitation and/or ascending aortic aneurysms [7, 10, 16, 18, 20, 29]. A recent systematic review concluded that "durability limitations become apparent by the end of the first postoperative decade, in particular in younger patients" [28], and it was asked whether the Ross procedure is a "Trojan horse" [15]. As a result of these newer data, many centers appear to have stopped performing the Ross procedure.

In Lübeck, we have retained the subcoronary implantation of the pulmonary autograft, as originally described by Donald N. Ross in 1967 [22], and have tried to refine this technique. These results have been extensively published. For more detailed analyses, especially regarding the influence of

Table 1. Proposed criteria of an ideal valve substitute

- Hemodynamic function as original valve; preserves interaction with surrounding structures
- Same macroscopic appearance and size as original valve
- Same histologic composition
- No antigenicity
- Viable
- Growth potential
- Non-thrombogenic
- Unrestricted quality of life (no audible valve sound; no need for medication; no restrictions regarding lifestyle including pregnancy, career, sports, etc.)
- Easy to implant with reproducible results
- No structural degeneration, stable long-term results

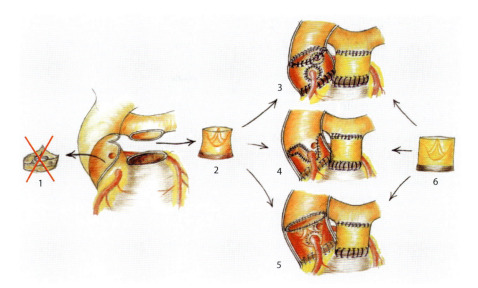

Fig. 1. Schematic drawing of the Ross procedure. The diseased aortic valve is resected (**1**). Then, the autologous pulmonary root including the valve is harvested from the right ventricular outflow tract (*RVOT*) (**2**). The autologous pulmonary valve can be implanted into the aortic position using different techniques

▌ Full root replacement: this technique was popularized by Stelzer and Elkins and is the technique most often used worldwide. The autologous pulmonary root is implanted in the aortic position (**3**). With this technique, reimplantation of the coronary arteries into the neoaortic root is necessary, but the geometry of the pulmonary root can be easily preserved in its new position

▌ Subcoronary implantation: this is the technique originally described by Ross and still preferred by the Luebeck group. The autologous pulmonary valve is implanted into the aortic root in a subcoronary position (**4**)

▌ Cylinder inclusion technique: this technique combines features from the other two techniques. It is technically the most demanding and is only rarely used (**5**)

▌ To complete the operation, the defect in the RVOT needs to be reconstructed, usually by implantation of a pulmonary allograft root (**6**)

technical issues, the German Ross registry (launched in 2002) [13] and the German-Dutch Ross registry (launched in 2007) were initiated. In this chapter, we review the experience gathered by the latter registry and give a personal appreciation on the implications and future perspectives.

Table 2. Centers participating in the German-Dutch Ross registry

- Department of Cardiac and Thoracic Vascular Surgery, University of Lübeck, Germany (Registry Site) (JFMB, TH, US, MM, HHS)
- Sana Herzchirurgische Klinik, Stuttgart, Germany (WH, JOB, JGR)
- Department of Cardiothoracic Surgery, Erasmus University Medical Center, Rotterdam, The Netherlands (AJJJCB, JJMT)
- Herzzentrum Bodensee, Konstanz, Germany (CAB)
- Department of Cardiovascular Surgery, German Heart Center, Munich, Germany (RL, JH)
- Department of Cardiovascular Surgery, Johann Wolfgang Goethe University, Frankfurt/Main, Germany (AM)
- Department of Cardiothoracic Surgery, University of Cologne, Germany (TW)
- Department of Cardiovascular Surgery, Robert Bosch Hospital, Stuttgart, Germany (UFWF)
- Department of Cardiothoracic Surgery, Friedrich Schiller University, Jena, Germany (MB, KFK)
- Department of Cardiac, Thoracic and Vascular Surgery, German Heart Center, Berlin (RH, MH)
- Department of Thoracic, Cardiac, and Vascular Surgery, Eberhard Karls University Tübingen, Germany (GZ)
- Department of Thoracic, Cardiac and Thoracic Vascular Surgery, Justus Maximilians University, Wuerzburg, Germany (AWG)

The German-Dutch Ross registry

Currently, 12 centers are participating in the registry (Table 2). For each patient, 61 preoperative, 43 surgical, and 15 postoperative variables are collected. The surgical technique is determined by the responsible surgeon at each center. At each follow-up visit, another 63 variables are collected, including detailed echocardiographic information. Details on the surgical techniques have been published elsewhere [5, 25].

As shown in Fig. 2, the numbers of Ross procedures per year in the participating centers appears to be stable. For this article, 1548 patients with a mean follow-up of 6.3 ± 4.0 years (min-max: 0.0–19.3 years; total follow-up 9707 patient-years) were analyzed. Patient characteristics are given in Table 3 and Fig. 3. Operative details are given in Table 4.

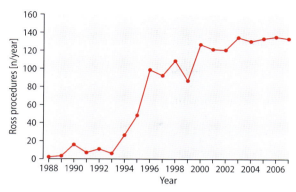

Fig. 2. The number of Ross procedures per year as performed by the centers grouped in the German-Dutch Ross registry is shown. So far, no reduction in the number of procedures performed is apparent. Data for 2008 are incomplete and not shown

Table 3. Patient characteristics[a]

Male/female (n)	1166/382
Age (years)	39 ± 16 (min–max: 0–71)
Valve lesion (n)	
– stenosis	314 (20.3%)
– regurgitation	429 (27.7%)
– combined stenosis+regurgitation	759 (49.0%)
– unknown	46 (3.0%)
Endocarditis (n)	
– acute	65 (4.2%)
– healed	178 (11.5%)
Valve morphology (n)	
– bicuspid	935 (60.4%)
– tricuspid	409 (26.4%)
– other	120 (7.8%)
– unknown	84 (5.4%)

[a] Values are expressed as mean ± standard deviation, or numbers of patients

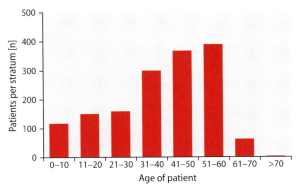

Fig. 3. The distribution of age at the time of the Ross procedure is shown by decades. Mean age was 39±16 years, but the largest group of patients are those in their sixth decade of life

Table 4. Operative details

■ **Technique (n)**	
– subcoronary (or root inclusion)	704 (45.5%)
– root replacement	844 (54.5%)
– with annular or STJ reinforcement	443 (52.5% and 28.6%, respectively)
■ **Cross-clamp duration (min)**	
– subcoronary	166±38
– root replacement	131±27 [a]
■ **ECC duration (min)**	
– subcoronary	207±39
– root replacement	172±46 [a]

[a] $p<0.01$; *STJ* sinotubular junction, *ECC* extracorporeal circulation
Values are expressed as mean±standard deviation, or numbers of patients

Results

The 30-day mortality was 1.4% (n=21). During the first 30 days, 104 patients needed surgical reexploration because of bleeding or pericardial effusion (6.7%) and 11 patients received a permanent pacemaker (0.7%). In addition, there were 12 cerebrovascular events (permanent, n=7; transient, n=5; overall 0.8%).

During follow-up, another 24 cerebrovascular events were observed (permanent, n=10; transient, n=14), resulting in a linearized rate of occurrence of 0.37%/patient-year including the perioperative period (0.27%/patient-year excluding the first 30 postoperative days).

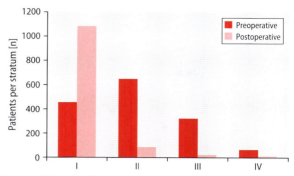

Fig. 4. Physical symptoms according to NYHA classification are shown 1) before the Ross procedure (solid red box), and 2) at the time of latest follow-up (6±4 years postoperatively; pink box). A remarkable clinical improvement is apparent. *NYHA* New York Heart Association

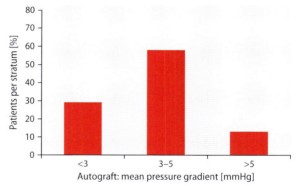

Fig. 5. The mean pressure gradient across the autograft at the time of latest follow-up is shown. Data are given in three intervals on the x-axis and as percentage on the y-axis. Overall, the mean pressure gradient was 3.8±3.2 mmHg

At the latest follow-up, a remarkable clinical improvement – as compared to preoperatively – is apparent in almost all patients (Fig. 4). The autograft (neoaortic valve) showed very good hemodynamic performance in systole (mean pressure gradient: 3.8±3.2 mmHg, Fig. 5). In diastole, trivial or mild autograft regurgitation is often found, but significant autograft regurgitation is rare (Fig. 6).

We observed a steep increase of the transvalvular pressure gradient across the allograft (neopulmonary valve) during the first 1–2 years; thereafter, the results appear to be stable. At latest follow-up, the mean gradient was 8.6±5.8 mmHg (Fig. 7), and trace or trivial regurgitation is a common finding (Fig. 8).

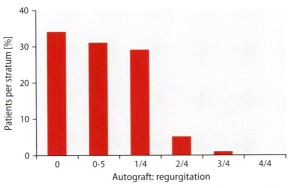

Fig. 6. Regurgitation across the autograft at the time of latest follow-up is shown. 0 denotes no regurgitation, 0.5 trivial, 1/4 mild, 2/4 mild-to-moderate, 3/4 moderate, and 4/4 severe regurgitation. Data on the y-axis are percentage of patients

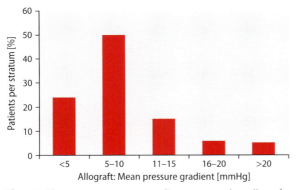

Fig. 7. The mean pressure gradient across the allograft at the time of latest follow-up is shown. Data are given in five intervals on the x-axis and as percentage of patients on the y-axis. Overall, the mean pressure gradient was 8.6 ± 5.8 mmHg

During follow-up, 135 patients were reoperated on either the auto- or allograft (linearized rate: 1.39%/patient-year; 12 patients needed reoperation on both valves). The reasons for reoperation are given in Table 5. When stratified according to the surgical technique, it became apparent that – during the period of observation – the reoperation rate was significantly higher for the root replacement technique without annular and/or reinforcement than for the subcoronary technique or for root replacement with annular and/or reinforcement (Fig. 9).

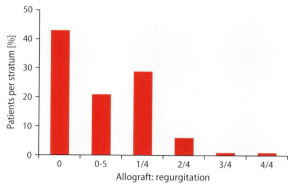

Fig. 8. Regurgitation across the allograft at the time of latest follow-up is shown. 0 denotes no regurgitation, 0.5 trivial, 1/4 mild, 2/4 mild-to-moderate, 3/4 moderate, and 4/4 severe regurgitation. Data on the y-axis are percentage of patients

Table 5. Reasons for reoperation [a]

Autograft failure (n)	77 (0.79%/patient-year)
– endocarditis	11 (14%)
– regurgitation	66 (86%)
– structural valve disease	22 (33% and 29%, respectively)
– nonstructural valve disease	44 (67% and 57%, respectively)
Allograft failure (n)	58 (0.58%/patient-year)
– endocarditis	12 (21%)
– stenosis	33 (57%)
– regurgitation	7 (12%)
– combined lesion	4 (7%)
– other	2 (3%)

[a] 12 patients were reoperated on the auto- as well as on the allograft

Discussion

The German-Dutch Ross registry demonstrates that the reoperation rates in the first postoperative decade are acceptably low. By the end of the first decade, however, the reoperation rate begins to rise, but mainly in patients who had full root implantation of the autograft without annular or STJ reinforcement. This finding suggests that technical details of the implantation play a major role for the fate of the allograft. It should be noted that those centers that report high reoperation rates predominantly used the full root technique, usually without any reinforcement [7, 10, 16, 18, 20, 29]. Taken

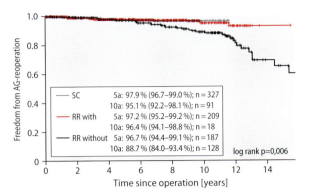

Fig. 9. Actuarial freedom from reoperation on the autograft is shown as stratified by technique. Subcoronary implantation (SC) and root replacement (R) with annular or STJ reinforcement yield similar results within the period of observation, whereas RR without annular or STJ reinforcement is associated with significantly lower freedom from reoperation (p = 0.006). This difference becomes apparent by the end of the first decade. *STJ* sinotubular junction

together, it can therefore be speculated that reoperations for autograft failure may – to some extent – be preventable. Several techniques for annular or STJ reinforcement have been described [5, 8].

It must be stressed that the mean follow-up in the registry is still rather short (6 ± 4 years). Therefore, all projections beyond the first postoperative decade are somewhat crude. The long-term results (mean follow-up: 20 years) of the original series of D.N. Ross himself are reported to be excellent, but there was no regular follow-up visit with echocardiography in all patients, the number of patients was not very high (n = 131), some basic data were missing, and the completeness of follow-up was < 95% [9]. Therefore, neither the experience reported herein nor the results of the original series should be considered proof that the pulmonary autograft can withstand aortic hemodynamics indefinitely, and patients should be informed that the "true long-term" results are still unknown.

The reasons for failure of the RVOT reconstruction are poorly understood. Since the RVOT is usually reconstructed using allograft valves, which were found to provoke a specific humoral and cellular immunologic response [14, 26], it is tempting to hypothesize that some kind of rejection may cause allograft failure. So far, however, clinical studies on this topic are inconclusive [1–3, 11, 12, 21, 24, 31], and clinical important pulmonary allograft failure is rare during the period of observation in adults undergoing the Ross procedure. Younger age was repeatedly shown to be associated with higher allograft failure rates, but the reason for this is unclear. An alternative explanation for allograft failure is that the methods used for sterilization and/or preservation can lead to a detrimental reaction [6, 17, 19, 30].

A limitation of the Registry is that only those patients who eventually received a Ross procedure are captured. Patients undergoing a Ross procedure are a highly selected group, and not all patients with aortic valve disease are candidates for the Ross procedure. Generally accepted contraindications are anatomic or structural defects of the pulmonary valve, connective tissue disorders (e.g., Marfan syndrome), severe calcification or unusual location of the coronary ostiae, chronic inflammatory disease (e.g., lupus erythematosus, juvenile rheumatoid arthritis) and severely reduced left ventricular function or any other disease that interferes with the possibility to recover from a long operation. In our experience, uncontrolled or poorly controlled hypertension should also be considered a contraindication. The Ross procedure is usually advocated to be of special interest to young patients. However, in the German-Dutch Ross registry many patients are >50 years at the time of operation. Some lines of evidence suggest that the results are even better than in younger patients [4, 23], and the "true long-term" results may not be as important in this group of patients. We therefore consider the Ross procedure a valuable option in this group of patients.

Conclusions

In experienced hands, the Ross procedure has a low perioperative risk and is an attractive alternative to conventional valve substitutes because of excellent hemodynamics and the low incidence of extracardiac complications (low thromboembolic risk; virtually no bleeding). Thus, the Ross procedure offers an unrestricted lifestyle and appears to be especially suited for very active patients and women who want to become pregnant.

There is a risk of reoperation on the auto- and allograft, and patients need to be informed that the long-term results (mainly second and third decade) are still unknown. However, the experience gathered in the German-Dutch Ross registry suggests that the probability of reoperation on the autograft is dependent on the surgical technique used. This means that reoperations for autograft failure may – to some extent – be preventable. The reasons for allograft failure are poorly understood, but are likely to be related to some kind of interaction between graft and host. More research on the reasons for allograft failure is needed.

References

1. Baskett RJF, Nanton MA, Warren AE, Ross DB (2003) Human leukocyte antigen-DR and ABO mismatch are associated with accelerated homograft failure in children: Implications for therapeutic interventions. J Thorac Cardiovasc Surg 126: 232–239
2. Bechtel JFM, Bartels C, Schmidtke C et al (2001) Anti-HLA class I antibodies and pulmonary homograft function after the Ross-procedure. Ann Thorac Surg 71: 2003–2007
3. Bechtel JFM, Bartels C, Schmidtke C et al (2001) Does histocompatibility affect homograft valve function after the Ross-procedure? Circulation 104 [suppl I]:I-25–I-28
4. Böhm JO, Botha CA, Hemmer W et al (2003) Older patients fare better with the Ross operation. Ann Thorac Surg 75:796–801
5. Böhm JO, Botha CA, Rein JG, Roser D (2001) Technical evolution of the Ross operation: midterm results in 186 patients. Ann Thorac Surg 71:S340–S343
6. Brockbank KGM, Lightfoot FG, Song YC, Taylor MJ (2000) Interstitial ice formation in cryopreserved homografts: a possible cause of tissue deterioration and calcification in vivo. J Heart Valve Dis 9:200–206
7. Brown JW, Ruzmetov M, Fukui T, Rodefeld MD, Mahomed Y, Turrentine MW (2006) Fate of the autograft and homograft following Ross aortic valve replacement: reoperative frequency, outcome, and management. J Heart Valve Dis 15:253–259
8. Carrel T, Schwerzmann M, Eckstein F, Aymard T, Kadner A (2008) Preliminary results following reinforcement of the pulmonary autograft to prevent dilatation after the Ross procedure. J Thorac Cardiovasc Surg 136:472–475
9. Chambers JC, Somerville J, Stone S, Ross DN (1997) Pulmonary autograft procedure for aortic valve disease: long-term results of the pioneer series. Circulation 96:2206–2214
10. de Kerchove L, Rubay J, Pasquet A et al (2009) Ross operation in the adult: long-term outcomes after root replacement and inclusion techniques. Ann Thorac Surg 87:95–102
11. Dignan R, O'Brien M, Hogan P et al (2003) Aortic valve allograft structural deterioration is associated with a subset of antibodies to Human Leucocyte Antigens. J Heart Valve Dis 12:382–391
12. Dignan R, O'Brien M, Hogan P et al (2000) Influence of HLA matching and associated factors on aortic valve homograft function. J Heart Valve Dis 9:504–511
13. Hanke T, Stierle U, Boehm JO et al (2007) Autograft regurgitation and aortic root dimensions after the Ross procedure: the German Ross Registry experience. Circulation 116 [Suppl I]:I251–I258
14. Hoekstra F, Knoop C, Vaessen L et al (1996) Donor-specific cellular immune response against human cardiac valve allografts. J Thorac Cardiovasc Surg 112:281–286
15. Klieverik LM, Takkenberg JJ, Bekkers JA, Roos-Hesselink JW, Witsenburg M, Bogers AJ (2007) The Ross operation: a Trojan horse? Eur Heart J 28:1993–2000
16. Kouchoukos NT, Masetti P, Nickerson NJ, Castner CF, Shannon WD, Dávila-Román VG (2004) The Ross procedure: long-term clinical and echocardiographic follow-up. Ann Thorac Surg 78:773–781
17. Legare JF, Lee TDG, Ross DB (2000) Cryopreservation of rat aortic valves results in increased structural failure. Circulation 102 [suppl III]:III75–III78

18. Luciani GB, Favaro A, Casali G, Santini F, Mazzucco A (2005) Reoperations for aortic aneurysm after the Ross procedure. J Heart Valve Dis 14:766–772
19. Nishizawa Y, Saeki K, Hirai H, Yazaki Y, Takaku F, Yuo A (1998) Potent inhibition of cell density-dependent apoptosis and enhancement of survival by dimethyl sulfoxide in human myeloblastic HL-60 cells. J Cell Physiol 174:135–143
20. Pasquali SK, Cohen MS, Shera D, Wernovsky G, Spray TL, Marino BS (2007) The relationship between neo-aortic root dilation, insufficiency, and reintervention following the Ross procedure in infants, children, and young adults. J Am Coll Cardiol 49:1806–1812
21. Pompilio G, Polvani G, Piccolo G et al (2004) Six-year monitoring of the donor-specific immune response to cryopreserved aortic allograft valves: implications with valve dysfunction. Ann Thorac Surg 78:557–563
22. Ross DN (1967) Replacement of aortic and mitral valves with a pulmonary autograft. Lancet 2:956–958
23. Schmidtke C, Bechtel JFM, Noetzold A, Sievers HH (2000) Up to seven years of experience with the Ross procedure in patients >60 years of age. J Am Coll Cardiol 36:1173–1177
24. Shaddy RE, Lambert LM, Fuller TC et al (2001) Prospective randomized trial of azathioprine in cryopreserved valved allografts in children. Ann Thorac Surg 71:43–48
25. Sievers HH, Hanke T, Stierle U et al (2006) A Critical Reappraisal of the Ross Operation. Renaissance of the subcoronary implantation technique? Circulation 114 [suppl I]:I504–I511
26. Smith JD, Ogino H, Hunt D, Laylor RM, Rose ML, Yacoub MH (1995) Humoral immune response to human aortic valve homografts. Ann Thorac Surg 60:S127–S130
27. Stelzer P, Jones DJ, Elkins RC (1989) Aortic root replacement with pulmonary autograft. Circulation 80 [Suppl III]:III209–III213
28. Takkenberg JJ, Klieverik LM, Schoof PH et al (2009) The Ross procedure: a systematic review and meta-analysis. Circulation 119:222–228
29. Takkenberg JJ, van Herweden LA, Galema TW et al (2006) Serial echocardiographic assessment of neo-aortic regurgitation and root dimensions after the modified Ross-procedure. J Heart Valve Dis 15:100–106 (discussion 106–107)
30. Tominaga T, Kitagawa T, Masuda Y et al (2000) Viability of cryopreserved semilunar valves: An evaluation of cytosolic and mitochondrial activities. Ann Thorac Surg 70:792–795
31. Yap CH, Skillington PD, Matalanis G et al (2008) Human leukocyte antigen mismatch and other factors affecting cryopreserved allograft valve function. Heart Surg Forum 11:E42–E45

Aortic valve repair and valve sparing root procedures

The bicuspid aortic valve

J. F. M. Bechtel, M. Misfeld, C. Schmidtke, H.-H. Sievers

The bicuspid aortic valve (BAV) is the most common congenital cardiac malformation. Despite being a seemingly simple and harmless anatomic variation, BAV is said to cause more morbidity than any other congenital cardiac defect [52]. BAV may lead to aortic valve stenosis (AS) or regurgitation (AR), endocarditis, an ascending aortic aneurysm, and/or devastating dissection or rupture. Although these potential consequences of BAV were first described long ago [19, 35, 36], only recently have clinicians become fully aware that the presence of a BAV poses a serious health risk. However, the so-called bicuspid aortic valve syndrome [14] is extremely heterogeneous with some patients having rapidly progressive valve and/or aortic disease, while some individuals with BAV remain free of complications throughout their lifetime. In this article, we review current concepts regarding etiology, pathomechanisms, diagnosis, and treatment of BAV with special emphasis on topics relevant for cardiac surgeons.

Etiology

Despite intensive research during recent years, the etiology and mechanisms leading to congenital BAV remain largely unknown. The process of valvulogenesis is complex and begins early during development of the heart [25]. Endothelial-mesenchymal transformation of the endocardium leads to development of endocardial cushions in the outflow tract and in the atrioventricular canal. All four valves are formed from elongations of the endocardial cushions, but cells from the neural crest appear to contribute to the development of the semilunar valves [22–24]. Experiments in Syrian hamsters indicate that a BAV does not result from fusion of two normally developed cusps, but from failure of the anlagen of the three cusps to separate [42]. Thus, involvement of genes and molecular mechanisms responsible for separation and further differentiation of the valve cushions in the etiology of BAV appears likely – and this may include genes encoding transcription factors, extracellular matrix proteins or signaling pathways that regulate cell proliferation, apoptosis, or differentiation. As such, the Notch signaling pathway, which is extremely conserved evolutionarily and contributes to the differentiation of various organs, has come into the focus of research. Several mutations in the NOTCH1 gene have been described in association with BAV [18, 28], but other chromosomal loci and genes have also been linked to BAV [12, 26, 29]. Thus, BAV syndrome appears to be heterogeneous not only with regard to the clinical phenotype, but also with respect to molecular and cellular events. It is tempting to hypothesize that BAV syndrome is the final common pathway for a variety of genetic defects. This would also serve as an explanation for associated cardiac and vascular malformations (displaced left coronary ostium, short left main artery; malalignment and dilatation of the noncoronary sinus; ventricular septal defect; ascending aortic aneurysm; coarctation of the aorta or aortic interruption; patent ductus arteriosus) which are often, but not always found.

Prevalence

The prevalence of BAV is usually given as 1–2%. This estimation is mainly based on older autopsy series [37], whereas most [20, 30, 33, 50], but not all [49] more recent echocardiographic studies suggest a prevalence of 0.5–1.0%. However, although three of these studies examined echocardiograms from more than 20 000 individuals, none of the studies was population-based. Men are usually found to be more frequently affected than women, but this is not consistent in all studies [21, 38].

While most cases of BAV appear to be sporadic, there is strong evidence of heritability in some families [7, 21]. These findings are often interpreted to show autosomal dominant inheritance with reduced penetrance [15, 17]. Screening of first-degree relatives of patients seems advisable – and is mandatory in relatives of patients who suffered aortic complications.

Diagnosis

Today, the diagnosis of BAV can usually be made with high reliability using echocardiography. It is essential to study the valve in both systole and diastole, as a tall raphe may be mistaken for a commissure. The systolic appearance is less deceptive as a BAV will show a characteristic abnormal fishmouth opening. However, in heavily calcified valves – either bicuspid or tricuspid – the echocardiographic appearance will be so abnormal that the number of cusps cannot be determined.

Table 1. Criteria of congenital BAV for discrimination from acquired bicuspid valves (postnatally fused tricuspid valve)

- One or two of the commissures are more or less malformed and obliterated, giving rise to a raphe; this malformation may be identified by the fact that
  - from the aorta, the highest point of the parallel attachments of two adjacent cusps is lower than at the other commissures
  - from the left ventricle, the commissural area presents as a indentation, not a space
- The free edge of the conjoint cusps is slightly larger than that of the opposite cusp
- The circumferential distances between the three commissures are not equal

The valve configuration is ultimately ascertained in the operating room (or during autopsy). Even then, distinguishing a congenital BAV from a tricuspid aortic valve with acquired fusion of two cusps may be very difficult in some cases, but can usually be achieved using the criteria outlined in Table 1.

Classification

Given the large spectrum of how a BAV can appear, a classification system is needed. A universally accepted classification system would help make comparisons between reports possible. In addition, there is some evidence that the exact valvular configuration might be of relevance with regard to the degree of associated aortic disease [40], the chances for aortic valve reconstruction, or for doing a Ross procedure.

Several classification systems have been described in the literature but have not been widely adopted and did not allow concise, easily applicable classification and coding. We have recently proposed a classification system that takes into account morphology, spatial position, and valvular function. It allows description of valves that are commonly called unicuspid, monocuspid, or unicommissural, and it can be extended to tricuspid or quadricuspid valves [48] (Fig. 1).

The classification system distinguishes three categories, the most important category being the number of raphes (0 to 2). This main category is called "type" and is complemented with two subcategories: the first representing the spatial position of the raphes (or the orientation of the free edge of the cusps in type 0, respectively) and the second subcategory representing the functional status of the valve (no dysfunction, AS, AR, or a combination of both). Thus, the classification may be coded into three blocks – type, spatial position, function. More subcategories may be added (e.g., presence or absence of ascending aneurysm), if needed.

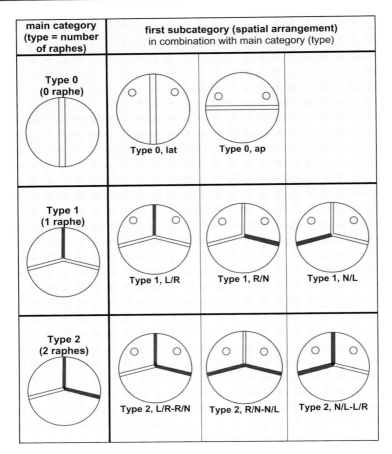

Fig. 1. Proposed classification system for bicuspid aortic valves (BAV). Schematic presentation as viewed from the surgeon's position with the left coronary sinus on the left side. The main category (type) and the first subcategory (spatial position) and their possible shapes are shown. Bold line in schematic drawings represents a raphe, which is the nonseparated or conjoint segment of two underdeveloped cusps extending into the commissural area. Type 0 stands for a BAV with no raphe; Type 1 for BAV with one raphe; Type 2 for BAV with two raphes. The second subcategory is not depicted: BAV may have either no dysfunction (*no*), or may show stenosis (*S*), insufficiency (*I*), or both (*B*). Missing information is coded as "*X*".
ap anterior-posterior, *lat* lateral, *L* left coronary sinus, *R* right coronary sinus, *N* noncoronary sinus

Using this classification system, we found among 304 BAVs that type I (a BAV with one raphe, Fig. 2) is by far the most common configuration (88%), that the raphe was usually between the left and the right coronary sinus (L-R; 80% of type I BAVs), and that stenotic valves prevailed (55% of type I L-R). Type 2 (a BAV with 2 raphes, 5% of the sample examined; Fig. 3) was associated with a significantly higher proportion of ascending aortic aneurysms (p = 0.022; Fig. 4).

The bicuspid aortic valve ■ 93

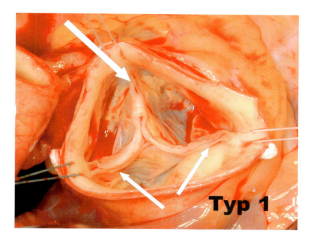

Fig. 2. Intraoperative picture of a bicuspid aortic valve type 1, L/R, I (see text and Fig. 1 for explanation). One raphe (large arrow) and two normal commissures (small arrows) are evident. Reprinted from [48]; with permission from the American Association for Thoracic Surgery

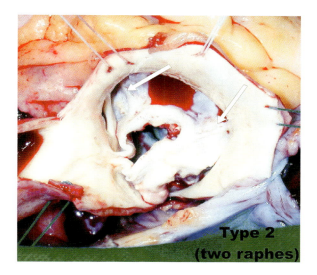

Fig. 3. Intraoperative picture of a bicuspid aortic valve type 2, L/R-R/N, S (see text and Fig. 1 for explanation). Two raphes (arrows) are evident, with developmental anlagen of three cusps with a high degree of stenosis. Reprinted from [48]; with permission from the American Association for Thoracic Surgery

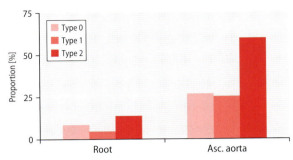

Fig. 4. Proportion of aneurysms of the aortic root or ascending aorta in relation to the type of bicuspid aortic valve (BAV). A BAV type 2 (valve with two raphes) was associated with a significantly ($P=0.022$) higher proportion of aneurysms. Reprinted from [48]; with permission from the American Association for Thoracic Surgery

Complications and treatment

It is estimated that at least one third of all individuals with BAV will suffer some kind of complication from it [52]. A recent study in 212 asymptomatic individuals with BAV found that about 42% will have had any cardiovascular event 20 years after diagnosis, and 27% will have had any cardiovascular surgery [27]. Another recent study on 642 adults with BAV, which had a shorter follow-up, found comparable rates [51]. In both studies, using contemporary strategies for surveillance and surgical techniques, the overall survival of the groups was excellent.

Valve-related complications must be distinguished from aortic complications, but both may occur in the same patient, either at the same time or successively.

Valve-related complications

In surgical series on the treatment of aortic valve lesions, in 50% or more of the cases BAV appears to be the underlying pathology. This is by far more common than its prevalence in the population and highlights the relevance of BAV. The most common fate of BAV seems to be development of stenosis [38, 41], and patients with stenotic BAV are about a decade younger than patients with stenotic tricuspid aortic valves. This is not a big surprise as it had been shown that all BAV are inherently stenotic from birth and subjected to highly abnormal stress during systole and diastole [39].

Aortic regurgitation (AR) is found in approximately 15% of patients with BAV [41]. AR may result from prolapse of the conjoined cusp, from fibrotic retraction, from cusp damage due to endocarditis, or from dilatation of the sinotubular junction or of the aortic root (or parts from it). Patients with BAV and AR are usually considerably younger than patients with AS and may reflect a subset of patients especially prone to aortic complications [17].

The frequency of endocarditis is reported to be alarmingly high in BAV patients (10–30% [17]), but more recent studies found lower numbers [27, 51]. Endocarditis prophylaxis is no longer routinely recommended in patients with BAV [32]. Taken together, it is believed that all BAV will eventually fail in some way if the patient lives long enough [17].

Aortic valve surgery in patients with a stenotic or regurgitant BAV is indicated if the usual criteria are fulfilled [3]. However, when to operate on the aortic valve if aortic surgery is indicated, is controversially discussed [17].

A significantly stenotic or regurgitant BAV will usually be replaced using standard techniques. An ongoing debate relates to the question whether a Ross procedure can be performed in patients with BAV arguing that the pulmonary root has the same embryologic origin as the aortic root and is prone to dilatation [8, 9]. In our experience, the presence of BAV is not a contraindication to the Ross procedure [44, 47].

Another controversy involves the value of reconstructive aortic valve surgery which has gained more and more interest in recent years. Several techniques have been described for repair of regurgitant BAV in the absence or in presence of aortic aneurysms (Table 2, Figs. 5 and 6). We [13, 45] as well as others [4, 43] have reported good short- and mid-term re-

Table 2. Techniques for aortic valve repair*

- Exact identification of the lesion responsible for valve dysfunction (usually regurgitation); the lesion may be at the level of the sinotubular junction (STJ), on the cusps, at the annular level, or a combination of the three
- Repair of the lesion
  → on the STJ level
    – replacement with prosthesis
    – plication
  → on the cusp level
    – cusp plication
    – resection of raphe
    – partial replacement with pericardium
    – patch closure of defects
    – cusp debridement/shaving
    – reinforcement of free margin with GoreTex suture
    – subcommisural annuloplasty
  → on the annular level
    – valve sparing aortic root replacement (David/Yacoub techniques)
    – annuloplasty

* Combinations of techniques may be necessary. This list of techniques does not claim to be complete

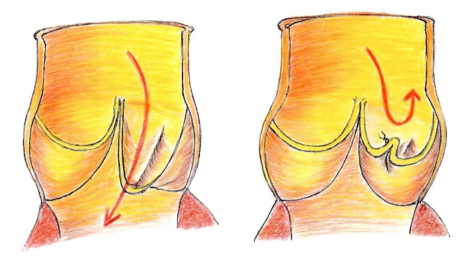

Fig. 5. Schematic drawing of cusp plication. On the left, there is regurgitation (arrow) because of prolapse of the larger, conjoined cusp along the raphe. On the right, the prolapse has been repaired by cusp plication at the raphe

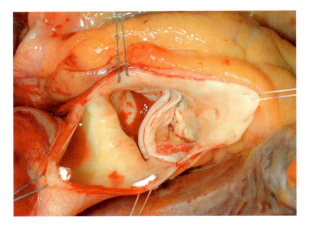

Fig. 6. Repair of a bicuspid aortic valve: reattachment of commissure. Intraoperative view of a type 0 (no raphe) bicuspid aortic valve. First subcategory: lateral; second subcategory: insufficiency. The valve had been regurgitant because of partial detachment of one commissure. As can be seen, this detachment has been repaired by reattachment of the commissure to the aortic wall. Sutures were passed through a small strip of PTFE

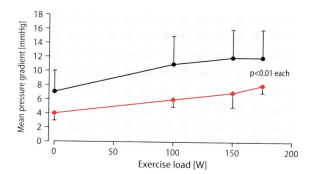

Fig. 7. Mean pressure gradient across the aortic valve during exercise. Patients with repaired bicuspid aortic valves (black circles, n=25) had higher pressure gradients than controls (red diamonds, n=20) at rest and during exercise, indicating a mild, subclinical obstruction caused by the reconstruction. However, the rise of the pressure gradients during exercise was comparable to that observed in the healthy volunteers. Data are from [45]

sults using these repair techniques (Fig. 7). Repair of regurgitant valves is increasingly used in our department. However, the long-term stability of these techniques remains unknown.

Aortic complications

The literature about the association of BAV and ascending aortic disease fills a complete library and mainly centers around the question whether there is an intrinsic aortic disease or whether the aortic pathology is caused by abnormal flow [39]. A detailed review of this discussion is beyond the scope of this article, but today most authorities believe that there is an intrinsic aortic disease in (most) patients with BAV [15, 17]. Although not necessarily evident on standard histopathologic examination [2], a closer look frequently detects aortic wall abnormalities [1, 16, 31]. Such abnormalities appear to vary with location (convexity vs. concavity) [5, 6, 11]; whether these asymmetries are related to flow patterns and as such are related to the morphology of the valve remains speculative.

Mid-ascending dilatation is found more often than root aneurysms [10, 48]. Impaired wall elasticity appears to be fundamental in aneurysm formation, and there is some evidence that ascending aortic elasticity can be measured noninvasively [34]. This might prove to be of great help in determining whether aortic replacement surgery is indicated. Generally, replacement of the ascending aorta is advised if the diameter exceeds 4.5–5.0 cm [15, 17], but more individualized recommendations appear possible [46]. The value of reduction ascending aortoplasty (instead of aortic replacement) has only been poorly studied so far.

Summary and outlook

The bicuspid aortic valve (BAV) is the most common congenital cardiac malformation. Most cases appear to be sporadic, but BAV can be inherited. The genetics of BAV are studied intensively, and some progress has been made. The phenotype of BAV varies widely, and the presence of BAV will probably be found to be the final pathway of several genetic defects.

BAV is of special interest to the cardiac surgeon because it frequently causes valvular and/or aortic complications. While eventual dysfunction of a malformed valve is not unexpected, the association of BAV and aortic disease is less self-evident. More research is needed to better understand this association and the underlying mechanisms.

At the moment, treatment of BAV and its complications is entirely surgical. With improving understanding of aortic valve function and refined surgical materials and techniques, reconstructive surgery in patients with regurgitant BAVs has become an attractive option. However, once the mechanisms that promote aortic dilatation and dissection in patients with BAV are better understood, conservative treatment might become possible and delay the need for aortic surgery – or even render it unnecessary.

References

1. Bauer M, Gliech V, Siniawski H, Hetzer R (2006) Configuration of the ascending aorta in patients with bicuspid and tricuspid aortic valve disease undergoing aortic valve replacement with or without reduction aortoplasty. J Heart Valve Dis 15:594–600
2. Bechtel JFM, Noack F, Sayk F, Erasmi AW, Bartels C, Sievers HH (2003) Histopathological grading of ascending aortic aneurysm: Comparison of patients with bicuspid versus tricuspid aortic valves. J Heart Valve Dis 12:54–61
3. Bonow RO, Carabello BA, Kanu C et al (2006) ACC/AHA 2006 guidelines for the management of patients with valvular heart disease: a report of the American College of Cardiology/American Heart Association Task Force on Practice Guidelines (writing committee to revise the 1998 Guidelines for the Management of Patients With Valvular Heart Disease): developed in collaboration with the Society of Cardiovascular Anesthesiologists: endorsed by the Society for Cardiovascular Angiography and Interventions and the Society of Thoracic Surgeons. Circulation 114:e84–e231
4. Boodhwani M, de Kerchove L, Glineur D et al (2009) Repair-oriented classification of aortic insufficiency: impact on surgical techniques and clinical outcomes. J Thorac Cardiovasc Surg 137:286–294
5. Choudhury N, Bouchot O, Rouleau L et al (2009) Local mechanical and structural properties of healthy and diseased human ascending aorta tissue. Cardiovasc Pathol 18:83–91

6. Cotrufo M, Della CA, De Santo LS et al (2005) Different patterns of extracellular matrix protein expression in the convexity and the concavity of the dilated aorta with bicuspid aortic valve: preliminary results. J Thorac Cardiovasc Surg 130:504–511
7. Cripe L, Andelfinger G, Martin LJ, Shooner K, Benson DW (2004) Bicuspid aortic valve is heritable. J Am Coll Cardiol 44:138–143
8. David TE, Omran A, Ivanov J et al (2000) Dilation of the pulmonary autograft after the Ross procedure. J Thorac Cardiovasc Surg 119:210–220
9. de Sa M, Moshkovitz Y, Butany J, David TE (1999) Histologic abnormalities of the ascending aorta and pulmonary trunk in patients with bicuspid aortic valve disease: clinical relevance to the Ross procedure. J Thorac Cardiovasc Surg 118:588–596
10. Della CA, Bancone C, Quarto C et al (2007) Predictors of ascending aortic dilatation with bicuspid aortic valve: a wide spectrum of disease expression. Eur J Cardiothorac Surg 31:397–404
11. Della CA, Quarto C, Bancone C et al (2008) Spatiotemporal patterns of smooth muscle cell changes in ascending aortic dilatation with bicuspid and tricuspid aortic valve stenosis: focus on cell-matrix signaling. J Thorac Cardiovasc Surg 135:8–18
12. Ellison JW, Yagubyan M, Majumdar R et al (2007) Evidence of genetic locus heterogeneity for familial bicuspid aortic valve. J Surg Res 142:28–31
13. Erasmi AW, Sievers HH, Bechtel JF, Hanke T, Stierle U, Misfeld M (2007) Remodeling or reimplantation for valve-sparing aortic root surgery? Ann Thorac Surg 83:S752–S756
14. Fedak PW (2008) Bicuspid aortic valve syndrome: heterogeneous but predictable. Eur Heart J 29:432–433
15. Fedak PW, David TE, Borger M, Verma S, Butany J, Weisel RD (2005) Bicuspid aortic valve disease: recent insights in pathophysiology and treatment. Expert Rev Cardiovasc Ther 3:295–308
16. Fedak PW, de Sa MP, Verma S et al (2003) Vascular matrix remodeling in patients with bicuspid aortic valve malformations: implications for aortic dilatation. J Thorac Cardiovasc Surg 126:797–806
17. Friedman T, Mani A, Elefteriades JA (2008) Bicuspid aortic valve: clinical approach and scientific review of a common clinical entity. Expert Rev Cardiovasc Ther 6:235–248
18. Garg V, Muth AN, Ransom JF et al (2005) Mutations in NOTCH1 cause aortic valve disease. Nature 437:270–274
19. Gore I, Seiwert VJ (1952) Dissecting aneurysm of the aorta; pathological aspects; an analysis of eighty-five cases. AMA Arch Pathol 53:121–141
20. Gray GW, Salisbury DA, Gulino AM (1995) Echocardiographic and color flow Doppler findings in military pilot applicants. Aviat Space Environ Med 66:32–34
21. Huntington K, Hunter AGW, Chan KL (1997) A prospective study to assess the frequency of familial clustering of congenital bicuspid aortic valve. J Am Coll Cardiol 30:1809–1812
22. Kappetein AP, Gittenberger-de Groot AC, Zwinderman AH, Rohmer J, Poelmann RE, Huysmans HA (1991) The neural crest as a possible pathogenetic factor in coarctation of the aorta and bicuspid aortic valve. J Thorac Cardiovasc Surg 102:830–836
23. Kirby ML, Waldo KL (1990) Role of neural crest in congenital heart disease. Circulation 82:332–340
24. Le Douarin NM, Teillet MA (1974) Experimental analysis of the migration and differentiation of neuroblasts of the autonomic nervous system and of neuroecto-

dermal mesenchymal derivates, using biologic cell marking techniques. Dev Biol 41:162–184
25. Maron BJ, Hutchins GM (1974) The development of the semilunar valves in the human heart. Am J Pathol 74:331–344
26. Martin LJ, Ramachandran V, Cripe LH et al (2007) Evidence in favor of linkage to human chromosomal regions 18q, 5q and 13q for bicuspid aortic valve and associated cardiovascular malformations. Hum Genet 121:275–284
27. Michelena HI, Desjardins VA, Avierinos JF et al (2008) Natural history of asymptomatic patients with normally functioning or minimally dysfunctional bicuspid aortic valve in the community. Circulation 117:2776–2784
28. Mohamed SA, Aherrahrou Z, Liptau H et al (2006) Novel missense mutations (p.T596M and p.P1797H) in NOTCH1 in patients with bicuspid aortic valve. Biochem Biophys Res Commun 345:1460–1465
29. Mohamed SA, Hanke T, Schlueter C, Bullerdiek J, Sievers HH (2005) Ubiquitin fusion degradation 1-like gene dysregulation in bicuspid aortic valve. J Thorac Cardiovasc Surg 130:1531–1536
30. Mohaved MR, Hepner AD, Ahmadi-Kashani M (2006) Echocardiographic prevalence of bicuspid aortic valve in the population. Heart Lung Circ 15:297–299
31. Nataatmadja M, West M, West J et al (2003) Abnormal extracellular matrix protein transport associated with increased apoptosis of vascular smooth muscle cells in marfan syndrome and bicuspid aortic valve thoracic aortic aneurysm. Circulation 108 Suppl 1:II329–II334
32. Nishimura RA, Carabello BA, Faxon DP et al (2008) ACC/AHA 2008 guideline update on valvular heart disease: focused update on infective endocarditis: a report of the American College of Cardiology/American Heart Association Task Force on Practice Guidelines: endorsed by the Society of Cardiovascular Anesthesiologists, Society for Cardiovascular Angiography and Interventions, and Society of Thoracic Surgeons. Circulation 118:887–896
33. Nistri S, Basso C, Marzari C, Mormino P, Thiene G (2005) Frequency of bicuspid aortic valve in young male conscripts by echocardiogram. Am J Cardiol 96:718–721
34. Nistri S, Grande-Allen J, Noale M et al (2008) Aortic elasticity and size in bicuspid aortic valve syndrome. Eur Heart J 29:472–479
35. Osler W (1866) The bicuspid condition of aortic valves. Trans Assoc Am Physicians 2:185–192
36. Peacock TB (1866) On malformations of the human heart. Churchill, London
37. Roberts WC (1970) The congenitally bicuspid aortic valve. A study of 85 autopsy cases. Am J Cardiol 26:72–82
38. Roberts WC, Ko JM (2005) Frequency by decades of unicuspid, bicuspid, and tricuspid aortic valves in adults having isolated aortic valve replacement for aortic stenosis, with or without associated aortic regurgitation. Circulation 111:920–925
39. Robicsek F, Thubrikar MJ, Cook JW, Fowler B (2004) The congenitally bicuspid aortic valve: how does it function? Why does it fail? Ann Thorac Surg 77:177–185
40. Russo CF, Cannata A, Lanfranconi M, Vitali E, Garatti A, Bonacina E (2008) Is aortic wall degeneration related to bicuspid aortic valve anatomy in patients with valvular disease? J Thorac Cardiovasc Surg 136:937–942
41. Sabet HY, Edwards WE, Tazelaar HD, Daly RC (1999) Congenitally Bicuspid Aortic Valves: A Surgical Pathology Study of 542 Cases (1991 Through 1996) and a Literature Review of 2715 Additional Cases. Mayo Clin Proc 74:14–26
42. Sans-Coma V, Fernández B, Durán AC et al (1996) Fusion of valve cushions as a key factor in the formation of congenital bicuspid aortic valves in Syrian hamsters. Anat Rec 244:490–498

43. Schäfers HJ, Aicher D, Langer F, Lausberg HF (2007) Preservation of the bicuspid aortic valve. Ann Thorac Surg 83:S740–S745
44. Schmidtke C, Bechtel M, Hueppe M, Sievers HH (2001) Time course of aortic valve function and root dimensions after subcoronary Ross procedure for bicuspid versus tricuspid aortic valve disease. Circulation 104 (Suppl):I21–I24
45. Schmidtke C, Poppe D, Dahmen G, Sievers HH (2005) Echocardiographic and hemodynamic characteristics of reconstructed bicuspid aortic valves at rest and exercise. Z Kardiol 94:437–444
46. Sievers HH (2004) Reflections on reduction ascending aortoplasty's liveliness. J Thorac Cardiovasc Surg 128:499–501
47. Sievers HH, Hanke T, Stierle U et al (2006) A Critical Reappraisal of the Ross Operation. Renaissance of the subcoronary implantation technique? Circulation 114[suppl I]:I-504–I-511
48. Sievers HH, Schmidtke C (2007) A classification system for the bicuspid aortic valve from 304 surgical specimens. J Thorac Cardiovasc Surg 133:1226–1233
49. Stefani L, Galanti G, Toncelli L et al (2008) Bicuspid aortic valve in competitive athletes. Br J Sports Med 42:31–35
50. Strader JR, Harrell TW, Adair A, Kruyer WB (2008) Efficacy of echocardiographic screening of pilot applicants. Aviat Space Environ Med 79:514–517
51. Tzemos N, Therrien J, Yip J et al (2008) Outcomes in adults with bicuspid aortic valves. JAMA 300:1317–1325
52. Ward C (2000) Clinical significance of the bicuspid aortic valve. Heart 83:81–85

From dynamic anatomy to conservative aortic valve surgery: the tale of the ring

E. Lansac, I. Di Centa

Introduction

Pure aortic insufficiency (AI) represents 9.5% of the surgical indications of valve surgery in western countries [53, 92]. Dilation of the aortic root and/or cusp prolapse are the most common causes of AI, characterized by pliable cusps that are macroscopically close to normal [29, 70]. Until recently, valve replacement was the only surgical option for AI. However, none of the current valve substitutes are ideal options, since mechanical valves require life-long anticoagulation and bioprosthetic valves present the risk of reoperation. Inspired by mitral experience, reconstructive methods have been developed to treat AI, based on sparing or repairing the native aortic valve, while replacing or stabilizing the other components of the aortic root [17, 24, 116]. Recent progresses in aortic valve-sparing techniques mirrors the evolving understanding of the functional anatomy of the aortic root complex which includes the cusps, the crown-shaped aortic annulus, the interleaflet triangles, and the sinuses of Valsalva [72, 77]. All "share a dynamic coordinated behaviour, which can be partially or completely restored in various repair or replacement procedures of the aortic root" [77]. Although mid-term results are encouraging, heterogeneousness of current valve-sparing techniques limits the widespread adoption of these procedures and reinforces the need for standardization and rigourous evaluation.

Anatomy of the aortic root

Descriptive anatomy

The ascending aorta may be defined as the ensemble of two distinct entities, separated by the sinotubular junction (STJ):

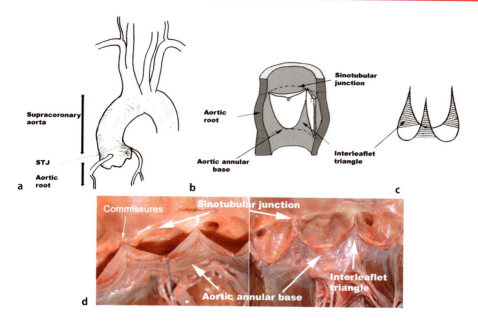

Fig. 1. Anatomy of the aortic root: **a** ascending aorta is separated by the sinotubular junction (STJ) into the supracoronary aorta and aortic root; **b** detailed components of the aortic root; **c** crown-shaped aortic annulus as a three-dimensional structure; **d** right: aortic root opened at commissural level between the right and left coronary sinuses, left: cusps resected, revealing their semilunar attachments. Reprinted from E. Lansac (2008) Chapter 10: Aortic aneurysms, new insight into an old problem. Ed. Universitaire de Liège, pp 199–233

- the aortic root, initial portion of the aorta that includes the aortic valve with its crown-shaped annulus, interleaflet triangles, and sinuses of Valsalva, and
- the supracoronary aorta extending above the STJ up to the brachiocephalic trunk (Fig. 1) [6, 72, 94, 103].

The sinuses of Valsalva are the expanded portions of the aortic root confined proximally by the concave attachments of each cusp and named accordingly (right, left, and noncoronary). The aortic annulus is not planar since it is formed by the semilunar insertion of the cusps that extend from their basal attachments within the left ventricle (aortic annular base) to their distal attachments at the STJ, forming the commissures. This three-dimensional structure of the aortic annulus may be rationalized into two functional diameters of the aortic root, ensuring proper valve function, namely the aortic annular base and the STJ [70, 103]. Echographic measurement of the aortic annulus corresponds to the aortic annular base diameter.

The aortic valve apparatus: a dynamic structure

Although the relationship between the sinuses of Valsalva and the aortic valve were intuitively illustrated by Leonardo da Vinci, the aortic valve has been regarded for a long time as a passive, trileaflet structure whose cusps open and close according to pressure differences between the left ventricle and aorta [94]. Several authors have questioned this simplistic view by showing that the expansion of the aortic root actively participates in aortic valve opening and precisely describe the three-dimensional deformational dynamics of the aortic root as a function of the different phases of the cardiac cycle [14, 21, 74, 94, 110, 111]. In an experimental study on sheep, aortic root volume increases by a total of $33.7 \pm 2.7\%$ with maximal changes occurring at the commissural level during systole in order to maximize ventricular ejection [72]. The aortic root is the junction between the left ventricle (LV) and the systemic circulation. The thin cusps separate two compartments with different hemodynamic systems. The first, the LV compartment, is situated below the cusps and includes the sigmoid-shaped cusp attachment line, the interleaflet triangles, and the commissures. These structures are related to the LV hemodynamics. The second, aortic compartment, is situated above the cusps and includes the sinuses of Valsalva, the STJ, and ascending aorta, and is related to aortic and coronary flow dynamics [72, 103].

Expansion of the aortic root starts during isovolumic contraction, initiating at the base and commissures, followed by the STJ, and then the ascending aorta reaching its maximum expansion during the first third of ejection (Fig. 2a, b). Therefore, significant aortic root expansion ($37.7 \pm 2.7\%$ of volume increase) occurs prior to ejection and initiates aortic cusp separation under minimal leaflet stresses. The preejectional expansion of the aortic root is due to commissural and annular base expansion resulting from volume redistribution in the LV outflow tract via the interleaflets triangles [21, 95].

Furthermore, aortic root expansion is asymmetric and induces a dynamic tilting of the aortic valve throughout the cardiac cycle. In systole, the LV outflow tract is aligned with the ascending aorta in order to maximize ejection. As soon as the valve starts to close, this angle tilts back and behaves as a shock absorber, to reduce stresses on the cusps [73] (Fig. 2c, d).

The shape of the aortic valve orifice remains speculative. Thubrikar et al., followed by Higashidate et al., described it as being initially stellate, then triangular, and finally circular at its maximum opening [51, 109–111]. Three-dimensional sonomicrometry with a high data sampling rate (200 to 800 Hz) showed that the shape of the aortic valve orifice progressed from initially stellate to triangular, then circular, and finally clover shaped at maximum opening [74] (Fig. 3). At that time, the cusps' free edge area exceeded the commissural area by $+16.3 \pm 2.0\%$. This behavior of the valve cusps might explain cases of early cusp deterioration following reimplantation of the aortic valve within a tubular conduit without sinuses of Valsalva

From dynamic anatomy to conservative aortic valve surgery: the tale of the ring

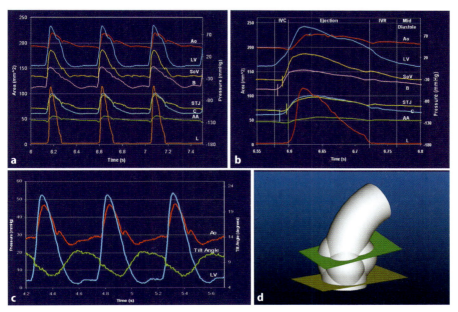

Fig. 2. Changes at each level of the aortic root time related to left ventricular and ascending aorta pressures in one sheep, **a** during three cardiac cycles and **b** detail of one cardiac cycle. **c** Dynamic changes of tilt angle of the aortic root time related to left ventricular and aortic pressures. **d** Diagram of the tilt angle between the basal and commissural planes of the aortic root at end-diastole. *Ao* aortic pressure, *LV* left ventricular pressure, *SoV* sinuses of Valsalva, *B* annular base, *STJ* sinotubular, *C* commissures, *AA* ascending aorta, *L* leaflet. Reprinted from E. Lansac (2008) Chapter 10: Aortic aneurysms, new insight into an old problem. Ed. Universitaire de Liège, pp 199–233

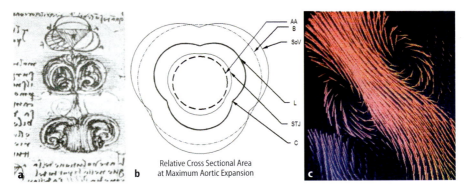

Fig. 3. Shape of the aortic valve orifice and vortices: **a** clover-shaped aortic annular base and vortices drawn by Leonardo da Vinci, **b** cross-sectional area diagram of the aortic root at maximum expansion during ejection (sonomicrometry) showing the clover-shaped orifice of the aortic valve. **c** Normal aortic ejectional flux imaged with MRI, in late systole, showing vortices in the sinuses of Valsalva. *C* commissures, *STJ* sinotubular junction, *L* leaflets, *SoV* sinus of Valsalva, *B* base, *AA* ascending aorta. Fig. 3c reprinted with permission from [63]; © American Heart Association

[41, 77]. Cusp displacement beyond the commissural level would result in cusp impact against the wall of the cylindrical prosthetic conduit. Indeed the bulging shape of the sinuses of Valsalva prevents contact between the cusps and aortic wall. They induce formation of vortices that initiate valve closure during ejection, thus, avoiding valve regurgitation [11, 63, 93].

Echocardiographic anatomy of the normal aortic root

Analysis of aortic root anatomy and function relies on the study of the following parameters: root diameters (aortic annular base, sinuses of Valsalva, STJ, and supracoronary aorta), valve coaptation, and aortic root motion [96].

Recent echocardiographic studies show the STJ to be larger than the aortic annular base with a STJ/aortic annular base ratio of 1.2 (Table 1) [9, 57, 64, 67, 79, 86, 96, 106, 113].

Correlations between aortic root diameter and body surface area for the adult population remain controversial, ranging from 1 to 92% (mean 44%) for the aortic annular base and from 32 to 44% (mean 39%) for the STJ [16, 66, 113–115]. Therefore, in surgical practice for the average adult population, it seems reliable and simpler to consider absolute values and to define an aortic annular base diameter larger than 25 mm and a STJ diameter larger than 30 mm as dilated.

Although aortic root expansion is well documented in experimental studies, few data are available on humans. Analysis of 183 normal echographies showed an aortic root expansion of 6.2% (2.5–9.6%) and of 5.7% (2.8–9.8%) at the aortic annular base and the STJ levels, respectively [28,

Table 1. Echographic analysis of normal and dystrophic aortic root diameters

	Normal aortic root [9, 57, 64, 67, 79, 86, 96, 106, 113]	Dystrophy of the aortic root	
		Aortic root aneurysms [3, 30, 33, 61, 70, 92, 101]	Isolated aortic insufficiency [70, 84, 98]
	Total n=665	Total n=700	Total n=595
■ Aortic annular base diameter (mm)	22.6 (20.5–24.5)	26.4 (25–27.5)	27.3 (27–28)
■ STJ diameter (mm)	27.4 (24.7–29.5)	45.3 (39.5–52.4)	31 (28–35)
■ Ratio STJ/aortic annular base	1.2	1.7	1.1

n number of patients, *STJ* sinotubular junction, values in parentheses denote ranges

61, 77, 79, 80, 94, 113]. However the measurement precision of a two-dimensional echocardiography or CT scan is on the order of 1–2 mm, which limits detection of differences between systole and diastole.

Anatomy of dystrophic aortic roots

Dystrophic aortic root (bicuspid or tricuspid valve) includes two phenotypes depending on the dilation of the sinuses of Valsalva:
- aortic root aneurysms (sinus of Valsalva > 45 mm);
- isolated AI (sinus of Valsalva < 40 mm) ± supracoronary aneurysms.

In all cases, at least one of the two functional diameters of the aortic root is dilated (STJ or aortic annular base) (Table 1) [3, 30, 33, 61, 70, 84, 92, 98, 101]. Therefore, dystrophy of the aortic root can be described as a "diameter disease" leading to inadequate coaptation of the aortic cusps. Cusp prolapse is often associated with root aneurysms and is the most common cause of isolated dystrophic AI.

Surgical treatment for aortic root aneurysm

Surgical indications for aortic root aneurysms are based on maximum aortic diameter (Table 2) [5, 108]. Two different surgical approaches are available, either
- radical, replacing the aortic valve and root, or
- conservative, replacing the aortic root while sparing or repairing the aortic valve.

Composite valve and graft replacement

Composite valve and graft replacement was first described by De Bono and Bentall in 1968 [12]. Although defined as the gold standard, its benefits have to be weighed against the risks of life-long anticoagulation. Indeed, the majority of patients with aortic root aneurysms are young, and although the risks of thromboembolism and bleeding in the presence of mechanical valves are low, their long life expectancy will increase the cumulative risk of valve-related morbidity and impact significantly the 10 years survival (Table 3) [7, 31, 38, 45, 46, 58, 84, 85, 90, 102].

Table 2. Surgical indications for aortic root aneurysms American College of Cardiology/American Heart Association (ACC/AHA) and European Society of Cardiology (ESC) guidelines [5, 108]

- **ACC-AHA 2006** [5]
  - Symptomatic aneurysms (Class IA)
  - $\varnothing \geq 50$ mm irrespective of AI grade (Class IC)
  - Aortic root increase in diameter ≥ 0.5 cm/year
  - $\varnothing \geq 45$ mm and AS or AI on a bicuspid valve (Class IC)
  - $\varnothing \geq 45$ mm in Marfan women desiring pregnancy
- **ESC 2007** [108]
  - Symptomatic aneurysms (Class IA)
  - $\varnothing \geq 55$ mm irrespective of AI grade (Class IIaC)
  - $\varnothing \geq 45$ mm in case of Marfan, aortic root increase in diameter ≥ 0.5 cm/year or familial history of aortic dissection (Class IC)
  - $\varnothing \geq 50$ mm in case of bicuspid valve when aortic root increase in diameter ≥ 0.5 cm/year or familial history of aortic dissection (Class IIaC)
  - $\varnothing \geq 40$ mm in Marfan women desiring pregnancy (Class IC)

$\varnothing$ diameter, *AI* aortic insufficiency, *AS* aortic stenosis

Aortic valve-sparing procedures

Owing to the improved understanding of aortic valve dynamics, conservative aortic valve surgery was developed based on reduction of the dilated aortic root diameter ($\pm$ cusp lesion), while preserving root dynamics with vortices (neosinuses of Valsalva) and expansibility (interleaflet triangles) [29, 70].

Two types of aortic valve-sparing operations were originally performed to treat root aneurysms: "remodeling" of the aortic root and "reimplantation" of the aortic valve. By reducing the sinotubular junction diameter and creating three neosinuses of Valsava with a scalloped Dacron tube graft sutured in the supravalvular position, the remodeling technique provides a physiological reconstruction of the root, but it does not address annular base dilation [116, 117]. Alternatively, reimplantation as an inclusion technique of the aortic valve within a cylindrical tube implanted in the subvalvular position reduces both the annulus and the sinotubular junction diameters to the detriment of root dynamics [22–27].

Results of main series of aortic valve sparing

These techniques spare the patient from anticoagulation and prosthetic valve morbidity with a 10-year survival rate ranging from 80.4 to 92% (mean 88.2%) (Table 4) [3, 22, 25, 30, 35, 36, 56, 59, 69, 87, 100, 117]. In both techniques with proper patient selection, the results up to 10 years are equally excellent (Tables 4 and 5). However, in earlier series of the remodeling technique, the reoperation rate was higher after type A aortic dissection and in patients with Marfan syndrome [68, 76, 78]. In the unselected population of the original remodeling series, up to 30% of patients presented recurrence of AI grade II or III [69, 78, 117]. The only risk factor for failure was a dilated native aortic annulus (diameter ≥25 mm) [47a, 69, 78]. Based on larger series, Schafers et al. recommend choosing the remodeling technique whenever the sinuses and STJ are enlarged and aortoventricular junction preserved in order to obtain more physiologic root dynamics; a larger diameter should be treated with the reimplantation procedure to secure the aortic root at the aortoventricular junction [3, 100].

Aortic root and valve dynamics after remodeling or reimplantation

In vitro studies. All studies show that the remodeling technique exhibits valve dynamics closest to those of the native aortic root. The recreation of the sinuses of Valsalva preserves vortex formation, as well as cusp opening and closing dynamics, thus, reducing cusp stress which theoretically improves their durability. The valve shows asymmetric motion after reimplantation. The cusp bending deformation index is increased with the reimplantation techniques and sinus prosthesis compared with the control and remodeling groups [36, 40, 44, 91].

In vivo studies. Leyh and colleagues clearly demonstrated that distensibility of the aortic root and a proper valve motion were better preserved after the remodeling than after the reimplantation technique [77]. They showed that reimplantation with a straight tube abolished root distensibility at all levels; the cusps took longer for closing, and systolic contact of at least one cusp against the tube graft was constantly found. Reconstruction of the sinuses may assure a sufficient gap to avoid any such contact between the open cusp and the Dacron wall, which is known to be responsible for cusp thickening and accelerated degeneration [8, 28, 79]. The presence of vortices inside the neosinuses of Valsalva preserves the slow closing displacement of the cusps and is associated with a valve motion similar to that of normal subjects [28, 79]. Although not significant, valve velocities after the remodeling procedure using the Valsalva graft (Gelweave Valsalva^{TM}, Vascutek, Inc.) are closer to normal than after reimplantation using the same graft [28].

Therefore, all dynamic studies suggest that cusp motion and flow patterns across the reconstructed aortic root are more physiologic
- after remodeling of the aortic root than after reimplantation of the aortic valve and
- after procedures using a prosthetic conduit fashioned with neosinuses of Valsalva than without.

Table 3. Results of main series of composite valve and graft replacement since 1999

	Dossche K 1999 [31]	Nieder-hauser 1999 [85]	Aomi 2002 [7]	Hagl 2003 [46]	Pacini 2003 [84]	Sioris 2004 [102]	Guilmet 2004 [45]	Radu 2007 [90]	Etz 2007 [38]	Kalkat 2007 [58]	Total[c]
Number	244	181	193	142	274	452	150	100	275	1962	3973
Age (years)	54±15	53	43.2±13.2	46	53.5	52.3±16.3	50±16	51	69±11	54	52.6
Marfan	14.8%	8.8%	46%	7%	12.8%	6%	24%	4%	1%	–	13.8%
Bicuspid	2.5%	–	–	46%	–	38%	–	31%	3%	–	24.1%
Valve type											81%
Mechanical	83.6%	100%	100%	88%	100%	43%	96%	100%	0%	100%	17.4%
Bioprosthesis	16.4%	–	–	12%	0%	42%	4%	0%	100%	–	
Acute dissection	13.5%	24%	30%	0%	6.6%	6%	3.3%	0%	5%	17%	10.5%
AC time (min)	130±43	–	–	142±31	106±32.4	106±36	–	117±49	181±48	–	130.3
Elective operative mortality	7.1%	6.6%[b]	5.6%[b]	0.7%	6%	4%[b]	0.6%	4%	2%	5.8%	3.7%
Median follow-up (months)	96	28[a]	70	42 (0–156)	62.7[a]	53±33.6[a]	94±65[a]	52±36[a]	43	49	60

Freedom from reop.	88.9% 10 y	69.4±9% 7 y	76.5±4.4% 10 y	–	98.8±1.2% 10 y	94±3% 10 y	–	100% follow-up	100% follow-up	97% follow-up	89.5% 10 y
Freedom from TE complications	97.7% 10 y	–	2% patient/y	99.3% follow-up	90.9±3.1% 10 y	92±2% 10 y	0.42% patient/y	74.7±6.4% 7 y	0.85% patient/y	–	91.3% 10 y
Freedom from HC	87.5% 10 y	–	–	93% follow-up	87.5±3.7% 10 y	83±4% 10 y	0.42% patient/y	87.7±5.8% 7 y	0.3% patient/y	–	90.3% 10 y
Freedom from endo- carditis	92.8% 10 y	–	–	98.6% follow-up	96.4±2% 10 y	96±2% 10 y	–	100% follow-up	100% follow-up	–	95.1% 10 y
Survival 5 years	76%	75.4±9% 7 y	–	95%	77.7%	87±5%	–	89.1±3.5%	74%	77%	82.2% 5 y
10 years	62%		71.5±4.4%	93% 8 y	63%	74±4%	85%	83.2±5.2% 7 y	–	70%	71% 10 y

[a] Mean follow-up; [b] Overall operative mortality including acute and elective mortality;
[c] Total corresponds to a summary of the present series, only when available data were comparable

TE thromboembolic; *AC* aortic cross-clamping time; *y* year; *op* operative; *reop* reoperation; *HC* hemorragic complications

Table 4. Latest publications of main series (>20 patients) of valve-sparing procedures

	Reimplantation					Remodeling		
	Obadia 2004 [87]	Kallenbach 2005 [59]	Di Bartolomeo 2006 [30]	David 2007 [25]	Total[a]	Yacoub 1998 [117]	Aicher 2007 [3]	Total[a]
Number	50	284	63	167	564	158	274	432
Age (years)	60±15	53±16	54.9±14.4	45±15	53.2	46.6	59±15	52.8
Marfan	2.5%	15%	9.5%	38%	16.2%	68%	1.8%	34.9%
Bicuspid	2.5%	6%	12.6%	9%	7.5%	–	11.3%	11.3%
Acute dissection	2%	3.5%	6.3%	14%	6.4%	31%	16.8%	23.9%
AC time (min)	99±15	131±32	128.8±27.6	140±35	124.7	–	83±17	83
Cusp repair	3%	6.3%	20.6%	21% resuspension	17.2%	0%	63%	31.5%
Elective op. mortality	0	1.3%	1.7%	1.2%	1.4%	0.97%±0.9%	3.1%	2%
Mean follow-up (months)	19	41±32 (0–130)	16.6±9.1	61.2±45.6	34.4	67.5 (1–213)	48±32.4	57.8
10 y Freedom from reoperation	–	87.1±4.5%	93.8±5.1%	95±3%	91%	89.5±0.5 10 y	96% 10 y	92.7%

	98% FU	97.1%	91.7±4.3% 3 y	94% 10 y	94% 10 y	63.4%	91% 10 y	87 to 91% 10 y
■ Freedom AI≥ grade II								
■ Freedom from TE complications	–	99.3%	100%	99.4%	99.6%	99.4%	100%	100%
■ Freedom from HC	–	100%	100%	99.4%	99.8%	100%	100%	100%
■ Freedom from endocarditis	–	98.5%	100%	–	99.2%	99.4%	99.6%	99.5%
■ Survival 5 y	92%	90.7%	94.7±2.9% 3 y	98%	93.6%	88% 5 y	91%	89.5%
10 y	96%	80.4±5.7%		92±3%	89.5%	–	87%	87%

[a] Total corresponds to a summary of the present series, only when available data were comparable

TE thromboembolic; *AC* aortic cross-clamping time; *y* year; *m* months; *AI* aortic insufficiency; *op* operative; *HC* hemorragic complications

Table 5. Main series reporting both remodeling and reimplantation results

	Schafers 1998 [100]		Lansac 2006 [69]		David 2006 [22]		Jeanmart 2007 [56]		Erasmi 2007 [36]		Total
	Remod.	Reimp.	Remod.	Remod. + annuloplasty	Remod.	Reimpl.	Remod.	Reimpl.	Remod.	Reimpl.	
Number	29	11	34	49	53	167	48	66	96	68	621
Age (years)	64±12	49±17	48.7±14.9	49.9±15.3	47.7±16	45.5±15	54±17	51±15	56±14.8	50.2±16	51.6
Marfan	0	27.3%	44%	32.6%	45%	38%	10.4%	6%	0	18%	22.1%
Bicuspid	12.2%	0	0	8.2%	0%	9%	22.9%	36.4%	13.5%	8.8%	11.1%
Acute dissection	41.4%	27.3%	0	0	10%	11%	0	0	22%	41%	11.3%
AC time (min)	87±25	112±32	114.7±27	125.2±28	104±26	115±27	98±31	110±25	135	159	116
Cusp repair	–	–	0	10.2%	50%	61%	47.9%	72.7%	22.9%	27.9%	36.6%
Elective op. mortality	0	0	2.9%	4%	1.9%	1.1%	2%	0	0	0	1.2%
Mean follow-up (months)	11		17.2±13.4	10.41±7.95	62.4±44.4		50±35		54±28	48.4±37.3	36.2

Freedom from reoperation	100%	86.4%	95.5%	93±4% 10 y	96±3% 10 y	97% 5 y	85% 5 y	89±4% (55±28 m)	98±2% (49±37 m)	94.5% 10y (93–96)
Freedom from AI ≥ grade II	88% 1 year	90%	95.5%	75%±10% 10 y	94%±4% 10 y	97% 5 y	83% 5 y	98.7%	100%	85% 10 y
Freedom from TE complications	–	100%	95.7%	92±3% 10y		–	–	100%	100%	92% 10y
Freedom from HC	–	100%			99%	–	–	100%	100%	99.5% (99–100)
Freedom from endocarditis	100%	100%			99.2%	100%		100%		99.8%
Survival										
5 y			97.7%		94±1%	87% 5 y	92% 5 y	92%	96%	89.5%
10 y	100%	100%			88±3%	–	–			88%

TE thromboembolic; *AC* aortic cross-clamping time; *y* year, *m* months; *AV* aortic valve; *op* operative; *Remod* Remodeling; *Reimpl* Reimplantation; *HC* hemorragic complications

Modification of original remodeling and reimplantation techniques

Multiple modifications of these original techniques have been proposed, aiming to combine the rationale of treating annular base dilation, while preserving root dynamics with vortices (neosinuses of Valsalva) and root expansibility (interleaflet triangles) [19, 23, 26, 28, 42, 49, 50, 52, 65, 81, 83, 97, 104, 105, 112, 119].

David et al. added an external Teflon strip on the aortomitral junction to the remodeling technique (David III) or oversized (+4 mm) the tube graft for the reimplantation technique (David IV) [23, 26]. The David V technique used an even larger graft size (+6–8 mm), which is "necked down" at both the bottom and the top ends to create graft pseudosinuses [81]. Many authors suggested different methods to customize the tube graft for the reimplantation or remodeling in order to provide better neosinuses of Valsalva. More recently De Paulis et al. designed the Valsalva graft (Gelweave Valsalva^{TM}, Vascutek, Inc.) with vertical pleats in the proximal section for reconstruction of the aortic root and with the standard horizontal pleats for ascending aorta replacement [28, 97, 112, 119]. Furthermore, multiple criteria and methods have been suggested to help determine graft size, such as annular base diameter (resulting in a tube graft diameter from –15 to +40% of annular base diameter), height of the cusp, distance between the commissures producing maximal coaptation of the cusps or even more complex formulae resulting in confusion and lack of standardization.

Towards a standardized and physiological approach to aortic valve-sparing procedures

The remodeling and the reimplantation techniques may be considered in a complementary rather than a competing fashion, thus, combining the advantages of each technique by adding an external subvalvular prosthetic ring annuloplasty to the physiological remodeling of the aortic root (Fig. 4). In order to standardize this physiological approach to valve sparing, we designed a calibrated expansible aortic ring (Extra Aortic, Fig. 5). The rationale for the design of the ring was based on a controlled reduction of the diameter of the native aortic annular base in diastole in order to increase cusp coaptation height, while maintaining systolic expansibility, with the goal of reducing cusp stress and optimizing left-ventricular ejection. The main steps of the surgical techniques are detailed in Fig. 6 [71].

The choice of the Valsalva graft is based solely on the measurement of the native aortic annular base internal diameter using Hegar's dilators (Fig. 6e). Diameter of the prosthetic aortic ring is undersized from one size.

Since May 2003, these standardized procedures were conducted in 114 patients with aortic root aneurysms [71]. Two patients required perioperative conversion (1.7%). Operative and follow-up data are summarized in Table 6.

From dynamic anatomy to conservative aortic valve surgery: the tale of the ring 117

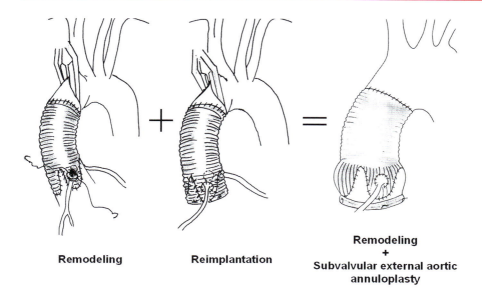

	Remodeling	Reimplantation	Remodeling + subvalvular external aortic annuloplasty
Reduction of sino-tubular junction Ø	+	+	+
Reduction of aortic annular base Ø	-	+	+
Re-creation of sinuses of Valsalva	+	±	+
Dynamics of the root (interleaflet triangles)	++	-	+

Fig. 4. Remodeling of the aortic root using a scalloped graft (Gelweave Valsalva™, Vascutek, Inc.): three neosinuses of Valsalva associated to an external subvalvular aortic annuloplasty, combining advantages of the original remodeling and reimplantation techniques

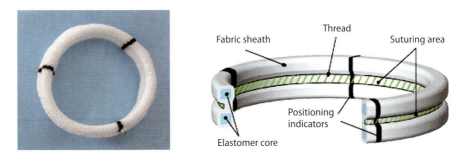

Fig. 5. Expansible ring composed of two separate rings covered by a polyester fabric sheath to provide a suturing area between the rings (Extra-Aortic™, CORONEO, Inc.). Black indicator marks on the ring are placed to guide suture placement. Reprinted from E. Lansac (2008) Chapter 10: Aortic aneurysms, new insight into an old problem. Ed. Universitaire de Liège, pp 199–233

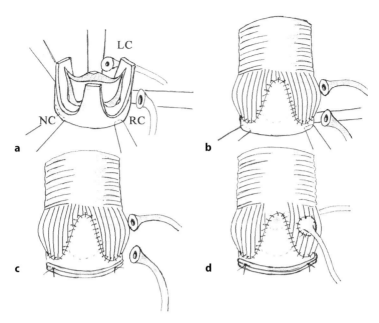

Criteria for choice of the expansible prosthetic rings

	Aortic annular base ⌀ (mm) Hegar Dilator			
	25–26	27–28	29–30	31–32
⌀ **Tube graft**	26	28	30	32
⌀ **Subvalvular ring**	23	25	27	29

Fig. 6. Surgical steps of remodeling of the aortic root associated to an external subvalvular aortic annuloplasty: **a** five "U" stitches are placed inside out as circumferentially in the subvalvular plane. Three stitches are placed 2 mm below the nadir of insertion of each cusp, and two stitches are placed below two of the three commissures at the base of the interleaflet triangles (no suture is placed at the base of the interleaflet triangle situated between the right and noncoronary sinuses to avoid potential injury to the bundle of His). First step of valve repair is performed by aligning adjacent cusp free edges. Excess of length is corrected by placating central stitches (5/0); **b** remodeling of the aortic root is standardized by scalloping a bulged graft (Gelweave Valsalva™, Vascutek, Inc.) with three symmetrical neosinuses using the linear demarcations on the tube. The heights of the neocommissures are cut up to the level of the bulging part of the graft. Cusp resuspension is re-evaluated in order to obtain an effective height of 8 mm; **c** the five anchoring "U" stitches are passed through the inner aspect of the prosthetic aortic ring and tied down externally in the subvalvular position; **d** final aspect of the neoaortic root after anastomosis of the coronary ostia (*NC* noncoronary, *RC* right coronary, *LC* left coronary); **e** criteria for choice of the prosthetic annuloplasty rings (Extra-Aortic™, CORONEO, Inc.) and tube graft (Gelweave Valsalva™, Vascutek, Inc.).

Table 6. Results of preliminary series of aortic annuloplasty

	Remodeling and subvalvular aortic annuloplasty	Double sub- and supravalvular aortic annuloplasty
■ Number of patients	114	17
■ Mean age (years)	53.2 ± 14.3 (24–81)	56.6 ± 15.9 (27–77)
■ Marfan syndrome	18 (15.8%)	0
■ Bicuspid valves	22 (19.3%)	4 (23.5%)
■ Mean preoperative AI grade	1.9 ± 0.9 (0–4)	3.2 ± 0.7 (2–4)
■ Aortic annulus diameter (mm)	27.7 ± 1.9 (26–37)	27.5 ± 0.7 (24–30)
■ Sinotubular junction diameter (mm)	44.8 ± 14.8 (34–79)	34 ± 5.8 (30–38)
■ Aortic cross-clamping time (min)[a]	129.3 ± 20.8 (81–187)	94 ± 16.9 (62–120)
■ Perioperative conversions	2 (1.7%)	1 (5.9%)
■ Associated valve repair	36 (31.6%)	12 (70.5%)
■ Operative mortality	4 (3.5%)	0
■ Postoperative aortic annulus diameter (mm)	20.4 ± 2.1 (16–25)	21.2 ± 2 (18–24)
■ Postoperative mean aortic gradient (mmHg)	8 ± 4 (0–13)	6 ± 2 (1.3–11)
■ Mean follow-up (months)	29.8 ± 4.8 (1–67)	27.3 ± 18.7 (2–57)
■ Reoperation for aortic valve replacement	6 (5.5%)	0
■ Transient thromboembolic events	2 (1.8%)	0
■ Hemorrhagic events	0	0
■ Aortic endocarditis	0	0
■ Survival at follow-up	106[b] (96.3%)	16[c] (94.1%)

[a] excluding patients with associated cardiac procedures (10 patients remodeling group, 4 patients in the double annuloplasty group)
[b] 4 deaths during follow-up
[c] 1 death during follow-up (pancreatic cancer)

Valve repair for isolated aortic insufficiency

Surgery is indicated for isolated AI in symptomatic patients and/or LV systolic dysfunction (EF < 50%, or end-systolic dimension > 55 mm or 25 mm/m^2) [5, 108].

Techniques for aortic valve repair have been documented for over 50 years [15, 107] and interest has been renewed with the spread of valve-sparing procedures. Series of isolated AI repair combine patients of heterogeneous indications and techniques. Overall, results of 372 patients are reported in the literature [34, 47, 48, 55, 75, 82]. Total aortic cross-clamping time averages 71.8 min (42.4–99.8 min). Operative mortality ranges from 0 to 2.5% (mean 0.9%). Incidence of thromboembolic events and infectious endocarditis is low for a mean follow-up of 32.1 months (13.8–50 months). The average 5-year freedom from reoperation ranges from 82 to 94.4% (mean 90.1%).

Techniques are based on the same principles associating treatment for valvular prolapse and aortic annular base dilation. Commissural annuloplasty is commonly used but remains an incomplete annuloplasty plicating only the interleaflets triangles. Other techniques of annuloplasty have been developed ranging from experimental prototypes to homemade ring devices lacking standardization [13, 39, 43, 47, 48, 54, 62].

Valve repair for isolated dystrophic AI should follow the same surgical principles as for aortic root aneurysm (treatment of the dilated diameters ± cusp lesion and preservation of aortic root dynamics). Therefore, we suggest a standardized approach performing a double sub- and supravalvular external annuloplasty preserving root dynamics, while protecting valve repair. The main steps of this surgical technique are detailed in Fig. 7 [71].

Seventeen patients with isolated dystrophic AI underwent a double sub- and supravalvular aortic annuloplasty [71]. One patients required perioperative conversion. Operative and follow-up data are summarized in Table 6.

Repair of cusp prolapse and bicuspid valve

Aicher et al. and El Khoury have reported excellent mid-term results from the association of cusp repair with an aortic valve-sparing procedure [2, 34]. There were no differences in operative mortality, survival, and freedom from aortic valve replacement or recurrence of AI when a cusp repair was added. Along with the alignment of the free edges of the cusp, Schafers et al. defined an intraoperative effective height ≥8 mm (difference between the central free margins and the aortic insertion lines at the cusp nadir) as a goal for aortic valve repair. A special calliper was designed to standardize this height measurement [99].

Repair of bicuspid valves provides very encouraging results. About 446 patients have been operated for isolated AI (52.9%), aortic root aneurysms (29.6%) or supracoronary aneurysms (17.5%). Operative mortality ranges from 0 to 1.2% (mean 0.4%); with a mean aortic cross-clamping time of 57.3 min (47–71 min). Freedom from reoperation at 5 years is 92% (87–97%) [4, 18, 31, 33, 98]. Schafers et al. showed no difference in valve stability after repair of bicuspid or tricuspid aortic valves [98]. In most cases,

From dynamic anatomy to conservative aortic valve surgery: the tale of the ring

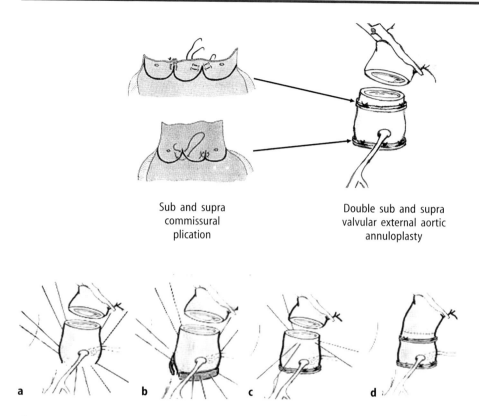

Fig. 7. Surgical steps of the double sub- and supravalvular external aortic annuloplasty: **a** after complete transsection of the aorta above the STJ, external dissection down to the base of the aortic annulus is performed, passing under the coronary arteries, without detaching them from the aortic wall. Five "U" stitches are placed from the inside out circumferentially in the subvalvular plane, as described in Fig. 6. Valve repair is then performed by aligning free edges of adjacent cusp. Cusp\ktau resuspension is completed in order to obtain an effective height of 8 mm on each cusp; **b** the subvalvular stitches are passed through the inner aspect of the "open" subvalvular prosthetic ring; **c** three U stitches are placed on the top of each commissure and the aortotomy is closed; **d** the commissural stitches are then passed through the inner aspect of a supravalvular aortic ring and tied at the STJ level

cusp repair is associated with aortic annular base reduction and aggressive management of the dilated aortic root [33, 98]. However, a reliable criterion for determining aortic root replacement remains controversial, especially when the aortic diameter is below 45 mm.

Lesional classification for aortic insufficiencies

As for mitral valve repair, functional classifications for AI are described [1, 29, 48]. We suggest a lesional classification in order to allow a better understanding of the mechanisms of AI and to standardize its surgical management towards a more reconstructive approach (Fig. 8) [70]. This classification relies on a systematic echocardiographic analysis of the regurgitant jet leading to define AI according to the anatomical lesions. In case of a central jet (Type I), the lack of valvular coaptation is related to dilation of at least one of the functional diameters of aortic root (STJ and/or aortic annular base). In case of an eccentric jet (Type II), the lack of valvular coaptation is related to the combination of a valvular lesion and the dilation of the aortic root (Fig. 8).

The design of a lesional classification led us to adapt the reconstructive techniques to each type of AI in a standardized approach. A subvalvular aortic annuloplasty is systematically performed using an external expansible aortic ring to reduce aortic annular base diameter. Depending on the phenotype of the aortic root, reduction of the STJ diameter will be achieved through a root remodeling (root aneurysm), a supracoronary graft (supracoronary aneurysm) or a supravalvular expansible annuloplasty ring (isolated AI).

In all cases, intraoperative transesophageal echocardiography remains critical in order to analyze the lesional mechanism of AI both pre- and postrepair. Any residual AI (grade >1) requires correction, because it is a risk factor for early and late failure of the repair [2, 56].

Conservative aortic valve surgery versus valve replacement: what do we know?

Few series have compared valve sparing with composite valve and graft replacement (Table 7) [10, 20, 27, 60, 89, 118]. Conclusions remain controversial since they were often based on comparisons of different operating time periods and learning curves periods. Overall, rates of thromboembolism, bleeding, and endocarditis after valve sparing seem lower than those reported for prosthetic valves. However, there is a lack of consistency in the way to report pre-, perioperative and follow-up results that prevent the ri-

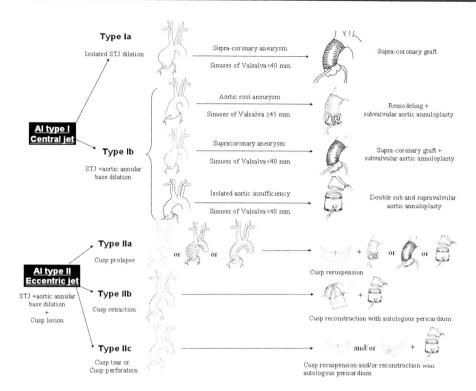

Fig. 8. Lesionnal classification for aortic insufficiency (AI) and adapted surgical strategies. STJ sinotubular junction. Reprinted from E. Lansac (2008) Chapter 10: Aortic aneurysms, new insight into an old problem. Ed. Universitaire de Liège, pp 199–233

gourous evaluation of both techniques. A current prospective international registry just provided 30-day morbidity and mortality data and shows equivalent results after a composite valve replacement or a valve-sparing procedure (despite various type of reimplantation) in a selected population of Marfan patients (National Marfans Foundation prospective aortic root replacement registry) [20].

Although reliable data comparing valve replacement and valve-sparing procedures are still needed, it has already impacted surgical strategies as being recently added in the ACC/AHA and ESC guidelines [5, 108]. In order to validate the indication for valve sparing versus replacement, patients with aortic root aneurysm and/or AI will be enrolled in France in the ongoing prospective multicenter CAVIAAR trial (Conservative Aortic Valve surgery for aortic Insufficiency and Aneurysm of the Aortic Root), over the next 5 years, comparing 130 patients with a standardized valve-sparing procedure using an expansible aortic annuloplasty ring versus 130 patients with a mechanical valve replacement (http://clinicaltrials.gov/ct2/show/NCT00478803).

Table 7. Results of main series comparing valve sparing with composite valve and graft replacement (CVG)

	Bassano 2001 [10]		de Oliveira 2003 [27]		Karck 2004 [60]		Zehr 2004 [118]		Coselli 2008 [20]		Patel 2008 [89]	
	Valve sparing	CVG	Valve sparing	CVG	Valve sparing	CVG	Valve sparing	CVG	Valve sparing	CVG	Valve sparing	CVG
Number	32	37	61	44	45	74	54	149	66	33	84	56
Age (years)	53±19	58±13	35±10	34±11	28±12	35±11	51±15	54±16	31±11	40±14	29.2±12.3	38.1±14.1
Marfan	12%	3%	100%	100%	100%	100%	30%	23%	100%	100%	100%	100%
Bicuspid	–	–	–	9%	2%	4%	15%	12%	–	–	1 (1.2%)	1 (1.2%)
Type of operation	Remod.	–	Reimpl. 63.9% Remod. 36.1%	Mech. 59% Biop. 20.4%	Reimpl.	Mech.	Reimpl. 85.1% Remod. 14.8%	Mech. 89.2% Biop. 9.8%	Reimpl. 98% fs 2%	Mech. 85% Biop. 15%	Remod. 40 (47.6%) Reimpl. 44 (52.4%)	Mech. 100%
Acute dissection	0	0	9 (15%)	6 (14%)	3 (7%)	17 (23%)	12 (6%)		6 (9%)	3 (9%)	7 (12.5%)	9 (16.1%)
AC time (min)	101±24	96±25	–	–	125±29	78±26	107±30	96±28	185±76	111±48	102.6±14.7	115.2±60.4
Op. mortality	0	5.4%	0	2.3%	0	6.7%	3.7%	4%	0	0	0	0
Reexploration for bleeding	12.5%	21.6%	8.2%	9%	4.4%	10.8%	4%	4%	7.5%	15.1%	0	3,6%
Follow-up	1021 pt/m	926 pt/m	49±38 m	75±54 m	30 m	114 m		7.3±6 y	30 days	30 days	8 y	8 y

From dynamic anatomy to conservative aortic valve surgery: the tale of the ring

Freedom from reop.	87.5%	100%	5 y 100% 10 y 100%	5 y 92±5% 10 y 75±9%	5 y 84±8%	92±3% 5 y	63% 5 y	96% 5 y	Early: 1 valve reoperation	0	90.4±4.3% 8 y	95.8±5.1% 8 y
Freedom from TE complications							97% 5 y	97% 5 y			98.8%	91%
Freedom from HC	82±8% 5 y	88±7% 5 y	100% 5 y 100% 10 y	89±5% 5 y 89±5% 10 y	97.8%	76%	–	73% 15 y	–		98.8%	91%
Freedom from endocarditis					100%	97.1%		99% 15 y	–	–	97.6% 100%	96.4%
Survival 5 y 10 y	100% follow-up	97.3% follow-up	96±3% 96±3%	92±5% 87±7%	96±4% –	89±4% –	93% 79%		–	–	100% 8 y	90.1%± 4.8% 8 y

CVG composite valve and graft replacement; *TE* thromboembolic; *AC* aortic cross-clamping; *Reimpl* reimplantation; *Remod* remodeling, *m* month; *y* year; *op* operative; *pt/m* patients/month; *fs* Florida Sleeve; *reop* reopration; *HC* hemorrage complications; *Mech* mechanical; *Biop* Bioprosthesis

Conclusions

Conservative aortic valve surgery carries the hope that cumulative valve-related morbidity and mortality would be lower than in prosthetic valve replacement surgery, which still represents the surgical "gold standard" and the most performed procedure. The evolution of valve-sparing and repair techniques mirrors the evolving understanding of aortic root and valve dynamics. Principles for conservative aortic valve surgery have been refined, based on treatment of lesions (dilation of the aortic annular base and STJ and/or cusp lesions) and preservation of the dynamics of the aortic root in order to improve the durability of the repair. Considering these issues, an expansible aortic annuloplasty represents a useful adjunct to standardize a physiological approach to conservative aortic valve surgery. However, objective long-term evaluation is needed to validate evidence that repairing the aortic valve is better than replacing it.

References

1. Acar C, Jebara V (1995) Reconstructive surgery of the aortic valve. In: Textbook of acquired Heart Valve Disease. ICR Publishers, pp 853–859
2. Aicher D, Langer F, Adam O, Tscholl D, Lausberg H, Schäfers HJ (2007) Cusp repair in aortic valve reconstruction: does the technique affect stability? J Thorac Cardiovasc Surg 134:1533–1538
3. Aicher D, Langer F, Lausberg H, Bierbach B, Schäfers HJ (2007) Aortic root remodeling: ten-year experience with 274 patients. J Thorac Cardiovasc Surg 134:909–915
4. Alsoufi B, Borger MA, Armstrong S, Maganti M, David TE (2005) Results of valve preservation and repair for bicuspid aortic valve insufficiency. J Heart Valve Dis 14:752–758, discussion 758–759
5. American College of Cardiology/American Heart Association Task Force on Practice Guidelines; Society of Cardiovascular Anesthesiologists; Society for Cardiovascular Angiography and Interventions; Society of Thoracic Surgeons; Bonow RO, Carabello BA, Kanu C et al (2006) ACC/AHA 2006 guidelines for the management of patients with valvular heart disease: a report of the American College of Cardiology/American Heart Association Task Force on Practice Guidelines (writing committee to revise the 1998 Guidelines for the Management of Patients With Valvular Heart Disease): developed in collaboration with the Society of Cardiovascular Anesthesiologists: endorsed by the Society for Cardiovascular Angiography and Interventions and the Society of Thoracic Surgeons. Circulation 114:e84–e231
6. Anderson RH, Devine WA, Ho SY, Smith A, Mc Kay R (1991) The myth of the aortic annulus: the anatomy of the subaortic outflow tract. Ann Thorac Surg 52: 640–646
7. Aomi S, Nakajima M, Nonoyama M, et al (2002) Aortic root replacement using composite valve graft in patients with aortic valve disease and aneurysm of the ascending aorta: twenty years' experience of late results. Artif Organs 26:467–473

8. Aybek T, Sotiriou M, Wohleke T, Miskovic A, Simon A, Doss M, Dogan S, Wimmer-Greinecker G, Moritz A (2005) Valve opening and closing dynamics after different aortic valve-sparing operations. J Heart Valve Dis 14:114–120
9. Babaee Bigi MA, Aslani A (2007) Aortic root size and prevalence of aortic regurgitation in elite strength trained athletes. Am J Cardiol 100:528–530
10. Bassano C, De Matteis GM, Nardi P, Buratta MM, Zeitani J, De Paulis R, Chiariello L (2001) Mid-term follow-up of aortic root remodelling compared to Bentall operation. Eur J Cardiothorac Surg 19:601–605
11. Bellhouse B, Bellhouse F (1969) Fluid mechanics of model normal and stenosed aortic valves. Circulation Res 25:693–704
12. Bentall HH, De Bono A (1968) A technique for complete replacement of the ascending aorta. Thorax 23:338–339
13. Bouchot O, Chaput M, Demers P, Bouchard D, Cartier R (2005) Aortic Root Remodeling And A Full Ring Aortic Annuloplasty. SHVD meeting
14. Brewer RJ, Deck JD, Capati B, Nolan SP (1976) The dynamic aortic root: its role in aortic valve function. J Thorac Cardiovasc Surg 72:413–417
15. Cabrol C, Cabrol A, Guiraudon G, Bertrand M (1966) Treatment of aortic insufficiency by means of aortic annuloplasty. Arch Mal Coeur Vaiss 59:1305–1312
16. Capps SB, Elkins RC, Fronk DM (2000) Body surface area as a predictor of aortic and pulmonary valve diameter. J Thorac Cardiovasc Surg 119:975–982
17. Carpentier A (1983) Cardiac valve surgery – the "french correction". J Thorac Cardiovasc Surg 86:323–337
18. Casselman FP, Gillinov AM, Akhrass R, Kasirajan V, Blackstone EH, Cosgrove DM (1999) Intermediate-term durability of bicuspid aortic valve repair for prolapsing leaflet. Eur J Cardiothorac Surg 15:302–308
19. Cochran RP, Kunzelman KS (2000) Methods of pseudosinus creation in an aortic valve-sparing operation for aneurysmal disease. J Card Surg 15:428–433
20. Coselli JS, Sundt TM, Miller DC, Bavaria JE, LeMaire SA, Connolly HM, Dietz HC, Milewicz DM, Palmero LC, Wang XL, Volguina IV (2008) Valve-Sparing versus Valve Replacement Techniques for Aortic Root Operations in Marfan Patients: Interim Analysis of Early Outcome. AATS meeting
21. Dagum P, Green GR, Nistal FJ, Daughters GT, Timek TA, Foppiano LE, Bolger AF, Ingels NB Jr, Miller DC (1999) Deformational dynamics of the aortic root: modes and physiologic determinants. Circulation 100:II54–II62
22. David T, Feindel CM, Webb GD et al (2006) Long term results of aortic valve sparing operations for aortic root aneurysm. J Thorac Cardiovasc Surg 132:347–354
23. David TE (1999) Aortic valve repair for management of aortic insufficiency. Adv Card Surg 11:129–159
24. David TE (2005) Sizing and tailoring the Dacron graft for reimplantation of the aortic valve. J Thorac Cardiovasc Surg 130:243–244
25. David TE, Feindel CM (1992) An Aortic Valve-sparing operation for patients with aortic incompetence and aneurysm of the ascending aorta. J Thorac Cardiovasc Surg 103:617–622
26. David TE, Feindel CM, Webb GD, Colman JM, Armstrong S, Maganti M (2007) Aortic valve preservation in patients with aortic root aneurysm: results of the reimplantation technique. Ann Thorac Surg 83:S732–S735, discussion S785–S790
27. de Oliveira NC, David TE, Ivanov J, Armstrong S, Eriksson MJ, Rakowski H, Webb G (2003) Results of surgery for aortic root aneurysm in patients with Marfan syndrome. J Thorac Cardiovasc Surg 125:789–796
28. De Paulis R, De Matteis GM, Nardi P et al (2002) Analysis of valve motion after the reimplantation type of valve-sparing procedure (David I) with a new aortic root conduit. Ann Thorac Surg 7:53–57

29. de Waroux JB, Pouleur AC, Goffinet C, Vancraeynest D, Van Dyck M, Robert A, Gerber BL, Pasquet A, El Khoury G, Vanoverschelde JL (2007) Functional anatomy of aortic regurgitation: accuracy, prediction of surgical repairability, and outcome implications of transesophageal echocardiography. Circulation 116(11 Suppl):I264–I269
30. Di Bartolomeo R, Pacini D, Martin-Suarez S, Loforte A, Dell'amore A, Ferlito M, Bracchetti G, Bozzetti G (2006) Valsalva prosthesis in aortic valve-sparing operations. Interact Cardiovasc Thorac Surg 5:294–298
31. Doss M, Sirat S, Risteski P, Martens S, Moritz A (2008) Pericardial patch augmentation for repair of incompetent bicuspid aortic valves at midterm. Eur J Cardiothorac Surg 33:881–884
32. Dossche KM, Schepens MA, Morshuis WJ, de la Riviere AB, Knaepen PJ, Vermeulen FE (1999) A 23-year experience with composite valve graft replacement of the aortic root. Ann Thorac Surg 67:1070–1077
33. El Khoury G, Vanoverschelde JL, Glineur D, Pierard F, Verhelst RR, Rubay J, Funken JC, Watremez C, Astarci P, Lacroix V, Poncelet A, Noirhomme P (2006) Repair of bicuspid aortic valves in patients with aortic regurgitation. Circulation 114:I610–I616
34. El Khoury G, Vanoverschelde JL, Glineur D, Poncelet A, Verhelst R, Astarci P, Underwood MJ, Noirhomme P (2004) Repair of aortic valve prolapse: experience with 44 patients. Eur J Cardiothorac Surg 26:628–633
35. El Khoury GA, Underwood MJ, Glineur D, Derouck D, Dion RA (2000) Reconstruction of the ascending aorta and aortic root: experience in 45 consecutive patients. Ann Thorac Surg 70:1246–1250
36. Erasmi A, Sievers HH, Scharfschwerdt M, Eckel T, Misfeld M (2005) In vitro hydrodynamics, cusp-bending deformation, and root distensibility for different types of aortic valve-sparing operations: remodeling, sinus prosthesis, and reimplantation. J Thorac Cardiovasc Surg 130:1044–1049
37. Erasmi AW, Sievers HH, Bechtel JF, Hanke T, Stierle U, Misfeld M (2007) Remodeling or reimplantation for valve-sparing aortic root surgery? Ann Thorac Surg 83:S752–756, discussion S785–S790
38. Etz CD, Homann TM, Rane N, Bodian CA, Di Luozzo G, Plestis KA, Spielvogel D, Griepp RB (2007) Aortic root reconstruction with a bioprosthetic valved conduit: a consecutive series of 275 procedures. J Thorac Cardiovasc Surg 133:1455–1463
39. Frater R (1986) Aortic valve insufficiency due to aortic dilatation: correction by sinus rim adjustment. Circulation 74:136–142
40. Furukawa K, Ohteki H, Cao Z, Doi K, Narita Y, Minato N, Itoh T (1999) Does dilatation of the sinotubular junction cause aortic regurgitation? Ann Thorac Surg 68:949–954
41. Gallo R, Kumar N, Al Halees Z, Duran C (1995) Early failure of aortic valve conservation in aortic root aneurysm. J Thorac Cardiovasc Surg 109:1011–1012
42. Gleason TG (2005) New graft formulation and modification of the David reimplantation technique. J Thorac Cardiovasc Surg 130:601–603
43. Gogbashian A, Ghanta RK, Umakanthan R, Rangaraj AT, Laurence RG, Fox JA, Cohn LH, Chen FY (2007) Correction of aortic insufficiency with an external adjustable prosthetic aortic ring. Ann Thorac Surg 84:1001–1005
44. Grande-Allen KJ, Cohran RP, Reinhall PG et al (2000) Re-creation of sinuses is important for sparing the aortic valve: a finite element model. J Thorac Cardiovasc Surg 119:753–763
45. Guilmet D, Bonnet N, Saal JP et al (2004) Long term survival with the Bentall button operation in 150 patients. Arch Mal Coeur Vaiss 97:83–91
46. Hagl C, Strauch JT, Spielvogel D, Galla JD, Lansman SL, Squitieri R, Bodian CA, Griepp RB (2003) Is the Bentall procedure for ascending aorta or aortic valve re-

placement the best approach for long-term event-free survival? Ann Thorac Surg 76:698–703, discussion 703

47. Hahm SY, Choo SJ, Lee JW, Seo JB, Lim TH, Song JK, Shin JK, Song MG (2006) Novel technique of aortic valvuloplasty. Eur J Cardiothorac Surg 29:530–536

47a. Hanke T, Charitos EI, Stierle U, Robinson D, Gorski A, Sievers HH, Misfeld M (2009) Factors associated with the development of aortic valve regurgitation over time after two different techniques of valve-sparing aortic root surgery. J Thorac Cardiovasc Surg 137:314–319

48. Haydar HS, He GW, Hovaguimian H, Mc Irvin DM, King DH, Starr A (1997) Valve repair for aortic insufficiency: surgical classification and techniques. Eur J Cardiothorac Surg 11:258–265

49. Hess PJ Jr, Klodell CT, Beaver TM, Martin TD (2005) The Florida sleeve: a new technique for aortic root remodeling with preservation of the aortic valve and sinuses. Ann Thorac Surg 80:748–750

50. Hetzer R, Komoda S, Komoda T (2008) Remodeling of aortic root by annular reconstruction and plication of sinuses of valsalva. J Card Surg 23:49–51

51. Higashidate M, Tamiya K, Toshiyuki B, Yasaharu I (1995) Regulation of the aortic valve opening: in vivo dynamic of aortic valve orifice area. J Thorac Cardiovasc Surg 110:496–503

52. Hopkins RA (2003) Aortic valve leaflet sparing and salvage surgery: evolution of techniques for aortic root reconstruction. Eur J Cardiothorac Surg 24:886–897

53. Iung B, Baron G, Butchart EG, Delahaye F, Gohlke-Barwolf C, Levang OW, Tornos P, Vanoverschelde JL, Vermeer F, Boersma E, Ravaud P, Vahanian A (2003) A prospective survey of patients with valvular heart disease in Europe: The Euro Heart Survey on Valvular Heart Disease. Eur Heart J 24:1231–1243

54. Izumoto H, Kawazoe K, Kawase T, et al (2002) Subvalvular circular annuloplasty as a component of aortic valve repair. J Heart Valve Dis 11:383–385

55. Izumoto H, Kawazoe K, Oka T, Kazui T, Kawase T, Nasu M (2006) Aortic valve repair for aortic regurgitation: intermediate-term results in patients with tricuspid morphology. J Heart Valve Dis 15:169–173

56. Jeanmart H, de Kerchove L, Glineur D, Goffinet JM, Rougui I, Van Dyck M, Noirhomme P, El Khoury G (2007) Aortic valve repair: the functional approach to leaflet prolapse and valve-sparing surgery. Ann Thorac Surg 83:S746–S751

57. Jondeau G, Boutouyrie P, Lacolley P, et al (1999) Central pulse pressure is a major determinant of ascending aorta dilation in Marfan syndrome. Circulation 99:2677–2681

58. Kalkat MS, Edwards MB, Taylor KM, Bonser RS (2007) Composite aortic valve graft replacement: mortality outcomes in a national registry. Circulation 116:I301–I306

59. Kallenbach K, Karck M, Pak D, Salcher R, Khaladj N, Leyh R, Hagl C, Haverich A (2005) Decade of aortic valve sparing reimplantation: are we pushing the limits too far? Circulation 112:I253–I259

60. Karck M, Kallenbach K, Hagl C, Rhein C, Leyh R, Haverich A (2004) Aortic root surgery in Marfan syndrome: Comparison of aortic valve-sparing reimplantation versus composite grafting. J Thorac Cardiovasc Surg 127:391–398

61. Kazui T, Izumoto H, Nasu M, et al (2004) Perioperative changes in dynamic aortic root morphology after Yacoub's root remodeling and concomitant aortic annuloplasty. Interactive Cardiovascular and Thoracic Surgery 3:465–469

62. Kazui T, Tsuboi J, Izumoto H, Nakajima T, Ishihara K, Kawazoe K (2007) Aortic root remodeling with aortic annuloplasty: mid-term results. Circ J 71:207–210

63. Kilner PJ, Yang GZ, Mohiaddin RH, Firmin DN, Longmore DB (1993) Helical and retrograde secondary flow patterns in the aortic arch studied by three-directional magnetic resonance velocity mapping. Circulation 88:2235–2247

64. Kim M, Roman MJ, Cavallini MC, Schwartz JE, Pickering TG, Devereux RB (1996) Effect of hypertension on aortic root size and prevalence of aortic regurgitation. Hypertension 28:47–52
65. Kollar A (2007) Valve-sparing reconstruction within the native aortic root: integrating the Yacoub and the David methods. Ann Thorac Surg 83:2241–2243
66. Krovetz LJ (1975) Age-related changes in size of the aortic valve annulus in man. Am Heart J 90:569–574
67. La Canna G, Maisano F, De Michele L, Grimaldi A, Grassi F, Capritti E, De Bonis M, Alfieri O (2009) Determinants of the degree of functional aortic regurgitation in patients with anatomically normal aortic valve and ascending thoracic aorta aneurysm transesophageal doppler echocardiography study. Heart 95:130–136
68. Lansac E, Di Centa I, Varnous S, Rama A, Jault F, Duran CMG, Acar C, Pavie A, Gandjbakhch I (2005) External aortic annuloplasty: a usefull adjunct to valve sparing procedure. Ann Thorac Surg 79:356–358
69. Lansac E, Di Centa I, Bonnet N, Leprince P, Rama A, Acar C, Pavie A, Gandjbakhch I (2006) Aortic prosthetic ring annuloplasty: a useful adjunct to a standardized aortic valve-sparing procedure? Eur J Cardiothorac Surg 29:537–544
70. Lansac E, Di Centa I, Raoux F, Al Attar N, Acar C, Joudinaud T, Raffoul R (2008) A lesional classification to standardize surgical management of aortic insufficiency towards valve repair. Eur J Cardio Thorac Surg 33:872–880
71. Lansac E, Di Centa I, Raoux F, Raffoul R, El Attar N, Rama A, Acar C, Nataf P (2006) Aortic annuloplasty: towards a standardized approach of conservative aortic valve surgery. Multimed Man Cardiothorac Surg http://mmcts.ctsnetjournals.org/cgi/content/full/2007/0102/mmcts.2006.001958
72. Lansac E, Lim HS, Shomura Y, Lim KH, Rice Nt, Goetz W, Duran C (2002) A four-dimensional study of the aortic root dynamics. Eur J Cardiothorac Surg 22:497–503
73. Lansac E, Lim HS, Shomura Y, Lim KH, Rice NT, Goetz WA, Duran CM (2005) Aortic root dynamics are asymmetric. J Heart Valve Dis 14:400–407
74. Lansac E, Lim HS, Shomura Y, Rice NT, Lim KH, Yoe JH, Acar C, Oury JH, Duran CMG (2001) The mechanisms of aortic valve opening and closure. J Am Coll Cardiol 37(suppl A):475A
75. Lausberg HF, Aicher D, Kissinger A, Langer F, Fries R, Schäfers HJ (2006) Valve repair in aortic regurgitation without root dilatation–aortic valve repair. Thorac Cardiovasc Surg 54:15–20
76. Leyh RG, Fischer S, Kallenbach K, et al (2002) High failure rate after valve-sparing aortic root replacement using the "remodelling technique" in acute type A aortic dissection. Circulation 106:I229–I233
77. Leyh RG, Schmidtke C, Sievers HH, Yacoub MH (1999) Opening and closing characteristics of the aortic valve after different types of valve-preserving surgery. Circulation 100:2153–2161
78. Luciani GB, Casali G, Tomezzoli A, Mazzucco A (1999) Recurrence of aortic insufficiency after aortic root remodeling with valve preservation. Ann Thorac Surg 67:1849–1852
79. Maselli D, Montalto A, Santise G, et al (2005) A normogram to anticipate dimension of neo-sinuses of valsalva in valve-sparing aortic operations. Eur J Cardiothorac Surg 27:831–835
80. Matsumori M, Tanaka H, Kawanishi Y, Onishi T, Nakagiri K, Yamashita T, Okada K, Okita Y (2007) Comparison of distensibility of the aortic root and cusp motion after aortic root replacement with two reimplantation techniques: Valsalva graft versus tube graft. Interact Cardiovasc Thorac Surg 6:177–181
81. Miller DC (2007) Valve-sparing aortic root replacement: current state of the art and where are we headed? Ann Thorac Surg 83:S736–S739

82. Minakata K, Schaff HV, Zehr KJ, Dearani JA, Daly RC, Orszulak TA, Puga FJ, Danielson GK (2004) Is repair of aortic valve regurgitation a safe alternative to valve replacement? J Thorac Cardiovasc Surg 127:645–653
83. Morishita K, Murakami G, Koshino T, Fukada J, Fujisawa Y, Mawatari T, Abe T (2002) Aortic root remodeling operation: how do we tailor a tube graft? Ann Thorac Surg 73:1117–1721
84. Nash PJ, Vitvitsky E, Li J et al (2005) Feasibility of valve repair for regurgitant bicuspid aortic valves an echocardiographic study. Ann Thorac Surg 79:1473–1479
85. Niederhauser U, Kunzli A, Genoni M, Vogt P, Lachat M, Turina M (1999) Composite graft replacement of the aortic root: long-term results, incidence of reoperations. Thorac Cardiovasc Surg 47:317–321
86. Nistri S, Sorbo MD, Marin M, Palisi M, Scognamiglio R, Thiene G (1999) Aortic root dilatation in young men with normally functioning bicuspid aortic valves. Heart 82:19–22
87. Obadia JF, Abdullatif Y, Henaine R, Chavanis N, Saroul C, Barthelet M, Andre-Fouet X, Raisky O, Robin J, Ninet J (2004) Replacement of the ascending aorta with conservation of the aortic valve. Arch Mal Coeur Vaiss 97:1183–1187
88. Pacini D, Ranocchi F, Angeli E, Settepani F, Pagliaro M, Martin-Suarez S, Di Bartolomeo R, Pierangeli A (2003) Aortic root replacement with composite valve graft. Ann Thorac Surg 76:90–98
89. Patel ND, Weiss ES, Alejo DE, Nwakanma LU, Williams JA, Dietz HC, Spevak PJ, Gott VL, Vricella LA, Cameron DE (2008) Aortic root operations for Marfan syndrome: a comparison of the Bentall and valve-sparing procedures. Ann Thorac Surg 85:2003–2010
90. Radu NC, Kirsch EW, Hillion ML, Lagneau F, Drouet L, Loisance D (2007) Embolic and bleeding events after modified Bentall procedure in selected patients. Heart 93:107–112
91. Ranga A, Bouchot O, Mongrain R, Ugolini P, Cartier R (2006) Computational simulations of the aortic valve validated by imaging data: evaluation of valve-sparing techniques. Interact Cardiovasc Thorac Surg 5:373–378
92. Roberts WC, Ko JM, Moore TR, Jones WH 3rd (2006) Causes of pure aortic regurgitation in patients having isolated aortic valve replacement at a single US tertiary hospital (1993 to 2005). Circulation 114:422–429
93. Robicksek F (1991) Leonardo da Vinci and the sinuses of Valsalva. Ann Thorac Surg 52:328–335
94. Robicsek F, Thubrikar MJ (1999) Role of sinus wall compliance in aortic leaflet function. Am J Cardiol 84:944–946
95. Rodríguez F, Green GR, Dagum P, Nistal JF, Harrington KB, Daughters GT, Ingels NB, Miller DC (2006) Left ventricular volume shifts and aortic root expansion during isovolumic contraction. J Heart Valve Dis 15:465–473
96. Roman MJ, Devereux RB, Niles NW, Hochreiter C, Kligfield P, Sato N, Spitzer MC, Borer JS (1987) Aortic root dilatation as a cause of isolated, severe aortic regurgitation. Prevalence, clinical and echocardiographic patterns, and relation to left ventricular hypertrophy and function. Ann Intern Med 106:800–807
97. Ruvolo G, Fattouch K (2009) Aortic valve-sparing root replacement from inside the aorta using three Dacron skirts preserving the native Valsalva sinuses geometry and stabilizing the annulus. Interact Cardiovasc Thorac Surg 8(2):179–181
98. Schäfers HJ, Aicher D, Langer F, Lausberg HF (2007) Preservation of the bicuspid aortic valve. Ann Thorac Surg 83:S740–S745; discussion S785–S790
99. Schäfers HJ, Bierbach B, Aicher D (2006) A new approach to the assessment of aortic cusp geometry. J Thorac Cardiovasc Surg 132:436–438

100. Schäfers HJ, Fries R, Langer F et al (1998) Valve-preserving replacement of the ascending aorta: remodeling versus reimplantation. J Thorac Cardiovasc Surg 116:990–996
101. Settepani F, Szeto WY, Pacini D, De Paulis R, Chiariello L, Di Bartolomeo R, Gallotti R, Bavaria JE (2007) Reimplantation valve-sparing aortic root replacement in Marfan syndrome using the Valsalva conduit: an intercontinental multicenter study. Ann Thorac Surg 83:S769–S773; discussion S785–S790
102. Sioris T, David TE, Ivanov J, Armstrong S, Feindel CM (2004) Clinical outcomes after separate and composite replacement of the aortic valve and ascending aorta. J Thorac Cardiovasc Surg 128:260–265
103. Sutton JP III, Ho SY, Anderson RH (1995) The forgotten interleaflet triangles: a review of the surgical anatomy of the aortic valve. Ann Thorac Surg 59:419–427
104. Svensson LG (2003) Sizing for modified David's reimplantation procedure. Ann Thorac Surg 76:1751–1753
105. Takamoto S, Nawata K, Morota T (2006) A simple modification of "David-V" aortic root reimplantation. Eur J Cardiothorac Surg 30:560–562
106. Tamás E, Nylander E (2007) Echocardiographic description of the anatomic relations within the normal aortic root. J Heart Valve Dis 16:240–246
107. Taylor WJ, Thrower WB, Black H, Harken DE (1958) The surgical correction of aortic insufficiency by circumclusion. J Thorac Surg 35:192–205
108. The task force on the management of valvular heart disease (2007) Guidelines for the management of valvular heart disease of the European Society of Cardiology. Eur Heart J 28:230–268
109. Thubrikar M, Bosher LP, Nolan SP (1979) The mechanism of opening of the aortic valve. J Thorac Cardiovasc Surg 77:863–870
110. Thubrikar M, Harry L, Nolan SP (1977) Normal aortic valve function in dogs. Am J Cardiol 40:563–568
111. Thubrikar M, Heckman JL, Nolan SP (1993) High speed cine-radiographic study of the aortic valve leaflet motion. J Heart Valve Dis 2:653–661
112. Urbanski PP, Zhan X, Frank S, Diegeler A (2009) Aortic root reconstruction using new vascular graft. Interact Cardiovasc Thorac Surg 8(2):187–190
113. Varnous S, Lansac E, Acar C et al (2003) Echographic study of the aortic diameters: implication for graft size in aortic valve sparing operation. Meeting of the society of heart valve disease, June 2003, Paris, France
114. Vasan RS, Larson MG, Levy D (1995) Determinants of echocardiographic aortic root size. The Framingham Heart Study. Circulation 91:734–740
115. Westaby S, Karp RB, Blackstone EH et al (1984) Adult human valve dimensions and their surgical significance. Am J Cardiol 53:552–556
116. Yacoub M, Fagan A, Stassano P, Radley-Smith R (1983) Result of valve conserving operations for aortic regurgitation [abstract]. Circulation 68(suppl):III321
117. Yacoub MH, Gehle P, Chandrasekaran V, Birks EJ, Child A, Radley-Smith R (1998) Late results of a valve sparing operation in patients with aneuryms of the ascending aorta and root. J Thorac Cardiovasc Surg 115:1080–1090
118. Zehr KJ, Orszulak TA, Mullany CJ, Matloobi A, Daly RC, Dearani JA, Sundt TM 3rd, Puga FJ, Danielson GK, Schaff HV (2004) Surgery for aneurysms of the aortic root: a 30-year experience. Circulation 110:1364–1371
119. Zehr KJ, Thubrikar MJ, Gong GG, Headrick JR, Robicsek F (2000) Clinical introduction of a novel prosthesis for valve-preserving aortic root reconstruction for annuloaortic ectasia. J Thorac Cardiovasc Surg 120:692–698

Yacoub/David techniques for aortic root operation: success and failures

J. F. M. Bechtel, H. H. Sievers, T. Hanke, E. I. Charitos,
C. Schmidtke, E. G. Kraatz, U. Stierle, M. Misfeld

The aortic valve is a complex structure which functions perfectly in systole and diastole and under a wide range of hemodynamic conditions. Even today, no valve prosthesis can match the function of the native aortic valve. This is – at least partly – due to the fact that the aortic valve is not just an outlet whose cusps do move passively in the blood stream. Rather, the aortic valve – which consists of three cusps attached to the wall of the aortic root – interacts with the aortic root and the left ventricular outflow tract. During the cardiac cycle, the aortic root undergoes complex movements that precede and aide opening and closing of the aortic valve [2, 3, 17, 18]. These complex interactions within the aortic root and throughout the cardiac cycle are not yet completely understood. The aortic valve cusps themselves are thin-walled pocket-like structures, made from specialized tissue with fibrous, elastic, nervous, and muscular properties [13, 16, 21]. No such thin, but at the same time strong and non-thrombogeneic material can be produced in laboratories and even less by industrial processes.

It is against this background that valve-sparing aortic root operation has gained interest. In preserving the aortic valve cusps and trying to rebuild an aortic root, such techniques are theoretically appealing, and several groups have reported excellent short- and mid-term results [5, 9, 12, 14, 19]. However, no technique completely meets the complexity of the aortic valve/root function [7], rendering the durability of the repair somewhat questionable. We have reviewed our experience with valve-sparing aortic root operation and tried to identify factors associated with failure.

Techniques of valve-sparing aortic root replacement

There are basically two different types of procedures. With both techniques, the sinus of valsalvae are resected first; only a 3–4 mm rim of tissue to both sides of all commissures and along the attachment line of the cusps as well as the coronary ostiae are left in place. The aortic root is then replaced by a vascular graft. The aortic valve can be reimplanted into the vascular graft in a way described by David [4] (Fig. 1) or can be remo-

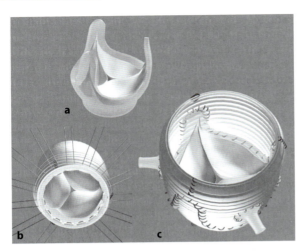

Fig. 1. Schematic drawing of the reimplantation (David) procedure. **a** The aortic root is resected first leaving only the crown-like attachments of the aortic valve cusps with 3–4 mm of surrounding tissue and the coronary ostiae in place. **b** The vascular graft is put over the aortic valve and secured below the aortic valve attachment with several U-stitches. **c** Then, the basal aortic valve attachment and the commissures are sewn into the graft with three continuous sutures. As the vascular graft has been left tubular, no pseudosinuses are created. Finally, the coronary ostiae have to be reimplanted into the graft. Reprinted from [1]; with permission from the Society of Thoracic Surgeons

deled into it (Yacoub technique [20]) – in this case, the graft first needs to be incised at its base so that the three commissures of the valve can be sewn into the three incisions (Fig. 2). This way, pseudosinuses within the vascular graft are created. The sinuses within the aortic root are considered important for aortic valve function and coronary perfusion. Several technical modifications of the David procedure have been described [12], some of them aimed at the creation of pseudosinuses. We have exclusively used the original technique.

Methods

Between 1994 and 2006, 192 patients had valve-sparing aortic root replacement (Yacoub technique, n = 108, David technique, n = 83) for either aortic root aneurysm and/or type A dissection. Prerequisite for valve-sparing aortic root operation were macroscopically intact cusps (either tricuspid or bicuspid) without calcifications, thickening, or fenestrations. The choice of the valve-preserving technique was merely surgeon related.

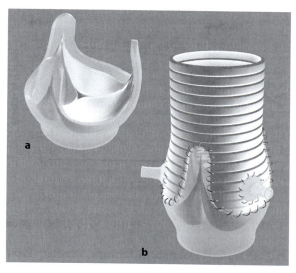

Fig. 2. Schematic drawing of the remodeling (Yacoub) procedure. **a** The aortic root is resected first leaving only the crown-like attachments of the aortic valve cusps with 3-4 mm of surrounding tissue and the coronary ostiae in place. **b** The vascular graft is incised at its base in such a way that the incisions match the height of the commissures – the graft now looks as if it has three "tongues". Then, the basal aortic valve attachment and the commissures are sewn into the graft and between the "tongues" with three continuous sutures. The three "tongues" of the vascular graft act as pseudosinuses. Finally, the coronary ostiae have to be reimplanted into the graft. Reprinted from [1]; with permission from the Society of Thoracic Surgeons

Follow-up data were acquired in our outpatient clinic or by the referring cardiologist. Completeness of follow-up was 100% for clinical variables and 95% for echocardiography. The mean duration of the echocardiographic follow-up was 3.1 ± 2.9 years (median: 2.3 years; minimum-maximum: 0.1–12.1 years). Total echocardiographic follow-up was 560 patient-years. Serial echocardiographic examinations (total number of examinations: n = 654; mean 3.6 ± 2.0 examinations per patient) were used for hierarchical multilevel modeling of the development of aortic regurgitation. For further details on echocardiography and analysis see [8].

Results

Patient characteristics and operative details are displayed in Table 1. There were 6 in-hospital deaths (Yacoub: n = 4 (3.7%); David: n = 2 (2.4%), p = 0.70). Note that none of the deaths in the Yacoub group occurred in elective patients.

Table 1. Patient characteristics. Reprinted from [8]; with permission from the American Association for Thoracic Surgery

	Yacoub	David	p
Male (%)	63	76	0.08
Age (years)	56 ± 14	49 ± 17	0.007
Ascending aortic aneurysm (%)	73	53	0.007
Aneurysm diameter (mm)	60 ± 13	59 ± 12	0.59
Type A dissection (%)	29	42	0.09
Marfan syndrome (%)	13	20	0.27
Bicuspid aortic valve (%)	14	11	0.69
Aortic regurgitation ≥ grade II (%)	43	59	0.04
Previous cardiac surgery (%)	3	4	0.98
CPB duration (min)	185 ± 45	221 ± 60	< 0.001
Aortic cross-clamp duration (min)	138 ± 39	165 ± 49	< 0.001
Open distal anastomosis (%)	65	68	0.78
– with partial arch replacement	33	26	0.38
– with total arch replacement	3	8	0.22
Vascular graft size (mm)	28 ± 2	29 ± 2	0.05
Concomitant cusp intervention (%)	13	19	0.35
Concomitant annulus intervention (%)	20	0	< 0.001
GRF glue used (%)	13	19	0.35

Values are expressed as mean ± standard deviation, or percentage of patients;
CPB cardiopulmonary bypass, *GRF* gelatine-resorcine-formol

The follow-up events as well as the results of the latest echocardiographic measurements are given in Tables 2 and 3. Fig. 3 shows the survival curve and Fig. 4 the actuarial freedom from valve-related reoperations. There have been 11 valve-related reoperations (Yacoub: n = 10; David: n = 1; p = 0.065).

For a more detailed analysis of the stability of the operative results, serial echocardiographic measurements were analyzed regarding changes in aortic regurgitation. As shown in Fig. 5, there is – on average – trace aortic regurgitation early postoperatively that slowly progresses with time (0.082 grades/year, i.e., after 10 years the aortic regurgitation is approximately one grade more than early after surgery. *Please note* that the values depicted are average values, and reoperated patients contribute to the figures. Aortic regurgitation *change is not* perceivable in most patients.). The initial regurgitation is higher with the Yacoub technique than with the David technique, but the annual increase is not significantly different. Further analyses showed that adding cusp interventions to the valve-sparing proce-

Table 2. Events during follow-up, hospital survivors[a]

	Yacoub	David
■ Thrombembolism (n)	3 (3%)	1 (1%)
■ Cerebrovascular accident (n)		
– transient, lasts < 24 h	0	1 (1%)
– transient, lasts more > 24 h	1 (1%)	0
– permanent	3 (3%)	4 (5%)
■ Bleeding (n)		
– minor	0	0
– major	1 (1%)	0
■ Myocardial infarction (n)	1 (1%)	0
■ Sepsis (n)	0	1 (1%)
■ Arrhythmias (n)	14 (13%)	5 (6%)
– requiring pacemaker implantation	3 (3%)	0

[a] There were no significant differences regarding the frequency of the events between the groups

Table 3. Echocardiographic data at the most recent follow-up examination[a]. Reprinted from [8]; with permission from the American Association for Thoracic Surgery

	Yacoub	David	p
■ Aortic root dimensions (mm)			
– annulus	23 ± 4	22 ± 3	0.13
– mid sinus	30 ± 4	26 ± 4	< 0.001
– sinutubular junction	25 ± 3	25 ± 4	1.00
– ascending aorta	30 ± 4	29 ± 3	0.13
■ Aortic valve area (cm^2)	3.0 ± 1.1	2.2 ± 0.8	< 0.001
■ Pressure gradient across LVOT (mmHg)			
– maximal	9 ± 1	13 ± 10	0.003
– mean	5 ± 5	6 ± 5	0.19
■ Aortic regurgitation (n)			
– none	15 (20%)	23 (47%)	0.003
– trivial	23 (31%)	11 (22%)	0.37
– mild	28 (37%)	12 (25%)	0.23
– ≥ grade II	9 (12%)	4 (6%)	0.42

[a] Values are expressed as mean ± standard deviation, or numbers of patients;
LVOT left ventricular outflow tract

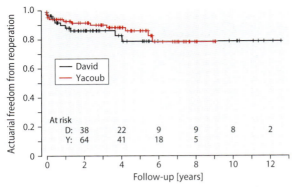

Fig. 3. Survival: Kaplan-Meier curve of all patients undergoing valve-sparing aortic root replacement, stratified by technique. Censored patient data are indicated by ticks to the curves. The curves do not differ (p=0.53)

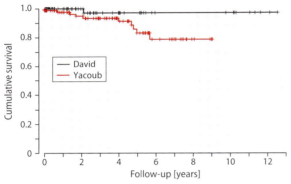

Fig. 4. Valve-related reoperations: actuarial freedom from valve-related reoperations in all patients undergoing valve-sparing aortic root replacement, stratified by technique. Censored patient data are indicated by ticks to the curves. The difference is not quite significant (p=0.065)

dure was associated with a significantly greater annual increase of the aortic regurgitation, irrespective of the technique used (Fig. 6). In addition, the Yacoub procedure appears to be not well suited in patients with Marfan syndrome (Fig. 7).

Discussion

Our data – along with those of other groups – show that good results can be achieved in a broad range of patients using valve-sparing aortic root replacement techniques and that the reoperation rates are acceptably low during the first decade after surgery. Our results also imply that there is

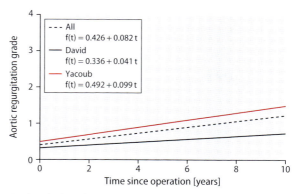

Fig. 5. Estimation of aortic regurgitation (AR) with time in patients undergoing valve-sparing aortic root replacement, stratified by technique. There is significant evidence that the mean intercept (AR at time=0) is higher for the Yacoub technique (p=0.013), but the annual progression rate of AR is not statistically significantly higher (p=0.061) with the Yacoub technique. *Note* that the values depicted are average values, and reoperated patients contribute to the figures. The aortic regurgitation *change is not* perceivable in most patients. Modified from [8]

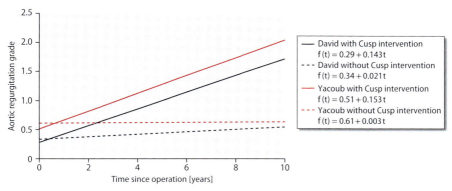

Fig. 6. Estimation of aortic regurgitation (AR) with time in patients undergoing valve-sparing aortic root replacement, stratified by technique and by use/non-use of concomitant cusp interventions (predominately central plication). There is no evidence that the mean intercepts differ depending on whether there were cusp interventions or not (p=0.38), but there was significant evidence of an increase in the annual progression rate of AR with cusp interventions for both surgical techniques (p<0.001). Adapted from [8]; with permission from the American Association for Thoracic Surgery

progression of aortic regurgitation with time. Thus, more reoperations have to be expected for the second decade. However, in-depth analysis revealed that technical details and the patient's underlying disease may have a significant impact on the progression of aortic regurgitation. Considering these factors may serve to improve the longevity of valve-sparing aortic root replacements.

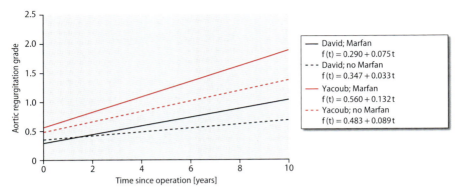

Fig. 7. Estimation of aortic regurgitation (AR) with time in patients undergoing valve-sparing aortic root replacement, stratified by technique and by presence or absence of Marfan syndrome. The difference in mean intercept between the Yacoub and the David technique is marginally significant (p = 0.049). The difference in annual progression rate of AR is not statistically significant (p = 0.10). However, the higher initial regurgitation plus the marginally higher progression rate of AR will result in meaningful differences between the techniques after a few years. Adapted from [8]; with permission from the American Association for Thoracic Surgery

What is the reason for the observed progression of aortic regurgitation with time? As said above, the aorta undergoes complex movements throughout the cardiac cycle. We have shown earlier that remodeling (Yacoub) restricts root movement less than the reimplantation (David) technique [10], but that no root replacement technique completely reproduces normal aortic valve and root dynamics [7] (Figs. 8 and 9). Distensibility of the root is restricted or even completely abolished and the bending deformation of the cusps themselves is increased. In addition, it is frequently observed that the cusps collide with the prosthetic wall during systole. Whether these factors promote the progression of aortic regurgitation remains speculative. Furthermore, the incisions into the vascular graft characteristic of the Yacoub technique may weaken the ability of the graft to prevent further dilatation of the aortic base annulus, e.g., in patients with Marfan syndrome.

Given the fact the aortic sinuses are believed to be important for valve function, modifications in the shape of the vascular graft may be helpful in limiting the burden on the cusps whenever a Yacoub procedure does not seem to be wise and the David technique is used. The DePaulis Valsalva graft (Vascutek) is already widely known [6, 15], but is has no separate sinuses of Valsalva; instead a segment with uniform circumferential dilatation is included in the graft. The sinus configuration, however, is preserved with the new UniGraft (Braun Melsungen), but there are no data available yet for judgment on this new prosthesis. However, as long as stiff materials, such as Dacron, are used for aortic grafts, no Windkessel function will be possible and normal aortic root function cannot be expected even with the best surgical techniques for aortic valve-sparing.

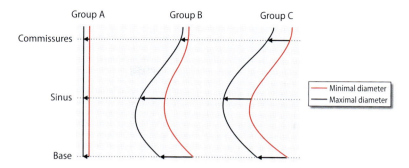

Fig. 8. Dimensional changes in the aortic root. Diagram of cyclic changes in dimensions derived from echocardiographic data at the base, sinus, and commisural levels. Note the reduced distensibility at all levels of the aortic root in patients who had a David procedure (group A), whereas movements in patients who had a Yacoub procedure (group B) closely mimics those in healthy volunteers (group C). Reprinted from [10]; with permission from the American Heart Association

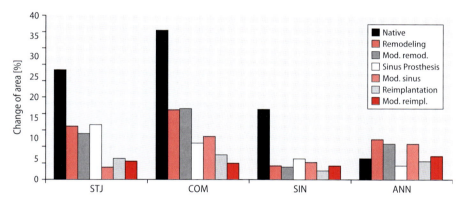

Fig. 9. Root distensibility of different valve-sparing techniques. Aortic root distensibility, expressed as diastolic-to-systolic change of area, was measured in vitro with three ultrasonic micrometric transceiver-receiver crystals each at the level of the sinutubular junction (*STJ*), at the mid-commisural level (*COM*), in the middle of each sinus (*SIN*) and at the annular level (*ANN*). Aortic root distensibility decreased – as compared to a native aortic root – in all surgical procedures examined. Reprinted from [8]; with permission from the American Association for Thoracic Surgery

We observed that cusp interventions were associated with a significantly more progressive increase of aortic regurgitation over time. Several factors may play an important role: unsuitable valve for either the valve-sparing or cusp intervention, secondary fibrotic retraction of the cusp margins after intervention, or improper surgical techniques. In addition, tissue properties of the aortic valve cusps (bicuspid with a more rigid cusp tissue vs. tricuspid with thin and vulnerable tissue) may play an important role. Because the immediate results seem favorable, there may be time-dependent factors that can adversely affect cusp function after the initial intervention. However, our results indicate that exact root reconstruction without cusp intervention is advisable. It should be noted that none of the patients who underwent reoperation had leaflet repair, which supports our opinion that leaflet repair per se does not necessarily lead to reoperation but seems to lead to increased development of aortic regurgitation over time. Our data were not sufficient to determine whether the observed increased rate of aortic regurgitation after concomitant cusp intervention could be attributed to unsuitable valve pathology or improper technique.

Conclusions

Valve-sparing aortic root replacement of either the Yacoub- or David-type can be performed safely in acute and elective settings and provide excellent valve function and low rates of thromboembolism in the majority of patients during the first postoperative decade. No anticoagulation is needed. However, our results also imply that there is slight progression of aortic regurgitation with time and that more reoperations may become necessary.

Given our results and analyses, we now predominantly use the David technique in enlarged roots (diameter >28 mm) and in patients with Marfan syndrome. It is crucial that valve-sparing aortic root replacement need to be performed after careful selection of the patient based on the underlying aortic disease and cusp anatomy. In addition the implantation into the vascular graft needs to be performed as perfect as possible. According to our analysis, the necessity of additional cusp interventions appears to have a negative effect on long-term valve function. We believe that considering these factors will improve the longevity of the procedures, but more data and a longer follow-up are necessary for final judgment of the durability of valve-sparing aortic root replacement, especially during the second postoperative decade and beyond.

References

1. Albes JM, Stock UA, Hartrumpf M (2005) Restitution of the aortic valve: what is new, what is proven, and what is obsolete? Ann Thorac Surg 80:1540–1549
2. Bellhouse BJ, Bellhouse FH (1968) Mechanism of closure of the aortic valve. Nature 217:86–87
3. Dagum P, Green GR, Nistal FJ et al (1999) Deformational dynamics of the aortic root. Modes and physiologic determinants. Circulation 100[suppl II]:II-54–II-62

4. David TE, Feindel CM (1992) An aortic valve-sparing operation for patients with aortic incompetence and aneurysm of the ascending aorta. J Thorac Cardiovasc Surg 103:617–621
5. David TE, Feindel CM, Webb GD, Colman JM, Armstrong S, Maganti M (2007) Aortic valve preservation in patients with aortic root aneurysm: results of the reimplantation technique. Ann Thorac Surg 83:S732–S735
6. De Paulis R, De Matteis GM, Nardi P et al (2002) One-year appraisal of a new aortic root conduit with sinuses of Valsalva. J Thorac Cardiovasc Surg 123:33–39
7. Erasmi A, Sievers HH, Scharfschwerdt M, Eckel T, Misfeld M (2005) In vitro hydrodynamics, cusp-bending deformation, and root distensibility for different types of aortic valve-sparing operations: remodeling, sinus prosthesis, and reimplantation. J Thorac Cardiovasc Surg 130:1044–1049
8. Hanke T, Charitos EI, Stierle U et al (2009) Factors associated with the development of aortic valve regurgitation over time after two different techniques of valve-sparing aortic root surgery. J Thorac Cardiovasc Surg 137:314–319
9. Kallenbach K, Baraki H, Khaladj N et al (2007) Aortic valve-sparing operation in Marfan syndrome: what do we know after a decade? Ann Thorac Surg 83:S764–S768
10. Leyh RG, Schmidtke C, Sievers HH, Yacoub MH (1999) Opening and closing characteristics of the aortic valve after different types of valve-preserving surgery. Circulation 100:2153–2160
11. Miller DC (2003) Valve-sparing aortic root replacement in patients with the Marfan syndrome. J Thorac Cardiovasc Surg 125:773–778
12. Miller DC (2007) Valve-sparing aortic root replacement: current state of the art and where are we headed? Ann Thorac Surg 83:S736–S739
13. Misfeld M, Chester AH, Sievers HH, Yacoub MH (2002) Biological mechanisms influencing the function of the aortic root. J Card Surg 17:363–368
14. Pacini D, Di Marco L, Suarez SM et al (2006) Aortic valve-sparing operations: early and midterm results. Heart Surg Forum 9:E650–E656
15. Pacini D, Settepani F, De Paulis R et al (2006) Early results of valve-sparing reimplantation procedure using the Valsalva conduit: a multicenter study. Ann Thorac Surg 82:865–871
16. Schoen FJ (2005) Cardiac valves and valvular pathology. Update on function, disease, repair, and replacement. Cardiovascular Pathology 14:189–194
17. Thubrikar MJ, Bosher LP, Nolan SP (1979) The mechanism of opening the aortic valve. J Thorac Cardiovasc Surg 77:863–870
18. Thubrikar MJ, Nolan SP, Bosher LP, Beck JD (1980) The cyclic changes and structure of the base of the aortic valve. Am Heart J 99:217–224
19. Volguina IV, Miller DC, Lemaire SA et al (2009) Valve-sparing and valve-replacing techniques for aortic root replacement in patients with Marfan syndrome: analysis of early outcome. J Thorac Cardiovasc Surg 137:641–649
20. Yacoub MH, Fagan A, Stassano P, Radley-Smith R (1983) Results of valve conserving operations for aortic regurgitation. Circulation [Suppl]:III-321
21. Yacoub MH, Cohn LH (2004) Novel approaches to cardiac valve repair: from structure to function: Part I. Circulation 109:942–950

Aortic annuloplasty

W. F. Northrup III, S. D. Rollins

Introduction

The word "annuloplasty" derives from the Latin word *anus* or *anulus* meaning "ring" [1, 2] and the Greek word *plastia* from *plastos* meaning "molded" [3]. The official definition of "annuloplasty" is "surgical reconstruction of an incompetent cardiac valve" [1]. More generally, it means "plastic repair of a cardiac valve by shortening the circumference of its annulus" [2]. However, in practical surgical situations, a valve annulus can either be enlarged or reduced. Accordingly, we will discuss reduction and augmentation aortic annuloplasty in this chapter.

The normal aortic annulus and root

The point has been appropriately made by Professor Robert Anderson that an understanding of cardiac anatomy is "truly a prerequisite for successful cardiac surgery." Moreover, he has argued that understanding cardiac anatomy "will be facilitated in the future if words are used in their generally accepted sense, and if artificial conventions are avoided" [4]. Unfortunately, some terms remain by convention that are probably too imbedded in our vocabulary to more appropriately modify. A good example is the convex portion of the very proximal aorta generally referred to as containing the "sinuses of Valsalva", despite the fact that Leonardo da Vinci not only described them anatomically, but also described the vortex created in them physiologically over 200 years before Valsalva's strictly anatomical posthumous description [5]. As suggested by Wells and Crowe [6], "this discovery should warrant the renaming of the sinuses of Valsalva to those of Leonardo."

The term *annulus* when applied to the aortic valve is somewhat misleading, inasmuch as the aortic valvar leaflets are not attached in the shape of a "ring" but in the shape of a 3-pointed crown spanning the entire vertical extent of the aortic *root* from the "basal ring" at the nadir of the sinuses to

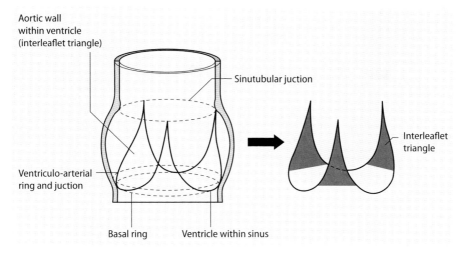

Fig. 1. Diagram of the aortic root. Reprinted with permission from [9]; © American Association for Thoracic Surgery

the commissures at the level of the sinutubular junction [7]. Although the attachment of the leaflets to the root occurs at the hinge point in a "definite fibrous structure" [8] or "collagenous condensation" [9], these fibrous thickenings are apparently not universally present [7] but are consistently thickest at the nadir of the semilunar attachments [9]. The aortic *root*, then, is essentially a cylinder supporting the leaflets and consisting of the leaflets themselves, the sinuses of Valsalva, and the interleaflet triangles extending from the proximal attachment of the valvar leaflets at the level of the ventriculoarterial junction (the "basal ring") to their distal attachments at the sinutubular junction (STJ) (Fig. 1). Strictly speaking, then, there are two literal "rings" of the aortic annulus – the basal ring proximally and the STJ distally. Conceptually, the aortic root is also "a bridge between the left ventricle and the ascending aorta" with the semilunar attachments of the leaflets creating a hemodynamic junction between the pressures of the left ventricle proximally and of the aorta distally [7].

Adding to the anatomic complexity of the aortic root is the aortic-mitral valvar continuity, often referred to as the aortic-mitral curtain [7], or simply as the aortic curtain or subaortic curtain, continuous at each lateral extremity with the right and left fibrous trigones (Fig. 2) [9]. The proportion of left ventricular muscle supporting the aortic root varies from 25–85% with an average of 47% [9]. The ventriculoarterial junction is a "straight circle" where the fibroelastic aortic wall joins with the supporting structures of the left ventricle [9]. Small fingerlike projections of collagen anchor the aortic root to the underlying myocardium [10].

Equally important to an understanding of the components of the aortic annulus is an understanding of adjacent structures that could be involved

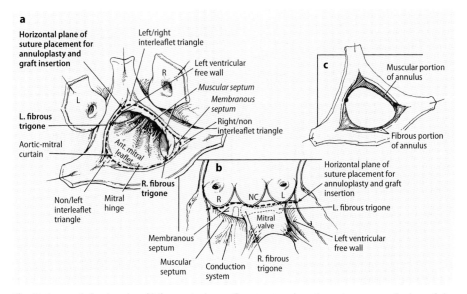

Fig. 2. Anatomic landmarks of left ventricular outflow tract and aortic root: **a** surgeon's view of the aortic root from the right side, **b** opened aortic root, and **c** approximately 55% of the left ventricular outflow tract is fibrous and 45% is muscular. Reprinted with permission from [82]; © American Association for Thoracic Surgery

in collateral damage with any sort of surgical modification of the annulus. The aortic root is contiguous with either the left or right atrium, the right ventricle, both coronary arteries, all the other cardiac valves, and the conduction system around its entire circumference except in the region of the left fibrous trigone, where it is contiguous with the transverse sinus outside the heart. Any opening in the aortic annulus, either surgical, traumatic or from endocarditis, can produce a communication between the left ventricular outflow tract (LVOT) and one of these contiguous structures, depending on the precise location of the communication in the short- or long-axis of the aortic root.

Histologically, the ratio of elastin to collagen in the aorta falls with increasing distance from the heart [11]. The elastic fibers, which are 90% elastin, represent more than 50% of the dry weight of the ascending aorta. They are organized into concentric elastic lamellae alternating with vascular smooth muscle cell layers [12]. Elastin is synthesized only in early life [12] with a half-life of more than 40 years [11].

Behind each leaflet lie the *aortic sinuses*, made up of the aortic wall. At the nadir of the left and right sinus, the annulus actually lies below the ventriculoarterial junction, incorporating a small crescent of ventricular muscle (Fig. 1). The noncoronary sinus is supported by the aortic-mitral curtain [7] (Fig. 2). Histologically, the sinuses are composed primarily of concentric elastic lamellae with a progressive decrease in the number of elastic lamellae and an increase in the amount of collagen between the elastic lamellae near the base of the sinus. In the proximal half of the sinus wall, the layer of elastic lamellae is restricted to the luminal side, disappearing at the base of the sinus [10].

Because the annulus is crown-shaped, there are three triangular extensions of the left ventricular outflow tract between each leaflet which extend the full height of the aortic root to the level of the STJ [7] (Fig. 1). Each of these *interleaflet triangles*, consisting of the aortic wall, occupies approximately 18% of the circumference of the aortic root and each one has a unique design. The right/left and non/right interleaflet triangles are bordered at the base by the myocardium of the interventricular septum. However, the non/right interleaflet triangle is also continuous with the membranous septum. The left/non interleaflet triangle is continuous with the aortic-mitral curtain and the left fibrous trigone (Fig. 2) [9, 10].

Histologically, the interleaflet triangles are composed primarily of circularly oriented collagen fibers with a very thin layer of elastic tissue on the luminal surface which is continuous with an elastic layer in the subendocardium of the ventricle. However, they are thinner and less collagenous than the attachments of the leaflets [9]. There are islets of elastic fibers in the collagenous interleaflet triangles on the luminal side which are not continuous with the elastic lamellae of the aortic wall. As the interleaflet triangle becomes thinner near its base, the elastic fibers disappear altogether [10].

In a study of 4636 aortic valves from donated human hearts intended for processing as allografts, the aortic annulus diameter averaged 23.1 ± 2.0 mm in men and 21.0 ± 1.8 mm in women [13]. These dimensions were confirmed in a study employing magnetic resonance imaging (MRI) with the mean annulus diameters of 22.4 ± 2.1 mm in men and 21.0 ± 2.1 mm in women during systole in the sagittal plane [14]. In the in vivo study, the mean indexed aortic valve area was 2.02 ± 0.52 cm^2/m^2 [13]. This value is in stark contrast to the current ACC/AHA Class I guidelines for surgical intervention on an obstructing aortic valve only when the indexed effective orifice area has fallen to 0.6 cm^2/m^2 [15] and the current definition of prosthesis-patient mismatch occurring only when the indexed effective orifice area falls to 0.85 cm^2/m^2 [16]. The long-term effects on the left ventricle of energy loss occurring with obstructing (or leaking) native or prosthetic valves are beginning to be more carefully studied [17, 18]. These data will likely encourage the development of annuloplasty techniques resulting in aortic roots which more closely approximate the normal geometry and physiology.

The normal aortic root is circumferentially and longitudinally *asymmetric*. The mean height from the base to the STJ varied from 19.6 ± 2.66 mm for the left sinus, to 21.7 ± 3.01 mm for the right sinus to 23.03 ± 2.49 for the noncoronary sinus in 10 cryopreserved human aortic roots. The mean leaflet attachments and free margin lengths corresponded to the asymmetry of the sinuses of Valsalva [19]. Reid [20], who appears to be the first to describe the STJ as a "ridge," found the mean ratio of the "inlet" radius to the "ridge" radius in 6 fixed human specimens to be 1.34 and accordingly described the aortic root as a "truncated cone." In another study of 10 cryopreserved aortic roots with a mean age of 39±12 years (range: 18–54) the base was 23.0±1.1 mm, the sinus of Valsalva was 23.7± 1.0 mm, the STJ was 19.3±0.9 mm, and the proximal aorta 1 cm above the STJ was 20.6±1.0 mm [21]. This normal truncated cone shape of the aortic root is confirmed in ovine models [20, 22, 23] and in the ox, pig, dog, and rabbit [20].

In ovine models, the aortic root tends to become more cylindrical during ejection due to a greater degree of dilatation of the sinotubular junction relative to the base of the aortic root [22, 23], most likely due to the preponderance of elastic tissue in the aortic root at the level of the STJ and the preponderance of collagen at the inlet. The relatively greater dilatation of the STJ compared to the ventriculoaortic junction has also been confirmed in humans with MRI [14] and multidetector computed tomography [24]. Although the sinuses of Valsalva are consistently larger than the sinotubular junction, the sinotubular junction tends to approximate the "annulus" (the ventriculoarterial junction at the nadir of sinus) when measured by transthoracic echocardiography and MRI in normal children and young adults, with the sinotubular junction actually being slightly larger [14, 25, 26]. These observations are obviously relevant to any aortic valve-sparing root replacement procedure designed to reproduce normal sinus dimensions in both short- and long-axis planes.

Although the aortic-mitral curtain has traditionally been considered rigid [27], it actually has a certain degree of flexibility, inasmuch as it normally bulges toward the mitral orifice during systole as the aortic root expands [8, 28]. Perhaps surprisingly, the aortic-mitral curtain itself also normally "expands" approximately 5–10% during systole in a canine and ovine model [28, 29]. Although Lansac et al. [28] did not believe that the change in length between the fibrous trigones was due to elasticity of the fibrous tissue, others have demonstrated a small degree of circumferential deformation in the noncoronary sinus in a similar model during early systole [22]. In another similar ovine study [30], the anterior mitral annulus dilated up to 11.2% in response to a 150% increase in afterload.

Moreover, by virtue of its inherent crimp [31], bovine and equine collagen have been shown to stretch 9% and 15%, respectively, during tensile stress-strain analysis [32], the collagen in porcine aortic and pulmonary valve cusps stretches roughly 12% and 10%, respectively, in the circumferential direction [33], and the collagen in human aortic valve cusps stretches roughly 10–12% in the circumferential direction [34]. In one study by Stradins et al. [35], circumferential stretch of human aortic and pulmonary valves was 18–19%. Clearly, collagen can stretch and the degree of stretch is related to the percentage of fibers crimped vs. the number of fibers straightened in response to a given stress [33].

Thus, although the fibrous skeleton of the heart has typically connoted a structure with a fixed dimension, it appears to have some normal inherent distensibility, which could become more pronounced with disease. The distensibility of the aortic annulus (at the ventriculoaortic junction), as defined by the percentage change in the systolic and diastolic diameter measured echocardiographically, was 4.5–12% (mean 7.5%) in a "normal aortic root." In patients with noncalcified aortic valve lesions it was 2.5–5.8% (mean 3.8%) [36].

The diseased aortic annulus and root

Aging

Changes in the diameter and molecular composition of the aorta occur with aging. In the in vivo study of 4,636 human hearts, the aortic "annulus" (measurement at the most proximal portion of the inlet of the aortic root) was demonstrated to increase with age [13]. In addition, Zhu et al. [26] reported in a study of 326 normal subjects with transthoracic echocardiography that the "annulus" (in imaging terminology) and the STJ both increase with age, with the STJ increasing relatively more than the annulus. The mean STJ/annulus ratio increased from 1.02 at age ≤20 years to 1.16 at age 51–60 years. These changes in diameter have also been noted in the aortic root. In the Framingham Heart Study of 1849 men and 2152 women, also using transthoracic echocardiography, the aortic root was shown to increase by 0.8 and 0.9 mm per decade for men and women, respectively [37]. These dimensional changes were confirmed by MRI in a study of 120 healthy volunteers with an increase of 0.9 and 0.7 mm per decade for men and women, respectively [14].

This aging process is the result of a change in the molecular composition of the aorta. Using finite element modeling, Grande et al. [38] demonstrated increased stiffness in the aortic root with age, with even greater stiffness in the leaflets. The collagen fibers in the valve leaflets become thicker and denser, losing their predominantly circumferential orientation. This leaflet stiffening over time results in a progressively decreased surface of coaptation [38]. Radial stretch of human aortic valve leaflets also decreases over time decreasing the surface area of leaflet coaptation, leading to possible aortic valve incompetence [34]. Age-related changes in the leaflet and root tissue result in a delayed and a slower rate of valve opening with a smaller magnitude of leaflet tip displacement as compared to normal. Stresses in the leaflet-root attachment and belly regions of the leaflets also increased progressively with aging creating a "balancing act of tissue stiffness and thickness on the leaflet stresses" [39].

While there appears to be an increase in the number of elastic fibers in the aorta [40], this is more than likely due to fragmentation of the elastin

[41]. In a study evaluating 100 normal aortas of various ages, elastin fragmentation, fibrosis, and medionecrosis were all correlated with advancing age. These changes were also more pronounced in the ascending aorta and the aortic arch [42]. In addition, the aorta becomes stiffer with age because the elastin not only becomes fragmented and degraded but is also replaced by much stiffer collagen [11, 12]. Moreover, both proteins also become stiffer due to cross-linking and calcification [11].

"Annuloaortic ectasia"/Marfan syndrome

Patients with annuloaortic ectasia demonstrate significant dilatation of the aortic root at all levels, including the ventriculoaortic junction, the sinuses of Valsalva, and the STJ. Moreover, there is a much greater distensibility during systole at all levels in the patients with annuloaortic ectasia compared to normal. Kazui et al. [43] used 64-row multidetector computed tomography in 5 patients with annulo-aortic ectasia and 25 normal controls to measure the diameters of all three levels of the aortic root during systole and diastole. Normal patients demonstrated 0.2%, 0.2% and 0.3% distensibility during systole, respectively, of the "annulus", sinuses of Valsalva and STJ; in contrast, the patients with annuloaortic ectasia demonstrated 15.3%, 4.8%, and 8.8% distensibility of these same levels, respectively. It is interesting that the greatest increase in distensibility in the patients with annuloaortic ectasia in this study occurred at the level of the ventriculoaortic junction, where the greatest concentration of collagen in the aortic root is present in the aortic-mitral curtain. It is believed that annular dilatation with annuloaortic ectasia from any cause only involves the fibrous component of the LVOT [44]. Assuming this hypothesis is true, any correction of annular dilatation should logically be aimed at the fibrous portion of the LVOT rather than the muscular portion, since specific structural abnormalities do not typically occur in the myocardium with these disorders.

The Marfan syndrome (MFS) is a specific form of annuloaortic ectasia. It is an autosomal dominant, multisytem disease with a mutation in the *FBN-1* gene that encodes the extracellular matrix glycoprotein, fibrillin-1 [45]. Fibrillin is an integral component of the microfibrils, linking vascular smooth muscle cells (VSMCs) to the surrounding elastic lamellae within the aortic media, allowing for the elasticity of the aortic wall. Fibrillin-1 also stabilizes the microfibril against degradation by matrix metalloproteinases (MMPs). Altered or deficient fibrillin results in a loss of these connections, which in turn produces impaired elasticity, smooth muscle cell apoptosis, destruction of the surrounding extracellular matrix by MMPs, and eventual aneurysm formation [46]. An additional component in the disruption of the extracellular matrix is a cytokine, transforming growth factor (TGF)β, which is thought to be normally inactivated by fibrillin [46]. Many of the multisystem manifestations of the MFS likely relate specifically to excess TGF-β signaling [47].

This combination of structural microfibril matrix abnormalities, dysregulation of matrix homeostasis mediated by excess TGF-β and abnormal cell-matrix interaction is responsible for the specific phenotypic features of the MFS aorta. Ongoing destruction of the elastic and collagen lamellae and medial degeneration result in progressive dilatation of proximal aortic segments [45]. The histological changes seen in the MFS aorta have been termed "cystic medial necrosis," although they have also been described in patients with a bicuspid aortic valve, aortic coarctation, tetralogy of Fallot and other conotruncal abnormalities [46]. Although the annulus dilates in MFS, the important measurement for surgical decision-making is at the level of the sinuses of Valsalva. In aortic valve-sparing operations on MFS patients, a reduction annuloplasty is typically accomplished with either the remodeling technique introduced by Yacoub [48] or reimplantation techniques introduced by David [49]. Annular stability appears to be more predictable with the reimplantation technique than with the remodeling technique, even if the remodeling technique is accompanied by an annuloplasty [50, 51]. This observation may be important in determining whether some sort of external buttress material needs to be added to an annuloplasty procedure in certain conditions.

Bicuspid aortic valve

Bicuspid aortic valves (BAV) are frequently associated with a dilated proximal aorta. The term "poststenotic dilatation" was originally used to refer to this finding [52]. This relationship of BAV to aortic dilatation is now recognized in the ACC/AHA 2006 Guidelines for the Management of Patients with Valvular Heart Disease with a new separate category *Bicuspid Aortic Valve with Dilated Ascending Aorta* created since the 1998 Guidelines were published [15]. Histologically, the pathology actually resembles that of the MFS aorta with cystic medial necrosis, loss of elastic fibers, increased apoptosis, and altered smooth muscle cell alignment [53]. The medial degeneration involves apoptosis of VSMCs, resulting in a decreased production of extracellular matrix proteins and elastin fragmentation which, in turn, results in a loss of structural support and elasticity. Fibrillin-1 deficiency results in a detachment of VSMCs from the elastin and collagen matrix. Differential expression of MMPs and tissue inhibitors of MMPs (TIMPs) result in an increased degradation of collagen and elastin [54]. Various lines of evidence also implicate perturbations of TGF-β in the aortopathy associated with a BAV [46].

This aortopathy appears to be present at birth even in the absence of valve dysfunction with a progressive dilatation over time [55], which also involves a loss of elasticity as measured by transthoracic echocardiography [56]. The prevalence of aortic dilatation with bicuspid aortic valve ranges from 7.5–57% at the annulus, 16–78% at the sinus level, and 15–79% at the sinotubular junction, and 35–68% at the proximal ascending aorta. Prevalence increases with age, beginning in childhood, continuing throughout life from 50% of those <30 years of age to up to 88% of those >80 years of age [54].

Four patterns of dilatation have been described in a cohort of 64 adults with BAV undergoing computed tomographic or magnetic resonance angiography and echocardiography with a mean age of 45±1 years, which frequently included the aortic root and aortic arch. The mean diameter of the ventriculoaortic junction ("aortic annulus") in the entire group was 28.1±0.7 mm [57], which is substantially dilated compared to normal [13] and would require a reduction annuloplasty for a normal-sized aortic allograft or pulmonary autograft implantation. In another study of 257 patients with BAV disease undergoing angiographic measurements at the ventriculoaortic junction ("aortic valve level"), the annulus and all components of the aortic root and ascending aorta were significantly larger in patients with aortic regurgitation compared to aortic stenosis. The mean annulus diameter was 24.8±3.4 mm in patients with stenosis and 27.9±3.3 in patients with regurgitation [58]. In the Mayo Clinic surgical pathology study of 542 cases of BAV, 19% had annuli greater than 3.5 cm. Annular dilatation, by this definition, occurred in 12% of pure stenosis, 68% of combined stenosis and regurgitation, and 94% of pure regurgitation. Annular dilatation was also generally associated with dilatation of the ascending aorta [59].

Although the pulmonary trunk demonstrates histopathological changes similar to those of the ascending aorta in patients with BAV [60, 61], the presence of a BAV, per se, is not generally felt to be a contraindication to the Ross procedure [62]. However, some surgeons have shown a higher degree of autograft failure in patients with primary aortic regurgitation [63–65] and aortic annular dilatation [64, 65], while others have not found either aortic regurgitation (AI) or annular dilatation to be a risk factor for late autograft failure [66–68]. For those surgeons who still perform the Ross procedure in patients with a dilated annulus, an annuloplasty is generally employed [64, 67, 69, 70].

Geometric mismatch without annuloplasty

After the simultaneous but independent introduction of the aortic allograft in 1962 by Dr. Donald N. Ross in London, UK [71] and Sir Brian G. Barratt-Boyes in Auckland, New Zealand [72], concerns began to surface about geometric mismatch between the homograft and the native aortic root and what to do about it. Yankah et al. [36] documented the significant negative impact on valve survival when the diameter of the homograft annulus was "undersized" in comparison to the recipient aortic annulus diameter by 3 mm. Annuloplasty was not employed; there was a perception of "the lim-

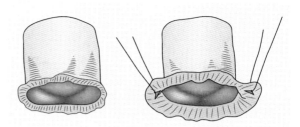

Fig. 3. *Left* Usual appearance of the harvested autograft with a small cuff of infundibular muscle. *Right* Autograft taken with a wider cuff of infundibular muscle when the native aortic annulus is larger than the pulmonary annulus. Reprinted with permission from [73]; © American Association for Thoracic Surgery

ited technical possibility to tailor all the three anatomic units of the aortic root" with the freehand subcoronary implantation technique which the authors preferred. Good long-term valve function, however, was demonstrated when the allograft was "matched or oversized" in relation to the host aortic annulus, presumably by providing "over 50% leaflet coaptation."

Reddy et al. [73] were reluctant to perform a reduction annuloplasty in the case of significant geometric mismatch with the Ross procedure in children, preferring rather to fill the gap with a larger skirt of RVOT muscle incorporated in larger suture bites (Fig. 3). (The authors actually describe a certain degree of annulus reduction in their description of one of the figures: "The autograft with a wide infundibular cuff is sutured to the larger aortic annulus with a running suture technique, which can be performed to exert a purse-string effect, allowing any residual geometric discrepancy to be compensated for by gradual reduction along the course of the entire suture line.")

There are, however, concerns about the structural integrity of a large muscle cuff on the pulmonary autograft. Possible devascularization of the subvalvular muscle cuff of the pulmonary autograft during its dissection has encouraged some surgeons to minimize the amount of remaining RVOT muscle on the autograft. For instance, Yacoub et al. [66, 70] purposely remove all but 2 mm of RVOT muscle in a scalloped fashion immediately beneath the cusp hinges of the pulmonary autograft, in part because of these concerns about viability and structural integrity of the muscle. Later follow-up of the pediatric Ross patients from Reddy's group [74] revealed 17% with moderate or severe aortic insufficiency within less than 7 years following surgery. Of the 7 patients requiring reoperation, all had echocardiographic findings of dilatation of all components of the aortic root, including the annulus. AI was the only predictor of autograft failure in this series by univariate analysis. In addition to the large cuff of RVOT muscle used "to compensate for the larger aortic root diameter without stretching the annulus of the autograft" in cases where the native aortic annulus exceeded the pulmonary annulus by ≥3 mm [73], absorbable suture was also employed [75]. Whether the larger muscle skirt or the absorbable sutures were responsible for the late annular dilatation in these patients is unknown.

Moreover, although AI is a risk for autograft dilatation in the hands of some surgeons [63–65, 74], it is not a risk factor for others who perform the Ross procedure [66, 67]. If late autograft dilatation occurs, it is not always clear whether it is due to the autograft or the aortic annulus. Furthermore, the reason for late annulus dilatation may not necessarily be a patient factor. In fact, it may be as much a surgeon factor, related to specific surgical techniques involving the pulmonary autograft, the aortic annulus, or both. Although the reasons for these differences in outcomes have not been definitively validated, it is likely that some technical nuances play an important role in long-term annulus stability, particularly inasmuch as some surgeons have not had significant problems with late autograft dilatation either by the root technique or by the subcoronary technique [67, 76].

In the case of the Ross procedure, the use of extra RVOT muscle to compensate for any geometric mismatch is not common practice. Most surgeons deal with a geometric mismatch by means of an annuloplasty.

Reduction aortic annuloplasty

Reduction aortic annuloplasty is employed when the aortic annulus is considered too large for a specific operation applied to the aortic root. A reduction annuloplasty of the aortic annulus is analogous in principle to an annuloplasty of a dilated mitral annulus, popularized by Professor Alain Carpentier of Paris, France in his numerous publications on the subject beginning in 1969 in the French literature [77] and in 1971 in the English literature [78]. His fundamental concept was to permanently return the diseased mitral or tricuspid annulus to its original size and shape. He coined the term "remodeling" to describe this process, employing a rigid "frame" to accomplish this result. His approach is mindful of Leonardo da Vinci's philosophical and scientific mantra captured in these two quotes: "those who are inspired by a model other than nature, a mistress above all masters, are laboring in vain" [79]; and "human ingenuity ... will never discover any inventions more beautiful, more appropriate or more direct than nature, because in her inventions nothing is lacking and nothing is superfluous" [80]. Carpentier's "back to nature" approach was supported by his careful analysis of the normal geometry of the mitral valve, which he was very careful to restore, at least in two dimensions. A few years later, he extended his annuloplasty concept to the aortic annulus, this time with a circular continuous "vertical mattress" running suture encompassing the entire aortic annulus, but without a "frame" [81]. Although he described the

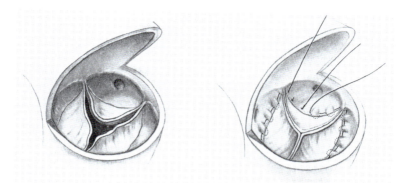

Fig. 4. Aortic annuloplasty with a circular continuous "vertical mattress" running suture. Reprinted with permission from [81]; © American Association for Thoracic Surgery

suture technique as "circular" it was not planar, following instead the entire span of the crown-shaped annulus from the commissures at the STJ to the nadir of each sinus at the ventriculoarterial junction (Fig. 4).

Annuloplasty math

Annuloplasty math is very simple. The degree of diameter reduction is directly related to the degree of circumferential reduction according to a 1:3 relationship of diameter to circumference by the formula: *circumference* = $\pi \times$ diameter. Accordingly, for every 1 mm of desired diameter reduction, 3 mm of circumference must be plicated. The amount of tissue plicated along the circumference of the aortic annulus is precisely equal to the interval of tissue within the loop of suture, which in turn is determined by the length and curvature of the needle. For example, a 12 mm bite of annulus with a single stitch will reduce the annulus diameter by 4 mm in only the time it takes to pass the needle and tie the suture.

Suturing techniques

Northrup and Kshettry [82] suggested several different suturing techniques in dealing with aortic annulus dilatation during allograft implantation, all with unpledgetted interrupted sutures. Figure-of-8 sutures were preferred when large plications were required. Other suturing techniques were employed when smaller plications were done, including "compression" sutures, horizontal mattress sutures (Fig. 5) and multiple simple interrupted sutures. Others have also used simple sutures, either with pledgets [83–86] or without pledgets [44, 87]. The type of suture is probably not very important since braided polyester suture is preferred by some [87] and monofilament polypropylene suture by others [86].

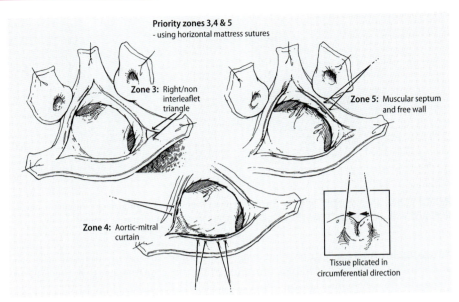

Fig. 5. Aortic annuloplasty method using horizontal mattress sutures. Reprinted with permission from [82]; © American Association for Thoracic Surgery

Subcommissural plication

The simplest annuloplasty is closure of one or more interleaflet triangles. Duran referred to this as a "commissual" annuloplasty [83], which he and his colleagues first described in 1988 in the treatment of rheumatic aortic insufficiency [88]. A "U" stitch was placed at the commissure with pledgets on the inside of the adjacent sinuses of Valsalva very close to the cusp insertion and extending 5–10 mm below the tip of each commissure depending on the amount of circumference plicated. Cosgrove et al. [84] popularized this technique as an adjunct to aortic valve repair for non-rheumatic cusp prolapse to increase the coapting surface of the cusps. David et al. [89] simply closed one or both of the interleaflet triangles of the noncoronary sinus with suture in cases when the aortic annulus was more than 2 mm larger than the pulmonary annulus during a Ross procedure. Eishi et al. [87] reported closing all 3 interleaflet triangles with unpledgeted 4-0 braided polyester "Z" stitches in cases of aortic annular dilatation during a Ross procedure.

Northrup and Kshettry [82] suggested three different priority zones among the three different interleaflet triangles during allograft implantation. The zone of first choice was always the left/non interleaflet triangle because it immediately faces the surgeon and is continuous with the sturdy aortic-mitral curtain. Moreover a large plication can be taken here, especially with the use of a figure-of-8 suture, without any risk of distorting the anterior mitral leaflet as long as the plication does not go below the interleaflet triangle. The right/left interleaflet triangle still seems to be a good second choice for a subcommissural plication since it has substantial collagen present in the interleaflet triangle. If engagement of the collagen with the plicating suture is important, as it intuitively seems to be, then it would be important not to take this plication too far below the top of the commissure where one would eventually encounter the myocardium of the ventricular septum. The third choice for a subcommissural plication would then be the non/right interleaflet triangle because of the presence of the conduction system at the inferior edge of the membranous septum (Figs. 2 and 5). Accordingly, a shallower bite is also in order at this zone. Kollar [90] has applied this technique of plicating all three interleaflet triangles in his valve-sparing procedures with pledgeted mattress sutures placed outside the aortic wall.

Intertrigonal plication

David [44, 49] has employed a partially circumferential reduction annuloplasty in cases of annulus dilatation when performing a remodeling type of valve-sparing aortic replacement and when performing a Ross procedure. The annuloplasty only involves the fibrous portion of the left ventricular outflow tract from the membranous septum to the left fibrous trigone. Horizontal mattress sutures of 4-0 polyester are placed from inside out in a single horizontal plane just below the aortic annulus and then either through a Dacron graft in the case of a valve-sparing procedure (Fig. 6) or a strip of polyester fabric placed outside the aortic root in the case of a Ross procedure (Fig. 7). Although in the case of the valve-sparing procedure, sutures are placed around the entire circumference of the subannular

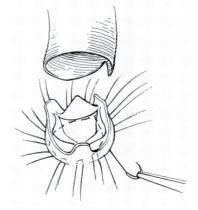

Fig. 6. Partially circumferential reduction annuloplasty, aortic valve-sparing operation. Reprinted with permission from [49]; © American Association for Thoracic Surgery

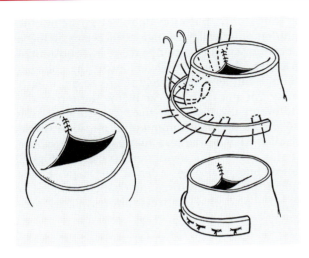

Fig. 7. Partially circumferential reduction annuloplasty using a strip of Dacron fabric. Reprinted with permission from [89]; © American Association for Thoracic Surgery

LVOT, the annular plication only occurs in the intertrigonal portion by taking smaller bites in the Dacron in this portion of the LVOT.

Sievers [91] uses a technique similar to David when performing a reduction annuloplasty during the subcoronary technique of the Ross procedure. Yacoub [70] performs a similar annuloplasty if necessary during the root replacement technique of the Ross procedure with an intertrigonal running "compression suture" woven in and out in the aortic-mitral curtain just beneath the left and nonaortic cusp hinges with a single monofilament suture tied externally. Stewart et al. [85] employed a variation of intertrigonal plication in 26 children undergoing a Ross procedure, using several horizontal mattress sutures to plicate a single area of the noncoronary sinus. Northrup and Kshettry [82] preferred separate small plications in the intertrigonal portion of the annulus when dealing with aortic annulus dilatation during aortic allograft implantation (Fig. 6), but also employed a circumferential external autologous pericardial buttress in the proximal suture line. Each stitch can be made in just the amount of time required to pass the needle and tie the suture. As long as the sutures stay in the aortic-mitral curtain and away from the hinge of the anterior mitral leaflet, there is no risk of distorting the mitral valve even with large plications.

Circumferential plication

As mentioned above, Carpentier [81] was the first to suggest a completely circumferential suture annuloplasty which followed the crown shape of the aortic annulus (Fig. 4). Izumoto et al. [92, 93] have utilized a similar annuloplasty concept following the entire vertical extent of the aortic annulus. They placed pledgeted horizontal mattress sutures in a row just *above* the

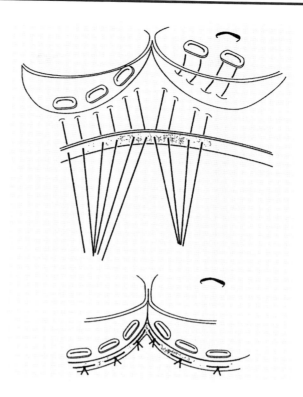

Fig. 8. Subvalvular circular annuloplasty technique. Reprinted with permission from [92]

hinge of the leaflets from inside the sinus out to back in just *below* the hinge of the leaflets *inside* the left ventricular outflow tract. The sutures were then placed through a PTFE strip 9 mm wide and 0.6 mm thick. Since the primary purpose of this annuloplasty was to "shorten the commissural annulus" the sutures were placed such that the interleaflet triangles were effectively closed (Fig. 8). This subvalvular circular annulplasty did not interfere with annulus motion during the cardiac cycle and, in conjunction with the remodeling procedure, restored near normal geometry and phasic motion. Ruvolo and Fattouch [94] performed a similar annuloplasty in patients with annulo-aortic ectasia undergoing a valve-sparing procedure with individual pledgeted mattress sutures placed immediately *below* the aortic annulus and brought up *behind* the cusp attachments to engage individual Dacron patches placed separately within each individual aortic sinuses. The mean aortic annulus diameter was accordingly reduced from 29 mm to 21 mm.

Other circumferential plication techniques in a "subvalvular" planar fashion have been reported. Elkins et al. [69] reported placing a double purse-string of 3-0 polypropylene suture in the plane of the nadir of the aortic sinuses in two patients with dilated aortic annuli undergoing a Ross

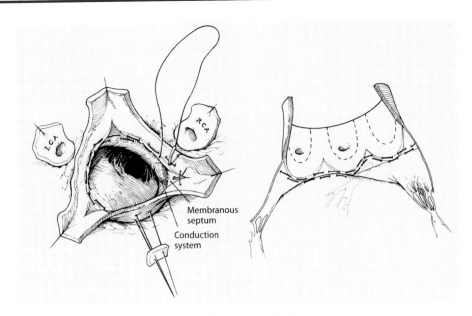

Fig. 9. Aortic annuloplasty with purse-string suture method

procedure. The suture was tied externally over a felt pledget in the noncoronary sinus with a sizer of a predetermined diameter placed through the aortic annulus (Fig. 9). In a total of 20 patients with dilated annuli, including these two patients, an external buttress of either Dacron, Teflon or pericardium was incorporated into the interrupted 4-0 polypropylene proximal suture line.

A circumferential piece of tubular Dacron graft has been employed as an annuloplasty buttress in three different manners. In the first example, David and Feindel [49] described an aortic valve-sparing operation for patients with annuloaortic ectasia entailing reimplantation of the aortic valve inside a tubular Dacron graft. Multiple 4-0 polyester mattress sutures were placed inside out immediately below the aortic valve. The sutures were planar in the fibrous portion of the left ventricular outflow tract and scalloped in the muscular portion (Fig. 6). The reduction annuloplasty was accomplished only in the fibrous portion by placing the sutures closure together in the graft than in the fibrous portion of the left ventricular outflow tract. A modification of this technique was reported by Gleason [95], whereby the lower suture line was *scalloped* in all three interleaflet triangles.

In another report [96], an annuloplasty of an annulus >35 mm was created by a series of horizontal mattress sutures placed from inside to outside the left ventricular outflow tract immediately below the level of the annulus and then passed through a 1 cm piece of a 34 mm Dacron graft from inside out. The Dacron graft was secured to the left ventricular out-

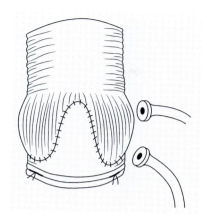

Fig. 10. Remodeling technique combined with a subvalvular external aortic annuloplasty using a prosthetic ring. Reprinted with permission from [98]; © European Association for Cardio-Thoracic Surgery

flow tract by tying the sutures over a 28 mm sizer, followed by insertion of a 25 mm aortic allograft within the Dacron graft.

In a third iteration, Lansac et al. [97] employed a similar technique using a very narrow *external* ring in the immediate subvalvular plane to reduce the annulus diameter in a small series of patients undergoing a remodeling type of valve-sparing procedure. The ring was originally fashioned from a "slice of the Dacron tube graft used to reconstruct the aortic root" and was anchored externally with five pledgeted 2-0 polyester horizontal mattress sutures placed inside out below the nadir of each cusp and at the base of the interleaflet triangles bordering the left coronary cusp (Fig. 10) [98]. More recently, Lansac [99] has developed an expansible ring with an elastomer core covered by knitted polyester fabric which has preserved the normal distensibility of the ventriculoarterial junction in an ovine model. This new device is currently being evaluated in a prospective trial comparing aortic valve-sparing to mechanical valve replacement.

Resection

In 1965, Barrett-Boyes [100] described excision of as much of the noncoronary sinus as necessary to deal with a geometric mismatch with the aortic annulus diameter 2 mm greater than the diameter of the aortic allograft. The author had a very keen understanding of the anatomy of the aortic root. His description of the details of this resection are worth repeating:

> "The excision must be carried through the base of the aortic cusp on to the mitral leaflet and this can nearly always be done without perforating this leaflet. As the base of the non-coronary cusp arises from the right fibrous trigone through which passes the bundle of His, the excision is centered slightly behind the deepest portion of the cusp remnant (towards the left rather than the right coronary orifice)

and, when a centimeter or more of the aortic root requires removal, this is therefore in a backward direction away from the trigone region. The deficiency so created is pear-shaped with its base on the mitral leaflet."

The defect was then closed with interrupted sutures.

Durham et al. [86] have performed a triangular resection of the dilated aortic annulus in young patients undergoing a Ross procedure. A vertical incision is made at the left/non commissure and carried down into the anterior mitral leaflet followed by excision of a triangular wedge large enough to produce an annulus diameter 2 mm less than the pulmonary autograft. The V-shaped defect is reapproximated with interrupted pledgeted horizontal mattress sutures over a calibrated dilator.

External buttress

Stable autograft dimensions by echocardiography up to 4 years have been demonstrated in Yacoub's Ross patients [76] despite the absence of any buttressing material at any level of the aortic root [70]. Similarly, Pigula et al. [101] demonstrated stable echocardiographic annulus diameters beyond 3 years in a series of pediatric Ross patients who had undergone some form of annulus reduction which was stabilized with either autologous pericardium or Teflon felt. Northrup and Kshettry [82] routinely incorporated an external autologous pericardial buttress in the proximal suture line of aortic allograft root implants. Elkins et al. [69] used an external buttress of Dacron, Teflon felt or pericardium to "fix" the annulus following a reduction annuloplasty and demonstrated stable Z values by echocardiography for up to 5.6 years. Luciani et al. [102] have also demonstrated that buttressing the suture lines at the annulus and sinotubular junction with glutaraldehyde-treated autologous pericardium is protective against pulmonary autograft dilatation with the root technique.

Based on these composite data, a geometric mismatch, particularly if the aortic annulus is larger than either the allograft or the autograft, seems to be best handled by a reduction annuloplasty. In some cases of the pulmonary autograft, it may also be appropriate to provide external support to the aortic root, either at the level of the ventriculoaortic junction, the sinuses or the STJ.

Augmentation annuloplasty

Occasionally, the aortic annulus must be enlarged either to avoid geometric mismatch during biological valve procedures such as the Ross procedure or aortic allograft implant or to avoid prosthesis-patient mismatch as originally described by Rahimtoola [103] and carefully studied in a variety of different aortic valve replacement procedures by Pibarot and colleagues at the Quebec Heart Institute [16, 104]. It is likely that annulus enlargement procedures will be employed more frequently in the future for routine prosthetic aortic valve replacement in view of recent data demonstrating progressive late excess mortality inversely proportional to age at surgery following implantation of mechanical valves and stented bioprostheses [105–108], especially with smaller sizes [107]. The specific techniques either enlarge the LVOT posteriorly in the fibrous portion of the aortic-mitral curtain or anteriorly in the muscular portion of the ventricular septum. It is important to be aware of the contiguous cardiac structures when performing these annulus enlargement procedures in order to avoid collateral damage or unintended communications.

Aortic-mitral curtain enlargement procedures

In 1970, Nicks et al. [109] described a technique for enlarging the aortic annulus by incising through the noncoronary sinus "across the aortic ring as far as the origin of the mitral valve" (Fig. 11). A piece of Dacron was sutured down to the "fibrous origin of the mitral ring" and on up as a con-

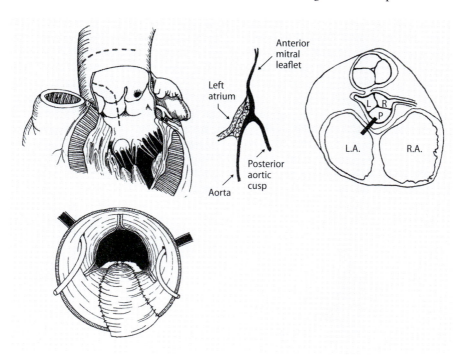

Fig. 11. Nicks technique for enlarging the aortic annulus. Reprinted with permission from [109], the BMJ Publishing Group

tinuous patch of the annulus and oblique aortotomy. In 1993, Yener et al. [110] reported a variation of the Nicks procedure in a single patient undergoing simultaneous replacement of the aortic and mitral valves, whereby the anterior mitral leaflet was reflected upward through the aortic annulus and used to patch the defect.

In 2007, Dhareshwar et al. [111] reported the Mayo Clinic's experience with aortic root enlargement in 249 of 2,366 patients undergoing aortic valve replacement from 1993-2001. The authors preferred the Nicks procedure specifically using a "teardrop-shaped patch of autologous or bovine pericardium" as patch material. They found a higher raw operative mortality in the root enlargement cohort (5.6% vs. 2.9%), but the procedure was not an independent risk factor for operative death by multivariate analysis. Hopkins [112] reported no technique-related mortalities in 196 patients undergoing a Nicks procedure with a "water droplet"-shaped patch of bovine pericardium allowing up to three prosthetic valve upsizings if the valve was tipped up to 15°. In 2005, Hopkins [113] described the use of a portion of the contiguous anterior mitral leaflet of the aortic allograft as patch material during a Nicks procedure.

In 1979, Manouguian and Seybold-Epting [114] created a variation of the Nicks operation with a transverse aortotomy by incising precisely down into the non/left commissure and carrying the incision "into the anterior mitral leaflet, maximally to its appositional portion" (Fig. 12). A 1 cm incision into the "initial portion of the anterior mitral leaflet" allowed for "an enlargement of the aortic ring of 15 mm." A single patch of Dacron or pericardium was used to close the defect in the same manner as with the Nicks procedure. The left atrium was typically entered with this maneuver because of its proximity and closed either by "simply including the cut edges of the atrium in the running suture lines with which the patch is sutured to the defect in the aortic leaflet of the mitral valve." With a deeper incision into the mitral leaflet "the defect between the left atrial wall and the patch must be closed with continuous sutures or with mattress sutures which also fix the sewing ring of the aortic prosthesis." Sometimes the obligatory incision in the left atrium with this deeper incision requires pericardial patch closure. The authors reported no impairment of mitral valve function with this procedure. Also in 1979, Rittenhouse et al. [115] de-

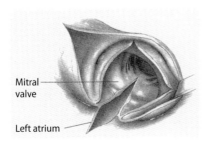

Fig. 12. Manouguian technique for enlarging the aortic annulus. Reprinted with permission from [138]; © Elsevier

scribed an identical technique with the incision "extended across the aortic annulus and down the center of the mitral valve leaflet to within 5 mm of the free edge."

In 2002, Molina [116] reported a double patch variation of a combination of the Nicks and Manouguian procedures using PTFE to patch the defect in the anterior mitral leaflet and aortic annulus and a Dacron patch in the aortotomy. The author claimed that the PTFE resulted in a more pliable and mobile mitral valve than with Dacron. In 2004, Okuyama et al. [117] reported on the application of the Manougian procedure in 30 patients with small aortic and mitral annuli undergoing simultaneous replacement of the aortic and mitral valves. The authors used an oval equine pericardial lined Dacron patch designed to enlarge the mitral annulus, a portion of the aortic-mitral curtain, the aortic annulus, and aorta in continuity. Hopkins [113] has described the use of the contiguous anterior mitral leaflet of the aortic allograft to patch the defect in the mitral valve and aortic-mitral curtain with the Manouguian procedure.

In 1993, Milsom and Doty [118] performed a variation of the Manougian procedure in three patients utilizing a portion of the contiguous anterior mitral leaflet of the aortic allograft as patch material for aortic annulus enlargement or nearly the entire allograft leaflet to replace the majority of a diseased anterior mitral leaflet. The use of the contiguous anterior mitral leaflet of the aortic allograft for aortic annulus enlargement has also been described more recently by Hopkins [113] and Yankah et al. [36]. The use of the mitral leaflet to replace damaged tissue in the aortic root was predictive of its eventual application particularly in extensive excavating native and prosthetic valve endocarditis involving the aortic annulus [119–121].

In 1997, Peterson et al. [122] reported on the Toronto General Hospital experience of 669 patients undergoing aortic annular enlargement from 1995–2005. A Nicks procedure (incision 2–5 mm below the aortic annulus) was used with a single teardrop-shaped patch of untreated autologous pericardium when the annulus was upsized by one. When the annulus was increased by two valve sizes, a Manouguian procedure (incision 10–15 mm below the annulus) was used with a double patch of untreated autologous pericardium. The second patch was used to close the obligatory defect in the contiguous left atrium, with the deeper incision below the aortic-mitral curtain and into the anterior mitral leaflet. The authors concluded that patch enlargement of the aortic annulus is a "safe adjunct to aortic valve replacement" based on a significant improvement in surgical mortality from 7.5% to 2.9% between the first and second halves of the decade under review.

In 1983, Nunez et al. [123] reported a variation of the Manouguian procedure by simply resecting the non/left commissure after a transverse aortotomy which results in "lateral spontaneous retraction of the edges" and a "wide separation of 15–22 mm." The authors avoided getting into the adjacent left atrium by blunt dissection between the media and adventitia of the aorta at the level of the left atrial attachment. In this case the defect was filled with Dacron patch "with a wide base." According to their description, the patch is anchored to the aortic-mitral curtain and the aortic wall, avoiding the anterior mitral leaflet. A later iteration combining aspects of the Nicks, Nunez, and Manouguian procedures was recently reported by Borowski and Kurt [124] who performed a subtotal resection of the noncoronary annulus and sinus extending "through the fibrous origin in the anterior leaflet of the mitral valve approximately 1 cm below the aortic annulus, without entering the left atrium." The commissures were left intact and the conduction system was avoided. The defect was filled with a "wedge-shaped" Dacron patch, allowing an upsize of 1 or 2 prosthetic valve sizes.

▮ Ventricular septum enlargement procedures (aortoventriculoplasty)

Anterior enlargement of the LVOT must necessarily take place in the muscular portion of the ventricular septum and is referred to as an aortoventriculoplasty. Enlargement through the membranous septum below the non/right interleaflet triangle, to the right side of the right coronary artery ostium, is an unacceptable option because it would result in damage to the conduction system and subsequent heart block. Accordingly, such an en-

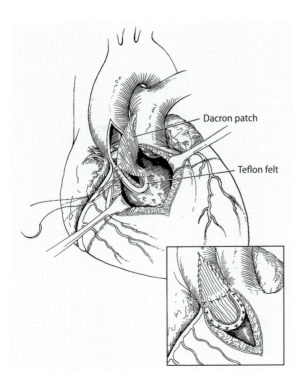

Fig. 13. Konno technique for enlarging the aortic annulus. A Dacron patch is being sutured to the defect in the ventricular septum and the prosthetic valve and used to close the aortotomy. Reprinted with permission from [127]; © American Association for Thoracic Surgery

Aortic annuloplasty   ▌   167

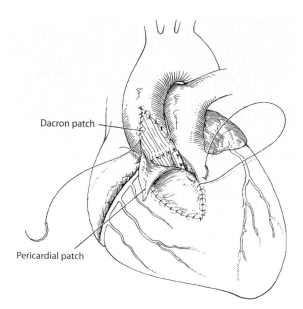

Fig. 14. Konno technique for enlarging the aortic annulus. A second patch of either Dacron or pericardium is sewn to the opening in the RVOT and the first patch. Reprinted with permission from [127]; © American Association for Thoracic Surgery

largement would have to be to the left of the origin of the right coronary artery.

In 1975, Konno et al. [125] described an aortic annulus enlargement procedure in two patients undergoing prosthetic aortic valve replacement with an incision into the anterior portion of the aorta "with an adequate sewing margin remaining to the left of the right coronary ostium" which was "extended downward into the upper portion of the ventricular septum" and the anterior wall of the right ventricle. The prosthetic valve was partially implanted as shown. A Dacron patch was sutured to the defect in the ventricular septum and the prosthetic valve and used to close the aortotomy (Fig. 13), while a second patch of either Dacron or pericardium was sewn to the opening in the RVOT and the first patch (Fig. 14). Also in 1975, Rastan and Koncz [126] independently described the identical procedure utilizing Dacron patches in four pediatric patients with tunnel-like subaortic stenosis. It has been estimated that 35–50% of the valve annulus is made up of the Dacron patch with such a procedure, allowing for nearly a doubling of size of the prosthesis [127].

Hopkins [128] has described using the contiguous anterior mitral leaflet of the aortic allograft as the ventricular septal patch during an aortoventriculoplasty. Since it is done as a root technique, there is no need for an aortic patch. The right ventricular free wall defect is simply closed with a pericardial patch.

In 1991, Yamaguchi et al. [129] described a variation of the Konno-Rastan procedure in conjunction with a Nicks procedure in two children with aortic stenosis. In both cases the annulus was enlarged by 9 mm, while avoiding the potential risk of a ventricular septal defect and damage to the septal coronary arteries. The anterior incision in the aortic annulus was "directed into the commissure between the right and left coronary cusps and carried downward across the aortic ring to near full thickness of the right ventricular wall as with the incision in the procedure of Konno and co-workers. Distinct from their procedure, however, the incision is stopped just before entering the right ventricular cavity and the interventicular septum." The defect was closed with a bifurcated teardrop-shaped Dacron patch similar to that used in an extended aortoplasty for supravalvular aortic stenosis. Otaki et al. [130] in 1997 employed the same "anterior aortotomy" in combination with either a Nicks or Manouguian "posterior enlargement" in three patients undergoing aortic valve replacement with aortic annuli 11–18 mm. The anterior incision was extended "to the ventricular septum through the commissure between the left and right coronary cusps; it did not reach the ventricular septum as in the Konno procedure." The mean increase in annular diameter after the posterior enlargement was 24%. A mean further increase after the anterior enlargement was 34%, for a total mean increase in annular diameter of 68%. The authors emphasize the advantages of the two-directional enlargement to not only allow for a more substantial annular enlargement than by a posterior enlargement alone but "a more central position to the prosthetic valve, and consequently more luminal and physiologic flow may be expected." Moreover, avoidance of the interventricular septal incision should minimize coronary injuries, endocarditis, residual shunts, and conduction disturbances.

In order to avoid the obvious disadvantages of the aortic allograft, mechanical valves, and bioprostheses in children with complex left heart obstruction, the Konno procedure was eventually combined with the pulmonary autograft procedure. In a series of 11 pediatric cases of the Ross-Konno procedure reported by Reddy et al. [131] in 1996 "the pulmonary autograft was harvested with an extension of infundibular free wall muscle attached to it" and "seated with the infundibular muscle extension fitting into the Konno incision in the interventricular septum." Despite the theoretical risk of devascularizing the RVOT conus muscle extension, no residual VSDs or abnormal function of either the left or right ventricle were reported by echocardiography during an 8.5 month mean follow-up.

In the same year, Starnes et al. [132] also employed the Ross-Konno procedure in eight children, but purposely avoided excision of any more than 5 mm of the RVOT conus muscle below the pulmonary valve during autograft harvest. The authors specifically stated that "no excess portion of the RVOT muscle was harvested to accommodate the completion of the septal ventriculoplasty." Moreover, "the incision of the conal septum, starting at the level of the intercoronary commissure, was carried *leftward* [italics ours] to avoid the conduction system". In 4 children, a relatively shallow septal incision was sufficient to open the subaortic area with the reconstruction completed with the short subpulmonary conal muscle skirt of the autograft. In the other 4 children who required a deeper incision in the septum, a Dacron patch was used in the manner of the classical Konno procedure. Mean echocardiographic follow-up of 13.5 months revealed normal right and left ventricular function with no residual VSDs with only one conduction disturbance. Elkins et al. [133] reported a series of 178 Ross patients under age 18 with only 11 Konno-type aortoventriculoplasties and no details on this small subgroup. The authors did comment on the 28 patients with complex LVOT obstruction where "left ventricular myomectomy or an aortoventriculoplasty has been effective in relief of the obstruction."

There appears to be a modest risk for rhythm and conduction disturbances after the Ross procedure. Pasquali et al. [134] reported on 47 patients who had a Ross procedure at a median age of 8.7 years. Twenty-two patients (47%) had complex left-side reconstructions, 18 of whom (82%) had a Konno procedure. At midterm follow-up with Holter monitoring one third of patients had rhythm and conduction disturbances, including sinus node dysfunction in 15%, atrioventricular block in 4% and ventricular tachycardia in 15%. However, the Konno procedure was not statistically related to the occurrence of any of these arrythmias or conduction disturbances. Although both patients who required a permanent pacemaker had a Konno procedure, one with a subaortic membrane resection, only 8% of patients undergoing either a Konno or subaortic membrane resection developed complete heart block.

Some surgeons apparently prefer to avoid a formal Konno operation and have apparently been successful in combining an alternative method for dealing with complex LVOT obstruction. Al-Halees et al. [135] in his report of 136 Ross procedures on children described a "modified Ross-Konno technique" where "part of the septum was actually cored out to completely open up the LVOT without creating a ventricular septal defect. In those patients the fibrous annulus of the aortic valve was often divided, and the cut was partially taken down to the septum. In all patients this resulted in complete relief of the obstruction …" Yacoub et al. [8] believe that an aortomyoplasty is "potentially destructive" and do not use it to accomplish LVOT enlargement.

Vouhe and Neveux [136] described a technique of dividing the aortic ring "through a vertical incision of the left anterior fibrous trigone." Fortunately, it is clear from their illustrations and descriptions that they were not really dealing with the left fibrous trigone, but with the intercoronary commissure and the right/left interleaflet triangle instead. On the other hand, Yacoub et al. [137] have described a technique for eliminating fixed subaortic LVOT obstruction by "mobilizing" the left and right fibrous trigones. By means of a combination of sharp and blunt dissection, the hinge mechanism that normally exists between the ventricular septum and the aortic-mitral curtain is freed up, allowing restoration of the normal backward movement of the aortic-mitral curtain during systole. The authors point out that the left fibrous trigone, unlike the rest of the circumference of the LVOT, is not related to a specific adjacent cardiac chamber, but is instead bounded by the transverse sinus outside of the heart. It is imperative that any incision made into the aortic annulus should never divide the left fibrous trigone.

Conclusion

The aortic annulus is a complex crown shaped three-dimensional collagenous structure beginning at the ventriculoaortic junction and spanning the entire aortic root up to the STJ in its longitudinal dimension to which three separate aortic valve leaflets are normally attached. In its circumferential dimension, it is contiguous with the roughly equal muscular and fibrous components of the LVOT at the proximal end and the ascending aorta distally. It is vulnerable to a variety of congenital and acquired diseases producing obstruction or regurgitation of blood flow at the level of the aortic valve. But it is also amenable to procedures which can relieve these perturbations by either reducing or enlarging its circumference in cases where there is a geometric mismatch between the aortic annulus and specific surgical procedures directed at salvage, repair or replacement of the aortic valve.

A critical understanding of the anatomy of the aortic annulus and adjacent structures is paramount to achieving a successful annuloplasty without causing collateral damage. Various techniques designed to accomplish either a reduction or augmentation annuloplasty are described in detail. Controversy still exists as to some specific technical details and particularly as to whether external buttressing materials are required to stabilize reduction annuloplasties and whether LVOT enlargement procedures can be done less invasively just as well by avoiding incisions into the anterior mitral leaflet and the ventricular septum. There appears to be a general trend toward restoration of more normal aortic root geometry and physiology with current annuloplasty techniques.

References

1. The American heritage Stedman's medical dictionary (2002) Houghton Mifflin Co, Boston
2. Dorland's Illustrated Medical Dictionary (2007) Saunders Elsevier, Philadelphia
3. The American heritage dictionary of the English language (2003) Fourth edition, Houghton Mifflin Company, Boston
4. Anderson RH, Wilcox BR (1995) Understanding cardiac anatomy: The prerequisite for optimal cardiac surgery. Ann Thorac Surg 59:1366–1375

5. Robicsek F (1991) Leonardo da Vinci and the Sinuses of Valsalva. Ann Thorac Surg 52:328–335
6. Wells FC, Crowe T (2004) Leonardo da Vinci as a paradigm for modern clinical research. J Thorac Cardiovasc Surg 127:929–944
7. Anderson, RH (2000) Clinical anatomy of the aortic root. Heart 84:670–673
8. Yacoub MH, Kilner PJ, Birks EJ et al (1999) The aortic outflow tract and root: a tale of dynamism and crosstalk. Ann Thorac Surg 68(Suppl):S37–S43
9. Sutton, JP, Siew YH, Anderson RH (1995) The forgotten interleaflet triangles: A review of the surgical anatomy of the aortic valve. Ann Thorac Surg 59:419–427
10. Hokken RB, Bartelings MM, Bogers AJJC et al (1997) Morphology of the pulmonary and aortic roots with regard to the pulmonary autograft procedure. J Thorac Cardiovasc Surg 113:453–461
11. Greenwald SE (2007) Ageing of the conduit arteries. J Pathol 211:157–172
12. Pezet M, Jacob MP, Escoubet B et al (2008) Elastin haploinsufficiencey induces alternative aging processes in the aorta. Rejuvenation Res 11:97–112
13. Capps SB, Elkins RC, Fronk DM (2000) Body surface area as a predictor of aortic and pulmonary valve diameter. J Thorac Cardiovasc Surg 119:975–982
14. Burman ED, Keegan J, Kilner PJ (2008) Aortic root measurement by cardiovascular magnetic resonance. Specification of planes and line of measurement and corresponding normal values. Circ Cardiovasc Imaging 1:104–113
15. Bonow RO, Carabello BA, Chatterjee K et al (2006) ACC/AHA 2006 practice guideline for the management of patients with valvular heart disease: Executive summary. J Am Coll Cardiol 48:598–675
16. Pibarot P and Dumesnil JG (2000) Hemodynamic and clinical impact of prosthesis-patient mismatch in the aortic valve position and its prevention. J Am coll Cardiol 36:1131–1141
17. Gerosa G, Tarzia V, Rizzoli G et al (2006) Small aortic annulus: The hydrodynamic performances of 5 commercially available tissue valves. J Thorac Cardiovasc Surg 131:1058–1064
18. Akins CW, Travis B, Yoganathan AP (2007) Energy loss for evaluating heart valve performance. J Thorac Cardiovasc Surg 136:820–833
19. Choo SJ, McRae G, Olomon JP et al (1999) Aortic Root Geometry: Pattern of differences between leaflets and sinuses of Valsalva. J Heart Valve Dis 8:407–415
20. Reid K (1970) The anatomy of the sinus of Valsalva. Thorax 25:79–85
21. Kunzelman KS, Grande KJ, David TE et al (1994) Aortic root and valve relationships. Impact on surgical repair. J Thorac Cardiovasc Surg 107:162–170
22. Dagum P, Green GR, Nistal FJ et al (1999) Deformational dynamics of the aortic root. Modes and physiologic determinants. Circulation 100(Suppl II):II-54–II-62
23. Lansac E, Lim HS, Shomura Y et al (2002) A four-dimensional study of the aortic root dynamics. Eur J Cardio-thorac Surg 22:497–503
24. Kazui T, Izumoto H, Yoshioka K et al (2006) Dynamic morphologic changes in the normal aortic annulus during systole and diastole. J Heart Valve Dis 15:617–621
25. Kaldararova M, Balazova E, Tittel P et al (2007) Echocardiographic measurements of the aorta in normal children and young adults. Bratial Lek Listy 108:437–442
26. Zhu D and Zhao Q (2008) Aortic valve annulus and sinus-tube joint diameters in normal adults of Chinese Han ethnic group. Chin Med J 121:1093–1095
27. van Rijk-Zwikker GL, Delemarre BJ, Juysmans HA (1994) Mitral valve anatomy and morphology: relevance to mitral valve replacement and valve reconstruction. J Card Surg 9(Suppl):255–261
28. Lansac E, Lim KH, Shomura Y et al (2002) Dynamic balance of the aortomitral junction. J Thorac Cardiovasc Surg 123:911–918

29. Glasson JR, Komeda MK, Daughters GY, Bolger AF, Tomizawa Y, Daughters GT II, Tye TL, Ingels NB Jr, Miller DC (1996) Three-dimensional regional dynamics of the normal mitral annulus during left ventricular ejection. J Thorac Cardiovasc Surg 111:574–585
30. Parish LM, Jackson BM, Enomoto Y, Gorman RC, Gorman JH III (2004) The dynamic anterior mitral annulus. Ann Thorac Surg 78:1248–1255
31. Schoen FJ (1997) Editorial: Aortic valve structure-function correlations: Role of elastic fibers no longer a stretch of the imagination. J Heart Valve Dis 6:1–6
32. Angele P, Abke J, Kujat R et al (2004) Influence of different collagen species on physico-chemical properties of crosslinked collagen matrices. Biomaterials 25: 2831–2841
33. Joyce EM, Liao J, Schoen FJ, Mayer JE, Sacks MS (2009) Funtional collagen fiber architecture of the pulmonary heart valve cusp. Ann Thorac Surg 87:1240–1249
34. Christie GW, Barratt-Boyes BG (1995) Age-dependent changes in the radial stretch of human aortic valve leaflets determined by biaxial testing. Ann thorac Surg 60: S156–S159
35. Stradins P, Lais R, Ozolanta I, Purina B, Ose V, Feldmane L, Kasyanov V (2004) Comparison of biomechanical and structural properties between human aortic and pulmonary valve. Eur J Cardiothorac Surg 26:634–639
36. Yankah AC, Klose H, Musci M et al (2001) Geometric mismatch between homograft (allograft) and native aortic root: a 14-year clinical experience. Eur J Cardiothorac Surg 20:835–841
37. Vasan RS, Larson, Levy D (1995) Determinants of echocardiographic aortic root size. Circulation 91:734–740
38. Grande KJ, Cochran RP, Reinhall PG et al (1999) Mechanisms of aortic valve incompetence in aging: A finite element model. J Heart Valve Dis 8:149–156
39. Singh R, Strom JA, Ondrovic L, Joseph B, VanAuker MD (2008) Age-related changes in the aortic valve affect leaflet stress distributions: Implications for aortic valve degeneration. J Heart Valve Dis 17:290–299
40. Dare AJ, Veinot JP, Edwards WD et al (1993) New observations on the etiology of aortic valve disease: A surgical pathologic study of 236 cases from 1990. Hum Pathol 24:1330–1338
41. Fleg JL (1986) Alterations in cardiovascular structure and function with advancing age. Am JCardiol 57:33C–44C
42. Schlatmann TJ, Becker AE (1977) Histologic changes in the normal aging aorta: Implications for dissecting aortic aneurysm. Am J Cardiol 39:13–20
43. Kazui T, Kin H, Tsuboi J, Yoshioka K, Okabayashi H, Kawazoe K (2008) Perioperative dynamic morphological changes of the aortic annulus during aortic root remodeling with aortic annuloplasty at systolic and diastolic phases. J Heart Valve Dis 17:366–370
44. David TE (1996) Remodeling the aortic root and preservation of the native aortic valve. Op Tech Cardiac Thorac Surg 1:44–56
45. Keane MG, Pyeritz RE (2008) Medical management of Marfan Syndrome. Circulation 117:2802–2813
46. Yetman AT, Graham T (2009) The dilated aorta in patients with congenital cardiac defects. J Am Coll Cardiol 53:461–467
47. Pearson GD, Devereux R, Loeys B et al (2008) Report of the National Heart, Lung, and Blood Institute and National Marfan Foundation Working Group on research in Marfan Syndrome and related disorders. Circulation 118:785–791
48. Sarsam LAJ, Yacoub M (1993) Remodeling of the aortic valve annulus. J Thorac Cardiovasc Surg 105:435–438

49. David TE, Feindel CM (1992) An aortic valve-sparing operation for patients with aortic incompetence and aneurysm of the ascending aorta. J Thorac Cardiovasc Surg 103:617–622
50. de Oliveira NC, David TE, Ivanov J, Armstrong S, Eriksson MJ, Rakowski H, Webb G (2003) Results of surgery for aortic root aneurysm in patients with Marfan syndrome. J Thorac Cardiovasc Surg 125:789–786
51. Miller DC (2003) Editorial. Valve-sparing aortic root replacement in patients with the Marfan syndrome. J Thorac Cardiovasc Surg 125:773–778
52. Holman E (1954) The obscure physiology of poststenotic dilatation; its relation to the development of aneurysms. J Thorac Surg 28:109–133
53. Fedak PW, Verma S, David TE, Leask RS, Weisel RD, Butany J (2002) Clinical and pathophysiological implications of a bicuspid aortic valve. Circulation 106:900–904
54. Tadros TM, Klein MD, Shapira OM (2009) Ascending aortic dilatation associated with bicuspid aortic valve. Pathophysiology, molecular biology, and clinical implications. Circulation 119:880–890
55. Beroukhim RS, Kruzick TL, Taylor AL, Gao D, Yetman AT (2006) Progression of aortic dilation in children with a functionally normal bicuspid aortic valve. Am J Cardiol 98:828–830
56. Nistri S, Sorbo MK, Basso C, Thiene G (2002) Bicuspid aortic valve: Abnormal aortic elastic properties. J Heart Valve Dis 11:369–373
57. Fazel SS, Mallidi HR, Lee RS, Sheehan MP, Liang D, Fleischman D, Herfkens R, Mitchell RS, Miller DC (2008) The aortopathy of bicuspid aortic valve disease has distinctive patterns and usually involves the transverse aortic arch. J Thorac Cardiovasc Surg 135:901–907
58. Bauer M, Gliech V, Siniawski H, Hetzer R (2006) Configuration of the ascending aorta in patients with bicuspid and tricuspid aortic valve disease undergoing aortic valve replacement with or without reduction aortaoplasty. J Heart Valve Dis 15:594–600
59. Sabet HY, Edwards WD, Tazelaar HD, Daly RC (1996) Congenitally bicuspid aortic valves: A surgical pathology study of 542 cases (1991 through 1996) and a literature review of 2,715 additional cases. Mayo Clin Proc 74:14–26
60. da Sa M, Moshkovitz Y, Butany J, David TE (1999) Histologic abnormalities of the ascending aorta and pulmonary trunk in patients with bicuspid aortic valve disease: clinical relevance to the Ross procedure. J Thorac Cardiovasc Surg 118:588–596
61. Niwa K, Perloff JK, Bhuta SM, Laks M, Drinkwater DC, Child JS, Miner PD (2001) Structural abnormalities of great arterial walls in congenital heart disease: light and electron microscopic analyses. Circulation 103:393–400
62. Takkenberg JJM, Klieverik LMA, Schoof PH, van Suylen RJ, van Herwerden LA, Zondervan PE, Roos-Hesselink JW, Eijkemans MJC, Yacoub JD, Bogers AJJC (2009) The Ross Procedure. A systematic review and meta-analysis. Circulation 119:222–228
63. Elkins RC, Thompson DM, Lane MM, Elkins CC, Peyton MD (2008) Ross operation: 16-year experience. J Thorac Cardiovasc Surg 136:623–630
64. da Costa FDA, Santos LR, Collatusso C, Matsuda CN, Lopes SAV, Cauduro S, Roderjan JG, Ingham E (2009) Thirteen years' experience with the Ross Operation. J Heart Valve Dis 18:84–94
65. David TE (2009) Editorial: Ross Procedure at the crossroads. Circulation 119:207–209
66. Yacoub MD, Klieverik LMA, Melina G, Edwards SER, Sarathchandra P, Bogers AJJC, Squarcia U, Sani G, van Herwerden LA, Takkenberg JJM (2006) An evaluation of the Ross Operation in adults. J Heart Valve Dis 15:531–539

67. anke T, Stierle U, Boehm JO, Botha CA, Bechtel JFM, Erasmi A, Misfeld M, Hemmer W, Rein JG, Robinson DR, Lange R, Horer J, Moritz A, Ozaslan F, Wahlers T, Franke UFW, Hetzer R, Hubler M, Aiemer G, Graf B, Ross DN, Sievers HH (2007) Autograft regurgitation and aortic root dimensions after the Ross Procedure. The German Ross Registry experience. Circulation 116(Suppl I):I-251–I-258
68. Favaloro RR, Roura P, Gomez C, Salvatori C (2008) Aortic valve replacement: Ten-year follow up of the Ross Procedure. J Heart Valve Dis 17:501–507
69. Elkins RC, Knott-Craig CJ, Howell CE (1996) Pulmonary autografts in patients with aortic annulus dysplasia. Ann Thorac Surg 1:1141–1145
70. El-Hamamsy I, Northrup WF III, Yacoub MH (2009) Anatomy-based surgical technique of the Ross procedure. In preparation
71. Ross DN (1962) Homograft replacement of the aortic valve. Lancet 2:487
72. Barratt-Boyes BG (1964) Homograft aortic valve replacement in aortic incompetence and stenosis. Thorax 19:131–150
73. Reddy VM, McElhinney DB, Phoon C, Brook MM, Hanley FL (1998) Geometric mismatch of pulmonary and aortic annuli in children undergoing the Ross procedure: Implications for surgical management and autograft funciton. J Thorac Cardiovasc Surg 115:1255–1263
74. Laudito A, Brook MM, Suleman S, Bleiweis MS, Thompson LD, Hanley FL, Reddy VM (2001) The Ross procedure in children and adults: A word of caution. J Thorac Cardiovasc Surg 122:147–153
75. Black MD, van Son JAM, Hanley FL (1995) Modified pulmonary autograft aortic root replacement: The sinus obliteration technique. Ann Thorac Surg 60:1434–1436
76. Carr-White GS, Afoke A, Birks EJ, Hughes S, O'Halloran A, Glennen S, Edwards S, Eastwood M, Yacoub MH (2000) Aortic root characteristics of human pulmonary autografts. Circulation 102(Suppl III):III-15–III-21
77. Carpentier A (1969) La valvuloplastie reconstitutive. Une nouvelle technique de valvuloplastie mitrale. Presse Med 77:251–253
78. Carpentier A, Deloche A, Dauptain J et al (1971) A new reconstructive operation for correction of mitral and tricuspid insufficiency. J Thorac Cardiovasc Surg 61:1–13
79. da Vinci, Leonardo, Codex Atlanticus, 387r
80. da Vinci, Leonardo, Windsor, 19115r
81. Carpentier A (1983) Cardiac valve surgery – the "French correction." J Thorac Cardiovasc Surg 86:323–337
82. Northrup WF III, Kshettry VR (1998) Implantation technique of aortic homograft root: Emphasis on matching the host root to the graft. Ann Thorac Surg 66:280–284
83. Duran CMG (1993) Present status of reconstructive surgery for aortic valve disease. J Card Surg 8:443–452
84. Cosgrove DM, Rosenkranz ER, Hendren WG, Bartlett JC, Stewart WJ (1991) Valuloplasty for aortic insufficiency. J Thorac Cardiovasc Surg 102:571–577
85. Stewart RD, Backer CL, Hillman ND, Lundt C, Mavroudis C (2007) The Ross operation in children: Effects of aortic annuloplasty. Ann Thorac Surg 84:1326–1330
86. Durham LA III, desJardins SE, Mosca RS, Bove EL (1997) Ross procedure with aortic root tailoring for aortic valve replacement in the pediatric population. Ann Thorac Surg 64:482–486
87. Eishi K, Nakajima S, Nakano K, Kosakai Y, Nakanishi N, Yagihara T, Takamoto S (1997) Pulmonary autograft implantation in the dilated aortic annulus. Ann Thorac Surg 63:1155–1158

88. Duran CMG, Alonso J, Gaite L, Alonso C, Cagigas JC, Marce L, Fleitas MG, Revuelta JM (1988) Long-term results of conservative repair of rheumatic aortic valve insufficiency. Eur J Cardio-thorac Surg 2:217–223
89. David TE, Omran A, Webb G, Rakowski H, Armstrong S, Sun A (1996) Geometric mismatch of the aortic and pulmonary roots causes aortic insufficiency after the Ross Procedure. J Thorac Cardiovasc Surg 112:1231–1239
90. Kollar A (2007) Valve-sparing reconstruction within the native aortic root: Integrating the Yacoub and David methods. Ann Thorac Surg 83:2241–2243
91. Sievers HH, Hanke t, Stierle U, Bechtel MF, Graf B, Robinson DR, Ross DN (2006) A critical reappraisal of the Ross operation. Renaissance of the subcoronary implantation technique? Circulation 114(Suppl I):I-504–I-511
92. Izumoto H, Kawazoe K, Kawase T, Kim H (2002) Subvalvular circular annuloplasty as a component of aortic valve repair. J Heart Valve Dis 11:383–385
93. Kazui T, Izumoto H, Nasu M, Kawazoe K (2004) Perioperative changes in dynamic aortic root morphology after yacoub's root remodeling and concomitant aortic annuloplasty. Interactive Cardiovasc Thorac Surg 3:465–469
94. Ruvolo G, Fattouch K (2009) Aortic valve-sparing root replacement from inside the aorta using three Dacron skirts preserving the native Valvsalva sinuses geometry and stabilizing the annulus. Interactive Cardiovasc Thorac Surg 8:179–181
95. Gleason TG (2005) New graft formulation and modification of the David reimplantation technique. J Thorac Cardiovasc Surg 130:601–603
96. Kasegawa H, Takahashi Y, Kawase M et al (1996) Reconstruction of dilated aortic annulus using short tubular Dacron graft for aortic root replacement by aortic homograft – A solution for size mismatch. J Heart Valve Disease 5:178–180
97. Lansac E, Di Centa I, Varnous S et al (2005) External aortic annuloplasty ring for valve-sparing procedures. Ann Thorac Surg 79:356–358
98. Lansac E, Di Centa ID, Bonnet N et al (2006) Aortic prosthetic ring annuloplasty: a susefula djucnt to a standardized aortic valve-sparing procedure? Eur J Cardio-thorac Surg 29:537–544
99. Lansac E, Di Centa ID, Raoux F et al (2008) An expansible aortic ring for a physiological approach of aortic valve repair. Circulation 118(Suppl 2):S858
100. Barrett-Boyes BG (1965) A method for preparing and inserting a homograft aortic valve. Brit J Surg 52:847–856
101. Pigula FA, Paolillo J, McGrath M, Gandhi SK, Myers JL, Rebovich B, Siewers RD (2001) Aortopulmonary size discrepancy is not a contraindication to the pediatric Ross operation. Ann Thorac Surg 72:1610–1614
102. Luciani GB, Casali G, Favaro A, Prioli MA, Barozzi L, Santini F, Mazzucco A (2003) Fate of the aortic root late after ross operation. Circulation 108(Suppl II):II-61–II-67
103. Rahimtoola SH (1978) The problem of valve prosthesis-patient mismatch. Circulation 58:20–24
104. Pibarot P, Dumesnil JG (2009) Prosthetic heart valves. Selection of the optimal prosthesis and long-term management. Circulation 119:1034–1048
105. Kvidal P, Bergstrom R, Horte LG, Stahle E (2000) Observed and relative survival after aortic valve replacement. J Am Coll Cardiol 35:747–756
106. Puvimanasinghe JPA, Takkenberg JJM, Eijkemans MJC, Steyerberg EW, van Herwerden LA, Grunkemeier GL, Habbema JDF, Bogers AJJC (2005) Prognosis after aortic valve replacement with the carpentier-Edwards pericardial valve: Use of microsimulation. Ann Thorac Surg 80:825–831
107. Mihaljevic T, Nowicki ER, Rjeswaran J, Blackstone EH, Lagazzi L, Thomas J, Lytle BW, Cosgrove DM (2008) Survival after valve replacement for aortic stenosis: Implications for decision making. J Thorac Cardiovasc Surg 135:1270–1279

108. van Geldorp MWA, Jamieson WRE, Kappetein AP, Ye J, Fradet GJ, Eijkemans MJC, Grunkemeier GL, Bogers AJJC, Takkenberg JJM (2009) Patient outcome after aortic valve replacement with a mechanical or biological prosthesis: Weighing lifetime anticoagulant-related event risk against reoperation risk. J Thorac Cardiovasc Surg 137:881–886
109. Nicks R, Cartmill T, Bernstein L (1970) Hypoplasia of the aortic root. The problem of aortic valve replacement. Thorax 25:339–346
110. Yener A, Ozdemir A, Sinav A, Yener N, Hauf E (1993) New technique to enlarge the aortic annulus. Ann Thorac Surg 55:1260–1261
111. Dhareshwar J, Sundt TM III, Dearani JA, Schaff HV, Cook DJ, Orszulak TA (2007) Aortic root enlargement: What are the operative risks? J Thorac Cardiovasc Surg 134:916–924
112. Hopkins RA (2006) Aortic annuloplasty with aortic root reconstruction to prevent patient-prosthesis mismatch. J Heart Valve Dis 15:488–493
113. Hopkins RA (2005) The small aortic root: Surgical techniques for annulus enlargement. In: Hopkins RA (ed) Cardiac reconstructions with allograft tissues 2005. Springer, New York
114. Manouguian S, Seybold-Epting W (1979) Patch enlargement of the aortic valve ring by extending the aortic incision into the anterior mitral leaflet. J Thorac Cardiovasc Surg 78:402–412
115. Rittenhouse EA, Sauvage LR, Stamm SJ, Mansfield PB, Hall DG, Herndon PS (1979) Radical enlargement of the aortic root and outflow tract to allow valve replacement. Ann Thorac Surg 27:367–373
116. Molina JE (2002) Enlargement of the aortic annulus using a double-patch technique: a safe and effective method. Ann Thorac Surg 73:667–670
117. Okuyama H, Hashimoto K, Kurosawa H, Tanaka K, Sakamoto Y Shiratori K (2005) Midterm results of Manouguian double valve replacement: Comparison with standard double valve replacement. J Thorac Cardiovasc Surg 129:869–874
118. Milsom FP, Doty DB (1993) Aortic valve replacement and mitral valve repair with allograft. J Card Surg 8:350–357
119. Dearani JA, Orszulak TA, Schaff HV, Daly RC, Anderson BJ, Danielson GK (1997) Result of allograft aortic valve replacement for complex endocarditis. J Thorac Cardiovasc Surg 113:285–291
120. Sabik JF, Lytle BW, Blackstone EH, Marullo AGM, Pettersson GB, Cosgrove DM (2002) Aortic root replacement with cryopreserved allograft for prosthetic valve endocarditis. Ann Thorac Surg 74:650–659
121. Yankah AC, Pasic M, Klose H, Siniawski HS, Weng Y, Hetzer (2005) Homograft reconstruction of the aortic root for endocarditis with periannular abscess: a 17-year study. Eur J Cardiothorac Surg 28:69–75
122. Peterson MK, Borger MA, Feindel CM, David TE (2007) Aortic annular enlargement during aortic valve replacement: Improving results with time. Ann Thorac Surg 83:2044–2049
123. Nunez L, Aguado MG, Pinto AG, Larrea JL (1983) Enlargement of the aortic annulus by resecting the commissure between the left and noncoronary cusps. Tex Heart Inst J 10:301–303
124. Borowski A, Kurt M (2008) A modification to the Manouguian Aortoplasty. Tex Heart Inst J 35:425–427
125. Konno S, Imai Y, Iida Y, Nakajima M, Tatsuno K (1975) A new method for prosthetic valve replacement in congenital aortic stenosis associated with hypoplasia of the aortic valve ring. J Thorac Cardiovasc Surg 70:909–917
126. Rastan H, Koncz J (1975) Aortoventriculoplasty. A new technique for the treatment of left ventricular outlow tract obstruction. J. Thorac Cardiovasc Surg 71:920–927

127. Misbach GA, Turley K, Ullyot DJ, Ebert PA (1982) Left ventricular enlargement by the Konno procedure. J Thorac Cardiovasc Surg 84:696–703
128. Hopkins RA (2005) Aortoventriculoplasty with aortic allograft. In: Hopkins RA (ed) Cardiac Reconstructions with allograft tissues 2005. Springer, New York
129. Yamaguchi M, Ohashi H, Imai M, Oshima Y, Hosokawa Y (1991) Bilateral enlargement of the aortic valve ring for malve replacement in children. New operative technique. J Thorac Cardiovasc Surg 102:202–206
130. Otaki M, Oku H, Nakamoto S, Kitayama H, Ueda M, Matsumoto T (1997) Two-directional aortic annular enlargement for aortic valve replacement in the small aortic annulus. Ann Thorac Surg 63:261–263
131. Reddy VM, Rajasinghe HA, Teitel DF, Haas GS, Hanley FL (1996) Aortoventriculoplasty with the pulmonary autograft: The Ross-Konno procedure. J Thorac Cardiovasc Surg 111:158–167
132. Starnes VA, Luciani GB, Wells WJ, Allen RB, Lewis AB (1996) Aortic root replacement with the pulmonary autograft in children with complex left heart obstruction. Ann Thorac Surg 62:442–449
133. Elkins RC, Lane MM, McCue C (2001) Ross operation in children: Late results. J Heart Valve Dis 10:736–774
134. Pasquali SK, Marino BS, Kaltman JR, Schissler AJ, Wernovsky G, Cohen MS, Spray TL, Tanel RE (2008) Rhythm and conduction disturbances at midterm follow-up after the Ross procedure in infants, children, and young adults. Ann thorac Surg 85:2072–2078
135. Al-Halees Z, Pieters F, Qadoura F, Shahid M, Al-Amri M, Al-Fadley F (2002) The Ross procedure is the procedure of choice for congenital aortic valve disease. J Thorac Cardiovasc Surg 123:437–442
136. Vouhe PR, Neveux JY (1991) Surgical management of diffuse subaortic stenosis: An integrated approach. Ann Thorac Surg 52:654–662
137. Yacoub M, Omuzo O, Riedel B, Radley-Smith R (1999) Mobilization of the left and right fibrous trigones for relief of severe left ventricular outflow obstruction. J Thorac Cardiovasc Surg 117:126–133
138. Doty DB (1997) Posterior enlargement of left ventricular outflow tract (Nicks-Nunez opration). In: Doty DB (ed) Cardiac surgery operative tehcnique 1997. Mosby-Year Book, St. Louis

Correction of aortic valve incompetence combined with ascending aortic aneurysm by relocation of the aortic valve plane through a short-length aortic graft replacement

R. Hetzer, N. Solowjowa, M. Kukucka, C. Knosalla, R. Röttgen

Introduction

Aortic aneurysms grow not only in diameter but also in length. In the ascending aorta, such elongation may cause aortic valve incompetence in an otherwise normal valve by dislocation of the aortic valve plane towards the left ventricle and subsequent valve dislocation, causing leaflet prolapse. Loss of the sinotubular junction by aneurysmal widening of the aortic root may further add to this mechanism.

A method is described for the correction of both aneurysm formation and aortic valve incompetence by relocating the displaced aortic valve annulus plane to its normal position. This is achieved by replacing the ascending aorta with a vascular graft considerably shorter than the original aorta and with a graft diameter the size of the inner aortic valve annulus, thus recreating a supravalvular narrowing at the site of the sinotubular junction.

Pathophysiological considerations

Longitudinal growth in aneurysmal disease affects the ascending aorta in an asymmetric fashion since this aortic segment is fixed to the pulmonary artery on the left side. Therefore, elongation is more pronounced on the right, "free" side, thus shifting the aortic valve annulus plane from its originally oblique position relative to the body long axis into a more parallel position (Fig. 1). The resulting dislocation of the otherwise normal aortic valve may lead to leaflet prolapse, in particular of the noncoronary leaflet, thus causing valve incompetence. This mechanism may be aggravated by loss of the supravalvular narrowing at the site of the sinotubular junction caused by aneurysmal aortic widening. It is well accepted that this narrowing above the aortic valve sinuses is essential for aortic valve leaflet coaptation and valve closure.

The method presented aims at relocating the aortic valve plane to its original position and orientation and restoring an adequate sinotubular junction.

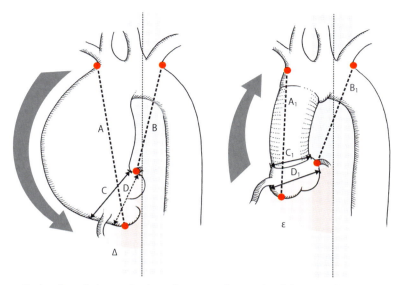

Fig. 1. Schematic drawing of the mechanism of asymmetric growth of the ascending aorta in aneurysmal disease and shift of the aortic root toward the left and to a position almost parallel to the vertebral column (left). "Relocation" of the aortic valve plane upwards and into a more oblique position by a relatively short ascending graft with a caliber equaling the inner diameter of the aortic valve, thus, creating a new sinotubular junction (right). The dimensions measured by CT scan are indicated: (A and A_1) from the deepest point of the noncoronary sinus to the inferior rim of the take-off of the brachiocephalic trunk; (B and B_1) from the left coronary ostium to the lateral rim of the take-off of the left subclavian artery; (C and C_1) the diameter at the presumed and the new sinotubular junction; (D and D_1) the diameter at the level of the coronary ostia; and the angles Δ and ε between the aortic root plane and the long axis of the vertebral column

Surgical technique

All operations were performed via median sternotomy and on total cardiopulmonary bypass with normothermia except in three patients with concomitant aortic arch replacement, in whom deep hypothermia (16 °C), low flow perfusion via the femoral artery and selective head perfusion via the brachicephalic trunk were applied. In the cases with isolated ascending aorta aneurysms, the aortic arch and the right atrium were cannulated and a left ventricular vent catheter was introduced via the right upper pulmonary vein. Except in the cases with concomitant arch replacement, the ascending aorta was clamped just below the take-off of the brachiocephalic trunc and the ascending aneurysm was incised in a longitudinal fashion; this incision was directed toward the noncoronary sinus to a point half way between the cranial tips of the neighboring commissures. The heart was arrested with blood cardioplegia infused via the coronary ostia and this cardioplegia infusion was repeated every 15 to 20 min. The aortic valve was carefully inspected and tested for potential competence. When the valve was found to be normal and the leaflets well coapting, the decision was made to preserve the valve. The inner diameter of the valve annulus was measured and a straight Dacron graft with a caliber equaling the inner diameter was chosen. This graft was sewn onto the aorta approximately 5 mm above the commissures with a continuous suture of 4-0 polypropylene. The competence of the aortic valve was tested by infusing blood cardioplegic solution into the graft under pressure and by pulling the aortic valve annulus toward the arch. When aortic valve competence was proven, the graft was then cut to appropriate length, which was considerably shorter than the original aorta, to a degree that aortic valve competence was maintained under cardioplegia pressure infusion. The distal anastomosis was sewn to the distal aorta with a 4-0 polypropylene running suture. The graft inclusion technique with wrapping of the aneurysmal wall around the implanted graft was used in all cases. Intraoperative transesophageal echocardiography (Fig. 2) was applied in all cases to document the degree of aortic valve incompetence and the morphology of the aortic root before and after the procedure.

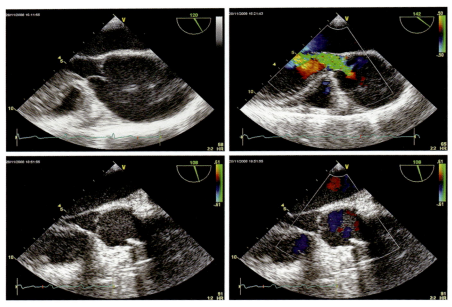

Fig. 2. Intraoperative transesophageal echocardiograms before and after the relocation procedure. The preoperative echo shows extensive ascending aortic aneurysm, loss of the sinotubular junction and normal valve leaflets (above left). The Doppler echo shows massive aortic incompetence (above right). After the procedure there is a new sinotubular narrowing at the proximal anastomosis of the graft (below left) and in Doppler studies there is no aortic incompetence (below right)

Routine investigations

Echocardiographic studies were performed in all patients before, during, and at long-term follow-up after the procedure. In 22 patients, computed tomography (CT) was performed before and after the operation, and the dimensions that were found important for this procedure were measured. The CT scans were performed with a Siemens Somatom Definition machine and the following parameters were measured in volume reconstruction CT data: distance from the noncoronary leaflet sinus to the ostium of the brachiocephalic trunc (A), distance from the deepest point of the left coronary ostium to the inferior rim of the ostium of the left subclavian artery (B), diameter of the sinotubular junction (C), diameter of the aortic root at the level of the coronary ostia (D), and the angle between the coronary ostial plane and the longitudinal plane of the spinal column (E). The data of these measurements are given in Table 1.

Patients

The initial series of this procedure as described here comprises 32 patients (17 men and 15 women). Ages ranged from 7 to 82 years (median 64 years). All had expanding ascending aortic aneurysms with aortic elongation and all had significant degrees of aortic valve incompetence. All patients survived the procedure; two patients died after discharge from the hospital from causes unrelated to the heart and to the procedure. Both these patients were older than 70 years. Follow-up was complete in all cases and follow-up time ranged from 1 to 128 months (median 29 months). Aortic

Table 1. Results of the dimensions measured in CT scans before and after the procedure in 22 cases. There was considerable but asymmetric shortening of the ascending aorta by graft replacement which was more pronounced on the right side (**A**) as compared to the left (**B**). The sinotubular junction became smaller, as determined by the graft at the proximal anastomosis (**C**). Even the diameter of the aortic root became smaller (**D**) and the angle between the aortic root plane and the longitudinal axis of the spine became wider (Δ, ε)

		Preop. (mm)	Postop. (mm)	Change (%)
A	NC sinus/rim of brachioceph. trunc	117.5 ± 10.8	96.5 ± 12.2	−22.0 ± 12.2
B	Left coron. ostium/rim left art. subclavia	100.4 ± 13.4	86.7 ± 12.8	−15.7 ± 9.2
C	⌀ sinotubular junction	47.7 ± 7.6	26.6 ± 2.3	−79.5 ± 21.7
D	⌀ aortic root at coronary ostia	43.9 ± 6.0	35.2 ± 3.9	−24.1 ± 13.0
Δ, ε	angle sagittal spine plane/aortic root plane	46.5 ± 8.3°	67.9 ± 13.3°	+32.3 ± 12.4

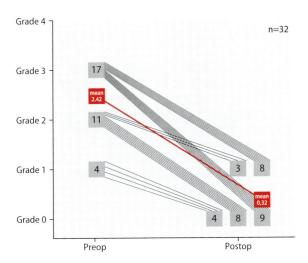

Fig. 3. Aortic valve incompetence (AI) determined by echocardiography. Most cases had AI grade 2 and 3 before the operation, with a mean of 2.42. After the operation, at the last follow-up, there were 11 cases with AI grade 1 and most had no measurable AI; mean was 0.32. There were three cases where AI went only from grade 2 to grade 1

valve incompetence regressed from a mean of 2.42 to 0.42 after the operation and to 0.32 at later follow-up (Fig. 3). Hitherto, there has been no case of a patient needing reoperation.

The CT measurements (Table 1) indicated considerable shortening of the distance between the aortic root and the aortic arch by a mean of 12% on the left side (dimension B) and by 19% on the right side (dimension A), thus proving the shift of the aortic root upwards and to a more "normal" oblique position relative to the long axis of the spinal column taken as a fixed structure for orientation. This is also proven by the widening of the angle between the transsectional plane of the aortic root and the spinal column by 21°. The creation of a sinotubular junction by the relatively small diameter of the graft (dimension C) also had the effect of a reduction of the width of the root itself at the level of the coronary ostia (dimension D), i.e., the widest extension of the sinuses.

Comments

The procedure described here was performed for the first time in 1998. This was in a case of ascending aortic aneurysm and aortic valve incompetence originally planned for ascending aortic and aortic valve replacement. During the operation, an entirely normal aortic valve with well coapting and tender leaflets was found. When trying to understand the reason for the valve dysfunction in this case, it was recognized that by elevating the valve at its noncoronary sinus the valve became competent. Simple supracoronary replacement of the ascending aorta with a graft shorter than the original ascending aorta itself in fact resulted in complete valve competence. Since this initial case, which showed favorable long-term results, a consecutive series of the relocation procedure has been added. The principle of the assumed mechanism and of the procedure was first mentioned in a review article in 2007 [1] and meanwhile oral presentation has been accepted for the 2010 annual meeting of the Society of Thoracic Surgeons [2].

The mechanism of prolapse of mainly the noncoronary leaflet by aortic lengthening and distortion of the aortic base follows a mechanism similar to aortic incompetence in acute type-A dissection when the inner layer of the aorta bearing one or two of the aortic valve commissures – usually the ones neighboring the noncoronary cusp – shifts toward the left ventricular cavity. In this setting, valve competence can be restored by "resuspension" of the aortic valve in combination with ascending aorta replacement.

For chronic aortic aneurysms, restoration of not only the location and orientation may be important but also the restoration of a sinotubular junction which is often flattened by the aneurysm. The aortic narrowing at the sinotubular junction, just above the aortic valve commissures, is of great importance for well-functioning coaptation of the valve leaflets and valve closure. This was recognized by Leonardo da Vinci [3] and several modern investigators [4–6].

In our technique, we determined the width of the sinotubular junction by the caliber of the implanted graft prosthesis, which was decided upon according to the inner diameter of the aortic valve annulus as measured during the operation.

In the combination of supracoronary ascending aneurysm and elongation of the aorta combined with aortic valve incompetence in a completely normal valve, the presented simple concept of "relocating" the aortic valve plane to its normal position and orientation by a relatively short ascending aortic graft enabled lasting valve competence to be restored, thus avoiding valve replacement or complicated valve repair procedures.

The restoration of a supravalvular narrowing at the site of the sinotubular junction is presumably important for valve closure. The effect of relocating the width of the root itself at the widest extension of the sinuses in a kind of "remodeling" of the aortic root was also shown. The procedure has not been attempted in bicuspid valves or in annulo-aortic ectasia of the Marfan type. However, it may well be that by further modifications of the technique those types of aortic root disease may be approached successfully in the future.

References

1. Hetzer R, Pasic M, Eichstädt H (2007) Chirurgie der Aorta ascendens und des Aortenbogens. Herzmedizin 24:175–182
2. Hetzer R, Mulahasanovic S, Solowjowa N, Röttgen R (2010) Succesful correction of aortic valve incompetence and ascending aortic aneurysm by relocation of the aortic valve plane through a short aortic graft replacement. Accepted for presentation at the 46th Annual Meeting of the Society of Thoracic Surgeons, Fort Lauderdale, FL, Jan 25–27, 2010
3. Keele KD, Pedretti C (eds) (1978–1980) Leonardo da Vinci: Corpus of the Anatomical Studies in the Collection of Her Majesty, the Queen, at Windsor Castle. Johnson Reprint, Harcourt Brace Jovanovich, London, New York
4. Demers P, Miller DC (2004) Simple modification of "T.-David-V" valve sparing aortic root replacement to create graft pseudosinuses. Ann Thorac Surg 78:1479–1481
5. Grande-Allen KJ, Cochran RP, Reinhall PG, Kunzelmann KS (2000) Re-creation of sinuses is important for sparing the aortic valve: a finite element study. J Thorac Cardiovasc Surg 119:753–763
6. Zehr KJ, Thubrikar MJ, Gong GG, Headrick JR, Robicsek F (2000) Clinical introduction of a novel prosthesis for valve-preserving aortic root reconstruction for annuloaortic ectasia. J Thorac Cardiovasc Surg 120:692–698

Using BioGlue to achieve hemostasis in aortic root surgery

S. A. LeMaire, J. S. Coselli

Rationale for using BioGlue

Aortic root operations involve the creation of fragile suture lines that become difficult to access once the repair is complete. Furthermore, these procedures involve working with aortic tissue that is extremely fragile, especially in patients with acute aortic dissection or connective tissue disorders. Consequently, securing hemostasis during these operations remains a significant challenge. In a multicenter study of 151 patients with Marfan syndrome who underwent aortic root replacement, 9% of patients required mediastinal reexploration to treat bleeding [34]. In another recent report, the incidence of bleeding requiring reoperation was 12.9% in a series of 132 patients who underwent root replacement with porcine aortic root xenografts [25].

There are many techniques and adjuncts used to prevent bleeding after aortic root surgery [11]. One adjunct that has been particularly useful is BioGlue (CryoLife, Inc., Kennesaw, GA, USA), a surgical adhesive composed of 45% purified bovine serum albumin and 10% glutaraldehyde, which mix within the delivery tip during application [36]. BioGlue reaches maximum bonding strength in 2 to 3 min and demonstrates excellent tensile and shear strengths. Because BioGlue is stored and used at room temperature and requires no solution preparation before use, it is rapidly available for use in the operating room. One drawback of BioGlue is that it requires a bloodless field to adhere, so it is not useful for controlling active bleeding.

Balancing potential benefits with risks

The decision to use BioGlue should be based on careful consideration of the agent's potential benefits and associated risks. Many groups have reported subjective benefits of using BioGlue to facilitate aortic repairs. BioGlue appears to improve hemostasis, strengthen weak tissues, provide anastomotic support, and enhance the durability of repair [10, 16, 30]; these benefits are especially pronounced in patients with marked tissue fragility, including those with connective tissue disorders or acute dissection. Additional purported early benefits of using BioGlue include reduced bleeding, decreased transfusion requirements, shortened operative times, and shortened hospital lengths of stay [7, 10].

Although BioGlue may offer benefits, it poses several potential risks that need to be considered [26]. Several reports suggest that BioGlue may severely injure the aortic tissue, ultimately leading to redissection or pseudoaneurysm formation [5, 13, 15, 21, 28, 29, 35]. Ngaage and colleagues [29], for example, recently reported nearly circumferential disruption of both the proximal and distal anastomoses after ascending aortic dissection repair. Reports after reoperations have described necrotic, fibrosed, and excessively thinned aortic tissue found at the site of adhesive application [5, 22, 28]. These complications may be the result of direct tissue toxicity, an intense local inflammatory response, or a mismatch between adhesive and tissue compliance. Azadani and colleagues [1] recently studied BioGlue's mechanical properties in the context of aortic root replacement and found that BioGlue's stiffness was at least 30 times greater than that of the other products tested, and its elasticity was significantly less than that of aortic tissue or commonly used aortic replacement conduits. In considering the clinical implications of their findings, the authors suggested that the high stiffness of BioGlue may cause elevated wall stress, which could weaken the tissue and lead to pseudoaneurysm formation.

When using BioGlue during root repair, surgeons should take extra care to avoid the phrenic nerves, because the glutaraldehyde component of BioGlue has been reported to be directly toxic to nerves [8, 18, 24, 33]. The concerns about toxicity to nerves also apply to cardiac conduction tissue [24]. BioGlue has also been linked to the development of vascular strictures and impaired aortic growth; therefore, it is not recommended for use during aortic root operations in children [5, 22].

Systemic embolization of adhesive fragments is another concern, especially given the proximity of the coronary ostia during aortic root repair. Several reports have raised concerns about adhesive leaking into the aortic lumen, resulting in embolization or valve dysfunction [2, 12, 17, 19, 20, 27]. Strokes and myocardial infarctions caused by polymerized glue emboli have been found on autopsy, and polymerized glue emboli have been extracted from patients with acute limb ischemia [4, 6, 17, 27]. There are several potential mechanisms by which adhesives may cause embolization, the most obvious of which is inadvertent direct spillage into the aortic lumen (despite precautions); this can result from technical error, so careful attention and proper training of the surgical team will minimize this risk. As originally suggested by Carrel and associates [6], glue can also leak into the aortic lumen through suture-line needle holes even when the glue is properly applied in accordance with the manufacturer's instructions [23]. Although the number of reported cases involving adhesive embolization remains low, the incidence of adhesive embolization may be underestimated, because adhesive embolization is rarely suspected as a cause when ischemic complications arise, and postmortem microscopy examinations are not routinely performed in patients who succumb to complications of aortic root repairs.

Given the well-documented risks involved in using BioGlue during aortic repairs, we do not recommend doing this routinely; however, during certain complex operations – especially in cases of acute aortic dissection – the benefits of using BioGlue may truly outweigh the risks. Thus, the risk-benefit ratio for using BioGlue should be carefully considered on a patient-by-patient basis. BioGlue should be used only when medically necessary to secure hemostasis and reinforce weak tissues. When the use of BioGlue is warranted by the clinical situation, several technical considerations can be applied to make the use of this product as safe as possible.

Technical aspects of using BioGlue during aortic root repair

The two principal clinical scenarios in which we use BioGlue are
- when repairing the acutely dissected aortic root and
- when performing valve-sparing or valve-replacing aortic root replacement [9].

In both situations, several technical steps and precautions can be taken to maximize efficacy and minimize complications associated with using this product.

When repairing the dissected aortic root, we use BioGlue to obliterate the false lumen and reinforce the fragile suture lines. Because blood interferes with tissue bonding, all clotted and fresh blood is removed from the false lumen to create a dry field. The dissecting membrane is carefully tacked to the outer wall with 6-0 sutures to keep the walls aligned during glue application. Moist sponges are used to protect adjacent structures, the aortic valve leaflets, and the coronary ostia from unintentional adhesive run-off during BioGlue application. The left main coronary artery can also be protected by the insertion of a red rubber catheter or another soft, flexible cannula to occlude the ostium [31]. To reduce the chance of glue leaking into the lumen while being applied to the suture line, it is important to temporarily stop the left ventricular sump suction [16, 23, 36].

Before BioGlue is applied, the applicator tip is primed to evacuate air and ensure the proper mixing of the components. This adhesive has a very low viscosity, making it difficult to fully control during application, particularly if it is rapidly released. Slowly releasing the glue during application tends to increase its initial viscosity and improve control. BioGlue is released so that a thin (approximately 2-mm) layer fills the false lumen, while spillage

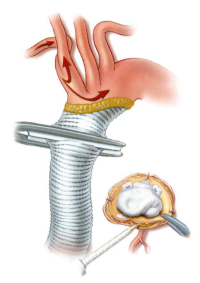

Fig. 1. Drawing illustrating the use of glue during repair of an acutely dissected aortic root. The arrows indicate the direction of arterial inflow from the cardiopulmonary bypass pump. In this case, a beveled hemi-arch repair has been performed during hypothermic circulatory arrest, while antegrade cerebral perfusion was delivered via a right axillary artery cannula. Glue is being used to obliterate the false lumen of the dissected aortic root. Note the fine sutures keeping the layers of the aorta aligned and the protective moist sponge covering the aortic valve and coronary ostia. Reproduced from LeMaire SA, Carter SA, Coselli JS (2008) Surgical adhesives. In: Coselli JS, LeMaire SA (eds) Aortic arch surgery: principles, strategies and outcomes. Wiley-Blackwell, Chichester, UK, p 244. Used with permission

outside the aorta or into the true lumen is carefully avoided (Fig. 1). Any spilled adhesive is rapidly evacuated with the wall suction (never with the cell saver or pump suctions). The walls of the aorta do not need to be pressed together; in fact, the goal is to maintain an even layer of glue between the tissue layers as it bonds to the aorta and polymerizes. After the glue has been allowed to set for 2 to 3 min, the protective sponges are removed. The true lumen and aortic valve leaflets are inspected to ensure that there is no glue there. Once the dissected layers of the aortic wall are reapproximated, the proximal anastomosis between the prosthetic graft and the sinotubular junction is performed. Rather than incorporating felt strips into the repair – a technique used by several surgeons [3, 32] – we often use pledgeted mattress sutures to circumferentially reinforce the anastomosis after completing the primary suture line. We then apply a thin layer of BioGlue to the outer surface of the distal suture line before removing the aortic clamp.

We occasionally also use BioGlue when performing aortic root replacement procedures. This is especially helpful in patients with severely weakened aortic tissue, such as those with connective tissue disorders. In these repairs, the glue is applied to the outer surface of the completed annular, aortic, and coronary suture lines to provide reinforcement and reduce bleeding. To avoid inadvertent coronary compression or kinking, care is taken to minimize the amount of glue placed around the coronary buttons [16].

Regardless of the type of the lesion being treated, although BioGlue is an excellent adjunct for creating a secure anastomosis, it is not helpful for controlling active bleeding once flow has been restored. In patients with active bleeding, we advocate using additional sutures to achieve hemostasis; after the bleeding has been controlled, adhesive can be used to strengthen the repair. In cases of severe bleeding that cannot be controlled by conventional means, BioGlue can be applied to a bleeding site during a brief period of hypothermic circulatory arrest [14].

Summary

BioGlue is one of the most widely used adhesives in aortic root surgery. Although there is limited objective evidence to support using BioGlue during aortic root operations, many surgeons have found that adhesives can be extremely useful as adjuncts for securing hemostasis, particularly in patients with acute aortic dissection. Because of the potential associated risks, BioGlue should be used only when medically necessary to facilitate hemostasis and reinforce weak tissues. There remains a critical need for new biocompatible adhesives that are nontoxic and rapidly achieve excellent bonding strength; such an adhesive would be an ideal adjunct for aortic root repairs.

Acknowledgments. The authors thank Scott A. Weldon, MA, CMI, and Carol P. Larson, CMI, for creating the medical illustration and Stephen N. Palmer, PhD, ELS, for invaluable editorial support.

References

1. Azadani AN, Matthews PB, Ge L, Shen Y, Jhun CS, Guy TS, Tseng EE (2009) Mechanical properties of surgical glues used in aortic root replacement. Ann Thorac Surg 87:1154–1160
2. Baciewicz FA Jr (2006) Mechanical aortic valve malfunction: an intraoperative BioGlue complication. J Thorac Cardiovasc Surg 131:761–762
3. Bavaria JE, Brinster DR, Gorman RC, Woo YJ, Gleason T, Pochettino A (2002) Advances in the treatment of acute type A dissection: an integrated approach. Ann Thorac Surg 74:S1848–1852

4. Bernabeu E, Castella M, Barriuso C, Mulet J (2005) Acute limb ischemia due to embolization of biological glue after repair of type A aortic dissection. Interact Cardiovasc Thorac Surg 4:329–331
5. Bingley JA, Gardner MA, Stafford EG, Mau TK, Pohlner PG, Tam RK, Jalali H, Tesar PJ, O'Brien MF (2000) Late complications of tissue glues in aortic surgery. Ann Thorac Surg 69:1764–1768
6. Carrel T, Maurer M, Tkebuchava T, Niederhauser U, Schneider J, Turina MI (1995) Embolization of biologic glue during repair of aortic dissection. Ann Thorac Surg 60:1118–1120
7. Chao HH, Torchiana DF (2003) BioGlue: albumin/glutaraldehyde sealant in cardiac surgery. J Card Surg 18:500–503
8. Chen YF, Chou SH, Chiu CC, Lin YT, Wang HJ (1994) Use of glutaraldehyde solution in the treatment of acute aortic dissections. Ann Thorac Surg 58:833–835
9. Coselli JS, LeMaire SA, Köksoy C (2000) Thoracic aortic anastomoses. Oper Tech Thorac Cardiovasc Surg 5:259–276
10. Coselli JS, Bavaria JE, Fehrenbacher J, Stowe CL, Macheers SK, Gundry SR (2003) Prospective randomized study of a protein-based tissue adhesive used as a hemostatic and structural adjunct in cardiac and vascular anastomotic repair procedures. J Am Coll Surg 197:243–252
11. Coselli JS, Conklin LD, LeMaire SA (2003) An effective strategy for optimizing hemostasis following aortic root replacement. J Vasc Br 2:183–186
12. Devbhandari MP, Chaudhery Q, Duncan AJ (2006) Acute intraoperative malfunction of aortic valve due to surgical glue. Ann Thorac Surg 81:1499–1500
13. Downing SW (2003) What are the risks of using biologic glues? Ann Thorac Surg 75:1063
14. Dunst KM, Antretter H, Bonatti J (2005) Control of suture hole bleeding after aortic valve replacement by application of BioGlue during circulatory arrest. Int Heart J 46:175–179
15. Erasmi AW, Sievers HH, Wolschlager C (2002) Inflammatory response after BioGlue application. Ann Thorac Surg 73:1025–1026
16. Fehrenbacher JW, Siderys H (2006) Use of BioGlue in aortic surgery: proper application techniques and results in 92 patients. Heart Surg Forum 9:E794–799
17. Guerrero MA, Cox M, Lumsden AB, Reardon M, Howell J (2004) Embolus of surgical adhesive to the extremities causing acute ischemia: report of two cases. J Vasc Surg 40:571–573
18. Hammond G (1994) Use of glutaraldehyde solution in the treatment of acute aortic dissections (invited commentary). Ann Thorac Surg 58:836
19. Hoschtitzky JA, Crawford L, Brack M, Au J (2004) Acute coronary syndrome following repair of aortic dissection. Eur J Cardiothorac Surg 26:860–862
20. Karimi M, Kerber RE, Everett JE (2005) Mechanical aortic valve malfunction: an intraoperative BioGlue complication. J Thorac Cardiovasc Surg 129:1442–1443
21. Kazui T, Washiyama N, Bashar AH, Terada H, Suzuki K, Yamashita K, Takinami M (2001) Role of biologic glue repair of proximal aortic dissection in the development of early and midterm redissection of the aortic root. Ann Thorac Surg 72:509–514
22. LeMaire SA, Schmittling ZC, Coselli JS, Undar A, Deady BA, Clubb FJ Jr, Fraser CD Jr (2002) BioGlue surgical adhesive impairs aortic growth and causes anastomotic strictures. Ann Thorac Surg 73:1500–1505
23. LeMaire SA, Carter SA, Won T, Wang X, Conklin LD, Coselli JS (2005) The threat of adhesive embolization: BioGlue leaks through needle holes in aortic tissue and prosthetic grafts. Ann Thorac Surg 80:106–110

24. LeMaire SA, Ochoa LN, Conklin LD, Schmittling ZC, Undar A, Clubb FJ Jr, Li Wang X, Coselli JS, Fraser CD Jr (2007) Nerve and conduction tissue injury caused by contact with BioGlue. J Surg Res 143:286–293
25. LeMaire SA, Green SY, Sharma K, Cheung CK, Sameri A, Tsai PI, Adams G, Coselli JS (2009) Aortic root replacement with stentless porcine xenografts: early and late outcomes in 132 patients. Ann Thorac Surg 87:503–512, discussion 512–513
26. Luthra S, Theodore S, Tatoulis J (2008) Bioglue: a word of caution. Ann Thorac Surg 86:1055–1056, author reply 1056–1057
27. Mahmood Z, Cook DS, Luckraz H, O'Keefe P (2004) Fatal right ventricular infarction caused by Bioglue coronary embolism. J Thorac Cardiovasc Surg 128:770–771
28. Mastroroberto P, Chello M, Onorati F, Renzulli A (2005) Embolisation, inflammatory reaction and persistent patent false lumen: is biological glue really effective in repair of type A aortic dissection? Eur J Cardiothorac Surg 27:531–532
29. Ngaage DL, Edwards WD, Bell MR, Sundt TM (2005) A cautionary note regarding long-term sequelae of biologic glue. J Thorac Cardiovasc Surg 129:937–938
30. Passage J, Jalali H, Tam RK, Harrocks S, O'Brien MF (2002) BioGlue Surgical Adhesive – an appraisal of its indications in cardiac surgery. Ann Thorac Surg 74: 432–437
31. Raanani E, Georghiou GP, Kogan A, Wandwi B, Shapira Y, Vidne BA (2004) 'BioGlue' for the repair of aortic insufficiency in acute aortic dissection. J Heart Valve Dis 13:734–737
32. Shiono M, Hata M, Sezai A, Negishi N, Sezai Y (2005) Surgical results in acute type A aortic dissection. Ann Thorac Cardiovasc Surg 11:29–34
33. Vasseur B, Hammond GL (1989) New technique for repair of ascending thoracic aortic dissections. Ann Thorac Surg 47:318–319
34. Volguina IV, Miller DC, Lemaire SA, Palmero LC, Wang XL, Connolly HM, Sundt TM III, Bavaria JE, Dietz HC, Milewicz DM, Coselli JS (2009) Valve-sparing and valve-replacing techniques for aortic root replacement in patients with Marfan syndrome: analysis of early outcome. J Thorac Cardiovasc Surg 137:641–649
35. Yoshitatsu M, Nomura F, Katayama A, Tamura K, Katayama K, Ihara K, Nakashima Y (2004) Pathologic findings of aortic redissection after glue repair of proximal aorta. J Thorac Cardiovasc Surg 127:593–595
36. Zehr KJ (2007) Use of bovine albumin-glutaraldehyde glue in cardiovascular surgery. Ann Thorac Surg 84:1048–1052

Endocarditis

Challenges in the surgical management of infective endocarditis

C.-A. Mestres, J.M. Miró

Introduction

Infective endocarditis (IE) is an uncommon disease. A key issue in IE is that it is still associated with significant morbidity and mortality [1]. It is uncommon as its current incidence rates vary between 2.4/100 000 and 11.6/100 000 population according to sources [2]. It is a very serious disease considering that early in the 21st century there is still significant risk involving the general population and hospital-admitted patients, which has remained almost unchanged for decades [3, 4]. Furthermore, despite advancements in medical and surgical treatment, hospital-acquired cases of IE have higher morbidity and mortality [4, 5].

The advent of surgical treatment of IE represented a major step forward after the introduction of antibiotics. This is obvious when reviewing the recent history of IE. From the early observations at the end of the 19th century by Osler [6] who has been continuously quoted since, remarkable changes have occurred leading to a better understanding of the disease and better treatment options. This has been very well depicted by Durack and Crawford [7] who stressed the need to reduce mortality by combining efforts. Currently, IE has to be considered a combined medical and surgical disease. This has been made possible by organizing multidisciplinary groups of professionals with shared interests in this uncommon, serious, and medically challenging disease.

At our institution, the Hospital Clinico Endocarditis Study Group has been functioning since 1979, including physicians who are experts in infectious diseases, microbiology, echocardiography, surgery and surgical pathology (Appendix 1). This has led to obtaining significant experience in diagnosis and treatment of this disease in an attempt to reduce mortality through a consensus case-by-case decision-making process (Fig. 1). More recently, a global initiative took form in 1999 as the International Collaboration on Endocarditis (ICE) [2], a worldwide group of investigators sharing common interests and tools like the Duke diagnostic criteria of IE [8]. These and some other departmental or interinstitutional working groups represent the underlying philosophy of a global approach to the patient.

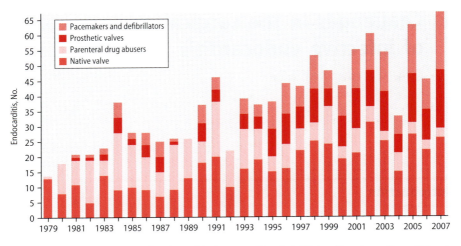

Fig. 1. Annual distribution of endocarditis by type. Hospital Clinico, Barcelona; No.= 989 episodes from 1979–2007

Appendix 1

Members of the Hospital Clinico Endocarditis Study Group

Infectious diseases	Cardiology	Cardiovascular surgery	Microbiology
J. M. Miró	J. C. Paré	C. A. Mestres	F. Marco
A del Río	C. Falces	R. Cartañá	M. Almela
C. Cervera	M. Azqueta	S. Ninot	M. T. Jiménez-deAnta
A. Moreno	M. Sitges	J. L. Pomar	
J. M. Gatell	L. I. Mont		
Other services	**Pathology**	**Experimental endocarditis lab**	**External collaborators**
D. Soy	N. Pérez	C. García de la María	G. R. Corey
M. Brunet	J. Ramírez	Y. Arnedo	V. Fowler
E. de Lazzari	T. Ribalta	M. E. Díaz	C. Cabell
			J. Gavaldà
			A. Pahissa

Current challenges in infective endocarditis

Infective endocarditis is a complex, challenging disease. If we assume that a challenge is "to stimulate especially by presenting difficulties" [9], then IE is a real challenge for all physicians involved in patient care. This is probably one of the best meanings of the word "challenge" and depicts quite well the problems seen daily with IE. Trying to look into the issues that make IE challenging, a few can be considered in different fields related to IE (Table 1). This includes mortality with or without surgical treatment. A summary then follows.

Conceptual challenges

The optimal diagnosis and management of patients suffering from IE requires a very high degree of suspicion due to the protean manifestations of the disease. Suspicion is a part of experience, and experience requires time. It is challenging to have knowledge disseminated in an appropriate way. Thus, the role of guidelines, which have to be dynamic, become important. Guidelines are meant to be information intended to advise people on how something should be done or what something should be [9] or a statement or other indication of policy or procedure by which to determine a course of action.

The good part is that they give an overview of the disease, they represent an organized approach, they try to define common pathways and unify criteria as help in the care of the patient. This has been extensively proved in the literature. However, there are always problems with guidelines. First, some people pretend them to be law. Second, despite the fact that they may represent an option looking for the best practice in a given problem, IE is an infrequent disease of which knowledge is still being accu-

Table 1. Mortality in infective endocarditis in different types of population by treatment groups; Hospital Clinic Barcelona: 989 episodes (1979–2007); ICE: 2781 episodes (2000–2005)

	Surgery Barcelona/ICE	Mortality Barcelona/ICE
IE in i.v. drug users	18/38%	11/10%
IE in general population	38/48%	31/17%
PV IE	46/49%	35/23%
Pacemaker/ICD IE	91/61%	12/10%
Overall	39/48%	25/18%

ICE International Collaboration in Endocarditis; *IE* infective endocarditis, *PV* prosthetic valve, *ICD* implantable-cardioverter defibrillator

Table 2. Summary of current knowledge and indications for surgery in infective endocarditis

▪ Congestive heart failure	Primary indication
▪ Uncontrolled infection	Rule out visceral involvement
▪ Vegetations and peripheral emboli	(risk < 1% after 1 week)
▪ Perivalvular infection	(10–40% NVE – 40–100% PVE)
▪ PVE	Surgery
▪ Fungal endocarditis	Surgery
▪ Neurological complications	Delayed surgery (> 30 d) according to recovery
▪ Timing of surgery	(Very complicated issue, yet to be decided…)

NVE native valve endocarditis, *PVE* prosthetic valve endocarditis

mulated from the perspective of daily clinical work, which is too scanty to construct large-size randomized trials. Currently, there are a number of society guidelines [10–13] aiming to summarize the best options from prevention to diagnosis and treatment; however, there are some differences in the way information is integrated by the practitioner. There are a number of different views and there is no consensus in some regards. A good example is the recent most modification of the prevention guidelines focusing on dental procedures [14–17].

Summarizing briefly, guidelines today confirm that cardiac surgery is the standard of care in certain subgroups of patients with active IE and that we are operating on more patients during the acute phase of IE due to a steady decrease in surgical mortality (Table 2). Despite this, indications and timing are difficult decisions. The way to make guidelines useful and profitable is still complex as there are a number of different approaches to them and the rate of adherence is not uniform [18].

▪ Timing

As a consequence of the intrinsic nature of the disease, a clear challenge in IE is the appropriate timing for a surgical intervention. This important problem has been addressed frequently in recent years. As stated earlier, experience and suspicion are important in the diagnosis of IE. Extensive clinical experience should help in determining the best moment to operate. Guidelines, of course, do fail in defining the best time for surgery. There are many factors influencing the surgical results, including the delay from the onset of symptoms to an accurate diagnosis, the patient's preoperative condition, the extent of anatomical destruction in a given region, etc. Therefore, taking all into account, it is unlikely that a correct decision with regard to appropriate timing would be reached in some subgroups of patients [19].

Table 3. Surgery for infective endocarditis – Group benefit

- NVE *S. aureus*
- NVE Coagulase-negative Staphylococci
- Congestive heart failure
- Aortic valve vegetations
- Perivalvular complications
- Sytemic embolization

NVE native valve endocarditis

Although indications for surgery are quite well defined today, the issue of timing for surgery is still a matter of controversy [20–24]. In fact, most papers refer to the indications for surgery as clearly stated by Olaison and Petterson [19]; however, there is no clear-cut conclusion as to what the appropriate timing is, thus, leaving substantial doubt about the correct decision, especially in patients with high surgical risk, risk that can be stratified in a number of ways, using different scores [25]. A recent contribution by Tleyjeh et al. [24] seems to suggest once again that a delay in surgery may be beneficial in terms of mortality but leaves open a number of questions that need further elucidation. Organizing prospective, randomized trials in IE is difficult. Although there is no doubt about the value of surgery in certain subgroups of patients (Table 3) [26, 27], no appropriate study has defined when a patient may benefit most from the operation. A recently published trial protocol underlines specific issues in this regard [28].

Special populations

HIV-infected patients

The subgroup of HIV-infected patients with IE continues to be of particular risk due to comorbidities and the eventual impact of the infection in patients who will eventually undergo an aggressive intervention like cardiac surgery. Our previous data showed that over the last 20 years there have been an increasing number of HIV-infected patients referred for cardiac surgery [29]. Very early data in a nationwide survey described a population at risk [30] and suggested that there may be no influence on the outcome of these patients due to surgery with cardiopulmonary bypass. At that time, there were also a number of ethical issues in terms of denying major surgery to advanced HIV-infected patients (with AIDS criteria or very immune suppressed (e.g., < 200 CD4+ T-cell count/mm^3)).

Intermediate data from our group disclosed that HIV-infected patients may have better outcome and prognosis than expected [29, 31]. Cardiopulmonary bypass did not impair the immune status of the patients as clearly assessed by CD4 count postoperatively [32]. These data included those of HIV-patients with IE but no intravenous drug abuse [33], an important fact if we take into account that almost on a universal basis it has been thought that IE was associated with drug abuse. Furthermore, medium-term follow-up also confirmed that HIV-infected patients on HAART have a more than acceptable survival at 10 years, between 35 and 40%.

Despite these positive outcomes, the problem still persists and the recent report by De Rosa et al. [34] warns about the persistence of the problem. Drug abuse continues to be a social problem with very strong medical implications due to the increased risk for infection, as is the case of IE. If patients undergo operations, the chance for reoperation does exist and cannot be neglected. Furthermore, around 40% of HIV-infected patients will develop left-sided IE, which carries a much worse prognosis than tricuspid or pulmonary valve involvement.

In addition, the issue of comorbidities has to be taken seriously. So far, previous publications from our group and from others suggest a lack of difference in terms of postoperative mortality and morbidity, especially in terms of surgical site infection. This was also the issue in a preliminary case-control study performed by us in HIV-infected patient with no IE [35], which was not extrapolated to the subgroup of HIV-infected patients with IE due to the difficulties in finding an appropriate population for comparison. A critical statement that is also supported by others [36] is that the level of immune suppression does not influence mortality unless the patient has developed AIDS. Because there is a high incidence of IE (10–12%) among HIV-infected patients with an associated high overall mortality of around 30%, every effort has to be made to cope with this risky population. So far, no patient has been denied surgery based on nonmedical reasons.

Liver cirrhosis

Liver cirrhosis is a very serious disease that, in advanced stages, has high mortality. Currently, for very advanced disease there is no other therapy than replacement therapy through liver transplantation [37, 38]. Our current level of knowledge indicates that patients with liver cirrhosis poorly tolerate major surgery, including intraabdominal or intrathoracic surgery in particular. Data from Filsoufi et al. [39] indicate that out of 27 patients with liver cirrhosis, who underwent major cardiac surgery at their institution, overall mortality was 26%, but when advancing into a major degree of severity for the liver disease, mortality rose to 67% in Child C class patients. Two patients were HIV-infected and 3 patients were operated on for acute IE. In addition, 9 patients underwent the operation off-pump, which we do believe is a different type of population, because the additional trauma of cardiopulmonary bypass is eliminated. In any case, this series by Filsoufi et al. [39] represents the largest cohort of patients operated on for cardiac conditions. The conclusion was that patients with advanced liver disease, Child C class, are at highest risk.

From our point of view, our current experience with liver cirrhosis patients seems to be similar in terms of risk. So far, we have experience with 19 patients undergoing 20 operations for acute IE out of a larger series of cardiac patients. These still unpublished data confirm that mortality is high in Child B and C patients, with the highest mortality being observed in the latter class (about 70%). In addition, postoperative morbidity is also significant, leading to a complex postoperative period. Data from the few papers published so far also seem to support that patient selection is, as usual, a key point for positive outcomes and we agree with this.

Patients with liver cirrhosis represent a challenge in the broadest sense of the word. Further analyses must be performed in order to elucidate the actual role of surgery in these patients, especially in IE considering the intrinsic high risk of IE patients. Because units specialized in the care of the liver patients have developed in the past two decades, initially caring for patients with gastrointestinal bleeding and later incorporating liver transplant patients, this special population represents a new subgroup of patients who will be referred for surgical evaluation.

Anatomical and technical issues

As stated earlier, mortality continues to be high in IE and possible causes include changes in the clinical pattern of the disease and the absence of adequate treatment [40, 41]. Adequate is a very wide term that describes a number of accepted possibilities to treat any condition. In the case of IE and despite all advances in microbiological and clinical diagnosis and advances in pharmacology leading to better antibiotic therapy, mortality remains high as previously discussed. Surgery is also not free from significant morbidity and mortality, and the factors influencing this have been discussed [2, 19].

A surgeon will definitely face many different conditions in a patient requiring an operation for IE, regardless of the valve location and number of valves involved. The truth is that the more extensive the local damage, the higher the risk and the worse the results, even in the best hands. Once again, the inability to organize controlled trials, the variability in the anatomic condition and extravalvular extension of tissue destruction due to infectious and inflammatory processes makes it extremely difficult to look for a uniform approach to patients with IE.

Typical examples of challenging cases in terms of anatomy are periannular complications. Perivalvular abscesses and aortocavitary fistulae represent very advanced and serious diseases as extravalvular extension confirm both a very aggressive pathogen like *S. aureus* and a delayed clinical diagnosis. Mortality and morbidity are definitely very high as has been our experience in the past with both anatomic conditions [42–45]. The situation is particularly worse in the setting of infected prosthetic valves [43], where the chances for adequate repair are slim with conventional valve replacement or repair techniques. The advent of aortic homografts [46–50] allowed for a technically successful repair in cases with no chances otherwise, despite complex techniques including extraanatomical reconstruction as suggested earlier by Danielson et al. [51]. In the aortic root, homografts [48, 50] and possibly autografts [52], despite being old techniques, continue to be extremely useful when there is extravalvular destruction. This, of course, does not necessarily guarantee a better final outcome, because the patient may eventually die from sepsis or other complications. However, the technical challenge can be better approached with such replacement devices. The results have to be looked at from the perspective of time and durability. The extraordinary results reported by Yankah [53] and Knosalla [54] confirm that the homografts play an important role in the management of challenging aortic roots, especially in prosthetic valve IE. However, a problem is the complexity of the disease and up to what extent some good results can be reproduced. If there is no such complex disease, good results have also been reported with other devices like stentless valves [55]. The underlying philosophy is that biological replacement devices seem to work extremely well, although no comparative studies have been performed with mechanical valves both in the short- and long-term.

Perivalvular complications originating in the mitral position are less frequent than in the aortic root. However, once they appear, the anatomical condition will pose difficulties to any surgeon, because the local destruction may extend into the fibrosa or a calcified annulus will become extremely difficult to treat. Although less frequent, technical complexity should not be neglected, and sometimes cumbersome and complex techniques like mitral valve replacement using the pulmonary autograft, also well known as the Ross II operation, are useful. Initially described in the setting of rheumatic valves [56–60], this technique may play a role in challenging situations in the mitral position [61].

The problem with the combination of perivalvular extension, mitral or aortic, in combination with multivalvular involvement may lead to the worse case scenario that can happen when looking at the anatomy. This is the destruction of the fibrous skeleton of the heart. This is does not occur frequently but is a dreaded complication of extravalvular extension in uni- or multivalvular involvement in IE. Some patients have such extensive destruction that it is technically almost impossible to manage. From our own experience, we can identify four patients with multiple destruction involving the fibrous skeleton in the setting of prosthetic valve IE. Three of them died perioperatively during attempted repair, despite the use of extensive debridement and homografts. One young 24-year-old male with three acute operations due to community-acquired methicillin-resistant *S. aureus* underwent orthotopic heart transplantation, while on a left ventricular assist device. Blood cultures were, of course, negative at the time of transplantation. He survived 2.5 years before he died from hyperacute rejection [62]. There are scanty reports on this subject [63, 64]; however, they demonstrate that in some cases, transplantation may be an alternative rather than a contraindication in the setting of IE. The key requirement is having negative blood cultures.

Risk stratification

To the list of challenges in IE that should be considered, we add the following: improving microbiological techniques (polymerase chain reaction, DNA testing, etc.), improving echocardiographic techniques (3D), identify vulnerable populations, increasing the awareness of the medical community, and preoperative risk assessment. There is no doubt that IE is still a very challenging disease from all perspectives, and we are still far from being successful in obtaining full control of the disease for, among them, the many reasons stated above.

In recent years, preoperative risk stratification has become popular in the cardiovascular surgery community [25]. Preoperative risk assessment is of crucial importance in high-risk patients; current risk scores tend to underestimate the risk of mortality in high-risk patients despite the fact that low- or medium-risk patients can easily be identified and matched. In Europe, the EuroSCORE has become the most popular risk stratification model, because it can handle the vast majority of adult cardiac surgery procedures; it has been validated in different populations and has been compared with other models that can be considered as competitors [65, 66]. Currently, it is accepted that risk models can be used to predict some outcomes, to determine quality assurance, and to educate individuals or departments in the monitoring of quality [67–70]. At our institution, we have been concerned with the extraordinary risk of some subgroups of patients with IE. This may sometimes not be easy to share with the patient or the relatives. However, using a specific tool, like risk models, may help in the decision-making process, especially when the surgical risk is considered to be unacceptable. As in most places in Europe, we have used the EuroSCORE for years and it has helped to identify the highest-risk candidates, been used to monitor surgical results, and to take uncomfortable decisions as to when to deny surgical treatment [71]. With a number of limitations, our study confirmed that the EuroSCORE model seems to work acceptably well in IE; these patients are usually in the high-risk area. There is still controversy as to when models may be trusted due to the dynamic nature of the surgical practice. This has been recently addressed by Choong et al. in an elegant editorial [72]. To what extent, this will help the physicians in defining what the real value of such models in IE is, remains to be confirmed.

Conclusions

Infective endocarditis is an infrequent and very serious disease. Despite a number of advances in all related disciplines, morbidity and mortality remain high. Surgical treatment is an integral part of the management of the patient with IE. This is a highly demanding disease with suboptimal results, thus, making it an unpopular medical and surgical problem, which requires a team approach. At the beginning of the 21st century, it should be considered a highly challenging problem with a number of still unanswered questions.

References

1. Cabell CH, Pond KK, Peterson GE et al (2001) The risk of stroke and death in patients with aortic and mitral valve endocarditis. Am Heart J 142:75–80
2. Cabell CH, Abrutyn E (2003) Progress toward a global understanding of Infective Endocarditis: Lessons from the International Collaboration on Endocarditis. In: Durack DT, Crawford MH (eds) Cardiology clinics – infective endocarditis. Saunders Company, Philadelphia, pp 159–166
3. Nissen H, Nielsen F, Frederiksen M et al (1992) Native valve endocarditis in the general population: 10-year survey of the clinical picture during the 1980s. Eur Heart J 13:872–877
4. Fernández-Hidalgo N, Almirante B, Tornos P, Pigrau C, Sambola A, Igual A, Pahissa A (2008) Contemporary epidemiology and prognosis of health care-associated infective endocarditis. Clin Infect Dis 15; 47:1287–1297
5. Fowler VG Jr, Miro JM, Hoen B, Cabell CH, Abrutyn E, Rubinstein E, Corey GR, Spelman D, Bradley SF, Barsic B, Pappas PA, Anstrom KJ, Wray D, Fortes CQ, Anguera I, Athan E, Jones P, van der Meer JT, Elliott TS, Levine DP, Bayer AS, ICE Investigators (2005) Staphylococcus aureus endocarditis: a consequence of medical progress. JAMA 22; 293:3012–3021
6. Osler W (1885) Gulstonian lectures on malignant endocarditis Lecture I. Lancet 1:415–418
7. Durack DT, Crawford MH (2003) Infective endocarditis. In: Durack DT, Crawford MH (eds) Cardiology clinics – infective endocarditis. Saunders Company, Philadelphia, pp xi–xiii
8. Durack DT, Lukes As, Bright DK (1994) New criteria for diagnosis of infective endocarditis: utilization of specific echocardiographic findings. Am J Med 96:200–209
9. Cambridge Advanced Learner's Dictionary (2009)
10. Vallés F, Anguita M, Escribano MP, Pérez Casar F, Pousibet H, Tornos P, Vilacosta I (2000) Guidelines of the Spanish Society of Cardiology on Endocarditis. Rev Esp Cardiol 53: 1384–1396
11. Horstkotte D, Follath F, Gutschik E, Lengyel M, Oto A, Pavie A, Soler-Soler J, Thiene G, Von Graevenitz A (2004) European Society of Cardiology Guidelines. Guidelines on prevention, diagnosis and treatment of infective endocarditis executive summary. The Task Force on Infective Endocarditis of the European Society of Cardiology. Eur Heart J 25:267–276

12. Baddour LM, Wilson WR, Bayer AS, Fowler VG Jr, Bolger AF, Levison ME, Ferrieri P, Gerber MA, Tani LT, Gewitz MH, Tong DC, Steckelberg JM, Baltimore RS, Shulman ST, Burns JC, Falace DA, Newburger JN, Pallasch TJ, Takahashi M, Taubert KA (2005) Infective endocarditis: diagnosis, antimicrobial therapy, and management of complications: A statement for healthcare professionals from the Committee on Rheumatic Fever, Endocarditis, and Kawasaki Disease, Council on Cardiovascular Disease in the Young, and the Councils on Clinical Cardiology, Stroke, and Cardiovascular Surgery and Anesthesia, American Heart Association: Endorsed by the Infectious Diseases Society of America. Circulation 111:e394–e434
13. Westling K, Aufwerber E, Ekdahl C, Friman G, Gårdlund B, Julander I, Olaison L, Olesund C, Rundström H, Snygg-Martin U, Thalme A; Werner M, Hogevik H (2007) Swedish guidelines for diagnosis and treatment of infective endocarditis. Scand J Infect Dis 39:929–946
14. Wilson W, Taubert KA, Gewitz M, Lockhart PB, Baddour LM, Levison M, Bolger A, Cabell CH, Takahashi M, Baltimore RS, Newburger JW, Strom BL, Tani LY, Gerber M, Bonow RO, Pallasch T, Shulman ST, Rowley AH, Burns JC, Ferrieri P, Gardner T, Goff D, Durack DT, American Heart Association Rheumatic Fever, Endocarditis, and Kawasaki Disease Committee, American Heart Association Council on Cardiovascular Disease in the Young, American Heart Association Council on Clinical Cardiology, American Heart Association Council on Cardiovascular Surgery and Anesthesia, Quality of Care and Outcomes Research Interdisciplinary Working Group (2007) Prevention of infective endocarditis: guidelines from the American Heart Association: a guideline from the American Heart Association Rheumatic Fever, Endocarditis, and Kawasaki Disease Committee, Council on Cardiovascular Disease in the Young, and the Council on Clinical Cardiology, Council on Cardiovascular Surgery and Anesthesia, and the Quality of Care and Outcomes Research Interdisciplinary Working Group. Circulation 116: 1736–1754
15. Johns J (2008) Prevention of endocarditis. The new guidelines. Heart Lung Circ 17(Suppl 4):S37–S40
16. Flückiger U, Troillet N (2008) New Swiss guidelines for the prevention of infective endocarditis. Rev Med Suisse 4:2134–2138
17. Zadik Y, Findler M, Livne S, Levin L, Elad S (2008) Dentists' knowledge and implementation of the 2007 American Heart Association guidelines for prevention of infective endocarditis. Oral Surg Oral Med Oral Pathol Oral Radiol Endod 106(6):e16–e19
18. Antunes MJ (2008) Guidelines in real life. Why are they not always enforced? Eur J Cardiothorac Surg 34:935–936
19. Olaison L, Petterson G (2003) Current best practices and guidelines. Indications for surgical intervention in infective endocarditis. In: Durack DT, Crawford MH (eds) Cardiology Clinics – infective endocarditis. Saunders, Philadelphia, pp 235–251
20. Reinhartz O, Herrmann M, Redling F, Zerkowski HR (1996) Timing of surgery in patients with acute infective endocarditis. Cardiovasc Surg (Torino) 37:397–400
21. Chamoun AJ, Conti V, Lenihan DJ (2000) Native valve infective endocarditis: what is the optimal timing for surgery? Am J Med Sci 320:255–262
22. Arzanauskiene R, Zabiela P, Benetis R, Jonkaitiene R (2002) Timing of surgery in infective endocarditis: impact on the outcome and recurrence. Medicina (Kaunas) 38(Suppl 2):238–242
23. F Delahaye, Célard M, Roth O, Gevigney G (2004) Indications and optimal timing for surgery in infective endocarditis. Heart 90:618–620

24. Tleyjeh IM, Steckelberg JM, Georgescu G, Ghomrawi HM, Hoskin TL, Enders FB, Mookadam F, Huskins WC, Wilson WR, Baddour LM (2008) The association between the timing of valve surgery and 6-month mortality in left-sided infective endocarditis. Heart 94:892–896
25. Nashef SA, Roques F, Michel P, Gauducheau E, Lemeshow S, Salamon R (1999) European system for cardiac operative risk evaluation (EuroSCORE) Eur J Cardiothorac Surg 16:9–13
26. Wang A, Pappas P, Anstrom KA, Abrutyn E, Fowler VG Jr, Hoen B, Miro JM, Corey R, Olaison L, MD, Stafford JA, Mestres CA, Cabell CH and the International Collaboration on Endocarditis Investigators (2005) The use and effect of surgical therapy for prosthetic valve infective endocarditis: A propensity analysis of a multicenter, international cohort. Am Heart J 150:1086–1091
27. Cabell CH, Abrutyn E, Fowler VG Jr, Hoen B, Miro JM, Corey R, Olaison L, Pappas P, Anstrom K, Stafford JA, Eykyn S, Habib G, Mestres CA, Wang A and ICE-MD Investigators, International Collaboration on Endocarditis Merged Database (ICE-MD) (2005) Use of surgery in patients with native valve infective endocarditis: Results from the International Collaboration on Endocarditis Merged Database. Am Heart J 150:1092–1098
28. San Román JA, López J, Revilla A, Vilacosta I, Tornos P, Almirante B, Mota P, Vilacorta E, Sevilla T, Gómez I, Del Carmen Manzano M, Fulquet E, Rodríguez E, Igual A (2008) Rationale, design, and methods for the early surgery in infective endocarditis study (ENDOVAL 1): a multicenter, prospective, randomized trial comparing the state-of-the-art therapeutic strategy versus early surgery strategy in infective endocarditis. Am Heart J 156:431–436
29. Miró JM, del Río A, Mestres CA (2002) Infective endocarditis in intravenous drug abusers and HIV-1 infected patients. Infect Dis Clin North Am 16:273–295
30. Aris A, Pomar JL, Saura E (1993) Cardiopulmonary bypass in HIV-positive patients. Ann Thorac Surg 55:1104–1108
31. Miró JM, del Río A, Mestres CA (2003) Infective endocarditis and cardiac surgery in intravenous drug abusers and HIV-1 infected patients. Cardiol Clin 21:167–184
32. Mestres CA, Chuquiure JE, Claramonte X, Muñoz J, Benito N, Castro MA, Pomar JL, Miró JM (2003) Long-term results after cardiac surgery in patients infected with the human immunodeficiency virus type-1 (HIV-1). Eur J Cardiothorac Surg 23:1007–1016
33. Losa JE, Miro JM, Del Río A, Moreno-Camacho A, Garcia F, Claramonte X, Marco F, Mestres CA, Azqueta M, Gatell JM; Hospital Clinic Endocarditis Study Group (2003) Infective endocarditis not related to intravenous drug abuse in HIV-1-infected patients: report of eight cases and review of the literature. Clin Microbiol Infect 9:45–54
34. De Rosa FG, Cicalini S, Canta F, Audagnotto S, Cecchi E, Di Perri G (2007) Infective endocarditis in intravenous drug users from Italy: the increasing importance in HIV-infected patients. Infection 35:154–160
35. Jiménez-Expósito MJ, Mestres CA, Claramonte X, Cartañá R, Josa M, Pomar JL, Mulet J, Miró JM; en representación del Grupo de Estudio de Endocarditis del Hospital Clínic-IDIBAPS (2006) Mortality and morbidity in HIV-infected patients undergoing coronary artery bypass surgery: a case control study. Rev Esp Cardiol 59:276–279
36. Smith DT, Sherwood M, Crisel R, Abraham J, Mansour C, Veledar E, Mondschein R, Lerakis S, Emory Endocarditis Group (2004) A comparison of HIV-positive patients with and without infective endocarditis: an echocardiographic study-the Emory Endocarditis Group experience. Am J Med Sci 328:145–149

37. Heuman DM, Abou-Assi SG, Habib A et al (2004) Persistent ascites and low serum sodium identify patients with cirrhosis and low MELD scores who are at high risk for early death. Hepatology 40:802–810
38. Cárdenas A, Ginés P (2008) Predicting mortality in cirrhosis – Serum sodium helps. N Eng J Med 359; 10:1060–1062
39. Filsoufi F, Salzberg SP, Rahmanian PB, Schiano TD, Elsiesy H, Squire A, Adams DH (2007) Early and late outcome of cardiac surgery in patients with liver cirrhosis. Liver Transpl 13:990–995
40. Mylonakis E, Calderwood SB (2001) Infective endocarditis in adults. NEJM 345: 1318–1330
41. Tornos P (2002) Are we managing our patients well? Rev Esp Cardiol 55:789–790
42. Anguera I, Miro JM, Evangelista A, Cabell CH, San Roman JA, Vilacosta I, Almirante B, Ripoll T, Fariñas MC, Anguita M, Navas E, Gonzalez-Juanatey C, Garcia-Bolao I, Muñoz P, de Alarcon A, Sarria C, Rufi G, Miralles F, Pare C, Fowler VG Jr, Mestres CA, de Lazzari E, Guma JR, Moreno A, Corey GR; Aorto-Cavitary Fistula in Endocarditis Working Group (2006) Periannular complications in infective endocarditis involving native aortic valves. Am J Cardiol 98:1254–1260
43. Anguera I, Miro JM, San Roman JA, de Alarcon A, Anguita M, Almirante B, Evangelista A, Cabell CH, Vilacosta I, Ripoll T, Muñoz P, Navas E, Gonzalez-Juanatey C, Sarria C, Garcia-Bolao I, Fariñas MC, Rufi G, Miralles F, Pare C, Fowler VG Jr, Mestres CA, de Lazzari E, Guma JR, del Río A, Corey GR, Aorto-Cavitary Fistula in Endocarditis Working Group (2006) Periannular complications in infective endocarditis involving prosthetic aortic valves. Am J Cardiol 98:1261–1268
44. Anguera I, Miro JM, Vilacosta I, Almirante B, Anguita M, Muñoz P, Roman JA, de Alarcon A, Ripoll T, Navas E, Gonzalez-Juanatey C, Cabell CH, Sarria C, Garcia-Bolao I, Fariñas MC, Leta R, Rufi G, Miralles F, Pare C, Evangelista A, Fowler VG Jr, Mestres CA, de Lazzari E, Guma JR; Aorto-cavitary Fistula in Endocarditis Working Group (2005) Aorto-cavitary fistulous tract formation in infective endocarditis: clinical and echocardiographic features of 76 cases and risk factors for mortality. Eur Heart J 26:288–297
45. Anguera I, Quaglio G, Miró JM, Paré C, Azqueta M, Marco F, Mestres CA, Moreno A, Pomar JL, Mezzelani P, Sanz G (2001) Aortocardiac fistulas complicating infective endocarditis. Am J Cardiol 87:652–654
46. Barratt-Boyes BG, Roche AH, Subramanyan R, Pemberton JR, Whitlock RM (1987) Long-term follow-up of patients with the antibiotic-sterilized aortic homograft valve inserted freehand in the aortic position. Circulation 75:768–777
47. Ross DN (1995) Evolution of the homograft valve. Ann Thorac Surg 59:565–567
48. Dearani JA, Orszulak TA, Schaff HV, Daly RC, Anderson BJ, Danielson GK (1997) Results of allograft aortic valve replacement for complex endocarditis. J Thorac Cardiovasc Surg 113:285–291
49. O'Brien MF, Harrocks S, Stafford EG, Gardner MA, Pohlner PG, Tesar PJ, Stephens F (2001) The homograft aortic valve: a 29-year, 99.3% follow up of 1022 valve replacements. J Heart Valve Dis 10:334–344
50. Yankah AC (2002) Forty years of homograft surgery Asian Cardiovasc Thorac Ann 10:97–100
51. Danielson GK, Titus JL, DuShane JW (1974) Successful treatment of aortic valve endocarditis and aortic root abscesses by insertion of prosthetic valve in ascending aorta and placement of bypass grafts to coronary arteries. J Thorac Cardiovasc Surg 67:443–449
52. Pettersson G, Tingleff J, Joyce FS (1998) Treatment of aortic valve endocarditis with the Ross operation. Eur J Cardiothorac Surg 13:678–684

53. Yankah AC, Pasic M, Klose H, Siniawski H, Weng Y, Hetzer R (2005) Homograft reconstruction of the aortic root for endocarditis with periannular abscess: a 17-year study. Eur J Cardiothorac Surg 28:69–75
54. Knosalla C, Weng Y, Yankah AC, Siniawski H, Hofmeister J, Hammerschmidt R, Loebe M, Hetzer R (2002) Surgical treatment of active infective aortic valve endocarditis with associated periannular abscess – 11 year results. Eur Heart J 21:490–497
55. Musci M, Siniawski H, Pasic M, Weng Y, Loforte A, Kosky S, Yankah C, Hetzer R (2008) Surgical therapy in patients with active infective endocarditis: seven-year single centre experience in a subgroup of 255 patients treated with the Shelhigh stentless bioprosthesis. Eur J Cardiothorac Surg 34:410–417
56. Lower RR, Stofer RC, Shumway NE (1961) Total excision of the mitral valve and replacement with the autologous pulmonic valve. J Thorac Cardiovasc Surg 42: 696–702
57. Ross DN (1967) Replacement of aortic and mitral valves with a pulmonary autograft. Lancet 2(7523):956–958
58. Ross DN, Kabbani S (1997) Mitral valve replacement with a pulmonary autograft: the mitral top hat. J Heart Valve Dis 6:542–545
59. Brown JW, Ruzmetov M, Rodefeld MD, Turrentine MW (2006) Mitral valve replacement with Ross II technique: initial experience. Ann Thorac Surg 81:502–507
60. Kabbani S, Jamil H, Nabhani F, Hamoud A, Katan K, Sabbagh N, Koudsi A, Kabbani L, Hamed G (2007) Analysis of 92 mitral pulmonary autograft replacement (Ross II) operations. J Thorac Cardiovasc Surg 134:902–908
61. Mestres CA, Ginel A, Cartana R, Pomar JL (1993) Cryopreserved homografts in aortic and mitral prosthetic endocarditis: expanding the use of biological tissues in complex cardiac infections. J Heart Valve Dis 2:679–683
62. Mestres CA, Cartañá R, García-Valentín A, Moreno A, Orrit J, Loma-Osorio P, Josa M, Azqueta M, Pérez-Villa F, Miró JM and the Hospital Clinico Endocarditis Study Group. Heart transplantation for acute complicated aortic root infective endocarditis (2005) Presented at the 8th International Symposium on Modern Concepts in Infective Endocarditis and Cardiovascular Infections. Charleston, SC (USA), May 22–24, Poster 49
63. Galbraith AJ, McCarthy J, Tesar PJ, McGiffin DC (1999) Cardiac transplantation for prosthetic valve endocarditis in a previously transplanted heart. J Heart Lung Transplant 18:805–806
64. Pulpón LA, Crespo MG, Sobrino M, Segovia J, Ortigosa J, Burgos R, Silva L, Serrano S, Artaza M, Téllez G (1994) Recalcitrant endocarditis successfully treated by heart transplantation. Am Heart J 127(4 Pt 1):958–960
65. Nashef SAM, Roques F Hammill BG, Peterson ED, Michel P, Grover FL, Wyse RK, Ferguson TB; EurpSCORE Project Group (2002) Validation of European System for Cardiac Operative Risk Evaluation (EuroSCORE) in North American cardiac surgery. Eur J Cardiothorac Surg 22:101–105
66. Gogbashian A, Sedrakyan A, Treasure T (2004) EuroSCORE: a systematic review of international performance. Eur J Cardiothorac Surg 25:695–700
67. Shahian DM, Blackstone EH, Edwards FH, Grover FL, Grunkemeier GL, Naftel DC, Nashef SA, Nugent WC, Peterson ED, STS workforce on evidence-based surgery (2004) Cardiac surgery risk models: a position article. Ann Thorac Surg 78: 1868–1877
68. Nilsson J, Ohlsson M, Thulin L, Höglund P, Nashef SA, Brandt J (2006) Risk factor identification and mortality prediction in cardiac surgery using artificial neural networks. J Thorac Cardiovasc Surg 132:12–19
69. Nashef SA (2007) Managing risk to improve cardiac surgical outcomes. Crit Care Resusc 9:323–326

70. Klein AA, Nashef SA (2008) Perception and reporting of cardiac surgical performance. Semin Cardiothorac Vasc Anesth 12:184–190
71. Mestres CA, Castro MA, Bernabeu E, Josa M, Cartaná R, Pomar JL, Miró JM, Mulet J; Hospital Clínico Endocarditis Study Group (2007) Preoperative risk stratification in infective endocarditis. Does the EuroSCORE model work? Preliminary results. Eur J Cardiothorac Surg 32:281–285
72. Choong CK, Sergeant P, Nashef SA, Smith JA, Bridgewater B (2009) The EuroSCORE risk stratification system in the current era: how accurate is it and what should be done if it is inaccurate? Eur J Cardiothorac Surg 35:59–61

Clinical results of the Shelhigh® stentless bioprosthesis in patients with active infective endocarditis:

8-year single center experience

M. Musci, Y. Weng, H. Siniawski, S. Kosky, M. Pasic, M. Hübler, A. Amiri, J. Stein, R. Meyer, R. Hetzer

Introduction

Despite improvements in medical care, the incidence of left-sided active infective endocarditis (AIE) has remained unchanged over the past few decades. As shown in a review of 26 publications on a total of almost 3800 patients treated between 1993 and 2003, it is reported to affect a median of 3.6–5.4/100 000 persons per year, increasing in individuals over 65 years old to 15.0/100 000 persons per year, with a male:female ratio of 2:1 [1]. This unchanging incidence may be explained by changes in both the spectrum of causative organisms and in the patients affected [2]. New groups at risk of endocarditis have emerged, for example, the increasingly aging population with heart valve sclerosis, patients with prosthetic valves, those exposed to nosocomial infections, hemodialysis patients, and intravenous drug abusers [3], while chronic rheumatic fever, which was a classic predisposing factor in the preantibiotics era, has become rare in industrialized

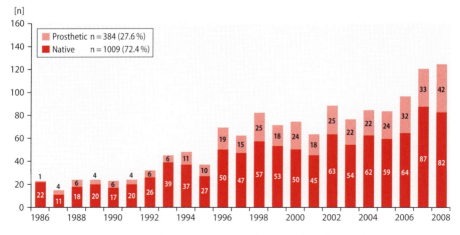

Fig. 1. Operations for native and prosthetic active infective endocarditis at the Deutsches Herzzentrum Berlin from May 1986 to December 2008

countries. These developments reflect our experience of continuing high numbers of patients who have to be operated on for AIE each year: between May 1986 and December 2008 a total of 1313 AIE patients were operated on at the Deutsches Herzzentrum Berlin, 72.4% (n = 1009) for native endocarditis and 27.6% (n = 384) for prosthetic endocarditis (Fig. 1).

To exclude the effects of different valve types on the outcome after an endocarditis operation, we analyzed a subgroup of patients with left-sided AIE (n = 297) in whom the same bioprosthesis (Shelhigh®) was implanted between February 2000 and December 2008. The retrospective study analyzed both prospectively updated data and patients recently operated upon.

The aim of this study was to investigate outcome after surgical therapy in these AIE patients, in particular, with regard to survival in relation to surgical urgency, valve position, the number of implanted valves, and abscess formation. Another objective was to analyze the reinfection rate of the implanted prostheses with regard to our previous findings in a larger group of patients over a longer period [4, 5].

Patients and methods

Patient population

An overview of the patient population is given in Table 1. Between February 2000 and December 2008, 297 patients with left-sided AIE (211 men, median age 60 years) received implantation of a Shelhigh® stentless valve prosthesis. In 213 (71.7%) patients, native valve endocarditis was present, while 84 (29.0%) had prosthetic valve endocarditis. A large proportion of patients were referred to our department in a condition of cardiac decompensation: 71 (23.9%) patients were intubated, 52 (17.5%) had protracted septic shock, and 77 (25.9%) required high doses of catecholamines. The operation was performed electively in 20 (6.7%), urgently in 184 (62.0%), and as an emergency procedure in 93 (31.3%) patients. S. aureus (23.6%) and Streptococci (18.5%) were the most common microorganisms found in the blood cultures. Follow-up was completed in all survivors by telephone contact with the patient, by analyzing standardized mail questionnaires sent to the patients, by consulting the population registry and by contacting peripheral hospitals.

The median follow-up time was 0.87 years (range 0 to 8.7 years), with 676.2 patient years.

The study population of 297 patients represents 22.6% of all patients operated on at our institution due to AIE over the past 20 years and 36.7% of all surgical endocarditis patients for the study period (n = 808).

Table 1. Patient population with left-sided endocarditis AIE

Period	2/2000–12/2008
Patients with AIE	n = 297
– Men	n = 211 (71.0%)
– Women	n = 86 (29.0%)
Age	
– Median	60 years
– Mean	57.4 years
– Range	17–85 years
Endocarditis	
– Native AIE	n = 213 (71.7%)
– Prosthetic AIE	n = 84 (28.3%)
Preoperative status	
– Intubation	n = 71 (23.9%)
– Septic shock	n = 52 (17.5%)
– High-dose catecholamines	n = 77 (25.9%)
Operation	
– Elective	n = 20 (6.7%)
– Urgent	n = 184 (62.0%)
– Emergency	n = 93 (31.3%)
Blood microorganisms	
– Staphylococci	n = 36 (12.1%)
S. aureus	n = 70 (23.6%)
– Streptococci	n = 55 (18.5%)
Viridans streptococci	n = 25 (8.4%)
– Enterococcus species	n = 33 (11.1%)
– Culture negative	n = 49 (16.5%)
– Others	n = 13 (4.4%)
– Unknown	n = 16 (5.4%)
Follow-up	
– Median	0.87 years
– Range	0–8.7 years
– Patient years	676.2 years
Indication	**No. of patients**
Progressive heart failure	244 (82.2%)
+ recurrent septic embolisms	111 (37.4%)
+ vegetations	178 (59.9%)
+ therapy-resistant septic infections	108 (36.4%)
Abscess formation	145 (48.8%)
– aortic	92 (30.9%)
– mitral	39 (13.1%)
– aortic + mitral	7 (2.4%)
Therapy-resistant septic infection	108 (36.4%)
Recurrent septic embolism	111 (37.4%)

AIE active infective endocarditis

Table 2. Numbers of Shelhigh® bioprostheses implanted and their position

Valve type	No.
■ **Single valve implantation**	**249**
– Aortic valve	125
– Aortic conduit	28
– Mitral valve	89
– Tricuspid valve	7
■ **Double valve implantation**	**66**
– Aortic and mitral valve	40
– Left- and right-sided implantation	8
– Others	18

■ Indications for surgery and operations performed

An overview of operative indications during the acute phase of AIE is given in Table 1. In general, patients developed a summary of indication for surgery during antibiotic treatment for AIE. The majority had to be operated on due to progressive heart failure in combination with recurrent septic embolisms, vegetations, or therapy-resistant infections. A total of 145 patients (48.8%) developed an abscess in the aortic and/or mitral valve. An overview of the number and the position of the Shelhigh® bioprostheses (n = 315) implanted is given in Table 2. A total of 43 patients received concomitant CABG operation.

■ Definition of active infective endocarditis

AIE was defined on the basis of vegetations or an abscess shown in the echocardiogram and accompanied by positive blood cultures or intraoperatively harvested valve cultures, on the basis of clinical evidence of persistent sepsis or recurrent septic embolism, or on the basis of the intraoperative diagnosis.

■ The Shelhigh® SuperStentless bioprosthesis

The aortic Shelhigh® SuperStentless bioprosthesis (Fig. 2) is made entirely of biological material and is a composite valve consisting of three individual porcine semilunar cusps. It is available in the sizes 21–31 mm. It is made from noncoronary cusps taken from three glutaraldehyde-fixed aortic valves that are congruent to each other and sewn together with cardiovascular sutures. The resulting composite trileaflet valve, which is covered with pericardium, has no stent and therefore an optimal opening area. It is

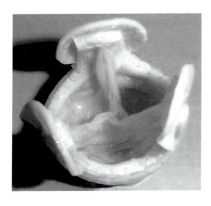

Fig. 2. The aortic Shelhigh® bioprosthesis (Modell NR-2000)

also free from mechanical parts and foreign material at the surface, which is favorable for implantation in patients with endocarditis. The valve has a very flexible ring situated between the valve tissue and the pericardial coat. The addition of three so-called struts gives the ring the character of a "skeleton" which simplifies the implantation process. As the framework is flexible, it is possible to implant the stentfree valve in the aortic position by placing a suture at the regular base of the annulus and an additional suture at the struts. The xenograft, which is coated with heparin, is conserved in glutaraldehyde at very low pressure (< 4 mmHg) and detoxified. This process eliminates residual glutaraldehyde and ensures stable cross-linking of the valve tissue. In addition, the valve is subjected to anticalcification treatment (the No-React® procedure). This is designed to reduce the reaction of the adjacent tissue and to limit valve calcification and tissue destruction in the long term [6, 7].

Statistical analysis

SPSS for Windows version 12.01 was used. Qualitative data are presented as number (n) and percent. For quantitative data means ± standard error were calculated. Analysis of survival and freedom from endpoints was performed according to Kaplan-Meier estimation. For comparison of survival in different patient groups, the Gehan test was used.

A logistic regression model was applied to investigate possible risk factors for early mortality (< 30 d). First all possible risk factors were evaluated with a univariate approach, followed by multivariate logistic regression with backward elimination procedure.

Survivors and nonsurvivors were compared by Pearson's χ^2 test or Student's t-test accordingly. A value of $P < 0.05$ was considered statistically significant.

Results

Overall survival and survival in relation to surgical urgency

The overall survival curves and the comparison between the patients operated on electively or urgently and those operated on in an emergency are given in Fig. 3. The 30-day, 1-, 3- and 5-year survival rates for the whole study population were 76.5%±2.7%, 59.9%±3.2%, 52.9±3.4%, and 46.8% ±4.0%, respectively.

We found a highly significant difference between the survival rates of patients with elective and urgent surgery vs. those operated on in an emergency: the 30-day, 1-, 3- and 5-year survival rates after elective and urgent operation were 87.3%±2.7%, 68.3%±4.0%, 61.8%±4.2%, and 53.7%±5.3%, respectively, in comparison to 59.2%±5.0%, 46.4%±5.1%, 38.8%±5.3%, and 36.5%±5.5% after emergency operation (p<0.0001). Analysis of the survival curve shows a clear difference between the two groups in the first 30 days.

There were 6 (2.3%) intraoperative deaths: 5 due to septic multiorgan failure and 1 due to myocardial failure. The main causes of the 60 (23.5%) early deaths (30 d) were septic multiorgan failure in 46 (76.6%), myocardial failure in 6 (10.0%), cerebral bleeding in 5 (8.3%), hemorrhagic shock in 2 (3.3%) cases, and pulmonary emboli in 1 (1.6%) case.

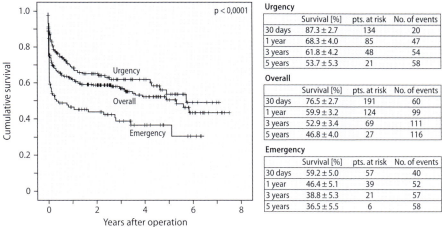

Fig. 3. Overall survival and survival in relation to surgical urgency in patients with active infective endocarditis after Shelhigh® implantation (n=255 patients)

Survival in relation to valve position and comparison of single versus double valve replacement

There was no significant difference between the survival rates of patients after aortic valve (AVR) or mitral valve replacement (MVR): the 30-day, 1-, 3- and 5-year survival rates after AVR were 76.3%±3.7%, 59.1%±4.4%, 55.6%±4.6%, and 46.4%±5.8%, respectively, in comparison to 80.7%± 5.0%, 67.9%±6.1%, 54.8%±7.1%, and 49.8%±8.0% after MVR (p=0.46). Compared to all study patients with single valve replacement, patients with double valve replacement (AVR and MVR) had a significantly worse survival rate: the 30-day survival rate after AVR and MVR was 60.7%±9.2% and for 1-, 3- and 5-years it remained at 40.4%±9.7% (p=0.0336).

Comparison of the survival curves of single versus double valve replacement showed a nonsignificant trend toward better survival after AVR alone (p=0.0728) and a highly significant better survival after MVR alone (p=0.0206) (Fig. 2), but the low risk for the double valve replacement group has to be taken into consideration. A clear difference is seen between the two groups in the first 30 days and in the period of between 1 month and 1 year.

Survival in relation to abscess formation

The survival curves in relation to abscess formation are shown in Fig. 4. From the study population, 145 (48.8%) showed abscess formation. Of these, 92 (30.9%) developed an isolated abscess of the aortic valve, 39

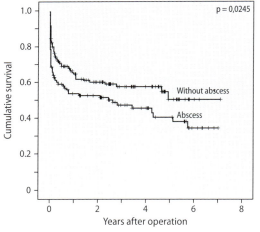

Fig. 4. Survival in relation to abscess formation in patients with active infective endocarditis after Shelhigh® implantation (n=255 patients)

(13.1%) patients of the mitral valve and 7 (2.4%) patients had abscess formation on both valves (Table 1). Comparing the groups with and without abscess, the figures for better survival in patients without an abscess were highly significant: the 30-day, 1-, 3- and 5-year survival rates for patients without abscess formation were 82.6% ± 3.2%, 64.6% ± 4.1%, 57.5% ± 4.5%, and 50.4% ± 6.2%, respectively, in comparison to 68.5% ± 4.4%, 53.7% ± 4.8%, 47.1% ± 5.1%, and 40.6% ± 5.6% in patients with abscess formation (p = 0.0245).

∎ Reinfection after Shelhigh® implantation

A total of 25 out of 297 patients (8.4%) developed reinfection following Shelhigh® implantation leading to reoperation. From these, there were only two early reinfections (< 60 d) at the 41st and 59th postoperative day (0.78%) with the same microorganism.

Fig. 5 shows the freedom from reoperation due to reinfection: the 30-day, 1-, 3- and 5-year rates were 100%, 94.4% ± 1.8%, 87.0% ± 3.2% and 83.8% ± 4.4%, respectively, for the whole population.

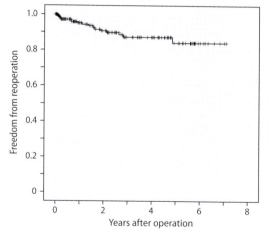

Fig. 5. Freedom from reoperation due to reinfection in patients with active infective endocarditis after Shelhigh® implantation (n = 255 patients)

Discussion

Survival and surgical urgency

For the risk stratification and survival in our study, it has to be taken into consideration that our hospital is a referral surgical center receiving patients who have already been treated medically elsewhere and sometimes coming for an operation as ultima ratio therapy. Our study shows that the survival of patients differs significantly depending on the surgical urgency. The difference in survival found between the patients operated on urgently but in stable condition and those in whom the operation was an emergency procedure due to unstable hemodynamics or septic shock reflects the aggressive nature of the disease but also shows that a large number of patients with endocarditis are referred too late for operation. These results suggest that early outcome can be improved if patients are operated upon before heart failure or septic shock develops. This is shown in the survival curve, where after the first 30 days the lines for urgent and emergency operation run parallel.

In addition, survival in patients after double valve replacement (aortic and mitral) was significantly worse than with single valve replacement. Better outcome could have been achieved, if the patients had been referred earlier for surgery. This view is also supported by the analysis of the 30-day mortality. Our results are in accord with those of two published studies in which Alexiou et al. found the hemodynamic status of the patient at the time of valve replacement to be one of the most important predictors for operative mortality [8], while Reinhartz et al. showed the optimal time for operation to be before hemodynamic instability or infiltration of the paravalvular tissue by the infection occurs [9].

Although rapid surgical treatment in patients with extensive endocarditic infection greatly influences their morbidity and mortality rate, the optimal time point for the operation is still controversially discussed in the literature [10, 11]. Because no randomized controlled trials have been conducted to clarify the role of surgery in the treatment of AIE patients and its optimal timing to improve outcomes, current practice guidelines for the surgical management of complex left-sided IE are largely based on results of observational studies and expert opinion [3, 11, 12]. Our results are consistent with those of published studies showing the benefit of surgical therapy. In a large, longitudinal, prospective cohort study to examine the impact of surgery, Aksoy et al. determined that surgical therapy in patients with left-sided AIE is a strong independent predictor of long-term survival. In this recently published study, the authors demonstrated that the use of surgery was independently predicted by age, the presence of heart failure, and an intracardiac abscess, concluding that these high-risk patients may reap the most benefit from early surgery and should be considered for early, aggressive surgical therapy [13]. Vikram et al. found in a large retrospective, observational cohort study of seven hospitals that valve surgery for patients with complex, left-sided native valve endocarditis was independently associated with reduced 6-month mortality, particularly evident among patients with moderate to severe congestive heart failure [14].

▌ Survival and abscess formation

Our study confirms previous reports that documented the association of periannular abscess complications with increased mortality and the need of surgery in almost all patients [15, 16]. In our study, abscess formation, which was found in 46% of patients, was not only associated with significantly decreased survival but also showed an association with early mortality in the univariate analysis (OR 2.16, 95% CI 1.21–3.85). These results are in accord with data published by the investigators of the International Collaboration on Endocarditis Merged Database, a cohort from 7 sites in 5 countries. They showed that, among 311 patients who had definite aortic valve AIE, 67 (22%) patients had a periannular abscess. These patients were more likely to undergo surgery (84% vs. 36%, p < 0.001), and their in-hospital mortality rate was higher (19% vs. 11%, p < 0.09). In this study, periannular abscess formation showed a nonsignificant trend towards an increased risk of death (OR 1.9, 95% CI 0.9 to 3.8) but failed to be an independent risk factor in multivariate analysis, in which S. aureus infection was independently associated with increased risk of death [17]. These results are confirmed by recently published studies in which S. aureus infective endocarditis is associated with high morbidity and mortality and a more severe prognosis compared with AIE caused by other pathogens [16, 18]. In our study, early nonsurvivors showed more infection with Staphylococcus species and a nonsignificant trend towards S. aureus infection.

▌ Clinical results of Shelhigh® bioprostheses

Our data show that Shelhigh® bioprostheses offer very good early and mid-term clinical results in patients with AIE. The low reinfection rate found with these valves is comparable to the results achieved at our institution in the treatment of endocarditis with cryopreserved homografts [19] although with a follow-up of 676 patient years the number of Shelhigh® patients having reached mid-term follow-up is still small and the results will need to be verified in the long-term course.

In June 2007, the FDA seized all finished devices at Shelhigh's manufacturing facility due to concerns of a potential risk of nonsterility (see press release FDA June 2007, homepage; *http://www.fda.gov*) but did not mandate a recall of the devices. In Germany, there was no government seizure but a voluntary distribution stop by the Shelhigh® company. In our study, no de novo infection due to possible nonsterility was found.

Study limitations

The present study is retrospective and nonrandomized, using prospectively updated data. Clinical endpoints such as exercise capacity and functional tests could not be assessed. There is a natural bias in the clinical assessment of the patient groups. Despite these limitations the present study represents a unique attempt to collect and analyze a single-center experience in the surgical treatment of AIE with the use of the Shelhigh® stentless bioprosthesis over a period of 8 years in a large group of patients.

Conclusions

The survival of patients differs significantly depending on the urgency of their operations. Better outcome could have been achieved if patients had been referred earlier for surgery. Compared to early survivors, nonsurvivors (< 30 d) showed clinical signs of cardiac decompensation and deterioration of the endocarditis suggesting that early outcome could be improved if patients are operated upon before heart failure or septic shock develops.

The low reinfection rate of Shelhigh® bioprostheses in AIE is promising and the satisfactory early and mid-term results achieved in patients with native and prosthetic endocarditis need to be verified in the long-term course.

Acknowledgments. We thank Ms. A. Benhennour for bibliographic assistance, Ms. K. Weber for photographic work, Ms. J. Stein for statistical work, and Ms. A. Gale for editorial assistance.

Conflict of interest. There is no financial relationship with any corporate sponsor that might relate in some way to the subject presented.

References

1. Moreillon P, Que YA (2004) Infective endocarditis. Lancet 363:139–149
2. Hoen B, Alla F, Selton-Suty C, Beguinot I, Bouvet A, Briancon S, Casalta JP, Danchin N, Delahaye F, Etienne J, Le Moing V, Leport C, Mainardi JL, Ruimy R, Vandenesch F (2002) Changing profile of infective endocarditis: results of a 1-year survey in France. JAMA 288:75–81
3. Cabell CH, Abrutyn E, Fowler VG, Jr., Hoen B, Miro JM, Corey GR, Olaison L, Pappas P, Anstrom KJ, Stafford JA, Eykyn S, Habib G, Mestres CA, Wang A

(2005) Use of surgery in patients with native valve infective endocarditis: results from the International Collaboration on Endocarditis Merged Database. Am Heart J 150:1092–1098
4. Musci M, Siniawski H, Knosalla C, Grauhan O, Weng Y, Pasic M, Meyer R, Hetzer R (2006) Early and mid-term results of the Shelhigh stentless bioprosthesis in patients with active infective endocarditis. Clin Res Cardiol 95:247–253
5. Siniawski H, Lehmkuhl H, Weng Y, Pasic M, Yankah C, Hoffmann M, Behnke I, Hetzer R (2003) Stentless aortic valves as an alternative to homografts for valve replacement in active infective endocarditis complicated by ring abscess. Ann Thorac Surg 75:803–808, discussion 808
6. Abolhoda A, Yu S, Oyarzun JR, Allen KR, McCormick JR, Han S, Kemp FW, Bogden JD, Lu Q, Gabbay S (1996) No-react detoxification process: a superior anticalcification method for bioprostheses. Calcification of bovine pericardium: glutaraldehyde versus No-React biomodification. Ann Thorac Surg 62:1724–1730
7. Abolhoda A, Yu S, Oyarzun JR, McCormick JR, Bogden JD, Gabbay S (1996) Calcification of bovine pericardium: glutaraldehyde versus No-React biomodification. Ann Thorac Surg 62:169–174
8. Alexiou C, Langley SM, Stafford H, Lowes JA, Livesey SA, Monro JL (2000) Surgery for active culture-positive endocarditis: determinants of early and late outcome. Ann Thorac Surg 69:1448–1454
9. Reinhartz O, Herrmann M, Redling F, Zerkowski HR (1996) Timing of surgery in patients with acute infective endocarditis. J Cardiovasc Surg (Torino) 37:397–400
10. Akar AR, Szafranek A, Alexiou C, Janas R, Jasinski MJ, Swanevelder J, Sosnowski AW (2002) Use of stentless xenografts in the aortic position: determinants of early and late outcome. Ann Thorac Surg 74:1450–1457, discussion 1457–1458
11. Tornos P, Iung B, Permanyer-Miralda G, Baron G, Delahaye F, Gohlke-Barwolf C, Butchart EG, Ravaud P, Vahanian A (2005) Infective endocarditis in Europe: lessons from the Euro heart survey. Heart 91:571–575
12. Horstkotte D, Follath F, Gutschik E, Lengyel M, Oto A, Pavie A, Soler-Soler J, Thiene G, von Graevenitz A, Priori SG, Garcia MA, Blanc JJ, Budaj A, Cowie M, Dean V, Deckers J, Fernandez Burgos E, Lekakis J, Lindahl B, Mazzotta G, Morais J, Smiseth OA, Vahanian A, Delahaye F, Parkhomenko A, Filipatos G, Aldershvile J, Vardas P (2004) Guidelines on prevention, diagnosis and treatment of infective endocarditis executive summary; the task force on infective endocarditis of the European society of cardiology. Eur Heart J 25:267–276
13. Aksoy O, Sexton DJ, Wang A, Pappas PA, Kouranly W, Chu V, Fowler VG Jr, Woods CW, Engemann JJ, Corey GR, Harding T, Cabell CH (2007) Early surgery in patients with infective endocarditis: a propensity score analysis. Clin Infect Dis 44:364–372
14. Vikram HR, Buenconsejo J, Hasbun R, Quagliarello VJ (2003) Impact of valve surgery on 6-month mortality in adults with complicated, left-sided native valve endocarditis: a propensity analysis. Jama 290:3207–3214
15. Choussat R, Thomas D, Isnard R, Michel PL, Iung B, Hanania G, Mathieu P, David M, du Roy de Chaumaray T, De Gevigney G, Le Breton H, Logeais Y, Pierre-Justin E, de Riberolles C, Morvan Y, Bischoff N (1999) Perivalvular abscesses associated with endocarditis; clinical features and prognostic factors of overall survival in a series of 233 cases. Perivalvular Abscesses French Multicentre Study. Eur Heart J 20:232–241
16. Fowler VG, Jr., Miro JM, Hoen B, Cabell CH, Abrutyn E, Rubinstein E, Corey GR, Spelman D, Bradley SF, Barsic B, Pappas PA, Anstrom KJ, Wray D, Fortes CQ, Anguera I, Athan E, Jones P, van der Meer JT, Elliott TS, Levine DP, Bayer AS (2005) Staphylococcus aureus endocarditis: a consequence of medical progress. JAMA 293:3012–3021

17. Anguera I, Miro JM, Cabell CH, Abrutyn E, Fowler VG Jr, Hoen B, Olaison L, Pappas PA, de Lazzari E, Eykyn S, Habib G, Pare C, Wang A, Corey R (2005) Clinical characteristics and outcome of aortic endocarditis with periannular abscess in the International Collaboration on Endocarditis Merged Database. Am J Cardiol 96:976–981
18. Hill EE, Vanderschueren S, Verhaegen J, Herijgers P, Claus P, Herregods MC, Peetermans WE (2007) Risk factors for infective endocarditis and outcome of patients with Staphylococcus aureus bacteremia. Mayo Clin Proc 82:1165–1169
19. Yankah AC, Pasic M, Klose H, Siniawski H, Weng Y, Hetzer R (2005) Homograft reconstruction of the aortic root for endocarditis with periannular abscess: a 17-year study. Eur J Cardiothorac Surg 28:69–75. Epub 2005 Apr 18

Double valve endocarditis and evolving paraannular abscess formation

H. Siniawski, M. Dandel, H. B. Lehmkuhl,
C. A. Yankah, R. Hetzer

Introduction

Active infective endocarditis (AIE), which was first described by Osler in 1885 [1], is still a pernicious disease although its clinical course and outcome have changed since the introduction of penicillin and other antibiotics. This made the disease treatable and mortality was dramatically lowered but recent decades have not brought about any further improvement in treatment [2]. Today the mortality rate varies between 15 and 40% [3–7], which is as high as in patients suffering from acute myocardial infarction complicated by heart failure [8, 9]. However, it should be mentioned that in some published series the surgical mortality is very low. This implies not only that the criteria by which patients are included in studies vary but also that there is something that could be done to improve the outcome of the disease. Because an important percentage of the patients demonstrate a disproportion between the objective state of the disease and their subjective symptoms [10], an improvement in visualization techniques such as magnetic resonance imaging [11] or computed tomography [12] – and especially the proper use of echocardiography [13] – could substantially improve diagnostic procedures. In "surgical cases" such an improvement helps to define the optimal window for surgical intervention and can lead to improved outcome. It is clear that, before the development of modern visualization techniques, root abscess was recognized only during surgery or in postmortem pathological investigations [14].

The different clinical presentations of endocarditis during the individual development of AIE [15] explain the use in the existing literature of the terms "chronic" and "acute" endocarditis in line with the course of clinical manifestation. The chronic type was previously considered to develop with delay and not to be severe in character. In this paper, the terms "acute" and "chronic" will not be applied because they are often misleading. The term "active infective endocarditis" (AIE) will be used to indicate virulence and progression, independent of the clinical situation. It includes all patients who had a positive blood culture in the 3 weeks before surgery (or positive culture of the excised valve) and the presence of macroscopically

typical lesions [16–19]. Echocardiographic investigations of AIE aim to answer the following important questions:
- How can we predict the clinical course of the disease in individual patients?
- How can we optimize treatment decisions, i.e., when can we state that medical treatment has been successfully completed and when is surgical support needed to improve clinical outcome?

Types of endocarditis

Native valve and prosthetic endocarditis

Native valve endocarditis should be treated differently from prosthetic endocarditis. Prosthetic endocarditis should be classified according to the type of prosthesis. The rate of infection is reported to be significantly lower in patients who have received homograft or Shelhigh valve implantation [20] and the course of infection seems not to be as dramatic as in other cases following valve replacement. Native valve endocarditis occurs when infection strikes the native valve. In most cases only valve structures are destroyed, which means that the inflammatory process is localized, and deeper parts of the heart are not involved. Most authors dealing with endocarditis suggest that the infected mitral valve be treated by "medical" means; however, at least 25% of these patients require additional surgery. Endocarditic lesions are often located on "preconditionally" changed valves. Preconditioning refers to general conditions that increase the risk of endocarditis. In our series the following preconditions were found as risk factors in 48% of the AIE patients: tooth extraction 32%, tonsillitis 18%, wound healing 11%, sepsis 11%, respiratory infection 7%, osteomyelitis 7%, cholecystitis 7%, skin abscess 4%, and HIV infection (as a preconditioning factor for right-sided endocarditis) 4% [21].

Prosthetic endocarditis

In prosthetic endocarditis visualization of the diseased structures is more difficult by echocardiography; on the other hand, the surgical option should be considered almost exclusively, once the diagnosis is certain.

Simple and destructive forms of endocarditis

From the practical and morphological viewpoints, native endocarditis can be classified on the basis of echocardiographic findings into the simple or the destructive form (prosthetic endocarditis is almost always destructive). This description helps to identify patients who require very early surgical treatment and distinguish them from those who need echocardiographic follow-up but in whom early surgery or surgery at all is probably not indicated. Simple endocarditis requires antibiotic treatment until the course of treatment is completed and surgical intervention should always be kept in mind if the classical indications are fulfilled.

The destructive form usually requires surgery before antibiotic treatment can be successfully performed. Any delay in surgery will promote the risk of devastating damage not only of the valves but also of surrounding tissue, including the myocardium.

Complication of simple endocarditis

The simple form of endocarditis can be complicated by the development of large vegetations that are a source of embolization. To avoid embolization, the size of any vegetation should be closely monitored and the risk of embolization should be assessed on the basis of the echocardiogram itself [22]. However, it should be kept in mind that in a small number of cases even small vegetations can produce severe clinical symptoms. The risk of embolization is substantially higher if the vegetations are larger than 1.0 cm (OR, 9; CI, 1.98–40.08; p = 0.004) [23]. It is important to note that stroke [24] (clinically manifested embolism) was an independent predictor of death (p < 0.0001).

Echocardiography with the transesophageal mode of insertion can help to assess other factors (extension of the abscess, valve regurgitations) influencing morbidity and mortality [25–28] and thus positively influence the result of the surgical or medical treatment [29].

The overall sensitivity of transthoracic investigation is not as accurate as that of transesophageal echocardiography [30] for vegetations, and ranges from 60% to 98% [31–33]. Right-sided localized vegetations, especially those larger than 2 mm in diameter [34] (which lie closer to the chest wall), are readily detected by TTE as well.

A vegetation per se can produce infection dissemination to peripheral organs [35] as well as infection extension into the heart muscle by coronary embolism or the phenomenon of "kissing vegetations" [36]. With kissing vegetations, infection spreads by contact with the anterior mitral valve leaflet in diastole, producing microdamage of the leaflet from the left ventricular side. This leads to total destruction of an important part of the mitral valve and mitral apparatus with all consequences, including the necessity of mitral valve surgery in patients who primarily suffered from aortic valve endocarditis.

The presence of vegetations is the result of multifactorial causes, including the virulence of microbes and the host reaction, which are modified by effective treatment. In the literature the risk of embolization in larger series is calculated to be between 34.1 [37] and 43% [38]. Some patients have more than one site of embolization and the three commonest sites in left-sided endocarditis are cerebral (62%), spleen (49%), and renal (22%). Fibroelastomas, usually small sized tumors, can mimic a vegetation and, being small, produce excessive embolic events [39]. The diagnosis of suspected fibroelastoma is very important because the tumor should be removed as soon as possible [40] when it is still small, to save patients from severe embolic complications such as blindness or hemiparesis. A full body scan is strongly advocated in patients suffering from AIE to exclude septic embolic events in other organs. "Silent" septic emboli in the brain or other vital organs can strongly affect the medical options. The medical team should be aware of the risk of complications in the course of the treatment of the "simple" or "benign" form of AIE and of the changing "clinical face" of endocarditis. The simple form can transform into the destructive form at any time. Any signs of such "turn over" should not be ignored. In such a situation the opinion of a second echocardiographer should be sought and abscess formation or extracardiac embolization should be suspected. In some cases, lack of clinical reaction during treatment can be affected by several factors, the most important being virulent microorganisms and/or microbes resistant to antibiotics but also a weak reaction of the host to infection. In such cases the decision in favor of surgery should be made without hesitation. It is important to search for peripheral embolization on the basis of ultrasonography or other modern techniques of visualization.

∎ Paravalvular abscess as the main sign of the destructive form of endocarditis

The diagnosis of paravalvular abscess as one of the distinguishing features of destructive endocarditis has long been based on surgical or necropsy findings [41], since preoperative clinical information is often misleading because the clinical manifestations of abscess formation are often not characteristic enough to prompt the diagnosis [107]. Today's echocardiographic techniques, particularly transesophageal echocardiography, have allowed diagnosis of abscess with high sensitivity and specificity, reaching 99% and 98.9%, respectively, at our institution [42]; similar results have been published elsewhere [43–48].

Diagnosis of the destructive form of endocarditis should warn physicians to refer a patient for surgical consultation at the right time.

Echocardiographic definition of abscess

New technology in ultrasound allows better definition of the abscess according to the sonographic appearance of the abscess content. An abscess should be assumed in ultrasonic investigation when an echodense area is visible – this is the first sign of an abscess (Figs. 1a and 2). This phase of abscess development is difficult to distinguish from the normal appearance of the cardiac structure in ultrasound. In the later course, a process of demarcation is strongly suggested by an echolucent area which is clearly visible in transthoracic echocardiography (TTE) or transesophageal echocardiography (TEE) and can be seen as a structure anatomically localized in the annulus (Figs. 1b and 3). In the next phase of development the cavity is opened and in two-dimensional echocardiography the flow appears inside the abscess cavity (color flow) after spontaneous rupture of the abscess, when the infected content is injected into the circulation. In such a case, a connection between the aorta and the abscess is established (Fig. 1c).

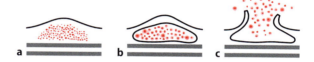

Fig. 1. Periannular abscess development: **a** infiltration, **b** demarcation process, **c** abscess cavity after rupture and emission of the contents into the circulation

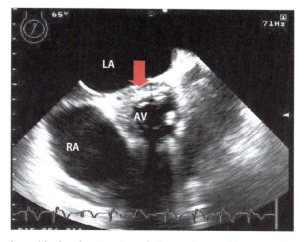

Fig. 2. Transesophageal investigation with the short section of the aortic root. The arrow indicates paravalvular abscess at the phase of infiltration (homogenous content) (*LA* left atrium, *AV* aortic valve, *RA* right atrium)

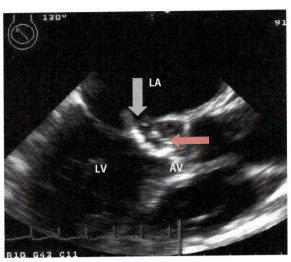

Fig. 3. Transesophageal long section of the aortic root and LV. The horizontal arrow indicates root abscess during second phase (nonhomogenous content) shortly after rupture into the left atrium. The second arrow indicates site of rupture of the abscess. (*LA* left atrium, *AV* aortic valve, *LV* left ventricle)

In the early phase of abscess development, its size is recognized as an important criterion of severity of the inflammation [49]. According to its extension, an abscess is classified on the basis of its appearance in the ultrasonic image. Three stages are advocated to distinguish sizes of abscess development in relation to the size of the aortic cusp:
- localized abscess
- circular abscess
- aortoventricular dehiscence.

A *localized abscess* is not larger than two aortic cusps and is small in size. Such an abscess should be described by reference to the nearest aortic cusp: "noncoronary" localization means that the abscess is located in the area of the noncoronary aortic cusp.

A *circular abscess* is defined as an abscess that is larger than or comparable in size to one half to two thirds of the annular circle without any signs of aortoventricular dehiscence.

Aortoventricular dehiscence is a separation (discontinuity) between the aorta and left ventricle of more than half of its circumference. Dehiscence in the ultrasonic image usually (but not always) means a wide echolucent area recognizable as a separation of structures. In approximately 20% of cases, the area of discontinuation is visible in echocardiography as an echolucent area between the aortic root and left ventricle.

Abscess classification according to stage of development

The stage of abscess is distinguishable during ultrasonic examination in TTE harmonic imaging and in TEE. One can postulate that periannular abscess formation is very similar to skin furuncle development. In the early stage of abscess (Stage I), infiltration is present which is visible as an isolated thickness in a very specific manner in the ultrasound (Fig. 1). Not seldom it appears in the ultrasound as an echodense area, which in some cases can be easily distinguished from the surrounding tissue, and is measurable. In general, the first stage is difficult to recognize even in the transesophageal investigation during the first examination; nevertheless sensitivity and specificity in our laboratory were 95.6 and 94.5%, respectively [42]. Stage II is characterized by an echolucent area or "nonhomogenous area" which means that echolucent spots are seen mixed with echodense areas in TEE. This stage correlates with the stage of skin abscess when fluctuation is present. The content of the abscess varies in consistency and ultrasonically presents as a nonhomogenous area created by the demarcation process. In this stage, the abscess can rupture and the infected content, sometimes more than 5 ml, will be injected into the blood, producing a septic reaction. In stage III, the echolucent area opens for flow, similar to stage II, but with visible color flow inside the cavity. This stage means that an abscess cavity is present and is "washed out" by the blood flow. In this way rupture of the abscess belongs to the stage of spontaneous healing (or healing after antibiotic therapy). In some cases this can be a sign that the process of local inflammation is completed, but the infected abscess content may seed new abscess areas in the peripheral organs.

However, large opened abscesses can cause dehiscence or pseudoaneurysms with the mechanism of ongoing infection or aseptically, and this process can and should be kept under surveillance by echocardiographic monitoring.

It seems that the presence of a large abscess in the first stage of development is not the optimal time for surgery (as is indeed also the case in skin abscesses) because of the lack of clear demarcation and adequate antibiotic pretreatment but also because the diagnosis may be uncertain. This hypothesis was tested in one preliminary study and the results of early surgery were not satisfactory [50].

Extension of infection from the aortic area

It should be stated that in one third of cases of the destructive form of endocarditis the inflammation process is not as straightforward as might be expected, even when medical treatment seems to be very effective. The inflammation can spread by local infiltration and not be limited to one area but spread to the next annulus (mitral or tricuspid) with all the consequences of destruction.

Double valve disease

Infective double valve disease seldom occurs as a primary lesion. Two thirds of the patients experience infection extension from primary aortic valve lesions. Extension of infection from the aortic valve can take several paths (Fig. 4). Anatomically the aortic valve with its annulus is located close to other valves and their valvular structures, tricuspid, mitral and pulmonary. If destruction takes place, these valves are at risk of secondary infection. In particular, the mitral valve is often involved in the destructive process. A fistula from the aortic annulus area may develop in the direction of the right atrium, right ventricle or left atrium. Independently in diastole, the vegetation may enter the coronary circulation producing abscess formation in the myocardium. The main processes responsible for infection are the following:

- *Jet lesion* (Hetzer) is the extension of infection through the infected blood stream. The infected blood coming from aortic regurgitation and impinging onto the left ventricular structures – usually the anterior mitral leaflet and its chordae – is able to cause ulceration and perforation (Fig. 5).
- *Local metastases* are formed by the extension of infection from the aortic root (abscess) deeper by direct contact, producing mitral annulus destruction and aortomitral dehiscence (Fig. 4). Such a complication is associated with poorer surgical results [51].
- *"Mitral kissing vegetations"* produce secondary involvement of the mitral valve in primary aortic valve endocarditis [36]. The mitral kissing vegetation is a vegetation that is attached to the aortic valve and flies and touches ("kissing") in diastole the anterior mitral leaflet, and can cause secondary damage of the ventricular side of the anterior mitral leaflet in

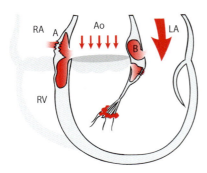

Fig. 4. The most characteristic path of extension seemed to be infection dissemination from the aortic area down to the other heart structures (*A*). Fistulas can extend into the right atrium or right ventricle, producing a septic ventricular defect, or all complications at the same time through mechanism of tissue infiltration. Fistulas can develop to the left side of the heart, to the left atrium, or the left ventricle (*B*)

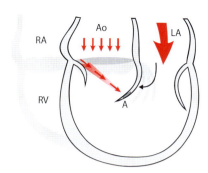

Fig. 5. Antidirectional propagation of infection from the aortic valve through diastolic regurgitant jet flow from a damaged aortic valve to the anterior mitral valve is known as "jet lesion" (A)

a similar way to infection extension by jet lesion. In practice, it is sometimes difficult to distinguish a jet lesion from a kissing vegetation lesion [42].

The route of extension of infection has a major influence on the mortality rate. Concomitant mitral valve operation in patients suffering from primary aortic valve infections raises the mortality rate if extension takes place through local metastases. Extension of the infection by a regurgitation jet does not increase mortality when double valve surgery is required because the reconstruction procedure is possible in the great majority of the cases. However, selection of the valve and the choice of a prosthesis resistant to bacterial invasion have a major impact on the results by reducing the risk of reinfection [52]. Extension of the infection into the mitral valve area is time-dependent, and adequate echocardiographic diagnosis should help to make the decision for surgery before disease extension occurs. In such cases precise two-dimensional echocardiography and color Doppler are extremely valuable in helping to identify the problem. It is important to note that destruction of the mitral valve itself is an indication for surgery even if the mitral regurgitation is not classified as hemodynamically important (grade 3 or 4).

■ Asymptomatic destruction of the heart structures after successful medical treatment of AIE

Silent progression of the lesions of the heart caused by microorganisms after successfully treated endocarditis should be distinguished from slow progression of the degenerative lesions. Such lesions can be the source of the next attack by microorganisms but also in themselves as *loci minoris resistentiae* of the tissue can cause progressive and silent development of valve disease or pseudoaneurysms. Since this process is silent or accompanied by only very minor clinical symptoms that may be ignored by patients, echocardiographic follow-up is mandatory even up to several years after completion of the treatment.

Primary mitral valve endocarditis

Approximately two thirds of left-sided native valve endocarditis primarily affect the aortic valve.

If the mitral valve is affected primarily, endocarditic valve lesions appear at the site of coaptation of the mitral leaflets, whereby primary mitral valve endocarditis can be recognized in the echocardiogram (Fig. 6). The early course of destruction of the mitral valve should be detected, when regurgitation may be minimal. However, the endocarditic lesions are often far more pronounced than is visible and such "small lesions" should be investigated very carefully as the destruction can be much more extended. In the later course, the vegetation and destruction can be so extensive that the mitral apparatus may be totally destroyed and patients are usually affected by embolic events. Primary mitral ring abscess affects the posterior part of the ring and should be distinguished from abscess extension from the aortic root.

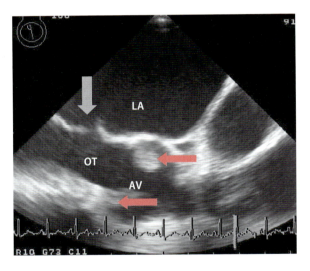

Fig. 6. Transesophageal long section of the aortic root and left ventricular outflow tract (OT). Horizontal arrow indicates aortic cusps with vegetations. Arrow on anterior mitral leaflet shows the jet lesion (*LA* left atrium, *AV* aortic valve, *OT* outflow tract)

Extension to the right side

Primary right-sided endocarditis (RSE) manifests differently and requires different treatment. RSE as an isolated lesion has a relatively benign prognosis with low inhospital mortality [53], and the surgical results are satisfactory. There are several preconditions bearing the risk of RSE development, including congenital heart defects [54], right heart catheterization [55], alcoholism, and sepsis [56]. However, in Western populations at least, it is predominantly a disease of intravenous drug abusers [57] where Staphylococcus aureus is the main microorganism involved [58]. Cardiac resynchronization therapy (CRT), which is probably the most rapidly developing medical option to treat patients with the end stage of dilated cardiomyopathy [59], has been noted in recent years as carrying the risk of cable infections in these severely ill patients [60]. Thus, a new challenge for the echocardiographer is to search pacemaker cables for the presence of vegetations in heart failure patients admitted with signs of infection [61].

Infection extension from the aortic valve, which produces left-right shunts and secondary RSE, requires a different strategy. In such a situation, surgery is needed before antibiotic treatment is completed, to improve the treatment results. Following these strategies, surgery of right-sided infective endocarditis with left-side involvement can be performed with good early, mid-term and long-term results [62]. Patients with involvement of the left side showed not only worse preoperative conditions but also a significantly poorer clinical outcome than those with isolated right-sided infective endocarditis. This strategy requires adequate and accurate monitoring of patients suffering from RSE on the basis of TEE [63], but for the follow-up TTE is advocated [64].

Three-dimensional echocardiography

Technological advances in ultrasonography equipment have resulted in a new modality, three-dimensional echocardiography. This modality provides a view that gives excellent imaging of the anatomical relations to surrounding structures [65].

From the surgical decision-making point of view, assessment of the dynamics of infection extension is generally of primary importance. Today's three-dimensional technology allows the location of the lesions and their relation to the cardiac structures to be assessed [66]. Unfortunately, infiltration and its extension cannot be assessed using this modality [67] as in classical two-dimensional echocardiography. This limitation reduces to some degree the utility of three-dimensional technology as a diagnostic tool in AIE.

Indications and timing for surgery

The classical indications for surgery, as described by Hetzer et al. [68], include the following: septic shock, septic emboli and persistent sepsis despite adequate antibiotic therapy, leading to kidney failure or congestive heart failure. The indications for surgery are fulfilled when prolonged infection persists despite treatment [69] or when there is resistance to antibiotic therapy. What makes surgery difficult? Severe destruction of the annular and periannular structures of the aortic, mitral and tricuspid valve by infection extension can produce technical problems that can be managed only in each situation individually, giving surgeons satisfaction when success is reached [70–79]. From the classical viewpoint, the value of echocardiography in the diagnosis of complications (such as secondary mitral valve involvement in the pathological process) is well established [80–84]. However, we have to consider other practical options and concentrate not only on the assessment of existing complications but also on the aim of echocardiography, which is *to predict the risk of complications as precisely as possible to find out the exact window of opportunity when a patient will benefit from surgery.* As stated previously, AIE is a malignant disease because prediction of the clinical course is not easy, as reported by Wallace et al. [85]. They identified 22 clinical, echocardiographic, and laboratory markers available within 48 h after admission and found that conventional prognostic factors in their study did not appear to predict outcome early during hospital admission. Nor did they help to select patients for surgery or to assess the optimal timing of surgery. This underlines the fact that a single echocardiographic investigation will not help significantly and that serial echocardiography with the aim of "critical vision" of each case is fundamental. Under such circumstances the value of echocardiography and the contribution of the echocardiographer who performs the investigation in selecting patients for surgery are of primary importance. The efficiency (accuracy, specificity, and sensitivity) of identification of destruction and prediction of the disease by assessment of the paths of infection propagation is very precise in experienced hands. For example, the size of vegetations [86] gives information about the risk of embolization [87].

The echocardiographer should have the clear aim of identifying patients who need reconstructive surgery [88] as the highest priority. If surgery is performed early for mitral valve repair [89–92] or reconstruction surgery, the operative mortality is lower and the operation provides satisfactory freedom from recurrent infection and freedom from repeat operation. Avoiding the implantation of foreign material means that anticoagulation is not necessary, and this is an important achievement. In general, a delay in surgical treatment has a very great influence on mortality and morbidity (reinfection, reversibility of congestive heart failure, cardiogenic shock) in patients suffering from extended infection [93].

Netzer et al. demonstrated that early aggressive treatment can have a strong influence on reducing mortality and is the best predictor of good long-term outcome [94] in patients without congestive heart failure which can be regarded as a factor of the time passed since the first symptoms developed (fever). It should not be forgotten that surgery after sterility of the surgical field is achieved reduces the risk of reinfection, which per se carries high mortality. It is also true that surgical correction of the severely destroyed heart by experienced surgeons is possible and mortality is not always elevated in such patients [68]. However, devastating destruction of the two valves requiring double valve surgery with reconstructive procedures of the roots and aorta carries a higher risk of mortality [50]. There is another important factor influencing mortality, which is hemodynamic instability.

Surgery is superior to medical treatment alone when AIE is complicated by heart failure [95]; in this situation the mortality rate has been reported as 51% compared with 14% in stable patients (OR, 0.22; 95% CI, 0.09–053; p = 0.001). On the other hand, as has been stated, destructive endocarditis complicated by shock is associated with a substantial mortality rate reaching 30% and should be treated surgically without delay as an ultima ratio measure to save the patient's life. Are we able to assess the risk of decompensation and, in the most severe form, hemodynamic shock?

Hemodynamic shock in AIE is a form of mixed vasodilatory shock and cardiogenic shock: vasodilatory shock, in which hypotension [96, 97] occurs as a result of failure of the vascular smooth muscle to constrict, and cardiogenic shock, in contrast characterized by profound vasoconstriction in the peripheral circulation because the systolic ejected volume of the heart is strongly reduced [98]. In all forms of vasodilatory shock that have been examined, plasma catecholamine concentrations are markedly increased [99–101], with activation of the renin–angiotensin system which indicates failure of the smooth muscle to keep tension. This makes this hemodynamic situation so difficult to survive for patients, and surgical correction of the destroyed parts of the valves with excision of the infected area is the only chance to save the patient's life. Prolonged medical treatment in one series published by our institution had a prominent negative influence on surgical results because of the rising risk of shock development (OR 11.00, p 0.005) [102]. In general, urgent surgery has the same impact on the surgical results (OR 11.00, p 0.001) [103]. Patients suffering from mixed (cardiogenic and septic) shock had an extremely high surgical mortality rate of 38.8% [104].

Is it possible to predict the risk of such grave hemodynamic complications on the basis of echocardiography? The hemodynamic state of patients can be followed on the basis of complete echocardiographic investigation, in which color Doppler helps to assess the severity of valve incompetence, which is one of the most important predictors of the development of low cardiac output syndrome. Assessment of the grade of valve regurgitation of patients suffering from AIE is critical. As described above, the endocarditic lesions at the beginning show a lack of demarcation and the continuity of the tissue seems to be complete. In fact the destruction may be severe but the function of the valves is partially protected and the regurgitation jet is not pronounced. In such cases the classical criteria of regurgitation published by Helmcke's group [105] can be misleading and are not adequate. The presence of any kind of jet, even a small one, is of primary importance and all small "color spots" can identify destruction of the heart structures and should be well defined by the echocardiographer and never ignored. The first further concept of color jet propagation, "A large jet means great regurgitation" is still true but the opposite, "a small jet means slight regurgitation," is in many cases untrue. It is advocated that this rule be remembered for the phenomenon of regurgitation assessment on the basis of convergence methods and estimation of vena contracta.

Despite these limitations of the color Doppler method, when the investigator is aware of these problems it can help not only in the precise estimation of regurgitant lesions but also in the estimation of the extent of endocarditic destruction and, thus, help to predict the risk of hemodynamic failure.

It seems to be true that if destructive endocarditis is treated surgically in good time, before any complications arise, the mortality rate can be as low as approximately 8% [106].

Conclusions

Echocardiographic investigation in experienced hands and performed serially allows us to define the extension of inflammatory processes in the heart with great sensitivity and specificity and can explain worsening of the hemodynamics, but it can also *predict* the dynamics of the illness [107].

During the course of treatment, echocardiographic monitoring of the size of vegetations [86] is mandatory to assess the risk of embolization [108]. All other complications, such as dissemination of destruction or any other form of blood or tissue expansion of inflammation, can be and should be followed by echocardiographic investigation to enable optimal timing of surgery [109].

Echocardiography can help to distinguish the dynamic form of destruction, which happenings within only a few days, from the more "stable" development of valve destruction. The destructive form of endocarditis requires definition of the exact window of opportunity when a patient will benefit from surgery.

The timing of the investigations is crucial in assessing the dynamic course of development. The echocardiographer's highest priority should be to select patients who require reconstructive surgery [110]. Prediction of the endocarditis is based on assessment of the presence or absence of vegetation formation and destruction development. Careful follow-up is required to recognize the tendency towards local and general infection extension. Knowledge and experience of these phenomena in ultrasonography are required to define and predict the probable course of active infective endocarditis in each individual patient.

■ **Acknowledgment.** The authors thank Anne M. Gale (Editor in the Life Sciences) for assistance in writing this article.

References

1. Osler W (1885) The Gulstonian lectures on malignant endocarditis. BMJ I:467–470, 522–526, 577–579
2. Peters PJ (2005) Infective endocarditis. Journal of Diagnostic Medical Sonography 21(3):192–204
3. Netzer ROM, Zollinger E, Seiler C, Cerny A (2000) Infective endocarditis: clinical spectrum, presentation and outcome. An analysis of 212 cases 1980–1995. Heart 84:25–30
4. Lowes JA, Hamer J, Williams G et al (1980) 10 Years of infective endocarditis at St. Bartholomewás Hospital: analysis of clinical features and treatment in relation to prognosis and mortality. Lancet I:133–136
5. Karchmer AW (1997) Infective endocarditis. In: Braunwald E (ed) Principles of Internal Medicine. Saunders, Philadelphia, pp 1077–1104
6. Hricak V, Kovacik J, Marks P, West D, Kromery V Jr (1999) Aetiology and outcome in 53 cases of native valve staphylococcal endocarditis Postgrad Med J 75:540–543
7. Cabell CH, Jollis JG, Peterson GE, Corey GR, Anderson DJ, Sexton DJ et al (2002) Changing patient characteristics and the effect on mortality in endocarditis. Arch Intern Med 162:90–94
8. Maisch B (1989) Klinik der infektiösen Endokarditis. Internist 30:483–491
9. Califf RM, Bengston JR (1994) Cardiogenic shock. N Engl J Med 330:1724–1730
10. Schön HR, Fuchs CJ, Schömig A, Blömer H (1994) Die infektiöse Endokarditis im Wandel. Analyse eines Krankheitsbilds im letzten Jahrzehnt. Z Kardiol 83:31–37
11. Jeang MK, Fuentes F, Gately A, Byrnes J, Lewis M (1986) Aortic root abscess: initial experiences using magnetic resonance imaging. Chest 89:613–615
12. Cowan JC, Patrick D, Reid DS (1984) Aortic root abscess complicating bacterial endocarditis: demonstration by computed tomography. Br Heart J 52:591–593
13. Enriquez-Sarano M, Nkomo VT, Michelena H (2008) Principles and practice of echocardiography in cardiac surgery. Card Surg Adult 3:315–348
14. Sheldon WH, Golden A (1951) Abscesses of the valve rings of the heart, a frequent but not well recognized complication of acute bacterial endocarditis. Circulation 4:1–12
15. Prendergast BD (2006) The changing face of infective endocarditis. Heart 92(7):879–885
16. Doukas G, Oc M, Alexiou C et al (2006) Mitral valve repair for active culture positive infective endocarditis. Heart 92:361–3

17. Alexiou C, Langley SM, Stafford H et al (2000) Surgical treatment of infective mitral valve endocarditis: predictors of early and late outcome. J Heart Valve Dis 9:327–334
18. Mullany CJ, Chua YL, Schaff HV et al (1995) Early and late outcome after surgical treatment of culture-positive active endocarditis. Mayo Clin Proc 70:517–525
19. Livesey S A (2006) Mitral valve reconstruction in the presence of infection (editorial). Heart 92(3):289–290
20. Siniawski H, Lehmkuhl H, Weng Y, Pasic M, Yankah C, Hofmann M, Behnke I, Hetzer R (2003) Stentless aortic valves as an alternative to homografts for valve replacement in active infective endocarditis complicated by ring abscess. Ann Thorac Surg 75(3):803–808
21. Siniawski H (2006) Clinical features in patients suffering from AIE with aortic root abscess. In: Hetzer R (ed) Active infective aortic valve endocarditis with infection extension. Clinical features, perioperative echocardiographic findings and results of surgical treatment. Fortschritte der Herz-, Thorax- und Gefäßchirurgie. Steinkopff, Darmstadt, pp 45–46
22. Habib G (2006) Management of infective endocarditis. Heart 92(1):124–130
23. Thuny F, Disalvo G, Belliard O (2005) Risk of embolism and death in infective endocarditis: prognostic value of echocardiography. Circulation 112:69–75
24. Thuny F, Avierinos J-F, Tribouilloy C, Giorgi R, Casalta J-P, Milandre L, Brahim A., Nadji G, Riberi A, Collart F et al (2007) Impact of cerebrovascular complications on mortality and neurologic outcome during infective endocarditis: a prospective multicentre study. Eur Heart J 28(9):1155–1161
25. Jaffe WM, Morgan DE, Pearlman AS, Otto CM (1990) Infective endocarditis, 1983–1988: echocardiographic findings and factors influencing morbidity and mortality. J Am Coll Cardiol 15:1227–1233
26. Wann LS, Hallam CC, Dillon JC, Weyman AE, Feigenbaum H (1979) Comparison of M-mode and cross-sectional echocardiography in infective endocarditis. Circulation 60:728–733
27. Mintz GS, Kotler NM, Segal BL, Parry WR (1979) Comparison of two-dimensional and M-mode echocardiography in the evaluation of patients with infective endocarditis. Am J Cardiol 43:738–744
28. Martin RP, Meltzer RS, Chia BL, Stinson EB, Rakowski H, Popp RL (1980) Clinical utility of two-dimensional echocardiography in infective endocarditis. Am J Cardiol 46:379–385
29. Stewart JA, Silimperi D, Harris P, Wise NK, Fraker TD Jr, Kisslo, JA (1980) Echocardiographic documentation of vegetative lesions in infective endocarditis: clinical implications. Circulation 61:374–380
30. Daniel WG, Mugge A, Grote J, Hausmann D, Nikutta P, Laas J, Lichtlen PR, Martin RP (1993) Comparison of transthoracic and transesophageal echocardiography for detection of abnormalities of prosthetic and bioprosthetic valves in the mitral and aortic positions. Am J Cardiol 71:210–215
31. Mugge A, Daniel WG, Frank G, Lichtlen PR (1989) Echocardiography in infective endocarditis: reassessment of prognostic implications of vegetation size determined by the transthoracic and the transesophageal approach. J Am Coll Cardiol 14:631–638
32. Shapiro SM, Young E, De Guzman S, Ward J, Chiu CY, Ginzton LE, Bayer AS (1994) Transesophageal echocardiography in diagnosis of infective endocarditis. Chest 105:377–382
33. Shively BK, Gurule FT, Roldan CA, Leggett JH, Schiller NB (1991) Diagnostic value of transesophageal compared with transthoracic echocardiography in infective endocarditis. J Am Coll Cardiol 18:391–397

34. Roy P, Tajik AJ, Guiliani ER, Schattenberg TT, Gau GT, Frye RL (1976) Spectrum of echocardiographic findings in bacterial endocarditis. Circulation 53:474–482
35. Habib G (2003) Embolic risk in subacute bacterial endocarditis: role of transesophageal echocardiography. Curr Cardiol Rep 5:129–136
36. Piper C, Hetzer R, Körfer R, Bergmann R, Horstkotte D (2002) The importance of secondary mitral valve involvement in primary aortic valve endocarditis: the mitral kissing vegetation. Eur Heart J 23:79–86
37. Thuny F, Di Salvo G, Belliard O et al (2005) Risk of embolism and death in infective endocarditis: prognostic value of echocardiography. A prospective multicenter study. Circulation 112:744–754
38. Steckelberg JM, Murphy JB, Ballard D, Bailey K, Tajik AJ, Taliercio CP, Giuliani ER, Wilson WR (1991) Emboli in infective endocarditis: the prognostic value of echocardiography. Ann Intern Med 114:635–640
39. Sun JP, Asher CR, Yang XS, Cheng GG, Scalia GM, Massed AG, Griffin BP, Ratliff NB, Steward WJ, Thomas JD (2001) Clinical and echocardiographic characteristics of papillary fibroelastomas: a retrospective and prospective study in 162 patients. Circulation 103:2687–2693
40. Shapiro LM (2001) Cardiac tumors: diagnosis and management. Heart 85:218–222
41. Berlin JA, Abrutyn E, Strom BL et al (1995) Incidence of infective endocarditis in the Delaware Valley, 1988–1990. Am J Cardiol 76:933–936
42. Siniawski H (2006) Value of perioperative echocardiography. In: Hetzer R (ed) Active infective aortic valve endocarditis with infection extension. Clinical features, perioperative echocardiographic findings and results of surgical treatment. Fortschritte der Herz-Thorax-und Gefäßchirurgie. Steinkopff, Darmstadt, p 31
43. Ivert TS, Dismukes WE, Cobbs CG, Blackstone EH, Kirklin JW, Bergdahl LA (1984) Prosthetic valve endocarditis. Circulation 69:223–232
44. Calderwood SB, Swinski LA, Waternaux CM, Karchmer AW, Buckley MJ (1985) Risk factors for the development of prosthetic valve endocarditis. Circulation 72: 31–37
45. Vlessis AA, Hovaguimian H, Jaggers J, Ahmad A, Starr A (1996) Infective endocarditis: ten-year review of medical and surgical therapy. Ann Thorac Surg 61: 1217–1222
46. Mugge A, Daniel WG, Frank G, Lichtlen P (1989) Echocardiography in infective endocarditis: reassessment of prognostic implications of vegetation size determined by the transthoracic and transesophageal approach. J Am Coll Cardiol 14:631–638
47. Erbel R, Rohmann S, Drexler M, Mohr-Kahaly S, Gerharz CD, Iversen S, Oelert H, Meyer J (1988) Improved diagnostic value of echocardiography in patients with infective endocarditis by transoesophageal approach: a prospective study. Eur Heart J 9:43–53
48. Marcus RH, Heinrich RS, Bednarz J, Lupovitsch S, Abruzzo J, Borok R, Vandenberg B, Kerber RE, Piccione W, Yoganathan AP, Lang RM (1998) Assessment of small-diameter aortic mechanical prostheses. Physiological relevance of the Doppler gradient, utility of flow augmentation, and limitations of orifice area estimation. Circulation 9:866–872
49. Chirillo F, Pedrocco A, De Leo A, Bruni A, Totis O, Meneghetti P, Stritoni P (2005) Impact of harmonic imaging on transthoracic echocardiographic identification of infective endocarditis and its complications. Heart 91(3):329–333
50. Siniawski H (2006) Clinical outcome after surgery in patients suffering from root abscess. In: Hetzer R (ed) Active infective aortic valve endocarditis with infection extension. Clinical features, perioperative echocardiographic findings and results of surgical treatment. Fortschritte der Herz-, Thorax- und Gefäßchirurgie. Steinkopff, Darmstadt, p 32

51. Wong CM, Oldershaw P, Gibson DG (1981) Echocardiographic demonstration of aortic root abscess after infective endocarditis. British Heart Journal 46:584–586
52. Siniawski H, Grauhan O, Hofmann M, Pasic M, Weng Y, Yankah C, Lehmkuhl H, Hetzer R (2004) Factors influencing the results of double-valve surgery in patients with fulminant endocarditis: the importance of valve selection. Heart Surgery Forum 7(5):1–6, doi:10.1532/HSF98.20041075
53. Hecht SR, Berger M (1992) Right-sided endocarditis in intravenous drug users: prognostic features in 102 episodes. Ann Intern Med 117:560–566
54. Bashore TM (2007) Adult congenital heart disease: right ventricular outflow tract lesions. Circulation 115:1933–1947
55. Pronovost P, Needham D, Berenholtz S et al (2006) An intervention to decrease catheter-related bloodstream infections in the ICU. N Engl J Med 355:2725–2732
56. McGee DC, Gould MK (2002) Preventing complications of central venous catheterization (review article). N Engl J Med 348:1123–1133
57. Moss R, Munt B (2003) Injection drug use and right sided endocarditis. Heart 89:577–581
58. Nadji G, Remadi JP, Coviaux F, Mirode AA, Brahim A, Enriquez-Sarano M, Tribouilloy C (2005) Comparison of clinical and morphological characteristics of Staphylococcus aureus endocarditis with endocarditis caused by other pathogens. Heart 91:932–937
59. Shah PK (2005) Preservation of cardiac extracellular matrix by passive myocardial restraint: an emerging new therapeutic paradigm in the prevention of adverse remodeling and progressive heart failure. Circulation 112:1245–1247
60. Denton MD, Digumarthy SR, Chua S, Colvin RB (2006) Case records of the Massachusetts General Hospital. Case 20-2006: an 84-year-old man with staphylococcal bacteremia and renal failure. N Engl J Med 354:2803–2813
61. Kranidis A, Filippatos G, Kouloris S, Charitos C, Sioula E (2003) Pacemaker endocarditis with sizeable vegetation and intermittent fever. Echocardiography 20:295–296
62. Musci M, Siniawski H, Pasic M, Grauhan O, Weng Y, Meyer R, Yankah CA, Hetzer R (2007) Surgical treatment of right-sided active infective endocarditis with or without involvement of the left heart: 20-year single center experience. Eur J Cardiothorac Surg 32:118–125
63. San Roman JA, Vilacosta I, Zamorano JL, Almeria C, Sanchez-Harguindey L (1993) Transesophageal echocardiography in right-sided endocarditis. J Am Coll Cardiol 21:1226–1230
64. Berger M, Delfin LA, Jelveh M, Goldberg E (1980) Two-dimensional echocardiographic findings in right-sided infective endocarditis. Circulation 61:855–861
65. El Muayed M, Chandrasekar Burjonroppa S, Croitoru M (2005) Added accuracy with 3D echocardiographic imaging of valvular vegetations. Echocardiography 22:361–362
66. Lang RM, Mor-Avi V, Sugeng L et al (2006) Three-dimensional echocardiography: the benefits of the additional dimension. J Am Coll Cardiol 48:2053–2069
67. Asch FM, Bieganski SP, Panza JA, Weissman NJ (2006) Real-time 3-dimensional echocardiography of intracardiac masses. Echocardiography 23:218–224
68. Hetzer R, Deyerling W, Borst HG (1984) Herzklappenchirurgie bei aktiver infektiöser Endokarditis. In: Gahl K (ed) Infektiöse Endokarditis. Klinik, Diagnostik, Therapie. Steinkopff, Darmstadt, pp 148–176
69. Oakley CM, Hall RJC (2001) Endocarditis: problems of patients being treated for endocarditis and not doing well. Heart 85:470–474
70. Braimbridge MV (1969) Cardiac surgery and bacterial endocarditis. Lancet 1:1307–1309

71. Buckley MJ, Mundth ED, Daggett WM, Austen WG (1971) Surgical management of the complications of sepsis involving the aortic valve, aortic root and ascending aorta. Ann Thorac Surg 12:291–399
72. Gonzalez-Lavin L, Liese M, Ross DN (1970) The importance of "jet lesion" in bacterial endocarditis involving the left heart. J Thorac Cardiovasc Surg 59:185–192
73. Gonzalez-Lavin L, Scappatura E, Liese M, Ross DN (1970) Mycotic aneurysm of the aortic root, a complication of aortic valve endocarditis. Ann Thorac Surg 9:551–556
74. Okies JE, Bradshau MMW, Williams TW (1973) Valve replacement in bacterial endocarditis. Chest 63:898–904
75. Shumacker HB (1972) Aneurysm of the aortic sinuses of Valsalvae due to bacterial endocarditis with special reference to their operative management. J Thorac Cardiovasc Surg 63:896–903
76. Hetzer R, Dalichau H, Borst HG (1975) Herzklappenchirurgie bei bakterieller Endocarditis. Thoraxchirurgie 23:427–430
77. Hetzer R, Oelert H, Borst HG (1981) Surgery for prosthetic valve endocarditis (Abstract). J Cardiovasc Surg 22:458
78. Hetzer R, Papagiannakis N, Dragojevic D, Oelert H, Gahl K, Borst HG (1981) Decision making aspects in valve surgery for active bacterial endocarditis. In: Birks W, Ostermeyer J, Shulte HD (eds) Cardiovascular Surgery. Springer, Berlin Heidelberg New York, pp 108–113
79. Hetzer R (1981) Prosthetic valve endocarditis. In: Boerhave (ed) Causes of Infectious Endocarditis. Leiden
80. Easaw J, El-Omar M, Ramsey M (2000) Perivalvar abscess of the mitral valve annulus with perforation owing to infective endocarditis. Heart 83:261
81. Espinosa-Caliani JS, Montijano A, Melero JM, Montiel A (2000) Pseudoaneurysm in the mitral-aortic intervalvular fibrosa: a cause of mitral regurgitation. Eur J Cardiothorac Surg 17:757–759
82. Mihaljevic T, Byrne JG, Cohn LH, Aranki SF (2001) Long-term results of multivalve surgery for infective multivalve endocarditis. Eur J Cardiothorac Surg 20:842–846
83. Gillinov M, Diaz R, Blackstone EH, Pettersson GB, Sabik JF, Lytle BW, Cosgrove DM (2001) Double valve endocarditis. Ann Thorac Surg 71:1874–1879
84. Tleyjeh IM., Ghomrawi HMK., Steckelberg JM. et al (2007) The impact of valve surgery on 6-month mortality in left-sided infective endocarditis Circulation 115: 1721–1728
85. Wallace SW, Walton BI, Kharbanda KR, Hardy R, Wilson AP, Swanton H (2002) Mortality from infective endocarditis: clinical predictors of outcome. Heart 88:53–60
86. Rohmann S, Erbel R, Darius H et al (1991) Prediction of rapid versus prolonged healing of infective endocarditis by monitoring vegetation size. J Am Soc Echocardiogr 4:465–474
87. Di Salvo G, Habib G, Pergola V et al (2001) Echocardiography predicts embolic events in infective endocarditis. J Am Coll Cardiol 37:1669–1676
88. Zegdi R, Debièche M, Latrémouille C et al (2005) Long-term results of mitral valve repair in active endocarditis. Circulation 111:2532–5236
89. Feringa HH, Shaw LJ, Poldermans D, Hoeks S, van der Wall EE, Dion RA, Bax JJ (2007) Mitral valve repair and replacement in endocarditis: a systematic review of literature. Ann Thorac Surg 83(2):564–570
90. Iung B, Rousseau-Paziaud J, Cormier B et al (2004) Contemporary results of mitral valve repair for infective endocarditis. J Am Coll Cardiol 43:386–392
91. Doukas G, Oc M, Alexiou C et al (2006) Mitral valve repair for active culture positive infective endocarditis. Heart 92:361–363

92. Dreyfus G, Serraf A, Jebara VA et al (1990) Valve repair in acute endocarditis. Ann Thorac Surg 49:706–711
93. Wallace SM, Walton BI, Kharbanda RK, Hardy R, Wilson AP, Swanton RH (2002) Mortality from infective endocarditis: clinical predictors of outcome. Heart 88:53–60
94. Netzer RO, Altweg SC, Zollinger E, Täuber M, Carrel T, Seiler C (2002) Infective endocarditis: determinants of long term outcome. Heart 88:61–66
95. Vikram HR, Buenconsejo J, Hasbun R, Quagliarello VJ (2003) Impact of valve surgery on 6-month mortality in adults with complicated, left-sided native valve endocarditis. JAMA 280:3207–3214
96. Wilson RF, Thal AP, Kindling PH, Grifka T, Ackerman E (1965) Hemodynamic measurements in septic shock. Arch Surg 91:121–129
97. Suffredini AF, Fromm RE, Parker MM et al (1989) The cardiovascular response of normal humans to the administration of endotoxin. N Engl J Med 321:280–287
98. Dole WP, O'Rourke RA (1983) Pathophysiology and management of cardiogenic shock. Curr Probl Cardiol 8:1–72
99. Sylvester JT, Scharf SM, Gilbert RD, Fitzgerald RS, Traystman RJ (1979) Hypoxic and CO hypoxia in dogs: hemodynamics, carotid reflexes, and catecholamines. Am J Physiol 236:H22–H28
100. Benedict CR, Rose JA (1992) Arterial norepinephrine changes in patients with septic shock. Circ Shock 38:165–172
101. Cumming AD, Driedger A, McDonald JWD, Lindsay RM, Solez K, Linton AL (1988) Vasoactive hormones in the renal response to systemic sepsis. Am J Kidney Dis 11:23–32 [Erratum (1988) Am J Kidney Dis 11:363]
102. Sinawski H, Pasic M, Hetzer R (2005) Risk factors influencing outcome after surgical treatment of destructive endocarditis. Eur J Cardiothorac Surg 28:510
103. Musci M, Siniawski H, Pasic M, Weng Y, Loforte A, Kosky A, Yankah C, Hetzer R (2008) Surgical therapy in patients with active infective endocarditis: seven-year single centre experience in a subgroup of 255 patients treated with the Shelhigh W stentless bioprosthesis. Eur J Cardiothorac Surg 34:410–417
104. Siniawski H (2006) Patients suffering from AIE complicated by vasoactive shock. In: Hetzer R (ed) Active infective aortic valve endocarditis with infection extension. Clinical features, perioperative echocardiographic findings and results of surgical treatment. Fortschritte der Herz-Thorax-und Gefäßchirurgie. Steinkopff, Darmstadt, p 33
105. Helmcke F, Nanda NC, Hsiung MC, Soto B, Adey CK, Goyal RG, Gatewood RP Jr (1987) Color Doppler assessment of mitral regurgitation with orthogonal planes. Circulation 74:175–183
106. Sasaki Y, Suehiro S, Shibata T et al (2000) Early surgery for active infective endocarditis. Jpn J Thorac Cardiovasc Surg 48:568–573
107. Chambers J (1999) Should we ever treat the echo rather than the patient? Heart 82:652–653
108. Di Salvo G, Habib G, Pergola V et al (2001) Echocardiography predicts embolic events in infective endocarditis. J Am Coll Cardiol 37:1669–1676
109. Tleyjeh IM, Ghomrawi HMK, Steckelberg JM et al (2007) The impact of valve surgery on 6-month mortality in left-sided infective endocarditis. Circulation 115:1721–1728
110. Zegdi R, Debièche M, Latrémouille C et al (2005) Long-term results of mitral valve repair in active endocarditis. Circulation 111:2532–2536

Aortic root abscess: reconstruction of the left ventricular outflow tract and allograft aortic valve and root replacement

C. A. Yankah, M. Pasic, H. Siniawski, Y. Weng, R. Hetzer

Introduction

Active infective aortic endocarditis complicated by abscess formation remains a life-threatening disease and continues to challenge cardiovascular surgeons. Sir William Osler first described endocarditis in the Gulstonian lectures at the Royal College of Physicians in 1885 as a malignant disease that is in all its forms a mycotic process. An aortic root abscess can be diagnosed very early at its onset by transthoracic and transesophageal echocardiography with a sensitivity and specificity of 98 and 100%, respectively [1–3]. If after diagnosis, during antibiotic therapy, associated complications occur, such as burrowing abscess formation and fistulous communication between the aorta and the right atrium or the right ventricle, interventricular septum, aneurysm of the sinus Valsalva, pseudoaneurysmal formation of an abscess cavity and mitral incompetence, then urgent surgical intervention is mandatory, otherwise fatal cardiovascular complications are imminent [1–5].

Based on the pioneering surgical clinical work by Wallace in 1965 to replace the infected aortic valve, other surgeons followed suit by treating other cardiac valves affected by active infective endocarditis with different types of prosthetic valve replacements (Table 1) [6–11]. The surgical results of aortic root abscesses treated with prosthetic valves varied and were associated with high rates of early recurrent infection and mortality and, therefore, were not very satisfactory. Consequently, in 1972 Donald Ross introduced the use of the aortic allograft, which is a completely biological tissue

Table 1. Surgery for endocarditis – historical developments

Wallace [6]	1963	Prosthetic AVR
Robicsek [7]	1967	Prosthetic MVR
Ross [15]	1984	Homograft AVR
Oswalt [10]	1992	P. Autograft ARR
Acar [8]	1992	Homograft MVR
Pomar & Mestres [9]	1993	Homograft TVR

for replacing the infected aortic valve. Allograft tissue is permeable to serum antibiotics and is therefore resistant to infection. It became popular because it has the physiological attribute of being non-thrombogenic; therefore, it requires no long-term anticoagulation and has superior hemodynamic performance [12–18]. Somerville, Lau, and Donaldson reported a series of patients with aortic root abscesses who underwent successful aortic root replacement with allografts in 1982 and 1984 and proved the concept of biological reconstruction of the left ventricular outflow tract (LVOT) for the surgical treatment of aortic root abscesses [12–15]. Prior to this revolutionary surgery for aortic root abscesses, a freehand subcoronary aortic valve replacement technique with an allograft was introduced for treating noninfected aortic valve diseases by Dr. Donald Ross and Sir Brian Barratt-Boyes, independently of each other, in 1962 [16–18]. The surgical procedure with allograft aortic root replacement (ARR) or freehand subcoronary valve replacement (FAVR) was technically demanding; therefore, it was confounded by learning curve periods without tutorial guidance [19–22].

For over 44 years since the introduction of surgical treatment of active infective endocarditis by Wallace [6], the valve of choice for treating aortic root abscesses has been controversial [23–33, 35–44]. In the light of this uncertainty, a clinical study was conducted at our institution between 1988 and 2005 to evaluate 161 patients with aortic root abscesses who underwent aortic valve and root replacement with cryopreserved allografts. The study was designed to evaluate 30-d survival, the long-term survival after discharge, and freedom from reinfection and valve-related reoperation. The paper also addresses the following question: How does the allograft aortic root replacement (ARR) or the freehand subcoronary valve replacement (FAVR) procedure help to convince the surgeon faced with a patient with endocarditis with periannular abscess requiring urgent surgery that the right treatment has been chosen?

Methods

A total of 203 patients, who were operated on between January, 1988, and December, 2003, were enrolled in the study. The clinical study period extended to 2005, whereby the evaluation was divided into three periods: 1988 to 1991, 1988–2000, and 1988–2005 and reported [31–33, 56]. Ad interim 46 additional patients with active infective aortic valve endocarditis who were not included in the study have been operated (Table 2).

Of the 203 study patients, 161 who had periannular aortic root abscess underwent freehand aortic valve (FAVR, n=78) and aortic root (ARR, n=83) replacement. The clinical and follow-up study was approved by the institution and consent was obtained from the patients. Preoperative char-

Table 2. Surgery for acute infective endocarditis. Distribution of valve replacements. Deutsches Herzzentrum Berlin, 1986–2007

	Aortic	Mitral	Tricuspid	Two valves	Total
Prosthetic valves	194	130	–	65	389
Xenografts	186	111	10	38	345
Allografts	249[a]	–	–	–	249
Shelhigh	134	61	8	54	257
Elan	6	–	–	–	6

AIE active infective endocarditis, [a] 1988–2007

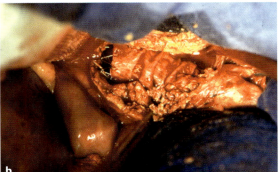

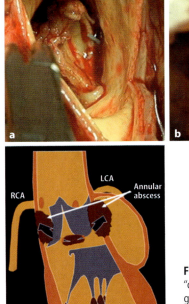

Fig. 1. a Stented prosthetic valve endocarditis. **b** Infected "composite" aortic valve prosthesis and ascending aortic graft. **c** Drawing of a circular periannual abscess formation in the aortic root

acteristics of the study population are shown in Table 3. There were 34 females (21.1%) and 127 (78.9%) males with a mean age of 53.1 years (range 2–82 years). Endocarditis of the native valve was found in 80 (49.7%) patients and of the prosthetic valve in 81 (50.3%); of the prosthetic valves, 49 (60.5%) were mechanical and 32 (39%) bioprosthetic (Fig. 1). Annular abscess formation was confined to the noncoronary sinus in 23 (14.2%), right coronary sinus in 16 (9.9%), left coronary sinus in 23 (14.3%), aortic mitral septum in 8 (5%), and ventricular septum in 8 (5%). Dehiscence of the

Table 3. Two hundred and three patients with active infective aortic valve endocarditis with and without aortic root abscess, 1988–2005

Patients with aortic root abscess	161
Age:	Mean 53.1 + 15.6 years
	Range 2–82 years
Gender:	Female 34
	Male 127
NYHA	II 17 III 63 IV 81 (44 cardiogenic shock)
AV-block	3 (2.7%)
Operative category:	
Urgent	80
Emergency	81
Freehand	
AVR	78 (48.4%)
ARR	83 (51.6%)
Follow-up 5.0 ± 4.3 years, 810 pt-years, 17 years maximum, 100% complete	
Aortic periannular abscess:	161
NVE:	80
PVE:	81
	49 (60.5%) Mechanical
	32 (39.5%) Bioprostheses
Aortic-ventricular discontinuity:	83
Abscess confined to the sinuses:	NC: 23, LC: 23, RC: 16
Aortic-mitral sept.	19
Aortic-atrial fistula	11
Jet lesion AML	27
Pseudoaneurysm	13

ventriculoarterial junction (ventriculoaortic dehiscence) caused by circular abscess formation was found in 83 patients (51.5%).

The most common microorganisms responsible were Staphylococcus (S. epidermidis: 34, S. aureus: 13) in 47 patients followed by Enterococcus in 23 and Streptococcus in 39 (Table 4). Additional procedures were replacement of the ascending aorta in 8 patients, mitral valve repair in 27, mitral valve replacement in 9, tricuspid valve reconstruction in 3, and coronary artery bypass graft (CABG) operation in 10. Follow-up totaled 810.8 patient-years (mean: 5.3 years) and was 100% complete.

Table 4. Surgery for acute infective endocarditis. Distribution of major responsible microorganisms. Deutsches Herzzentrum Berlin, 1986–2007

Microorganisms	No. of patients	Abscess formation	
		N	%
■ Staphylococcus	61	47[a]	79
■ Streptococcus	52	39	75
■ Enterococcus	27	23	85

[a] 34 S. epidermidis, 13 S. aureus

Table 5. Patients with intractable active infective aortic valve endocarditis who were bridged to heart transplantation

Patient	Age	Diagnosis	Microbiology	Abscess
■ BR	14	NVE	Negative	yes
■ CM	11	NVE	S. aureus	yes
■ FB	48	PVE	Negative	yes
■ GW	38	NVE	S. aureus	no

Preoperative complications were congestive heart failure, 100 (62%); septic/cardiogenic shock, 44 (27.3%); cerebral embolism, 19 (11.8%); peripheral embolism, 2 (1.2%); renal embolism, 3 (1.9%); spleen embolism, 3 (1.9%); pseudoaneurysm, 13 (8.1%); mitral valve dysfunction, 36 (22.4%); and tricuspid valve dysfunction, 3 (1.9%).

Four patients aged 14–48 years developed biventricular failure and were bridged with mechanical circulatory support for heart transplantation (Table 5).

■ The aortic root

The topographic anatomy of the aortic root and the anatomic relationship of the cardiac valves with the conducting system are shown in Fig. 2.

■ Pre- and postoperative monitoring and diagnostics

After the clinical diagnosis of active infective native and prosthetic endocarditis has been made, the patient remains under antibiotic therapy and close clinical observation in order to detect as early as possible the ensuing aortic root abscess formation by transthoracic echocardiography which is confirmed by transesophageal echocardiography [1–3]. The sensitivity and

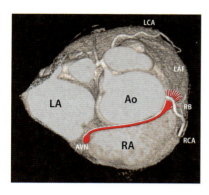

Fig. 2. Anatomic relationship of the cardiac valves and of the conducting system. The bundle of His

specificity for the detection of an abscess preoperatively by transesophageal echocardiography are 98 and 100%, respectively [3, 28]. Whole body computed tomography and ultrasound scanning are used to look for metastatic abscesses and ischemia in the abdominal organs (liver, spleen, kidney), skeletal bone, and brain. Large liver and spleen metastatic abscesses measuring more than 2 cm in diameter are treated by computed tomography-guided percutaneous puncture with drainage which is performed by the radiologist, while cerebral abscesses are treated by neurosurgeons. Small abscesses are treated with antibiotics and closely observed by sonographic scanning [28]. Previously, coronary angiography was performed in patients beyond 50 years of age or in cases with a positive troponin test, which suggests ongoing myocardial infarction. Currently, a preoperative 64-slice computed tomographic coronary angiography is performed to exclude a significant coronary artery disease or septic embolism, in particular when a large leaflet vegetation is present with symptoms of angina (Fig. 3).

The following concomitant procedures were performed: closure of ventricular septal defect, n = 8 (5%); mitral valve repair, n = 27 (16.8%); mitral

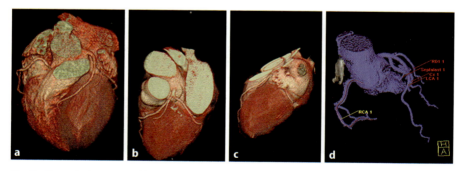

Fig 3. Computed tomographic coronary angiograms. **a** Right and left coronary arteries. **b** Left main coronary artery and its branches, the left anterior descending and the circumflex arteries. **c** The left anterior descending coronary artery. **d** An overview of the coronary arteries

valve replacement, n = 9 (5.6%); tricuspid valve repair, n = 3 (1.9%); coronary bypass grafting, n = 11 (6.8%); and replacement of the ascending aorta n = 8 (5%). Postoperatively 15 (9.3%) patients received intraaortic counterpulsation for low cardiac output and one patient needed a biventricular assist device and was bridged successfully to heart transplantation.

Current indications for allograft valve and root replacement

The indication for allograft aortic valve and root replacement is regarded as given
- in children and young adults,
- in women of child-bearing age,
- with active bacterial native and prosthetic aortic valve endocarditis with aortic root abscess, especially, aortic-ventricular discontinuity,
- with fungal endocarditis,
- with infected composite ascending aortic graft,
- following repeated "bland" periprosthetic leaks,
- according to patients' special wishes with refusal of long-term anticoagulant therapy and acceptance of the risk of reoperation [27, 32].

Surgical techniques

Operative steps

A complete median sternotomy is performed followed by free mobilization of the heart. This involves dissection of the aorta up to the arch, the innominate artery and innominate vein, the main pulmonary artery, and the inferior and superior vena cavae. The aorta is cannulated in the region of the ascending aorta and the aortic arch after administration of heparin. Bicaval venous cannulae are inserted when additional tricuspid and mitral valve reconstruction is anticipated. Otherwise, a double-stage venous cannula is inserted via the right atrium. The left ventricle is vented via a right superior pulmonary vein approach. Cardiopulmonary bypass is established at normothermia and the ascending aorta is then cross clamped. A transverse aortotomy is performed 2 cm above the sinotubular junction. The left and right coronary ostia are intubated with coronary cannulae, and antegrade blood cardioplegic solution is administered to induce cardioplegic cardiac arrest. Intermittent antegrade blood cardioplegia is performed every 20 min.

After myocardial protection, the infected native or prosthetic valve is excised and the foreign materials are removed followed by extensive debridement of the infected and necrotic tissues and the abscess cavity. The particles of the necrotic tissue are removed with a dry sponge and the local area is disinfected with polyvidon iodine for 3 min. This radical approach ensures elimination of biofilm bacteria and decolonization of the biofilm, thus, supporting the therapeutic effect of the serum and tissue antibiosis [12–15, 23–33].

The native aortic annulus is sized and an allograft of appropriate size for aortic root replacement is determined and selected for thawing. Ad interim when concomitant coronary artery bypass grafting (CABG) is anticipated with the saphenous vein or the left internal mammary artery, the distal coronary anastomosis is performed. A thawed, cryopreserved allograft aortic cylinder with flexible leaflets which is free from atheroma is prepared for the replacement of the native aortic valve in a subcoronary implantation technique or as a root replacement (Fig. 4).

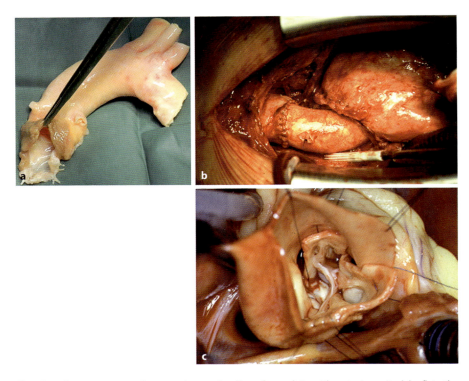

Fig. 4. a Long segment of composite aortic allograft conduit with anterior mitral leaflet, the arch, and the supraaortic branches. **b** Completed procedure of aortic root replacement as a freestanding root with reimplantation of the coronary arteries. See details of the implantation techniques in the next chapter. **c** Subcoronary implantation of scalloped aortic allograft with retention of the noncoronary sinus wall and the anticipated second row of the proximal suture

Implantation techniques

The implantation technique chosen for the aortic allograft depends on the pathology and geometry of the aortic root and the size of the available aortic allograft as well as the surgeon's preference [24, 33, 34].

Reconstruction of the left ventricular outflow tract

An equine pericardial patch is used to reconstruct the right and left coronary supra- and infraannular abscess cavity and ventricular septum defect to allow anatomic insertion of the allograft [16–33].

After reconstruction of the component parts of the left ventricular outflow tract (LVOT), the allograft cylinder is inserted anatomically as a root replacement. In a situation where a small annular abscess is present, a free-hand subcoronary valve replacement (FAVR) with an aortic allograft is performed [16, 21, 22, 24–26, 31–33].

Aortic root replacement

Aortic root replacement is preferred when there is extensive abscess formation and destruction of the aortic root.

Lower (proximal) suture line. The lower suture line is performed by placing two-color multiple interrupted sutures at the native aortic annulus with 4-0 polypropylene (Prolene) buttressed by glutaraldehyde-fixed equine pericardial pledgets when the aortic annulus has not been destroyed by the abscess. Otherwise it begins at the base of the abscess cavity beneath the noncoronary sinus at the native mitral annulus with the interrupted sutures in healthy tissue below the abscess cavity in the native left ventricular outflow tract, working up toward the level of the aortic annulus at the noncoronary sinus without tension or distortion. The lower suture line is completed by placing single interrupted mattress sutures on the remaining circumference of the aortic annulus. Multiple interrupted sutures are placed along the subvalvular skirt of the allograft beginning at the aortic anterior mitral leaflet which was fashioned to fit the anticipated lower line below the abscess cavity of the aortic mitral fibrous septum [24, 33].

The allograft cylinder is inverted into the left ventricular outflow tract to allow reliable tying down of the sutures, then the allograft is carefully pulled out of the left ventricular outflow tract. Direct side-to-end anastomosis of the native left and right coronary arteries with the circumcised left and right coronary ostia of the allograft is performed. In a situation where destruction of the aortic root is present, the coronary ostia are dissected and circumcised as buttons for reimplantation.

Distal suture line. The distal end of the allograft (the sinotubular junction) is anastomosed with the native ascending aorta end-to-end by continuous suture technique using 4-0 polypropylene beginning at the posterior wall, reinforcing the suture line with the surrounding tissue of the native aortic wall. The sinotubular junction, which is usually 90% of the size of the aortic annulus, is geometrically matched to the native ascending aorta (Fig. 4) [24, 31–33].

Freehand subcoronary aortic valve replacement

After the lower proximal suture line is completed and the knots tied, the right and the left commissural posts are temporarily attached 2 cm above the native commissures with stay sutures. This procedure gives the surgeon an overview of the coaptation of the valve leaflets. The remaining right and left scalloped sinus walls are then attached to the adjacent native sinus walls beginning at the midpoint of the left coronary ostium and leading up to the commissural post using a double-arm 4-0 polypropylene suture. The right sinus wall is anastomosed to the adjacent right native sinus wall using a double-arm 4-0 polypropylene running suture at the midpoint below the right coronary ostium in the same manner up to the top of the commissure to meet the other suture. At the top of the commissure the two suture materials are tied down to fix the commissural post. The other half of the left subcoronary suture line is continued using the other half of the double-arm 4-0 polypropylene as a running suture up to the top of the noncoronary sinus wall and is tied down.

The right subcoronary suture line is continued with the other half of the double-arm 4-0 polypropylene as a running suture to the top of the noncoronary sinus wall and tied down. At the closure of the aortotomy the allograft noncoronary sinus is incorporated and attached to the native noncoronary sinus wall. If necessary, the allograft noncoronary sinus is used to enlarge the native noncoronary sinus wall as suggested by Ross and by Nicks in his technique using the autologous pericardium [16, 18, 46].

The completed procedure of aortic root replacement as a freestanding root with reimplantation of the coronary arteries as described by Ross is shown in Fig. 4.

Postprocedurally intraoperative echocardiography is performed to verify complete closure of the ventricular septum defect and competent valve performance (Fig. 5). After closure of the aortotomy, the proximal aortic saphenous vein anastomoses are performed. The aortic clamp times for ARR and FAVR techniques were 70–263 min (mean 123 min) and 44–260 min (mean 110 min) and the postoperative bleeding was 125–2700 ml (mean 1024.6 ml) and 100–3025 ml (mean 883 ml), respectively.

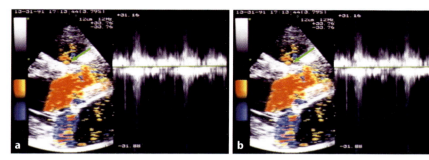

Fig. 5. a Preoperative echocardiogram demonstrating a ventricle septum defect caused by abscess formation. **b** Postprocedural echocardiogram demonstrating complete closure of the ventricle septum defect

Technical considerations for reducing postoperative allograft valve dysfunction

There are some technical operative factors which may influence the early and late outcome of the surgical management of aortic root abscess with and without dehiscence of the ventricular arterial junction (ventricular aortic dehiscence) with an allograft. Technical causes for reoperation may be associated with the following:

- incomplete resection of abscess cavity and necrotic tissues might cause reinfection, anastomic rupture and formation of a pseudoaneurysm,
- the use of a low quality or undersized aortic allograft may postoperatively cause an abnormally high gradient and early structural valve deterioration,
- continuous running sutures of the proximal anastomosis may cause anastomotic rupture in the presence of persistent infection,
- subaortic annular implantation of the aortic allograft can create compression and supravalvular stenosis of the allograft and subsequent high pressure gradients.
- Reduction aortic annuloplasty by plication of the trigona or annulorrhaphy of large aortic annulus as described by Carpentier and Elkins [54, 55] by placing two rows of purse-string sutures around the annulus of > 29 mm to down-size should be avoided because it may cause a catastrophic suture rupture in the presence of a persistent local infection.
- The mini-root replacement (inclusion technique) which incorporates the allograft within the native ascending aorta for infraanular aortic root abscess reduces the size of the outflow tract by 2 mm in diameter. The space between the native and allograft walls collects blood which induces organized hematoma and late calcification, thus, adding stress to the valve leaflets. Subsequently, structural valve deterioration develops with higher gradients. This is a serious pathology with a high reoperative risk.

- An undersized allograft will cause an abnormally high gradient and tension to the valve leaflets, furthermore, promoting an outward extension of the peripheral commissures at the sinotubular junction of a scalloped allograft and create central valve incompetence.
- Hemostasis as described by Ross is facilitated by reinforcing the proximal suture line with a glutaraldehyde-fixed pericardial strip placed within the suture loop of the lower suture line as they are tied down.
- This technique also prevents progression of annular dilation, particularly in patients with annuloectasia.
- The noncoronary sinus wall can be used to enlarge the aortic root as in the Nicks procedure, thus, creating a new noncoronary sinus and avoiding squeezing of the allograft when closing the aortotomy [16, 18, 46].

Data collection and postoperative follow-up

Patients were examined at our Institution or were contacted by means of telephone interview and mailed questionnaire. Further patient data were obtained from hospital records, family doctors, and cardiologists. Patients with unknown addresses could be tracked through the district or state registry, and the registry of births and deaths.

Follow-up of hospital survivors was complete in 100% of the patients who were available for analysis at a mean of 5.5 years and 1125 patient-years. They underwent routine echocardiographic studies at 3 and 9 months after operation and thereafter annually. Thirty patients were reoperated upon for all causes during the postoperative follow-up period at a mean of 1.2 years (range: 1 day–4.35 years). Eleven homografts were explanted due to recurrent infection (7 early, 4 late between 2 months and 4.6 years), 2 due to structural valve deterioration (2 and 4 years) and 17 due to nonstructural deterioration (130 days and 6.9 years). Transthoracic Doppler echocardiography was performed in uniform manner and the evaluations were comparable at the different institutions. The postoperative echocardiographic investigations performed during the study period until December 30, 2003, were documented and analyzed. If a patient had undergone more than one echocardiographic or clinical evaluation, the result of the most recent investigation was reported. Recurrent infection and structural and nonstructural valve deterioration of the aortic homograft were diagnosed preoperatively by echocardiographic studies and confirmed at the time of explantation.

Statistical methods

Tabular data are summarized by the mean and standard deviation for continuous variables and by percentages for categorical variables. Events are defined as valve-related complications, death, or other occurrences and determined by Kaplan-Meier actuarial analysis [15]. Differences in actuarial freedom between groups of patients are determined using the log-rank test. Differences in prognostic variables between two groups were evaluated by t-tests for continuous variables and the X^2 or Fisher exact test for categoric variables. Predictors of events during follow-up were identified by means of Cox's proportional hazards regression [45]. All variables were investigated for association with hospital death, overall death and valve-related complications in univariate and multivariate analysis.

Results

Hospital mortality

Early (30 day) mortality was 9.3% for urgent and 14.3% for emergency surgery. Forty-four (54%) of the emergency patients were in cardiogenic shock. Low output syndrome, congestive heart failure or both was the cause of 50% of the early deaths. The other causes of death were sepsis, multiorgan failure, cardiorespiratory failure, and renal failure. Staphylococcal infection was not an independent risk factor for operative death; although the incidence was higher than that of enterococcal and streptococcal endocarditis, the difference did not reach statistical significance (hazard ratio: 0.860; confidence interval, 95% confidence limits: 0.476–1.554, P < 0.69). Table 6 represents univariate Cox regression predicting risk factors for reoperation. Table 7 shows a summary of institutional results on early mortality.

Table 6. Cox regressional analysis of predictors for operative death

Variables	Risk ratio	95% Confidence interval	P-value
Staph. infection	0.87	0.48–1.55	0.62
Enterococcal infection	0.75	0.32–1.74	0.50
Streptococcal infection	0.90	0.49–1.66	0.75
Preoperative abscess	1.37	0.78–2.45	0.275
Reoperation	0.35	0.13–0.98	0.05
Reinfection	0.25	0.03–1.8	0.17
Implantation technique	0.71	0.42–1.20	0.20
Concomitant CABG	1.88	0.68–5.19	0.23
MV procedures	1.55	0.84–2.89	0.16

Table 7. Surgical results of active infective native and prosthetic valve endocarditis according to type of valve replacement. A review of the literature

Source	Years	30-d Mortality (%)		Reinfection/PL (%)	
		Allo/PA	Prosthesis	Allo PA	Prosthesis
Knosalla et al. [56]	11	8.5	23.5	3.2	27.1
Petrou et al. [24]	11	8.3		4.5	
Haydock et al. [25]	15	17	20.7	na	na
Yankah et al. [33]	17	9.3		4.3	
d'Udeckem et al. [23]	8		13		11.4
Niwaya et al. [29]	13	17	20	3	12.5
Niwaya et al. [29][a]	13	12		3	

[a] Ross operation
PL paravalvular leak, na not available

Late mortality

There were 9 (5.6%) late deaths. The actuarial patient survival at 15 and 20 years was 63% and 58%, respectively (Fig. 6). Recurrent endocarditis was not a predictive factor for late operative death (hazard ratio: 0.249; confidence interval, 95% confidence limits: 0.034–1.800, P<0.174). Long-term results of other authors are summarized in Table 8.

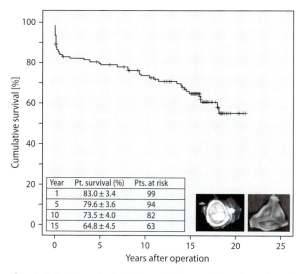

Fig. 6. Patient survival at 15 and 20 years after allograft aortic valve and root replacement

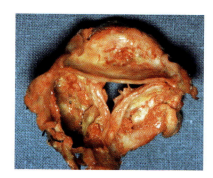

Fig. 7. Explanted allograft 15 years after subcoronary aortic valve replacement

Table 8. Comparison of surgical results of active infective native and prosthetic valve endocarditis according to technique for reconstruction of the LVOT and type of valve replacement

Procedure	FU years	Freedom from reinfection %	Survival %
Pericardium & prosth. Valve [25]	8	76	64
Pericardium/Dacron & prosth. Valve [25]	10	73	na
Allograft + AML [25]	15	24	na
	10	81	na
	15	72	50
Allograft + AML [24]	10	97	78
Allograft + AML [56]	11	96	82.1
Pericardium & prosth. Valve [56]	11	64.7	72
± Pericardium & allograft + AML [25]	17	72	70.4
Pericardium & prosth. Valve [25]	8	76	64
Ross procedure [25]	5	na	88

AML anterior mitral leaflet

Early and late complications

Reoperation

Of the 161 patients with aortic root abscess, there were 30 allograft explantations (Table 9). Seven (4.3%) early and 23 (14.3%) late allograft explantations of allograft valves were performed. Five early explantations were associated with the freehand subcoronary aortic valve and two with the aortic root replacement techniques. The surgical results of the 203 patients with and without aortic root abscess are shown in Table 10.

Three of the four patients with intractable heart failure were successfully bridged to heart transplantation. The fourth patient died while on mechanical circulatory support (Table 11).

Table 9. Allograft aortic valve and root replacement for aortic root abscess. Causes for reoperation and replacement of allograft (n=30/161)

	Early	Late
■ Residual/Recurrent infection	7	4
■ Paravalvular leak	5	–
■ Pseudoaneurysm		
■ Residual abscess cavity	1	2
■ AS (technical)	7	–
■ Residual VSD	1	–
■ Residual Ao-RA fistula	1	–
■ SVD	–	2

VSD ventricle septum defect, *SVD* structural valve deterioration

Table 10. Causes of reoperation by implantation technique: freehand AVR and ARR for active infective aortic endocarditis, n=43/203

	Freehand AVR				Aortic root replacement			
Causes for Reop	N	N	%	CI	N	%	CI	p value
■ NSVD	17	10	58.8	45.4–82.0	7	41.2	17.2–54.6	0.045
■ SVD	4	2	50.0	15.0–85.0	2	50.0	15.0–85.0	
■ Residual/Reinf.	11	9	81.8	55.2–95.3	2	18.2	4.70–44.8	0.0001
■ Early	7	6	85.7	48.7–97.4	1	14.3	2.60–51.3	
■ Late	4	3	75.0	37.6–96.4	1	25.0	3.60–62.5	

CI confidence interval, 95% confidence limits; *SVD/NSVD* structural and nonstructural valve deterioration, died: 4/43 (9.3%)

Table 11. Results of patients with intractable active infective aortic valve endocarditis who were bridged to heart transplantation

Patient	1st Op	2nd Op	3rd Op	Results [a]	Follow-up
■ BR	Allograft RR	ECMO	Htx	Alive	16 years
■ CM	Allograft RR	BVD	anticip Htx	Died	2 d
■ FB	Xenogr RR	BVD	Htx	Alive	4 years
■ CM	Stented AVR	IABP/RVAD	Htx	Died	3 mos

[a] Causes of death: (1) Sepsis & bleeding, (2) Sepsis and MOF

The 23 late reoperations were associated with the freehand subcoronary aortic valve replacement technique in 16 (9.9%) and the aortic root replacement technique in 7 (4.3%) patients. Table 12 shows various types of devices used to replace the aortic allograft at reoperation. The mean follow-up until reoperation was 1.2 years (range: 1 day–4.4 years). Actuarial freedom from explantation for all causes at 17 years was 72.7%. Undersized allografts measuring < 2 mm less than the native aortic annulus were revealed as an independent risk factor for reoperation in the patients with aortic periannular root abscess (hazard ratio: 0.146; confidence interval, 95% confidence limits: 2.263–10.990, P < 0.0001) (Fig. 8). Eleven allograft explantations were caused by residual/recurrent infection (ARR: 4, FAVR: 7). Causes of reoperation and type of replacement of allograft are shown in Tables 9, 10, and 12. Table 13 represents univariate Cox regression predicting risk factors for reoperation.

Allograft explantation in relation to implantation technique: aortic root replacement

Nine (10%) reoperations (2 early and 7 late) were carried out in 83 patients (4 recurrent infection, 4 nonstructural, and 1 structural valve deterioration) who underwent aortic root replacement (Table 10). The actuarial freedom from reoperation at 17 years for ARR was 82.5% (hazard ratio: 2.36; confidence interval, 95% confidence limits: 1.08–5.15). The root technique was not immune to developing early structural or nonstructural deterioration when an undersized allograft was used.

Allograft explantation in relation to implantation technique: freehand subcoronary aortic valve replacement

Of the 78 patients with the freehand aortic valve replacement (FAVR) technique, 21 (26.9%) underwent reoperation: 5 early and 16 late postoperatively. Recurrent infection occurred in 7, nonstructural valve deterioration in 13 patients and structural valve deterioration in 1 patient (Table 10). The actuarial freedom from reoperation at 17 years for the FAVR technique was 63.7% (hazard ratio: 2.36; confidence interval: 1.08–5.15). The freehand scalloped homograft technique for AVR was not an independent risk factor for a reoperation (hazard ratio: 0.477; confidence interval, 95% confidence limits: 0.202–1.123, P < 0.090) unless the allograft was undersized (Table 13).

Structural valve deterioration

Early structural valve deterioration resulting in valve incompetence required explantation in two young patients 2 and 4 years postoperatively (Tables 10 and 14). Actuarial freedom from explantation of allografts for structural valve deterioration at 17 years was 48% for undersized allografts (Fig. 8). Fig. 9 demonstrates actuarial freedom from allograft explantation for structural valve deterioration by age group.

Table 12. Prosthesis of choice for replacement of allografts after reinfection, structural and nonstructural valve deterioration (n=43)

Bioprostheses stentless	stented	Type of re-replacement Prostheses mechanical	Allografts	Total
3	5	21	14	43

Hospital deaths: 4/43 (9.3%)

Table 13. Univariate Cox regression predicting factors for reoperation

Variables	Risk ratio	95% Confidence interval	P value
■ Reinfection	14.34	6.30–32.91	0.0001
■ Preoperative abscess	2.03	0.86–4.78	0.11
■ Undersized	0.31	1.53–7.17	0.001
■ FAVR	2.19	0.88–5.49	0.09

FAVR freehand subcoronary aortic valve replacement

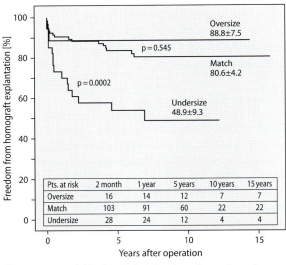

Fig. 8. Actuarial (Kaplan-Meier) freedom from allograft reoperation and explantation as determined by geometric match between the allograft and native annulus size. Reproduced with permission from Elsevier; Yankah et al. (2001) Eur J Cardiothorac Surg 20:839

Table 14. Allograft aortic root replacement for aortic root abscess. Freedom from valve-related complications (n = 161)

	1 year	5 years	15 years
■ SVD	100	97.3 ± 1.6	96.0 ± 2.0
■ TE & bleeding	100	100	100
■ Reinfection	95.1 ± 1.7	91.6 ± 2.4	91.6 ± 2.4
■ Reoperation	86.1 ± 4.3	77.7 ± 5.3	73.2 ± 6.1
– FAVR	83.8 ± 4.6	69.0 ± 6.0	63.5 ± 6.7
– ARR	88.5 ± 4.1	86.3 ± 4.6	82.9 ± 5.5
■ V-R mortality	95.9 ± 1.8	92.1 ± 2.5	92.1 ± 2.5

TE thromboembolism, *FAVR* freehand subcoronary aortic valve replacement, *ARR* aortic root replacement, *V-R* valve related, *SVD* structural valve deterioration

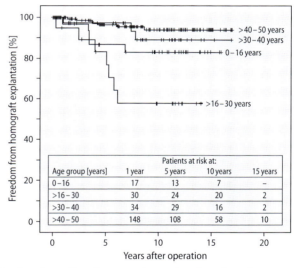

Fig. 9. Actuarial (Kaplan-Meier) freedom from allograft reoperation and explantation after structural valve deterioration by age group

Nonstructural valve deterioration

Seventeen (10.5%) patients required reoperation for nonstructural valve deterioration. Four (2.5%) of these cases were associated with aortic root and 13 (8.1%) with freehand subcoronary aortic valve replacement.

Thromboembolism and bleeding

Neither thromboembolism nor bleeding was observed among the 123 survivors [12].

Residual/recurrent infection and paravalvular leaks

Residual/recurrent infection and paravalvular leaks caused reoperation in 11 patients (7 (4.3%) early and 4 (2.5%) late postoperatively with one operative death). The actuarial freedom from explantation for residual/recurrent infection and aortic allograft paravalvular leaks was 91.64% at 10 years with no further events at 17 years (Table 14). Early or late allograft

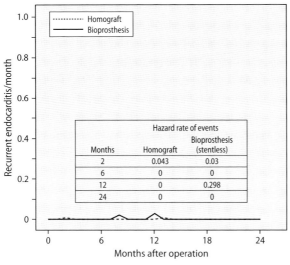

Fig. 10. Hazard function for recurrent endocarditis after replacement of infected aortic valves with allografts and stentless bioprostheses

Table 15. Incidence of prosthetic valve endocarditis. A review of the literature

Author	Valve type	Incidence
Yankah et al. [33]	Mitroflow	1.4%
Neville et al. [58]	CE-P	2.4%
Bach et al. [43]	Freestyle stentless	2.5%
David et al. [57]	Hancock II	2.7%
O'Brien et al. [60]	Allograft	0.1%
Yankah et al. [22]	Allograft	0.9%

CE-P Carpentier-Edwards Perimount

recurrent infection was not a predictive factor for operative death in the patients with periannular aortic abscess (hazard ratio: 1.37, confidence interval, 95% confidence limits, 0.78–2.45). Hazard function for a recurrent infection after replacement of infected aortic valve with allograft und stentless xenograft is shown in Fig. 10. The incidence of prosthetic valve endocarditis reported in the literature is summarized in Table 15.

Discussion

The first challenge of an aortic root abscess is a rescue operation, i.e., implanting into an infected aortic root a valve which has the potential to resist infection, a low transvalvular gradient to allow rapid left ventricular recovery of a compromised septic heart, and offers high patient survival. These conditions have to take precedence over other factors such as the surgeon's preference for a particular valve type or its anticipated durability.

Pre- and postoperative transesophageal and transthoracic echocardiography study of patients with acute infective endocarditis is a gold standard for diagnosis and for detecting cardiac complications, such as intracardiac communications by burrowing abscess, periannular and paraprosthetic abscess, or pseudoaneurysmal formation of an abscess cavity. The sensitivity and specificity for the detection of abscess preoperatively by transesophageal echocardiography were 98 and 100%, respectively [3, 28]. A pseudoaneurysm is caused by rupture or dehiscence of an anastomosis in the area of abscess cavity due to persistent local infection creating a communication between the systemic circulation and the abscess cavity [27, 33, 35]. These early cardiac and extracardiac complications can be well detected by transesophageal echocardiography and sonography to allow early intervention, therefore, offering better prognosis to the patient. When liver or spleen abscesses of more than 2 cm diameter are present, they are treated by computed tomography-guided percutaneous puncture with drainage if possible by the radiologist, while cerebral abscesses are treated by neurosurgeons. Small abscesses are treated with antibiotics and closely observed by sonography [26, 28, 31–33]. A preoperative 64-slice computing tomographic coronary angiography is useful for excluding significant coronary artery disease or septic coronary artery embolism.

When a small annular abscess is present, the subcoronary implantation technique with retention of the noncoronary sinus wall as described by Ross can be used. This technique offers stability to the commissural posts and therefore ensures adequate valve leaflet coaptation and reduces the probability of distortion and failure of the allograft which is associated with valve incompetence. The noncoronary sinus wall is used when necessary also for enlarging the aortic root [16, 18, 46]. This Ross technique is used for the implantation of stentless bioprostheses [41–43]. The potentials for valve distortion during allograft implantation especially when there is an extensive periannular aortic root abscess, can be avoided by maintaining the cylindrical shape of the aortic allograft and inserting it as a root replacement. The natural replacement of aortic root by an allograft and reimplantation of the circumcised coronary arteries as buttons followed by distal anastomosis to the native ascending aorta was first introduced by Donald Ross in 1972 [15–18]. This operation technique was initially used for reconstruction of a tunnel-type left ventricular outflow tract obstruction and was then adopted for treating aortic root abscesses. The original procedure was described by Hugh Bentall and Antony de Bono in 1968 [47]. They implanted a composite Dacron tube graft to replace the aortic root followed by direct implantation of the coronary arteries into the Dacron tube graft and used the native ascending aorta to wrap around the graft tube. The coronary artery reimplantation can be performed directly without circumcising the coronary artery particularly when there is no extensive root infection with necrotic tissues.

The fact that the aortic allograft and pulmonary autograft restore the anatomic and the physiologic units of the LVOT, thus, providing a low transvalvular gradient [48], have biological attributes similar to those of a natural valve in resisting infection, and are non-thrombogenic supports our choice for allograft valve tissue for managing active endocarditis complicated with annular abscess [12–15, 17, 24–26, 29–33, 56]. The limiting factor is that the aortic allograft does not have the potential to grow like the pulmonary autograft. It is weakly antigenic, like the glutaraldehyde-treated xenografts, but requires no immunosuppression in a clinical setting because the complication of immunosuppression would outweigh the benefits of the allograft, while ABO compatibility as claimed previously is for logistic reasons an option in adult patients [49, 50].

Our study provides data and outcome of 161 very sick patients with aortic root abscesses who were referred late for a rescue procedure. There was a higher incidence of abscess formation in patients with mechanical valves (60%) than in those with bioprostheses (40%). The most frequent biofilm microorganisms responsible for infection were staphylococcus (30% of all infections), streptococcus (25%), and enterococcus (13%). Among the patients with staphylococcal endocarditis associated with root abscess, 72% were infected by Staphylococcus epidermidis, which is widely respected as a very virulent organism. Although the incidence of staphylococcal endocarditis was higher than that of enterococcal and streptococcal endocarditis, the difference in operative risk/mortality did not reach statistical significance (hazard ratio: 0.860, confidence interval, 95% confidence limits: 0.476–1.554). This supports the fact that all biofilm bacteria can cause abscess formation, because they possess surface sensing systems that induce intracellular signals powerful enough to result in transcriptional and morphological changes for tolerating rapid environmental changes in nutrient availability, carbohydrate source, and pH [51–54]. This knowledge and information should, therefore, modulate echocardiographic and therapeutic decision-making in terms of the likelihood that biofilm bacteria will require early medical/surgical therapy before a periannular aortic root abscess develops.

Several technical modifications of the implantation technique of allografts and autografts have been suggested to improve surgical results.

- Geometric matching of the sinotubular junction: when performing the distal anastomosis of the allograft with the native ascending aorta, the sinotubular junction, which is usually 90% of the size of the aortic annulus, can be tailored to match the native ascending aorta.
- Hemostasis as described by Ross is facilitated by reinforcing the proximal suture line with glutaraldehyde-fixed pericardial strip placed within the suture loop of the lower line of sutures as they are tied down.
- This technique also prevents progression of annular dilation, particularly in patients with annuloectasia.
- Annulorrhaphy as described by Elkins and Northrup is performed by placing two rows of purse-string sutures around the annulus to downsize it [54, 55]. Further reduction annuloplasty can be performed by plicating the three interleaflet fibrous trigona with a pledgeted 3-0 polypropylene suture.

Clinical reports claimed that the type of valve used to replace the infected aortic valve may not be as important as radical debridement of infected and necrotic tissues and resection of the abscess [12–15, 24–33]. The study identified and confirmed the technique of radical debridement to eliminate the biofilm bacteria from the infected tissues. The following aspects which could improve the surgical management of aortic root abscess were established:

- radical debridement and resection of the infected and necrotic tissues,
- curetting of slimy endothelial surfaces of the aortic root. Curetting was reserved for the region of the interventricular septum below the right coronary artery and the membranous ventricular septum instead of resection in order to avoid A-V block. Three patients needed postoperative pacemaker implantation for A-V block.
- Local disinfection to decolonize the biofilm bacteria in order to enhance the effective antibiotic therapy.
- Avoidance of undersized allografts.
- Avoidance of aortic root tailoring.
- Use of antibiotic permeable cryopreserved aortic allografts which slowly release antibiotics into the site of implantation to resist infection.
- Use of sutures pledgeted with glutaraldehyde-fixed equine pericardium.
- Monitoring of intravascular and intracavitary catheters for local contamination and infection.
- Postoperative antibiotic therapy for 2–6 weeks with sensitivity tests and CRP monitoring.

The incidence of recurrent allogaft infection ranges from 1–4% which is lower than the 8–11% rate for prostheses [3, 23–25, 27–36, 56]. In further analysis, it has been shown that the incidence of early (<60 days) and late (>60 days) recurrent infection of allografts and autografts was 0–4% and 1–3%, as compared to 4% and 3% for stentless bioprostheses [3, 10, 11, 23, 24, 26, 29, 32]. Reinfection was the most common event in the first 6–12 weeks postoperatively [3, 25, 33]. The linearized rate of recurrent infection was 0.9%/pt-year in our study. Actuarial freedom from reinfection for allografts at 11 years and 17 years was 78–96% and 72%, as compared to 72% and 76% at 8 and 11 years for prosthetic valves, respectively [24, 33, 56]. The above data indicate that the aortic allograft tissue is more protective against recurrent infection than the prosthetic valves [23, 25, 31, 65]. The protective potential of allografts against infection is also demonstrated by the incidence of 0.1–0.9% allograft infection after primary ARR and AVR in a sterile aortic root. This is somewhat lower than that of stentless and stented bioprostheses (1.4–2.7%); see Table 13 [10, 11, 22, 33, 41, 43, 57, 58].

The aortic root replacement technique was used in 52% of this series. The subvalvular muscular skirt and the aortic anterior mitral leaflet of the allograft were used to exclude and exteriorize the abscess cavities and infected tissues of the left ventricular outflow tract from the blood circulation. The ARR technique allows reimplantation of the circumcised coronary artery buttons even in a destroyed aorta and, therefore, obviates the need for an extracardiac aortic coronary vein bypass. Patients undergoing allograft ARR have shown freedom from structural valve deterioration (SVD) of 82.9% and 56% at 17 and 25 years, respectively. The technique has proved to be superior when compared with the freehand subcoronary aortic valve replacement technique which has 63.5% and 15% freedom from SVD at 17 and 25 years [33, 61].

The allografts of the two implantation techniques, ARR and FAVR, showed neither dilatation nor aneurysmal pathology and did not present coronary ostial calcification or stenosis during the follow-up. Undersized allograft and aortic root tailoring were identified as incremental risk factors for early valve dysfunction and reoperation especially when performing the freehand subcoronary aortic valve replacement. Patients with undersized allograft and tailored aortic root who underwent freehand AVR had 48 and 13% freedom from reoperation at 10 and 15 years, respectively [37, 61].

The operative risk increases in patients with prosthetic valve endocarditis, native aortic root infection with burrowing abscess, and poor left ventricular function [32, 33, 35, 56, 60]. The recently reported 30-day mortality was 8–17%; for prosthetic valve endocarditis it was 8–23% [23–25, 33, 56]. NYHA class IV and cardiogenic shock at the time of surgery were predictive factors for the high early mortality [4, 5, 24, 28]. The mid-term survival of patients with prosthetic valves at 11 years was 64%. The 20-year survival of allograft patients in our series was 58%. Late death was 5.6%.

In other series the survival of allograft patients at 15, 20, and 25 years was 48%, 35%, and 26%. There was a significant difference in survival among patients with different implantation techniques of allografts. Others reported long-term survival of 71% for patients with a root replacement at 15 and 20 years, while for patients with subcoronary implantation it was 45%, 33%, and 23% at 15, 20, and 25 years, respectively [61].

According to the above results, the survival rate of patients with ARR technique is more favorable than that with prosthetic valves. An explanation of the difference in results might be related to the high rate of reinfection and hemodynamic performance of the prostheses. If one compares the survival of patients with degenerative aortic disease undergoing AVR with xenografts, the results are similar to those of allograft patients with similar aortic pathology [24, 59–61, 63, 66, 73]. Concomitant coronary artery bypass graft operation and mitral valve procedures were not predictive risk factors for operative death. Reoperative hospital death rate after replacement of reinfected allograft in our series was 9.3% and comparable to that of other reports. Recurrent endocarditis was the most common cause of death [23, 24, 28].

Owing to the limited availability of allografts in all sizes, the implanting surgeon may be tempted to use an undersized allograft or to tailor the aortic root to accommodate an allograft which is larger than the native aortic root. This scenario opens up an option for the use of stentless bioprostheses, preferably pericardial-covered, when the proper allograft size is not available. Long-term results of stentless bioprostheses are not available for comparison, but 20-year actuarial freedom from SVD for stented bioprostheses was 61–70% [60–68]. Bioprostheses in patients >65 years offer similar advantages in durability as the allograft [59–64, 69–72]. The actuarial freedom from reoperation for structural valve deterioration for stentless bioprostheses at 10 years in patients at a mean age of 73 and under 60 years with a sterile aortic root was 97.0% and 76.4%, respectively. The incidence of prosthetic valve endocarditis was 4.5% [43]. Data from mid-term clinical studies have shown that bioprostheses are potentially good alternatives to allografts. The major cause of reoperations after implantation of the Medtronic Freestyle stentless bioprosthesis was nonstructural valve dysfunction [41]. The role of the bioprosthesis as a complimentary biological valve replacement for surgical treatment of aortic valve endocarditis may become established. The long-term results of patients with active infective aortic valve endocarditis who were treated with stentless bioprostheses are yet to be determined [3, 41, 43, 74].

The three cases of bridge to heart transplantation in these series following lack of myocardial recovery confirm the reports of others that more aggressive myocardial support may be helpful in endocarditis patients with end-stage myocardial failure without septicemia [33, 75].

Inferences

The aortic allograft offers excellent results of root replacement technique and has a number of technical advantages (biological reconstruction of LVOT). The allograft heals in place and has demonstrated a low rate of re-infection because of its resistance to infection, and therefore a low reoperation rate [76].

As a natural valve, it has a very low gradient which offers rapid myocardial functional recovery of the septic heart and, thus, high patient survival. The low rate of early valve-related mortality and morbidity endorses its significant role as a rescue procedure. There is conflicting evidence on the benefits conferred on allograft patients after the 10th postoperative year compared with treatment with a bioprosthetic valve. Patient survival was higher than in patients with prostheses. Durability was high in endocarditis patients and patients under 60 years of age. There were no thromboembolic events and no need for anticoagulation. The impact of decellularized allograft tissue for repopulation of autologous cells to form biocompatible tissue and, therefore, enhance durability in younger age groups is yet to be established [77, 78].

Recommendations for cardiologists, surgeons, and patients

Close echocardiographic studies and early referral of patients with acute endocarditis and signs of periannular abscess formation are warranted. The valve of choice for replacing the infected native and prosthetic aortic valve in endocarditis with periannular aortic root abscess is the aortic allograft as root replacement and alternatively the stentless bioprosthesis, preferably the pericardial-covered prosthesis. For endocarditis without an abscess, any available valve substitute can be used. The patient should be well informed about the risk of prosthetic infection and the necessity of antibiotic prophylaxis for any intervention after discharge (Table 16).

Table 16. Prosthesis of choice for valve replacement in patients with infective aortic valve endocarditis

■ Periannular abscess:	Aortic allograft
	Stentless bioprosthesis (preferably pericardial-covered)
■ Without abscess:	Any available valve substitute
■ Antibiotic prophylaxis:	Any intervention after discharge

Early referral of patients with acute endocarditis presenting echocardiographic features of periannular abscess is mandatory for urgent surgery

Conclusions

We conclude that aortic root abscesses can be managed with excellent results by radical debridement and resection of all infected and necrotic tissues and local disinfection.

Allograft aortic root replacement is the preferential procedure for aortic periannular abscesses, whereas the freehand subcoronary aortic valve replacement may be used for an isolated annular abscess. The aortic allograft is, by virtue of its permeability to serum antibiotics, resistant to biofilm bacterial infection.

The aortic root replacement technique, although surgically demanding, has shown a low reoperative rate, and low early and late mortality.

The procedure is a rescue operation for very sick patients, which offers low valve-related morbid events, and better survival and prognosis.

An undersized or geometrically mismatched aortic allograft is predictive for a high rate of reoperation and should be avoided.

In the absence of an appropriate size allograft a stentless bioprosthesis should be considered. Explantation of the allograft root after structural valve deterioration is a challenging operation and demands surgical expertise and experience to be performed at a low risk.

Acknowledgments. The authors are grateful to Anne M. Gale, ELS, for editorial assistance, Julia Stein, MSc, for statistical assistance, Astrid Benhennour for bibliographic support, and Carla Weber for providing the graphics.

References

1. American College of Cardiology; American Heart Association Task Force on Practice Guidelines (Writing Committee to revise the 1998 guidelines for the management of patients with valvular heart disease); Society of Cardiovascular Anesthesiologists, Bonow RO, Carabello BA, Chatterjee K, de Leon AC Jr, Faxon DP, Freed MD et al (2006) ACC/AHA 2006 guidelines for the management of patients with valvular heart disease. Circulation 114:e84–e231
2. Horstkotte D, Follath F, Gutschik E, Lengyel M, Oto A, Pavie A, Soler-Soler J, Thiene G, von Graevenitz A, Priori SG, Garcia MA, Blanc JJ, Budaj A, Cowie M, Dean V, Deckers J, Fernández Burgos E, Lekakis J, Lindahl B, Mazzotta G, Morais J, Oto A, Smiseth OA, Lekakis J, Vahanian A, Delahaye F, Parkhomenko A, Filipatos G, Aldershvile J, Vardas P, Task Force Members on Infective Endocarditis of the European Society of Cardiology, ESC Committee for Practice Guidelines (CPG), Document Reviewers (2004) Guidelines on prevention, diagnosis and treatment of infective endocarditis executive summary; the task force on infective endocarditis of the European society of cardiology. Eur Heart J 25:267–276
3. Siniawski H, Lehmkuhl H, Weng Y, Pasic M, Yankah C, Hoffman M, Behnke I, Hetzer R (2003) Stentless aortic valves as an alternative to homografts for valve

replacement in active infective endocarditis complicated by ring abscess. Ann Thorac Surg 75:803–808
4. Aksoy O, Sexton DJ, Wang A, Pappas PA, Kourany W, Chu V, Fowler VG Jr, Woods CW, Engemann JJ, Corey GR, Harding T, Cabell CH (2007) Early surgery in patients with infective endocarditis: a propensity score analysis. Clin Infect Dis 44:364–372
5. Vikram HR, Buenconsejo J, Hasbun R, Quagliarello VJ (2003) Impact of valve surgery on 6-month mortality in adults with complicated, left-sided native valve endocarditis: a propensity analysis. JAMA 290:3207–3214
6. Wallace AG, Young WG, Osterhout S (1965) Treatment of acute bacterial endocarditis by valve excision and replacement. Circulation 31:450–453
7. Robicsek F, Payne RB, Daugherty HK, Sanger PW (1967) Bacterial endocarditis of the mitral valve treated by excision and replacement. Ann Surg 166:854–857
8. Acar C, Iung B, Cormier B, Grare P, Berrebi A, D'Attellis N, Acar J, Carpentier A (1994) Double mitral homograft for recurrent bacterial endocarditis of the mitral and tricuspid valves. J Heart Valve Dis 3:470–472
9. Pomar JL, Mestres CA (1993) Tricusüid valve replacement using a mitral homograft. Surgical technique and initial results. J Heart Valve Dis 2:125–128
10. Oswalt JD (1993) Pulmonary autograft for aortic endocarditis. J Heart Valve Dis 2:380–384
11. Oswalt JD (1997) Pulmonary autograft for aortic valve endocarditis. In: Yankah CA, Hetzer R, Yacoub MH (eds) Cardiac allografts. Steinkopff/Springer, Darmstadt New York, p 179
12. Somerville J, Ross D (1982) Homograft replacement of aortic root with reimplantation of coronary arteries. Results after one to five years. Br Heart J 47:473–482
13. Lau JK, Robles A, Cherian A, Ross D (1984) Surgical treatment of prosthetic endocarditis. Aortic root replacement using a homograft. J Thorac Cardiovasc Surg 87: 712–716
14. Perelman MJ, Sugimoto J, Arcilla RA, Karp RB (1989) Aortic root replacement for complicated bacterial endocarditis in an infant. J Pediatr Surg 24:1121–1123
15. Donaldson RM, Ross DM (1984) Homograft aortic root replacement for complicated prosthetic valve endocarditis. Circulation 70(Suppl I):I-178–I-181
16. Ross D (1964) Homotransplantation of the aortic valve in the subcoronary position. J Thoracic Cardiovasc Surg 47:713–719
17. Barratt-Boyes BG (1964) Homograft aortic valve replacement in aortic incompetence and stenosis. Thorax 19:131–150
18. Ross D (1991) Technique of aortic valve replacement with a homograft: orthotopic replacement. Ann Thorac Surg 52:154–156
19. Jones EL (1989) Freehand homograft aortic valve replacement. The learning curve: a technical analysis of the first 31 patients. Ann Thorac Surg 48:26–32
20. Doty JR, Salazar JD, Iiddicoat JR, Flores JH, Doty DB (1998) Aortic valve replacement with cryopreserved aortic allograft: ten-year experience. J Thorac Cardiovasc Surg 115:371–380
21. Barratt-Boyes BG, Christie GW (1994) What is the best bioprosthetic operation for the small aortic root?: allograft, autograft, porcine, pericardial? Stented or unstented? J Card Surg 9(2 Suppl):158–164
22. Yankah CA, Klose H, Musci M, Siniawski H, Hetzer R (2001) Geometric mismatch between homograft (allograft) and native aortic root: a 14-year clinical experience. Eur J Cardiothorac Surg 20:835–841
23. d'Udekem Y, David TE, Feindel CM, Armstrong S, Sun Z (1997) Long-term results of surgery for active infective endocarditis. Eur J Cardiothorac Surg 11:46–52
24. Petrou M, Wong K, Albertucci M, Brecker SJ, Yacoub MH (1994) Evaluation of unstented aortic homografts for the treatment of prosthetic aortic valve endocarditis. Circulation 90(Part 2):II-198–II-204

25. Haydock D, Barratt-Boyes B, MacedoT, Kirklin JW, Blackstone E (1992) Aortic valve replacement for active infectious endocarditis in 108 patients. J Thorac Cardiovasc Surg 103:130–139
26. Schmidtke C, Dahmen G, Sievers HH (2007) Subcoronary Ross procedure in patients with active endocarditis. Ann Thorac Surg 83(1)36–39
27. Miller DC (1990) Predictors of outcome in patients with prosthetic valve endocarditis and potential advantages of homograft aortic root replacement for prosthetic ascending aortic valve-graft infections. J Card Surg 5:53–62
28. David TE (1997) Surgical management of aortic root abscess. J Card Surg 12:262–269
29. Niwaya K, Knott-Craig CJ, Santangelo K, Lane MM, Chandrasekaran K, Elkins RC (1999) Advantage of autograft and homograft valve replacement for complex aortic valve endocarditis. Ann Thorac Surg 67(6):1603–1608
30. Tingleff JF, Pettersson G (1995) Expanding indications for the Ross operation. J Heart Valve Dis 4(4):352–363
31. Yankah CA, Hetzer R (1987) Valve selection and choice in surgery of endocarditis. J Cardiac Surg 2(Suppl):209–220
32. Yankah CA, Klose H, Petzina R, Musci M, Siniawski H, Hetzer R (2002) Surgical management of acute aortic root endocarditis with viable homograft: 13-year experience. Eur J Cardiothorac Surg 21:260–267
33. Yankah CA, Pasic M, Klose H, Siniawski H, Weng Y, Hetzer R (2005) Homograft reconstruction of the aortic root for endocarditis with periannular abscess: a 17-year study. Eur J Cardiothorac Surg 28:69–75
34. Anderson RH (2000) Anatomy: clinical anatomy of the aortic root. Heart 84:670–673
35. Vogt PR, von Segesser LK, Niederhauser U, Genoni M, Kunzli A, Schneider J, Turina MI (1997) Emergency surgery for acute infective aortic valve endocarditis: performance of cryopreserved homografts and mode of failure. Eur J Cardiothorac Surg 11:53–61
36. McGiffin DC, Galbraith AJ, O'Brien MF, McLachlan GJ, Naftel DC, Adams P, Reddy S, Early L (1997) An analysis of valve re-replacement after aortic valve replacement with biologic devices. J Thorac Cardiovasc Surg 113(2):311–318
37. Smedira NG, Blackstone EH, Roselli EE, Laffey CC, Cosgrove DM (2006) Are allografts the biologic valve of choice for aortic valve replacement in nonelderly patients? Comparison of explantation for structural valve deterioration of allograft and pericardial prostheses. J Thorac Cardiovasc Surg 131:558–564
38. Barratt-Boyes BG, Christie GW, Raudkivi PJ (1992) The stentless bioprosthesis: surgical challenges and implications for long-term durability. Eur J Cardiothorac Surg 6(Suppl 1):S39–S43
39. Albert A, Florath I, Rosendahl U, Hassanein W, Hodenberg EV, Bauer S, Ennker I, Ennker J (2007) Effect of surgeon on transprosthetic gradients after aortic valve replacement with Freestyle stentless bioprosthesis and its consequences: A follow-up study in 587 patients. J Cardiothorac Surg 2:40
40. Ali A, Halstead JC, Cafferty F, Sharples L, Rose F, Coulden R, Lee E, Dunning J, Argano V, Tsui S (2006) Are stentless valves superior to modern stented valves? A prospective randomized trial. Circulation 114(1 Suppl):I535–I540
41. Ennker J, Albert A, Rosendahl U, Ennker IC, Dalladaku F, Florath I (2008) Ten-year experience with stentless aortic valves: Full-root versusu subcoronary implantation. Ann Thorac Surg 85:445–453
42. Bach DS, Cartier PC, Kon ND, Johnson KG, Deeb GM, Doty DB (2002) Impact of implant technique following freestyle stentless aortic valve replacement. Ann Thorac Surg 74:1107–1114
43. Bach DS, Kon ND, Dumesnil JG, Sintek CF, Doty DB (2005) Ten-year outcome after aortic valve replacement with the Freestyle stentless bioprosthesis. Ann Thorac Surg 80:480–487

44. Emery RW, Erickson CA, Arom KV, Northrup WF 3rd, Kersten TE, Von Rueden TJ, Lillehei TJ, Nicoloff DM (2003) Replacement of the aortic valve in patients under 50 years of age: long-term follow-up of the St. Jude Medical prosthesis. Ann Thorac Surg 75:1815–1819
45. Cox DR (1972) Regression models and life tables. JR Stat Soc (B) 34:187–220
46. Nicks R, Cartmill T, Bernstein L (1970) Hypoplasia of the aortic root. The problem of aortic valve replacement. Thorax 25:339–346
47. Bentall H, De Bono A (1968) A technique for complete replacement of the ascending aorta.Thorax 23:338–339
48. Yankah CA, Sievers HH, Buersch JH, Radtcke W, Lange PE, Heintzen PH, Bernhard A (1984) Orthotopic transplantation of aortic valve allograft. Early hemodynamic results. Thorac Cardiovasc Surg 32:92–95
49. Yankah CA, Wottge H-U, Mueller-Hermelink HK, Feller AC et al (1987) Transplantation of aortic and pulmonary allografts, enhanced viability of endothelial cells by cryopreservation, importance of histocompatibility. J Cardiac Surg 2(Suppl): 209–220
50. Yacoub M, Rasmi NRH, Sundt TM, Lund O, Boyland E, Radley-Smith R, Khagani A, Mitchell A (1995) Fourteen-year experience with homovital homografts for aortic valve replacement. J Thorac Cardiovasc Surg 110:186–194
51. Fux CA, Wilson S, Stoodley P (2004) Detachment characteristics and oxacillin resistance of Staphylococcus aureus biofilm emboli in an invitro catheter infection model. J Bacteriol 186:4486–4491
52. Lemos JAC, Brown Jr TA, Burne RA (2004) Effects of Re1A on key virulence properties of planktonic and biofilm populations of Streptococcus mutans. Infect Immun 72:1431–1440
53. Jefferson KK (2004) What drives bacteria to produce a biofilm? Fed Eur Microbiol Soc Microbiol Lett 236:163–173
54. Carpentier A (1983) Cardiac valve surgery-The "French correction". J Thorac Cardiovasc Surg 86:323–337
55. Elkins RC (1996) Pulmonary autografts in patients with aortic annulus dysplasia. Ann Thorac Surg 61:1141–1145
56. Knosalla C, Weng Y, Yankah CA, Siniawski H, Hofmeister J, Hammerschmidt R, Loebe M, Hetzer R (2000) Homograft versus prosthetic valve for surgical treatment of aortic valve endocarditis with periannular abscess Eur Heart J 21:490–497
57. David TE, Armstrong S, Sun Z (1998) The Hancock II bioprosthesis at 12 years. Ann Thorac Surg 66(6 Suppl):S95–S98
58. Neville PH, Aupart MR, Diemont FF, Sirinelli AL, Lemoine EM, Marchand MA (1998) Carpentier-Edwards pericardial bioprosthesis in aortic or mitral position: a 12-year experience. Ann Thorac Surg 66(6 Suppl):S143–S147
59. Yankah CA, Pasic M, Musci M, Stein J, Detschades C, Siniawski H, Hetzer R (2008) Aortic valve replacement with the Mitroflow pericardial bioprosthesis: durability results up to 21 years. J Thorac Cardiovasc Surg 136:688–696
60. O'Brien MF, Harrocks S, Stafford EG, Gardner MA, Pohlner PG, Tesar PJ, Stephen F (2001) The homograft aortic valve: a 29-year, 99.3% follow up of 1,022 valve replacements. J Heart Valve Dis 10:334–345
61. Lund O, Chandrasekaran V, Grocott-Mason R, Elwidaa H, Mazhar R, Khaghani A, Mitchell A, Ilsev C, Yacoub MH (1999) Primary aortic valve replacement with allografts over twenty-five years: valve-related and procedure-related determinants of outcome. J Thorac Cardiovasc Surg 117:77–91
62. Myken PSU, Bech-Hansen O (2009) A 20-year experience of 1712 patients with the Biocor porcine bioprosthesis. J Thorac Cardiovasc Surg 137:76–81
63. Jamieson WR, Burr LH, Miyagishima RT, Germann E, MacNab JS, Stanford E, Chan F, Janusz MT, Ling H (2005) Carpentier-Edwards supra-annular aortic por-

cine bioprosthesis: clinical performance over 20 years. J Thorac Cardiovasc Surg 130:994–1000
64. Borger MA, Ivanov J, Armstrong S, Christie-Hrybinsky D, Feindel CM, David TE (2006) Twenty-year results of the Hancock II bioprosthesis. J Heart Valve Dis 15(1):49–56
65. Khan SS, Trento A, De Robertis M, Kass RM, Sandhu M, Czer LS, Blanche C, Raissi S, Fontana GP, Cheng W, Chaux A, Matloff JM (2001) Twenty-year comparison of tissue and mechanical valve replacement. J Thorac Cardiovasc Surg 122: 257–269
66. Eichinger WB, Hettich I, Ruzicka D, Holper K, Schricker C, Bleiziffer S, Lange R (2008) Twenty-year experience with the St.-Jude medical biocor prosthesis in the aortic position. Ann Thorac Surg 86:1204–1211
67. Yankah CA, Schubel J, Buz S, Siniawski H, Hetzer R (2005) Seventeen-year clinical results of 1037 Mitroflow pericardial heart valve prostheses in the aortic position. J Heart Valve Dis 14:172–180
68. Aupart MR, Mirza A, Mueresse YA, Sirinelli AL, Neville PH, Marchand MA (2006) Perimount pericardial bioprosthesis for aortic calcified stenosis: 18-year experience with 1133 patients J Heart Valve Dis 15:768–776
69. Puvimanasinghe JP, Takkenberg JJ, Edwards MB, Eijkemans MJ, Steyerberg EW, Van Herwerden LA, Taylor KM, Grunkemeier GL, Habbema JD, Bogers AJ (2004) Comparison of outcomes after aortic valve replacement with a mechanical valve or a bioprosthesis using microsimulation. Heart 90:1172–1178
70. Takkenberg JJ, Eijkemans MJ, van Herwerden LA, Steyerberg EW, Lane MM, Elkins RC, Habbema JD and Bogers AJ (2003) Prognosis after aortic root replacement with cryopreserved allografts in adults Ann Thorac Surg 75;5:1482–1489
71. Takkenberg JJ, Klieverik LM, Schoof PH, van Suylen RJ, van Herwerden LA, Zondervan PE, Roos-Hesselink JW, Eijkemans MJC, Yacoub MH and Bogers AJ (2009) The Ross procedure: A systematic review and meta-analysis. Circulation 119(2):222–228
72. Takkenberg JJ, Puvimanasinghe JP, Grunkemeier GL (2003) Simulation models to predict outcome after aortic valve replacement Ann Thorac Surg 75:1372–1376
73. Jamieson WR, Burr LH, Miyagishima RT, Janusz MT, Fradet GJ, Ling H, Lichtenstein SV (2003) Re-operation for bioprosthetic aortic structural failure – risk assessment. Eur J Cardiothorac Surg 24:873–887
74. Musci M, Siniawski H, Pasic M, Weng Y, Loforte A, Kosky S, Yankah C, Hetzer R (2008) Surgical therapy in patients with active infective endocarditis: seven-year single centre experience in a subgroup of 255 patients with the Shelhigh stentless bioprosthesis Eur J Cardiothorac Surg 34:410–417
75. Morgan JA, Park Y, Oz MC, Naka Y (2003) Device-related infections while on left ventricular assist device support do not adversely impact bridging to transplant or posttransplant survival ASAIO J 49(6):748–750
76. Mestres CA, Ginel A, Cartana R, Pomar JL (1993) Cryopreserved homografts in aortic and mitral prosthetic endocarditis: expanding the use of biological tissues in complex cardiac infections. J Heart Valve Dis 2:679–683
77. Bechtel JF, Gellissen J, Erasmi AW, Petersen M, Hiob A, Stierle U, Sievers HH (2005) Mid-term findings on echocardiography and computed tomography after RVOT reconstruction. Comparison of decellulaized (SynerGraft) and conventional allografts. Eur J Cardiothorac Surg 27(3):410–415, discussion 415
78. Dohmen PM, Konertz W (2008) Decellularized biologic tissue. Ann Thorac Surg 85(6):2163–2164

Implantation techniques of freehand subcoronary aortic valve and root replacement with a cryopreserved allograft for aortic root abscess

C. A. Yankah, M. Pasic, Y. Weng, R. Hetzer

Historical background

Prior to 1972, the surgical results of aortic root abscesses treated with prosthetic valves varied and, being associated with a high rate of early recurrent infection and mortality, were not very satisfactory. Consequently, in 1972 Donald Ross introduced the use of the aortic allograft, which is a completely biological tissue for replacing the infected aortic valve (see Figs. 2–7) [1–4]. This operation technique was initially used for reconstruction of a tunnel-type left ventricular outflow tract due to congenital obstruction and was then adopted for treating aortic root abscesses. The original procedure was described by Hugh Bentall and Antony de Bono in 1968 [5].

Replacement of the aortic valve for degenerative or congenital disease with an antibiotic treated refridgerated aortic allograft using the freehand subcoronary implantation technique was introduced by Dr. Donald Ross [6] and Sir Brian Barratt-Boyes [6], independently of each other in 1962. Barratt-Boyes used an aortic allograft with all three sinuses scalloped [7], whereas Ross used an aortic allograft with scalloped left and right sinuses, leaving the noncoronary sinus intact. The noncoronary sinus wall can be used when necessary for enlarging the aortic root. A similar technique using the autologous pericardium for aortic root enlargement during prosthetic aortic valve replacement was suggested by Nicks [8].

Surgical management of aortic root abscess

The techniques of biologic reconstruction of the left ventricular outflow tract with equine pericardium and allograft aortic valve and root replacement are depicted in detail in this chapter.

A thawed cryopreserved homograft aortic cylinder with flexible leaflets free from atheroma is used to replace the native aortic valve or the aortic root. The possibility of valve distortion during allograft implantation can be avoided by maintaining the cylindrical shape of the aortic allograft, inserting it as a root replacement and reimplanting the coronary arteries. The aortic root implantation technique with reimplantation of the coronary arteries also obviates extracardiac aortic coronary artery bypass. At the same time it prevents allograft root distortion and central valve incompetence.

Debridement and local disinfection of the aortic root

One of the major aspects of surgical management of aortic root abscesses is the radical debridement of the infected tissue, e.g., curetting of the slimy endothelial surfaces especially at the interventricular septum to avoid damage to the conducting system of His. Resection of the necrotic tissues is performed where necessary. Polyvidon iodine is applied to the infected tissue for 3 minutes to decolonize the biofilm bacteria and eliminate them. This ensures the therapeutic effect of the serum and allograft tissue antibiosis.

Pericardial reconstruction of the left ventricular outflow tract

The next step is the pericardial reconstruction of the periannular abscess cavities and closure of the ventricular septal defect. The aortic anterior mitral leaflet or the subvalvular muscular skirt of the composite aortic allograft facilitate the proximal lower suture line and anatomic reconstruction of the left ventricular outflow tract (LVOT) in the region of the aortic mitral fibrous septum, the noncoronary annulus, and the left coronary annulus (Figs. 1–3).

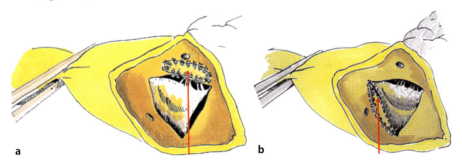

Fig. 1. a Schematic pericardial patch reconstruction of the right coronary periannular abscess cavity and closure of the ventricular septum defect. **b** Schematic pericardial patch reconstruction of the left coronary periannular abscess cavity

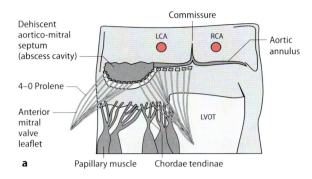

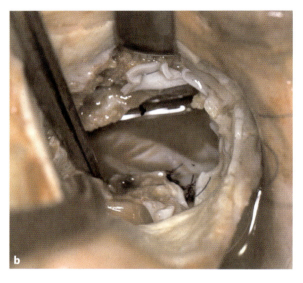

Fig. 2. a Schematic presentation of the anticipated proximal (lower) line below the infraannular abscess cavity in the region of the aortic mitral fibrous septum. *The lower line sutures*: Two-color multiple interrupted polypropylene (Prolene) 4-0 sutures buttressed by equine pericardial pledgets are placed at the base of the infraannular abscess cavity at the native mitral annulus and in the muscle of the left ventricular outflow tract in healthy tissue. The sutures are placed further toward the remaining circumference at the left and right coronary aortic annulus to complete the anticipated lower proximal line. **b** Reconstructed aortic mitral fibrous septum with a pericardial patch

Implantation techniques of freehand subcoronary aortic valve and root replacement 277

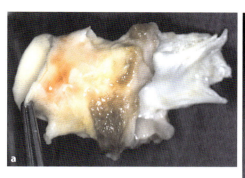
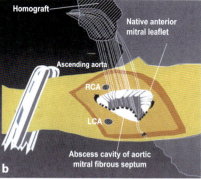
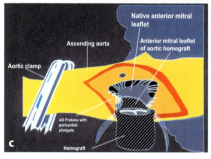

Fig. 3. a A short segment aortic allograft with anterior mitral leaflet. **b** The lower edge of the allograft aortic anterior mitral anterior leaflet (AML) is fed with two-colour multiple interrupted polypropylene (Prolene) 4-0 mattress sutures in such a fashion that they fit to the anticipated lower suture line below the infraannular abscess cavity. This technique ensures anatomic insertion of the allograft. **c** The allograft is lowered down with the AML in front of the abscess cavity in order to exclude the abscess cavity from the blood circulation. The sutures are tied down toward the noncoronary and right coronary annulus and fixed, thus excluding the abscess cavity from the LVOT. The sutures are placed further toward the remaining circumference at the left and right coronary aortic annulus to complete the circumference of the anticipated lower proximal line. The subvalvular muscular skirt of the allograft is then fed with the lower line sutures so that they fit to the anticipated proximal anastomosis with the native aortic annulus. The allograft cylinder is then inverted into the left ventricle to allow reliable tying down of the remaining sutures and to complete the fixation of the allograft. The technique allows the abscess cavity to drain into the pericardium

Aortic root replacement and reimplantation of the coronary arteries

The subvalvular muscular skirt and the anterior mitral leaflet of the allograft are fixed below and in front of the abscess cavity with two-color multiple interrupted 4-0 polypropylene mattress sutures. After placement of the proximal line sutures, the sutures at the anterior mitral leaflet are first tied down toward the aortic annulus, then the allograft is inverted into the LVOT to allow reliably tying down of the remaining sutures at the left and the right coronary annulus to complete the proximal anastomosis of the allograft. The same procedure is done at the left coronary periannular ab-

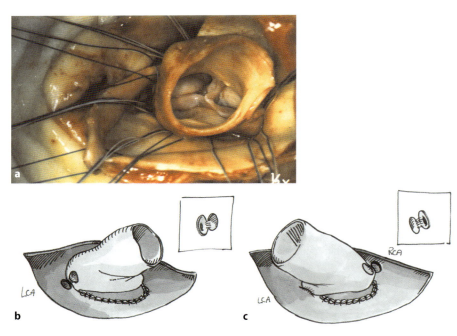

Fig. 4. a The allograft is carefully pulled out from the left ventricular outflow tract for reimplantation of the coronary arteries. The reimplantation of the coronary arteries is technically accomplished in two ways: 1. Anastomosis with a circumcised coronary arteries as buttons, 2. Direct anastomosis using a continuous interrupted 4-0 Prolene sutures. **b** Schematic reimplantation of the left coronary artery. The allograft is gently pushed caudally to allow a better view. Direct end-to-side anastomosis of the native left coronary artery with the adjacent aortic sinus at the site of the allograft left coronary ostium. **c** Schematic reimplantation of the right coronary artery. The allograft is gently pushed cranially to allow a better view. Direct end-to-side anastomosis of the native right coronary artery with the adjacent sinus at the site of the allograft right coronary ostium. Testing for the tightness of the proximal suture line. After testing of the tightness of the proximal line during the repeat induction of the blood cardioplegia the distal end-to-end anastomosis begins

scess cavity. After completion of the proximal anastomosis, the aortic allograft is everted into the aortic root and the adjacent coronary arteries are implanted directly onto the allograft aorta in end-to-side fashion with 4-0 polypropylene (Prolene) in a continuous running suture technique. In cases where extensive aortic root destruction is present, the coronary arteries are dissected and circumcised to allow a better view, while placing the sutures in viable tissue and proper reimplantation of the coronary arteries. The procedure exteriorizes the abscess cavity from the LVOT and the blood circulation (Figs. 3 and 4).

The distal allograft cylinder and the component sinotubular junction are then connected to match the native ascending aorta by continuous running suture. A review of the literature on the implantation technique of freehand allograft aortic valve and freestanding aortic root replacement root is presented in Fig. 5.

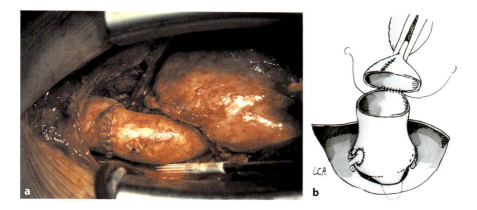

Fig. 5. a The distal end of the allograft (the sinotubular junction) is anastomosed with the native ascending aorta end-to-end by continuous suture technique using 4-0 polypropylene beginning at the posterior wall, reinforcing the suture line with the surrounding tissue of the native aortic wall. The sinotubular junction which is usually 90% the size of the aortic annulus is geometrically matched to the native ascending aorta. **b** Completed procedure of a total aortic root replacement as a freestanding root with reimplantation of the coronary arteries

Freehand subcoronary aortic valve replacement

After the lower proximal suture line is completed and the knots are tied down, the right and left commissural posts are temporarily attached 2 cm above the native commissures with stay sutures. This procedure will give the surgeon an overview of the coaptation of the valve leaflets. The remaining right and left scalloped sinus walls are then attached to the adjacent native sinus walls beginning at the midpoint of the left coronary ostium and leading up to the left commissural post using a double-arm 4-0 polypropylene suture. The right sinus wall is anastomosed to the adjacent right

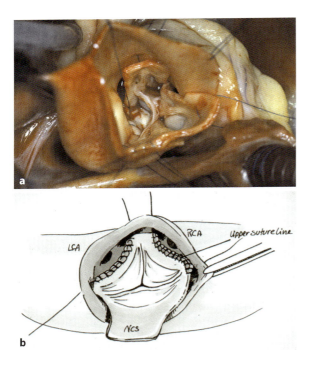

Fig. 6. Scalloped left and right sinuses of the aortic allograft as described by Ross with intact nonconcoronary sinus wall for freehand subcoronary aortic valve replacement. The technique reduces the probability of distortion of the allograft. The right and the left commissures are securely positioned with the intact noncoronary sinus wall of the allograft to provide adequate leaflet coaptation. **a** View of the anticipated second row suture line which begins below the midpoint of the coronary ostium with secured coaptation of the aortic valve leaflets. **b** Schematic presentation of completion of the two-row lower proximal suture line (the first row suture line is not visible) and the freestanding noncoronary sinus wall of the allograft. **c** Completed second row suture line below the left coronary artery ostium with adequate coaptation of the aortic valve leaflets

native sinus wall using a double-arm 4-0 polypropylene running suture at the midpoint below the right coronary ostium in the same manner up to the top of the left commissure to meet the previous suture. At the top of the commissure, the two suture materials are tied down to fix the left commissural post. The other half of the left subcoronary suture line is continued using the other half of the double-arm 4-0 polypropylene as a running suture up to the top of the noncoronary sinus wall and is tied down.

The other half of the right subcoronary suture line is continued with the other half of the double-arm 4-0 polypropylene as a running suture up to the top of the noncoronary sinus wall and tied down with a stay suture. At the closure of the aortotomy the allograft noncoronary sinus is incorporated and attached to the native noncoronary sinus wall. If necessary, the allograft noncoronary sinus is used to enlarge the native noncoronary sinus wall, as suggested by Ross [9] and by Nicks [8] in his technique using the autologous pericardium (Figs. 6 and 7).

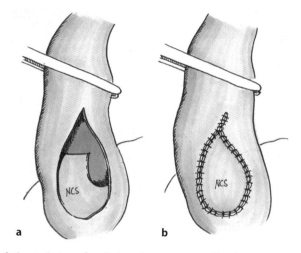

Fig. 7. Schematic presentation of the technique for closing the aortotomy. The freestanding noncoronary sinus wall of the allograft can be used for enlarging the aortic root, if necessary; otherwise it will be incorporated into the aortotomy closure and fixed to the native noncoronary sinus wall. **a** *Left:* Schematic presentation of the noncoronary sinus wall prior to closure of the aortotomy. **b** *Right:* Schematic presentation of the noncoronary sinus wall of the scalloped allograft. This is used to enlarge the native aortic noncoronary as described by Ross and to accommodate the noncoronary segment of the allograft comfortably in the aortic root without it being squeezed and causing central valve incompetence. The enlargement of the noncoronary sinus of a small aortic root was originally described by Nicks using pericardium after prosthetic aortic valve replacement

Comments

Postprocedural intraoperative transesophageal echocardiography provides information about coaptation of the valve leaflets and, therefore, the opening and closure mechanism of the competent aortic allograft valve and the transvalvular gradient. Intraoperative echocardiographic study rules out possible paravalvular leakage especially into the abscess cavity due to suture dehiscence (Fig. 8). The surgical procedure with allograft aortic root replacement (ARR) or freehand subcoronary valve replacement (FAVR) is

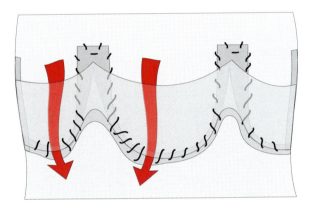

Fig. 8. Schematic presentation of suture dehiscence or rupture of the proximal suture line after freehand subcoronary allograft implantation

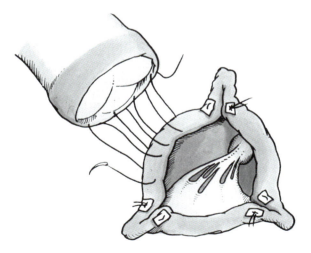

Fig. 9. Schematic presentation of reduction aortic annuloplasty by plication of the trigona

technically demanding; therefore, in its early development it was confounded by learning curve periods without tutorial guidance [9–23]. Long-term durability of the allograft valve for root and freehand subcoronary valve replacement in patients with endocarditis and degenerative aortic disease after 17–29 years has been reported by several authors [10, 26–28]. Reduction aortic annuloplasty by plication of the trigona or annulorrhaphy of the large aortic annulus as described by Carpentier and Elkins is associated with unfavorable results [15, 24, 27]. It should be avoided in the management of active infective aortic valve endocarditis (Figs. 9–11).

Owing to the limited availability of allografts in all sizes and current competing durability of bioprosthesis, the scenario opens up an option for the use of stentless bioprostheses, preferably pericardial-covered bioprostheses (Figs. 12–14). Data from mid-term clinical studies have shown that the bioprostheses are potentially good alternatives to allografts [30–34].

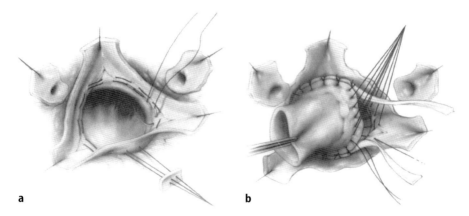

Fig. 10. Schematic presentation of reduction aortic annuloplasty originally described by Carpentier [24] and Elkins [25]. **a** Circumcised coronary buttons. Annulorrhaphy of large aortic annulus by placement of two rows of purse-string sutures around the annulus to down-size it. **b** Reinforcing of the proximal suture line with glutaraldehyde-fixed pericardial strip placed within the suture loop of the lower suture line as they are tied down, as suggested by Ross. Reproduced with permission from Elsevier; Elkins RC (1996) Ann Thorac Surg 61:1142

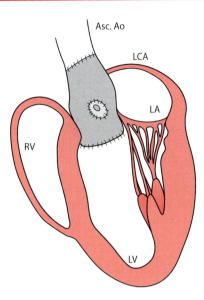

Fig. 11. Infraannular implantation of aortic allograft would create compression and supravalvular stenosis of the allograft and subsequent high pressure gradients. Undersized allograft will cause root distortion in an extensive aortic root abscess as well as tension on the proximal suture lines and postoperative high gradients and eventually suture dehiscence and paravalvular leaks, whereby blood from the LVOT would leak into the abscess cavity and develop pseudoaneurysm

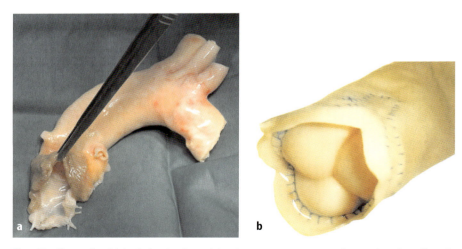

Fig. 12. Alternative biological valved conduits: Long segment composite aortic valve allograft and stentless valve bioprostheses. **a** Composite aortic allograft conduit with the anterior mitral leaflet, the aortic arch, and the supraaortic branches. **b** Long segment of Shelhigh composite porcine stentless bioprosthesis and bovine pericardial ascending aortic graft

Implantation techniques of freehand subcoronary aortic valve and root replacement   285

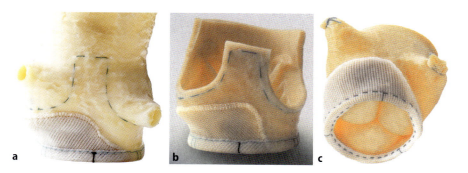

Fig. 13. Alternative biological valved conduits: **a** Edwards Prima Plus composite porcine stentless bioprosthesis, **b** Prima Plus Baxter, **c** St Jude Medical composite porcine stentless Toronto root

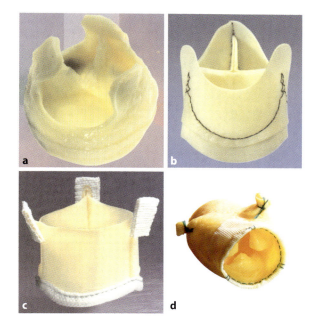

Fig. 14. Alternative biological valved conduits: **a** Vascutek-Elan stentless porcine aortic bioprosthesis, **b** Fabricated Sorin stentless bovine pericardial aortic bioprosthesis, **c** ATS 3F supraannular pericardial valve replacement, and **d** Medtronic freestyle composite stentless porcine bioprosthesis

References

1. Somerville J, Ross D (1982) Homograft replacement of aortic root with reimplantation of coronary arteries. Results after one to five years. Br Heart J 47:473–482
2. Lau JK, Robles A, Cherian A, Ross DN (1984) Surgical treatment of prosthetic endocarditis. Aortic root replacement using a homograft. J Thorac Cardiovasc Surg 87:712–716
3. Donaldson RM, Ross DN (1984) Homograft aortic root replacement for complicated prosthetic valve endocarditis. Circulation 70(Suppl I):I-178–I-81
4. Perelman MJ, Sugimoto J, Arcilla RA, Karp RB (1989) Aortic root replacement for complicated bacterial endocarditis in an infant. J Pediatr Surg 24:1121–1123
5. Bentall H, De Bono A (1968) A technique for complete replacement of the ascending aorta.Thorax 23:338–339
6. Ross D (1964) Homotransplantation of the aortic valve in the subcoronary position. J Thoracic Cardiovasc Surg 47:713–719
7. Barratt-Boyes BG (1964) Homograft aortic valve replacement in aortic incompetence and stenosis. Thorax 19:131–150
8. Nicks R, Cartmill T, Bernstein L (1970) Hypoplasia of the aortic root. The problem of aortic valve replacement. Thorax 25:339–346
9. Ross D (1991) Technique of aortic valve replacement with a homograft: orthotopic replacement. Ann Thorac Surg 52:154–156
10. Petrou M, Wong K, Albertucci M, Brecker SJ, Yacoub MH (1994) Evaluation of unstented aortic homografts for the treatment of prosthetic aortic valve endocarditis. Circulation 90(Part 2):II-198–II-204
11. Barratt-Boyes BG, Christie GW (1994) What is the best bioprosthetic operation for the small aortic root?: Allograft, autograft, porcine, pericardial? Stented or unstented? J Card Surg 9(2 Suppl):158–164
12. Jones EL (1989) Freehand homograft aortic valve replacement. The learning curve: a technical analysis of the first 31 patients. Ann Thorac Surg 48:26–32
13. Schmidtke C, Dahmen G, Sievers HH (2007) Subcoronary Ross procedure in patients with active endocarditis. Ann Thorac Surg 83(1):36–39
14. Doty JR, Salazar JD, liddicoat JR, Flores JH, Doty DB (1998) Aortic valve replacement with cryopreserved aortic allograft: ten-year experience. J Thorac Cardiovasc Surg 115:371–380
15. Yankah CA, Klose H, Musci M, Siniawski H, Hetzer R (2001) Geometric mismatch between homograft (allograft) and native aortic root: a 14-year clinical experience. Eur J Cardiothorac Surg 20:835–841
16. Niwaya K, Knott-Craig CJ, Santangelo K, Lane MM, Chandrasekaran K, Elkins RC (1999) Advantage of autograft and homograft valve replacement for complex aortic valve endocarditis. Ann Thorac Surg 67(6):1603–1608
17. Tingleff JF, Pettersson G (1995) Expanding indications for the Ross operation. J Heart Valve Dis 4(4):352–363
18. Barratt-Boyes BG, Christie GW, Raudkivi PJ (1992) The stentless bioprosthesis: surgical challenges and implications for long-term durability. Eur J Cardiothorac Surg 6(Suppl 1):S39–S43
19. Yankah CA, Hetzer R (1987) Valve selection and choice in surgery of endocarditis. J Cardiac Surg 2(Suppl):209–220
20. Yankah CA, Klose H, Petzina R, Musci M, Siniawski H, Hetzer R (2002) Surgical management of acute aortic root endocarditis with viable homograft: 13-year experience. Eur J Cardiothorac Surg 21:260–277

21. Yankah CA, Sievers HH, Buersch JH, Radtcke W, Lange PE, Heintzen PH, Bernhard A (1984) Orthotopic transplantation of aortic valve allograft. Early hemodynamic results. Thorac Cardiovasc Surg 32:92–95
22. Yankah CA, Wottge H-U, Mueller-Hermelink HK, Feller AC et al (1987) Transplantation of aortic and pulmonary allografts, enhanced viability of endothelial cells by cryopreservation, importance of histocompatibility. J Cardiac Surg 2(Suppl): 209–220
23. Yacoub M, Rasmi NRH, Sundt TM, Lund O, Boyland E, Radley-Smith R, Khagani A, Mitchell A (1995) Fourteen-year experience with homovital homografts for aortic valve replacement. J Thorac Cardiovasc Surg 110:186–194
24. Carpentier A (1983) Cardiac valve surgery-The "French correction". J Thorac Cardiovasc Surg 86:323–337
25. Elkins RC (1996) Pulmonary autografts in patients with aortic annulus dysplasia. Ann Thorac Surg 61:1141–1145
26. O'Brien MF, Harrocks S, Stafford EG, Gardner MA, Pohlner PG, Tesar PJ, Stephen F (2001) The homograft aortic valve: a 29-year, 99.3% follow up of 1,022 valve replacements. J Heart Valve Dis 10:334–345
27. Lund O, Chandrasekaran V, Grocott-Mason R, Elwidaa H, Mazhar R, Khaghani A, Mitchell A, Ilslev C, Yacoub MH (1999) Primary aortic valve replacement with allografts over twenty-five years: valve-related and procedure-related determinants of outcome. J Thorac Cardiovasc Surg 117:77–91
28. Yankah CA, Pasic M, Klose H, Siniawski H, Weng Y, Hetzer R (2005) Homograft reconstruction of the aortic root for endocarditis with periannular abscess: a 17-year study. Eur J Cardiothorac Surg 28:69–75
29. Albert A, Florath I, Rosendahl U, Hassanein W, Hodenberg EV, Bauer S, Ennker I, Ennker J (2007) Effect of surgeon on transprosthetic gradients after aortic valve replacement with Freestyle stentless bioprosthesis and its consequences: a follow-up study in 587 patients. J Cardiothorac Surg 2:40
30. Ennker J, Albert A, Rosendahl U, Ennker IC, Dalladaku F, Florath I (2008) Ten-year experience with stentless aortic valves: Full-root versusu subcoronary implantation. Ann Thorac Surg 85:445–453
31. Bach DS, Cartier PC, Kon ND, Johnson KG, Deeb GM, Doty DB (2002) Impact of implant technique following freestyle stentless aortic valve replacement. Ann Thorac Surg 74:1107–1114
32. Siniawski H, Lehmkuhl H, Weng Y, Pasic M, Yankah C, Hoffman M, Behnke I, Hetzer R (2003) Stentless aortic valves as an alternative to homografts for valve replacement in active infective endocarditis complicated by ring abscess. Ann Thorac Surg 75:803–808
33. Musci M, Siniawski H, Pasic M, Weng Y, Loforte A, Kosky S, Yankah C, Hetzer R (2008) Surgical therapy in patients with active infective endocarditis: seven-year single centre experience in a subgroup of 255 patients with the Shelhigh stentless bioprosthesis Eur J Cardiothorac Surg 34:410–417
34. Takkenberg JJ, Eijkemans MJ, van Herwerden LA, Steyerberg EW, Lane MM, Elkins RC, Habbema JD and Bogers AJ (2003) Prognosis after aortic root replacement with cryopreserved allografts in adults Ann Thorac Surg 75:1482–1489

Surgery for atrial fibrillation

Cryoablation for the treatment of atrial fibrillation in patients undergoing minimally invasive mitral valve surgery
Technique and recent results

J. Passage, M. A. Borger, J. Seeburger, A. Rastan, T. Walther, N. Doll, F. W. Mohr

Introduction

Atrial fibrillation (AF) is the most prevalent cardiac arrhythmia. The reported frequency is 0.5–1% in the general population, increasing with age to 10% in patients older than 80 years [22]. In patients undergoing mitral valve operations, the frequency of AF is reported to be as high as 60–80% [10].

Recurrent AF is classified according to the AHA/ACC guidelines into paroxysmal, persistent, and permanent [14]. More recently, Cox proposed a simpler classification into intermittent and continuous AF based on the clinical presentation and the electrophysiological basis of each type of AF [6].

Patients with AF have an increased long-term risk of stroke, heart failure, and all cause mortality. The mortality rate of patients with AF is reported to be double that of patients in normal sinus rhythm (SR) [14]. The risk of ischemic stroke is even higher in patients with rheumatic heart disease and concomitant AF – in the Framingham Heart Study the stroke risk was increased 17-fold compared with age-matched controls and attributable risk was 5 times greater than that in patients with nonrheumatic AF [14]. Given the aging population in the developed world, the treatment of AF and its complications results in significant current and future health care costs. Pharmacological treatment with or without electrical cardioversion cures AF in only a minority of patients with underlying structural heart disease [14]. For these reasons, surgical and percutaneous interventional strategies have been developed for the treatment of AF and are expected to steadily increase in frequency over time.

Surgical treatment options

The Cox MAZE procedure has been regarded as the gold standard of surgical therapy for AF since its development in 1987 [8]. It is based on the concept that multiple surgical incisions in both atria interrupt the macroreentry circuits that are thought to be the underlying mechanism of most types of AF [7]. However, the complex nature of the procedure and the lack of reproducibility of the original results by other groups have led to the development of alternative surgical strategies employing simpler lesion sets and/or alternative energy sources.

Cryoablation is, next to radiofrequency ablation (RF), the most frequently employed alternative method to create linear, continuous, transmural lesions. The efficacy of cryoablation has been known since the original description of its use in humans to create AV node block in 1977 [16]. Its mechanism is based on Boyle's law: refrigerated fluid – nitrous oxide in the older devices, argon or helium in newer devices – is delivered under high pressure to the inner lumen of an electrode with the tip maintained under vacuum. The rapid expansion of the gas as it reaches the tip induces cooling of the electrode to between –55 and –60 °C for nitrous oxide and down to –144 °C for argon. The lower temperature of the argon- or helium-based technology allows shorter ablation times. The end result is a line of frozen tissue at the ablated site.

The maturation of the so created lesions occurs in three phases. Phase 1: the formed ice crystals compress and distort cell membranes and intracellular organelles causing irreversible cell death within hours [26]. Phase 2: the infiltration of the ablated tissue by inflammatory cells leads to the development of edema and leads to apoptosis [3]. Phase 3: fibrosis develops due to the secretion of fibrin by inflammatory cells and capillary ingrowth. The end result is a fibrotic scar with preserved stromal scaffolding [19].

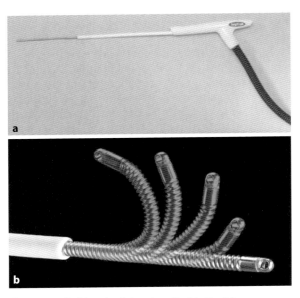

Fig. 1. Handheld probe (**a**) and malleable tip (**b**)

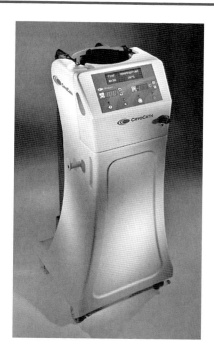

Fig. 2. Cryoablation control console

One of the most important advantages of cryoenergy, compared with hyperthermic energy sources such as radiofrequency, is the reduced risk of structural damage to adjacent structures [1, 11]. Collagen tissue and vasculature are unaffected and therefore the structural integrity of treated tissues is preserved [25]. A further significant advantage is the fact that endocardial thrombus formation at the site of cryoablation is reduced [18, 24].

The argon-based ATS CryoMaze surgical ablation system (formerly Surgi Frost system, CryoCath Technologies) has been used exclusively for all patients requiring endocardial AF ablation at our institution since 2004. It consists of a malleable handheld probe with a freezing segment of variable length of up to 10 cm (Fig. 1 a, b). At the console (Fig. 2), the time of ablation can be chosen and the temperature of the freezing segment is displayed via a thermocouple located at the tip of the probe. Temperatures of down to $-160\,°C$ can be achieved with this technology.

The CryoMaze system offers a number of potential advantages: first, the malleable freezing segment allows the probe to be bent into any shape necessary to create the required lesions, even in a more confined space such as during minimally invasive mitral valve surgery. Second, the creation of continuous lesions is simplified by the rapid freezing of the exposed segment of the probe after only a few seconds of activation. Care must be taken, however, to avoid tissue folding underneath of the probe, which can prevent transmurality of the lesions. The adhesive effect of the probe also

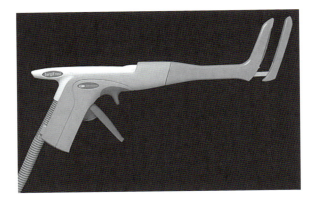

Fig. 3. Cryoablation clamp

allows the tissues to be lifted away from structures at risk of damage, such as the esophagus when creating lesions on the posterior wall of the left atrium or the phrenic nerve when creating lesions at the free edge of the atriotomy incision. Third, creation of a transmural lesion can be confirmed by visualization of frozen tissue on the epicardial side of the atrial wall while the probe is being applied endocardially.

The use of inert argon gas with extremely low temperatures allows the creation of transmural lesions in 1 min per treated segment, instead of the 2 min or longer that is required with nitrous oxide-based probes. A complete left atrial lesion set can therefore be performed in approximately 5–7 min, which is comparable to radiofrequency ablation techniques.

One drawback of cryoablation using the CryoMaze system is the fact that limited data are available to date on its efficacy during epicardial, beating heart application. The ability to create transmural lesions might be limited by the heat sink effect of intracardiac blood flow. A recent experimental study evaluated a new cryoclamp incorporating the above handheld probe using the same system (Fig. 3). The investigators found that the use of this cryoclamp in a canine model resulted in lesions with complete conduction block, while use of the linear hand held probe resulted in transmural lesions in only 85% of tissue sections [20]. Further clinical evaluation is required.

Minimal invasive MV surgery and cryoablation: current methods and results at the Leipzig Heart Center

Surgical technique and perioperative management

Our computerized database system was examined to identify all patients undergoing endocardial cryoablation for atrial fibrillation in combination with minimally invasive mitral valve (MV) surgery between January 2002

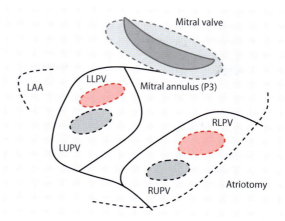

Fig. 4. Left atrial lesion set. Reprinted with permission from [12]; © American Association for Thoracic Surgery. (*LAA* left atrial appendage, *LLPV* left lower pulmonary vein, *LUPV* left upper pulmonary vein, *RLPV* right lower pulmonary vein, *PUPV* right upper pulmonary vein)

and December 2008. According to the new Cox classification [6], patients were classified into intermittent or continuous AF and analyzed separately.

Of the 1202 patients who underwent cryoablation at our institution during this time period, 406 (34%) underwent concomitant minimally invasive MV surgery and endocardial AF cryoablation and form the focus of this study. MV repair was performed in 308 patients (76%) and MV replacement in 98 (24%).

A minimally invasive approach via a right minithoracotomy is our procedure of choice for patients requiring isolated MV with or without tricuspid valve surgery. All patients received standard perioperative monitoring and a standard cardiac anesthesia. The femoral vessels were cannulated and cardiopulmonary bypass (CPB) was instituted with vacuum assistance (−30 to −50 mmHg) in order to achieve a flow of 2.0 to 2.5 L/min/m^2. Systemic temperature was lowered to 34 °C at the start of CPB and then rewarmed to 36 °C at the end of CPB. Myocardial protection was achieved with cold antegrade crystalloid cardioplegia. Techniques that were used to repair the MV have been described in detail elsewhere [13, 23].

The lesion set employed for the left atrial cryoablation is depicted in Fig. 4 [12]. The first lesion that was created was from the inferior aspect of the posterior mitral leaflet (P3) to the left lower pulmonary vein. This lesion was created first so that the annular tissue is no longer frozen when the annuloplasty sutures are placed. The left pulmonary veins are encircled next, connecting with the previous lesion. The right pulmonary veins are then isolated with a lesion connecting to the atriotomy. A further lesion is created across the roof of the left atrium connecting the lesions around the upper left and right pulmonary veins. In general, the left atrial appendage was obliterated only in patients with previous cerebrovascular events or in the presence of a thrombus. Right atrial ablation was performed only in patients with structural right heart pathology (e.g., atrial secundum defect or tricuspid valve lesions) or in patients with a past history of atrial flutter. In these cases, a lesion was created at the isthmus of the right atrium into the coronary sinus and to the tricuspid valve annulus.

Patients were monitored for recurrence of AF with continuous telemetry for a minimum of 48 consecutive hours postoperatively in our intensive care and/or intermediate care unit. A 12-lead ECG was also performed at least twice prior to discharge, or whenever signs or symptoms of AF occurred.

All patients who were taking beta-blockers preoperatively were continued on these medications postoperatively. Postoperative AF was treated aggressively with electrolyte replacement and optimization of amiodarone and/or beta blockade therapy. In addition, electrical cardioversion was attempted after correcting electrolyte abnormalities and establishing anti-arrhythmic medications. If cardioversion was unsuccessful after a minimum of two attempts, then patients were discharged on long-term warfarin and amiodarone therapy.

Clinical follow-up at 6 months was performed by either clinical examination during outpatient visit or telephone contact with patients and/or family members. Evaluation of postoperative rhythm was performed by contacting patients' family physicians or referring cardiologists. Rhythm status was confirmed by ECG in all patients, with a 24-h or 1-week Holter monitor being performed in patients who had symptoms suggestive of recurrent AF with a normal ECG.

Continuous variables are expressed as mean ± SD and categorical data as proportions throughout. All statistical analyses were performed using the JMP 7.0 statistical package (SAS Institute, Cary, NC, USA).

Results – perioperative

A total of 406 patients underwent minimally invasive MV surgery in combination with cryoablation. The preoperative characteristics are listed in Table 1 and intraoperative data are displayed in Table 2.

The overall perioperative mortality was 2.4% (10 patients). In none of the patients was the fatal outcome related to the ablation procedure. Major neurological complications occurred in 2.7%. The rate of new PPM implantation was 14.8% in the entire group. No major complications attributable to cryoablation, such as esophageal injury, phrenic nerve palsy or circumflex artery injury, were observed in any patient.

Sinus rhythm was present in 91.1% of patients at the end of the operation. At discharge, 315 patients (77.6%) were in sinus rhythm. Overall 315 cardioversions were performed in 185 patients according to the above outlined management protocol. Other perioperative outcomes are shown in Table 3.

Table 1. Preoperative characteristics of patients undergoing minimally invasive MV surgery and concomitant cryoablation for atrial fibrillation between 2002 and 2008

	Total	Intermittent AF	Continuous AF
Number of patients	406	180	226
Sex, female	198 (48.7%)	88 (48.9%)	110 (48.7%)
Age (years)	63.9 ± 10.6	63.7 ± 10.8	64.1 ± 10.3
BMI	25.9 ± 3.9	24.2 ± 3.2	26.4 ± 4.1
NYHA class	2.4 ± 0.7	2.4 ± 1.4	2.5 ± 1.3
Hypertension	249 (61.3%)	108 (60%)	141 (62.4%)
Diabetes	83 (20.3%)	22 (12.2%)	61 (27%)
Hypercholesterolemia	118 (29.1%)	51 (28.3%)	67 (29.6%)
History of embolism	22 (5.4%)	6 (3.3%)	16 (7.1%)
Pulmonary hypertension	119 (29.3%)	42 (23.3%)	77 (34.1%)
Duration of AF (years)	4.4 ± 3.6	3.9 ± 3.2	4.9 ± 3.9
LVEF (%)	59.4 ± 11.3	60.6 ± 11.4	58.6 ± 11.0
LA size (mm)	57.1 ± 10.8	55.7 ± 10.5	58.5 ± 10.7

BMI body mass index, *NYHA* New York Heart Association, *AF* atrial fibrillation, *LVEF* left ventricular ejection fraction, *LA* left atrium

Table 2. Intraoperative characteristics

	Total	Intermittent AF	Continuous AF
MV repair	308 (75.8%)	144 (80%)	164 (72.6%)
MV replacement	98 (24.2%)	36 (20%)	62 (27.4%)
Duration of surgery (min)	176 ± 47	174 ± 43	178 ± 50
CPB duration (min)	135 ± 41	134 ± 38	135 ± 42
Aortic clamp time (min)	84 ± 64	79 ± 30	79 ± 30
SR end of surgery	370 (91.1%)	167 (92.7%)	203 (89.8%)

MV mitral valve, *CPB* cardiopulmonary bypass, *SR* sinus rhythm

Long-term results

Six-month or more follow-up information was available in 316 patients (77.8%), with a mean duration of follow up of 241 ± 167 days. Ninety patients had either not yet reached 6 months postprocedure or were lost during follow-up. Of the patients with follow-up information, 292 (92.4%) were alive. Sinus rhythm was present in 208 surviving patients (71.2%).

Table 3. Early postoperative outcomes

■ ICU stay (days)	2.2 ± 7.8	1.8 ± 14.1	2.6 ± 9.5
■ Reoperation (bleeding)	35 (8.6%)	14 (7.8%)	21 (9.3%)
■ Renal failure	13 (3.2%)	5 (2.8%)	8 (3.5%)
■ ARDS	7 (1.7%)	3 (1.7%)	4 (1.8%)
■ Postop amiodarone	149 (36.7)	49 (27.2%)	100 (44.2%)
■ SR at discharge	315 (77.6%)	154 (85.6%)	161 (71.2%)
■ Atrial flutter	12 (2.9%)	4 (2.2%)	8 (3.5%)
■ III° heart block	10 (2.5%)	5 (2.7%)	5 (2.2%)
■ Cardioversion	185 (45.6%)	71 (39.4%)	114 (50.4%)
■ New PPM implantation	58 (14.3%)	28 (15.6%)	30 (13.3%)
■ TIA	7 (1.7%)	6 (3.3%)	1 (0.4%)
■ Stroke	11 (2.7%)	4 (2.2%)	7 (3.1%)
■ 30-day mortality	10 (2.4%)	2 (1.1%)	8 (3.6)

ICU intensive care unit, *ARDS* adult respiratory distress syndrome, *SR* sinus rhythm, *PPM* permanent pacemaker, *TIA* transient ischemic attack

Seventy-four patients (25.3%) were in AF. Atrial flutter or other rhythm was present in the remaining 3.5% of patients. No major neurological event occurred in the follow-up period. Mean NYHA class was 1.8 ± 0.7 and mean LVEF was 55 ± 13% at last follow-up.

■ Comment

Cryoablation has gained increasing popularity over the past few years. Next to RF ablation techniques, cryoablation is the most frequently performed ablation procedure. We have been using cryoablation at our institution almost exclusively for endocardial ablation since 2002, after observing a number of esophageal injuries that occurred with unipolar RF ablation [11].

The Cox MAZE procedure is still regarded as the benchmark against which all newer techniques have to be compared. However, the results for the Cox MAZE procedure are less impressive in patients undergoing concomitant mitral valve surgery, with freedom from AF rates that are far lower than the oft quoted 99% success rate for this procedure [9]. Izumoto and Raanani, for example, reported success rates of 75–82% in patients undergoing concomitant Cox MAZE procedures and MV surgery [17, 21]. Radiofrequency ablation achieves reported success rates of 70–80% in patients requiring concomitant mitral valve surgery [4, 27].

In comparison to other studies focusing on cryoablation during surgery for MV pathology, our results compare favorably. Ghavidel et al. reported a SR rate of 65% at 6 months with a nitrous oxide-based device [15]. A randomized trial comparing the effect of additional left atrial cryoablation to mitral valve surgery alone found a SR rate of 73% (22 of 30 patients) at 6 months follow-up in patients treated with cryoablation [5]. These investigators used the same device as used in our study and also employed a similar lesion set. One important difference, however, was that these investigators applied cryoablation epicardially on the beating empty heart. Baek et al. reported a SR rate of 84% at a mean follow-up of 26.6 months in a group of 170 patients with AF and rheumatic mitral valve disease undergoing Cryo-Maze and MV surgery [2].

Our study contained a high percentage of patients with continuous AF (55.7%). In addition, the relatively large mean left atrial size of 57 mm suggested an increased risk of failure of restoration of SR. In addition, biatrial lesion lines were performed in only a minority of patients. Despite these limitations, the success rate of SR 6-months postoperatively in our study was greater than 70%. Moreover, we did not observe a single case of serious complications related to cryoablation such as esophageal injury, phrenic nerve palsy or circumflex artery stenosis in over 400 patients. Indeed, we have not observed a single case of these potentially life-threatening complications in over 1200 cryoablation procedures that have been performed to date at our institution.

The rate of pacemaker implantation was fairly high in the current study (14.3%). A significant proportion of these patients required pacemakers because of unmasked sick sinus syndrome after ablation or other bradycardia syndromes. Complete heart block occurred in only 2.5% of the entire cohort. The reported incidence of pacemaker implantation after AF ablation ranges widely from just over 1% to 23% [2, 5], but is higher in patients requiring concomitant MV surgery.

In conclusion, the data from our study confirms the findings of other centers that cryoablation is a very safe and effective method for the treatment of AF in patients with MV disease and that the results with a minimally invasive approach are at least comparable with that of the conventional approach via a sternotomy. Since MV surgery alone in such patients is known to be associated with very low conversion rates to SR [5], and since endocardial cryoablation has an extremely good safety profile, we feel that it is prudent to offer all AF patients additional cryoablation when undergoing MV surgery.

References

1. Aupperle H, Doll N, Walther T, Kornherr P, Ullmann C, Schoon H-A, Mohr F W (2005) Ablation of atrial fibrillation and esophageal injury: Effects of energy source and ablation technique. J Thorac Cardiovasc Surg 130:1549–1554
2. Baek MJ, Chan YN, Sam SO, Chang HL, Jae HK, Hong JS, Sang WP, Wook SK (2006) Surgical treatment of chronic atrial fibrillation combined with rheumatic heart disease: effects of the cryo-maze procedures and predictors for late recurrence Eur J Cardiothorac Surg 30:728–736
3. Baust JG, Gage AA (2005) The molecular basis for cryosurgery. BJU Int 95(9): 1187–1191
4. Benussi S, Pappone C, Nascimbene S, Oreto G, Caldarola A, Stefano PL, Casati V, Alfieri O (2000) A simple way to treat chronic atrial fibrillation during mitral valve surgery: the epicardial radiofrequency approach. Eur J Cardiothorac Surg 17:524–529
5. Blomstroem-Lundqvist C, Johansson B, Berglin E et al (2007) A randomized double blind study of left atrial cryoablation for permanent atrial fibrillation in patients undergoing mitral valve surgery: the Swedish Multicentre Atrial Fibrillation study (SWEDMAF). Eur Heart J 28:2902–2908
6. Cox JL (2003) Atrial fibrillation: a new classification system. J Thor Cardiovasc Surg 126 (6):1686–1692
7. Cox JL, Canavan TE, Schuessler RB, Cain ME, Lindsay BD, Stone C (1991) The surgical treatment of atrial fibrillation: II Intraoperative electrophysiologic mapping and description of the electrophysiologic basis of atrial flutter and atrial fibrillation. J Thor Cardiovasc Surg 101:406–426
8. Cox JL, Boineau JP, Schuessler RB, Jaquiss RD, Lappas DG (1995) Modification of the Maze Procedure for atrial flutter and atrial fibrillation I. Rationale and surgical results J Thor Cardiovasc Surg 110:473–484
9. Cox JL, Ad N, Palazzo T, Fitzpatrick S et al (2000) Current status of the Maze procedure for the treatment of atrial fibrillation. Semin Thorac Cardiovasc Surgery 12(1):15–19
10. Deneke T, Khargi K, Grewe PH, Laczkovics A, von Dryander S, Lawo T, Muller KM, Lemke B (2002) Efficacy of an additional Maze procedure using cooled tip radiofrequency ablation in patients with chronic atrial fibrillation and mitral valve disease. Eur Heart J 23:558–566
11. Doll N, Borger MA, Fabricius A et al (2003) Esophageal perforation during left atrial radiofrequency ablation: Is the risk too high? J Thoracic Cardiovasc Surg 125:836–842
12. Doll N, Kiaii BB, Fabricius AM, Bucerius J et al (2003) Intraoperative left atrial ablation (for atrial fibrillation) using a new argon based cryocathter: early clinical experience. Ann Thor Surg 76:1711–1715
13. Falk V, Seeburger J, Czesla M et al (2008) How does the use of PTFE neochordae for posterior mitral valve prolapse (Loop technique) compare with leaflet resection? A prospective randomized trial. J Thoracic Cardiovasc Surg 136:1200–1206
14. Fuster V, Ryden L, Cannom D et al (2006) ACC/AHA/ESC 2006 Guidelines for the management of patients with atrial fibrillation: A report of the American College of Cardiology/American Heart Association Task force on practice guidelines Circulation 114:e257–e354
15. Ghavidel AA, Javadpour H, Shafiee M, Tabatabaie MB, Raiesi K, Hosseini S (2008) Cryoablation for surgical treatment of chronic atrial fibrillation combined with mitral valve surgery: a clinical observation. Eur J Cardiothorac Surg 33:1043–1048

16. Harrison L, Gallagher JJ, Kasell J et al (1977) Cryosurgical ablation of the A-V node-His bundle: a new method for producing A-V block. Circulation 55:463–470
17. Izumoto H, Kawazoe K, Kitahara H, Kamata J (1998) Operative results after the Cox/maze procedure combined with a mitral valve operation. Ann Thor Surg 66(3):800–804
18. Lustgarten DL, Keane D, Ruskin J (1999) Cryothermal ablation: mechanism of tissue injury and current experience in the treatment of tachyarrhythmia. Prog Cardiovasc 41:481–498
19. Manasse E, Colombo P, Roncalli M, Gallotti R (2000) Myocardial acute and chronic histological modifications induced by cryoablation. Eur J Cardiothorac Surg 17:339–340
20. Milla F, Skubas N, Briggs W et al (2006) Epicardial beating heart cryoablation using a novel argon-based cryoclamp and linear probe. J Thor Cardiovasc Surg 131:403–411
21. Raanani E, Albage A, Davit TE, Yau TM, Armstrong S (2001) The efficacy of the Cox/Maze procedure combined with mitral valve surgery: a matched control study. Eur J Cardiothorac Surg 19(4):438–442
22. Ryder KM, Bejamin EJ (1999) Epidemiology and significance of atrial fibrillation. Am J Cardiol 84(9A):131R–138R
23. Seeburger J, Borger MA, Falk V, Mohr FW (2008) Gore-Tex loop implantation for mitral valve prolapse: The Leipzig Loop Technique. Op Tech Thorac Cardiovasc Surg 13:83–90
24. Sie H, Beukema W, Elvan A et al (2003) New strategies in the surgical treatment of atrial fibrillation. Cardiovascular Research 58:501–509
25. Thibault B, Villemarie C, Talajic M et al (1998) Catheter cryoablation is a more effective and potentially safer method to create atrial conduction block: comparison with radiofrequency ablation. Pacing Clin Electrophysiol 21:944
26. Viola N, Williams MR, Oz MC et al (2002) The technology in use for the surgical ablation of atrial fibrillation. Semin Thor Cardiovasc Surg 14:198–205
27. Williams MR, Stewart JR, Bolling SF, Freeman S, Anderson JT, Argenziano M, Smith CR, Oz MC (2001) Surgical treatment of atrial fibrillation using radiofrequency energy. Ann Thor Surg 71:1939–1944

Minimally invasive endoscopic ablation on the beating heart in patients with lone atrial fibrillation

U. Rosendahl, J. Ennker

In the developed world between 1% and 1.5% of the population is suffering from atrial fibrillation [1]. Due to higher life expectancy, the prevalence of this disease will grow at least 3-fold in the next 50 years. Compared to many other diseases, the health and economic burden imposed by AF and AF-related morbidity is immense.

Atrial fibrillation is caused by various underlying diseases, ranging from genetic to degenerative origin. The most common and epidemiologically most prevalent conditions associated with AF are still hypertension and heart failure as both have been shown to initiate an arrhythmogenic milieu. The mechanism of atrial fibrillation is yet not identified; more than a

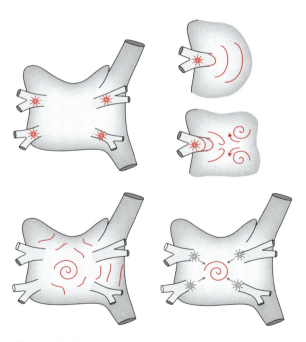

Fig. 1. Focal trigger initiate reentry, later, additional focal triggers act, and finally multiple reentry is perpetuated

few theories exist, but most of them can be joined essentially into the single focus hypothesis and the multiple sources hypothesis. Depending on the diversity of AF whether it is paroxysmal, intermittent, or persistent AF, these hypotheses have different levels of significance. Structural and electrophysiological properties of the atrial myocardium are altered by sustained AF, resulting in the atria becoming more susceptible to the initiation and maintenance of the arrhythmia. The foremost clinical significance of AF lies mainly in a 5-fold increased risk of stroke. Patients with AF who had a prior cerebral ischemia have a 10–12% risk of stroke per year [1]. In patients with lone AF the left atrial appendage is the site of thrombus in about 90% of cases. In this respect, novel mechanical approaches for the prevention of cardioembolic stroke have been invented: minimally invasive surgical isolation of the left atrial appendage, percutaneous left atrial appendage occluders, and carotid filtering devices.

Treatment of atrial fibrillation

The pharmacological approach is still the first choice in the treatment of most AF cases. But the interest towards nonpharmacological treatment of atrial fibrillation has considerably increased during the last decade; interventional procedures have been developed. Nowadays complete left lesion sets are feasible with good clinical results using percutaneous ablation methods. The surgical approach towards the treatment of AF is proving useful in a growing number of patients as well, being widely applied as a concomitant procedure in patients, not only undergoing mitral valve surgery anymore, but all kinds of cardiac procedures. The ability of resection or closing up the left atrial appendage in these procedures is probably more than advantageous regarding the most common hazard of AF, namely stroke. The development of new epicardial devices has launched the way to minimally invasive and thoracoscopic ablation approaches, which should give surgery a stronger role in the treatment of patients with lone AF, refractory to interventional ablation therapy or high thromboembolic risk.

Current surgical ablation practice

In 1991, when Cox developed the Maze procedure [2], His bundle ablation and pacemaker implantation were the only alternative non-pharmacological treatments of lone atrial fibrillation. However, owing to the extent of surgery and despite the progressive refinement and a 95% success rate, the

Maze operation never became popular. The 1-h cross-clamping time, 10% permanent pacemaker implantation, and a mortality of up to 1–2% were not acceptable for the treatment of atrial fibrillation [3].

The first indications of the prevailing function played by the left atrium in causing atrial fibrillation, prompted the proposal of simplified approaches only targeting the left atrium (LA) in 1996. Sueda was the first to describe a simple LA procedure to cure permanent AF in mitral valve patients with a 75% success rate [4]. Experience with cryo left atrial ablation in the treatment of lone AF showed an extremely high success rate in 93% of the patients [5]. The introduction of argon cryoenergy, radiofrequency (RF), and microwave surgical catheters allowed ablation procedures to be simplified further. The first reported experience of minimally invasive radiofrequency open-heart ablation of lone AF resulted in a success rate of up to 97%; however, esophageal perforation in 1% of the patients diminished the success [6]. Interest in lone AF surgery was renewed with the invention of epicardial ablation, which was first reported in 2000 [7]. Epicardial ablation allowed ablations to be performed without the use of cardiopulmonary bypass as off pump procedures on the beating heart. This was the start for minimally invasive surgical approaches to treat lone atrial fibrillation.

This paper describes the complete endoscopic microwave ablation of AF on the beating heart through a unilateral endoscopic approach. As the first working group, Saltman et al. published in 2003 their experience with a minimally endoscopic ablation through a bilateral thoracic approach, since then this method has been adopted by a growing number of surgeons [8, 9]. Later, La Meir et al. then moved towards an single right unilateral endoscopic method [10].

Totally endoscopic ablation

Totally endoscopic ablation is a stepwise approach, which is described as follows. First, three access ports are created on the right side of the chest: one camera and two working ports. The pericardium is opened above and parallel to the phrenic nerve in order to expose the pulmonary veins. Second, the pericardial reflections are dissected to enter into the transverse and oblique sinuses. Third, with the help of a bendable hook-like instrument, adopted from endoscopic liver surgery, the ablation catheter is guided through the sinuses and below the inferior vena cava towards the right atrial side. The device is then drawn around the base of left atrium. As soon as proper positioning of the device is established, a circumferential ablation line around the pulmonary veins is performed. The result is a complete ablation of the origins of the pulmonary veins from the left atrium in the form of a so-called box lesion.

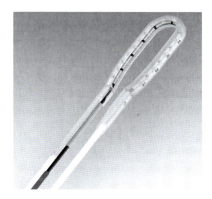

Fig. 2. Ablation tool for minimally invasive procedures

Patient inclusion criteria:

- Paroxysmal/persistent atrial fibrillation
- Highly symptomatic
- Failed numerous attempts of drug treatment
- Underwent at least one attempt of interventional catheter ablation which failed
- Has a small left atrium

Despite the above selection criteria, obviously most patients who do not meet one of the exclusion criteria might undergo endoscopic ablation therapy with different outcome regarding the cure of AF. As the method is not widely established yet and is to some extent in competition with catheter-based ablation methods, patient selection should be rigorous in order to achieve excellent results.

Patient exclusion criteria for the endoscopic approach:

- Previous cardiac surgery
- Left atrial thrombus
- Severe pulmonary malfunction

Preoperative diagnostics:

- Coronary angiography in all patients >40
- Transesophageal echocardiography (for exclusion of LA thrombus and valvular heart disease)
- Lung function test (single tube ventilation)
- Chest X-ray
- Routine blood tests

Surgical procedure

The patient is lying in a supine position. After deflating the right lung, a 5-mm port is inserted in the 4th intercostal space at the level of the anterior axillary line. Then, CO_2 is insufflated (Fig. 3).

Through this port a nonangled endoscope is inserted and the pericardium is inspected.

According to visualization, two further ports are inserted into the chest, first, in the 3rd intercostal space at the level of the anterior axillary line and, second, in the 5th intercostal space around the midclavicular line. The positioning of the ports tends to fluctuate, specifically with respect to height. As the ports are used for the instruments, they should be placed in order to allow an oblique handling of the pericardium rather than a rectangular approach. While placing these ports, it has to be kept in mind that one has to be able to pass the transverse sinus with the instruments. The phrenic nerve is located and the pericardium is opened 2 cm above and along the nerve. The pericardium is incised and the aorta and inferior vena cava are located (Fig. 4).

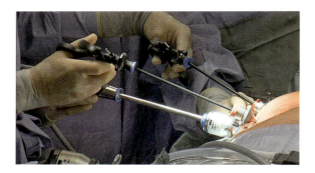

Fig. 3. Access via two accessory ports and one camera port

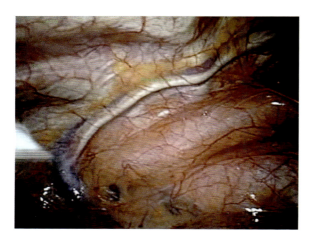

Fig. 4. After insufflation with CO_2, view of the pericardium prior to the incision

The pericardial reflections behind the superior and inferior vena cavae are dissected in order to obtain access to the transverse and oblique sinuses. Using blunt dissection after lifting the SVC upwards, the transverse sinus is entered. The endoscope is guided through the transverse sinus towards the left auricle, which can then be visualized. After the transverse sinus has been dissected, the oblique sinus needs to be opened up. Using blunt dissection, the thin layer of pericardium is divided and the oblique sinus is easily entered.

Ablation

In order to guide the ablation tool (which is fully flexible and cannot be steered) through the sinus, a guidance instrument is required. Several instruments are nowadays commercially available. A simple and cost effective instrument which has proved to be helpful is a bendable hook-like instrument, adopted from endoscopic liver surgery. This hook can be steered and bent from 0° to 360°. A major disadvantage is the size of the instrument. It cannot be passed through a port. Thus the instrumental port located toward the right of the camera port has to be removed in order to have an entryway for the ablation tool. The ablation catheter is then attached to the hook and passed through this incision into the right chest cavity. Under direct vision with the camera, it is then maneuvered into the transverse sinus by passing it under the superior vena cava (Fig. 5).

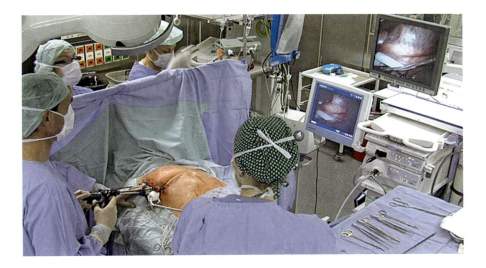

Fig. 5. Operational findings during endoscopic ablation

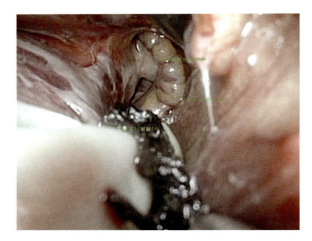

Fig. 6. Transverse sinus with view of left atrial appendage

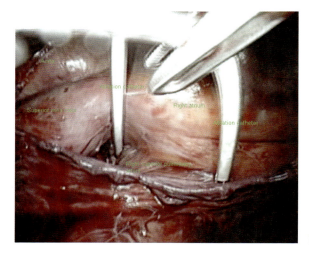

Fig. 7. Positioned ablation probe

The endoscope is passed into the transverse sinus and is kept in a position which allows visualization of the left atrial appendage. Under camera control, the hook with the ablation tool is then guided through the transverse sinus until it reaches the left auricle. Once it has reached the auricle, the hook is directed posterior of the auricle towards the diaphragmatic aspect of the pericardium (Fig. 6).

Once it is ensured that the ablation catheter is securely positioned below the left auricle and not on top of it, the hook is bent 360° and gently pushed forward until the tool appears under the inferior vena cava in the oblique sinus. Retrieval of the catheter is the most demanding part of the procedure, particularly if the heart or the left atrium is rather large. The ablation catheter is then removed from the guiding tool and completely pulled through the sinus until both ends reach each other. The correct position of the ablation catheter is confirmed with the endoscope. The tool is connected to the generator and stepwise ablation is carried out. In order enhance transmurality, the full ablation is carried out twice for each segment (Fig. 7).

After successful ablation, the catheter is removed and the ablation line, where possible, is checked with the endoscope. After insertion of temporary atrial and ventricular pacing wires, the pericardium is closed with two stitches. A chest tube is inserted, the wounds are closed appropriately. If the patient is in atrial fibrillation at this point of the operation, cardioversion is performed before the patient is extubated and awake.

Postoperative management

According to our protocol all patients are started on amiodarone 300 mg/d and warfarin immediately afterwards. Amiodarone is continued for 6 to 12 months, depending on the individual postoperative course. Warfarin is continued for 12 months, if stable sinus rhythm is apparent, then it is discontinued. Chest tubes are usually removed the next morning. If the immediate postoperative course was uneventful, patients are discharged after 48 hours.

Follow-up

The early reoccurrence of atrial fibrillation after surgical ablation is common. The literature and our own experience show an early reoccurrence rate within the first 6 months of about 50% (Fig. 8).

Patients therefore need to be followed up in regular intervals. In order to make the procedure worthwhile for the patient, a follow-up schedule with regular check-ups after 3-, 6-, 9-, and 12-months postoperation is mandatory. Thereafter, yearly follow-up has proven to be sufficient.

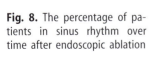
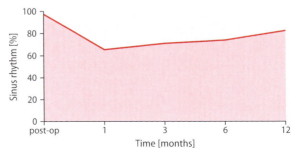

Fig. 8. The percentage of patients in sinus rhythm over time after endoscopic ablation

Future role of surgical ablation therapy for lone atrial fibrillation

Minimally invasive surgical ablation plays an important role in up to 20% of patients suffering from atrial fibrillation who do not respond to conventional medical treatment, are not candidates for percutaneous ablation, or have undergone percutaneous ablation unsuccessfully. Furthermore, if concomitant appendage obliteration could regularly be performed during the procedure, surgery for lone AF could have a rationale in the context of secondary prevention of stroke, where surgery could actually ameliorate prognosis. Data of controlled randomized studies are presently not available; hence the future of this surgical intervention depends on the experience of the surgeons and the cardiologist who refer the patients.

References

1. Ryder KM, Benjamin EJ (1999) Epidemiology and significance of atrial fibrillation. Am J Cardiol 84:131R–138R
2. Cox JL, Schuessler RB, D'Agostino Jr HJ, Stone CM, Chang BC, Cain ME, Corr PB, Boineau JP (1991) The surgical treatment of atrial fibrillation. III. Development of a definitive surgical procedure. J Thorac Cardiovasc Surg 101:569–583
3. Prasad SM, Maniar HS, Camillo CJ, Schuessler RB, Boineau JP, Sundt III TM, Cox JL, Damiano Jr RJ (2003) The Cox maze III procedure for atrial fibrillation: long-term efficacy in patients undergoing lone versus concomitant procedures. J Thorac Cardiovasc Surg 126:1822–1828
4. Sueda T, Nagata H, Shikata H, Orihashi K, Morita S, Sueshiro M, Okada K, Matsuura Y (1996) Simple left atrial procedure for chronic atrial fibrillation associated with mitral valve disease. Ann Thorac Surg 62:1796–1800
5. Todd DM, Skanes AC, Guiraudon G, Guiraudon C, Krahn AD, Yee R, Klein GJ (2004) Role of the posterior left atrium and pulmonary veins in human lone atrial fibrillation. Circulation 108:3108–3114
6. Doll N, Borger MA, Fabricius A, Stephan S, Gummert J, Mohr FW, Hauss J, Kottkamp H, Hindricks G (2003) Esophageal perforation during left atrial radiofrequency ablation: is the risk too high? J Thorac Cardiovasc Surg 125:836–842
7. Benussi S, Pappone C, Nascimbene S, Oreto G, Caldarola A, Stefano PL, Casati V, Alfieri O (2000) A simple way to treat atrial fibrillation during mitral valve surgery: the epicardial radiofrequency approach. Eur J Cardiothorac Surg 17:524–529
8. Saltman AE, Rosenthal LS, Francalancia NA, Lahey SJ (2003) A completely endoscopic approach to microwave ablation for atrial fibrillation. Heart Surg Forum 6(3):E38–E41
9. Salenger R, Lahey SJ, Saltmann AE (2004) The completely endoscopic treatment of atrial fibrillation: report on the first 14 patients with early results. Heart Surg Forum 7:E555–E558
10. La Meir M, De Roy L, Blommaert, D, Buche D (2007) Treatment of lone atrial fibrillation with a right thoracoscopic approach. Ann Thorac Surg 83(6):2244–2245

Hemodynamic evaluation of the bioprosthetic aortic valves

Evaluation of bioprosthetic valve performance as a function of geometric orifice area and space efficiency –
a reliable alternative to effective orifice area

J. SAUTER

Introduction

Performance comparisons among commercially available bioprosthetic valves are needlessly complicated by unreliable and complex parameters and exaggerated information from manufacturers. In addition to the issues surrounding the comparisons among valves, surgeons who are selecting the best fit for the patient on the operating table are hampered not only by the faulty parameters mentioned above but by selection tables based on these faulty parameters and by the often unachievable boundary between a proper match and an improper mismatch of the valve to the patient.

The surgeon can sidestep complexity and bias by acceptance of an essential tenet: The best patient outcome is achieved by fitting the patient with the largest flow area possible. The surgeon can observe flow area comparisons obtained by direct observation rather than abstract data derived from equipment-based algorithms. Specifically, direct observation enables valve comparisons on the basis of *geometric orifice area (GOA)* and *space efficiency*. To illustrate this simplified approach, comparisons among seven commercially available stented bioprosthetic valves will be made on the basis of these two characteristics.

The common approach to bioprosthetic valve evaluation

During aortic valve replacement surgery, cardiac surgeons are challenged to provide adequate perfusion to a body starved by a stenotic valve. The limitations of bioprosthetic valve prostheses make the restoration of adequate blood flow difficult for patients with normal body masses but even more difficult for obese patients who have outgrown the capacities of their hearts. No prosthetic heart valve can operate with the efficiency of the patient's original equipment. This means that, while prosthetic valves improve blood flow and stabilize the disease state, prosthetic valves nevertheless im-pose work on the heart. This work does not contribute to the heart's basic purpose, to pump blood for the perfusion of the tissue mass of the patient. Such imposed extra work is referred to as "work loss" or "energy loss".

Effective orifice area

In order to diminish this energy loss, the surgeon is faced with the perplexing task of selecting the prosthetic valve that most closely approximates the flow of the original healthy valve. To make this selection, the surgeon commonly turns to the concept of effective orifice area (EOA).

The EOA is the area of the invisible and narrowed control volume that "in effect" remains in the wake of forward flow energy losses (Fig. 1). Although EOA is expressed as a two-dimensional area (cm^2), EOA is considered a measure of performance. EOAs are directly related to and dependent on the opening area of the valve. The example illustrated in Fig. 1 depicts a mechanical valve. In the case of mechanical valves, the relationship between the EOA and the flow area is more complex because occluders (usually two leaflets) of varying sizes and opening angles obstruct the flow through the central orifice in ways that are difficult to interpret. The case for bioprosthetic valves is much simpler; bioprosthetic valves possess central and unobstructed openings such that the sizes of the openings alone determine the relative performances of the valves.

Doppler EOAs are calculated on the basis of the velocity-time integral (VTI) (Fig. 2) using the continuity theorem. The continuity equation simply states that the area at the inflow tract times the velocity time integral at that point equals the effective orifice area times the velocity time integral at the upstream narrowing of the valve. Since the EOA is the only un-

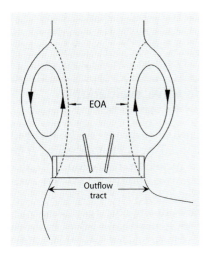

Fig. 1. Effective orifice area (EOA) is the narrowest area of the invisible control volume that "in effect" remains in the wake of forward flow energy losses

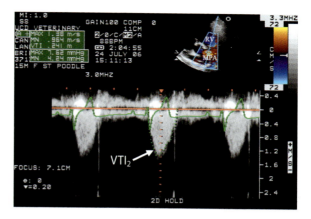

Fig. 2. Systolic ejection for an aortic valve is measured by Doppler as the change in velocity (y-axis) over time (x-axis). The echo technician outlines the edge of the velocity time curve with digital markers and the computer computes the area within the curve as the velocity-time integral

known, its value can be solved algebraically. Expressed mathematically, the continuity equation is:

$$EOA \times VTI_2 = A_{outflow\ tract} \times VTI_1$$

Solving for EOA:

$$EOA = (A_{outflow\ tract} \times VTI_1)/VTI_2$$

Despite the mathematical logic and high-tech equipment involved in the calculation of EOAs, time has demonstrated EOA to be an unreliable measure. For any given manufacturer's valve and any given size, effective orifice areas vary widely (Table 1).

Causes of the unreliability of in vivo EOA measurements have been summarized by Gillinov and colleagues [7]: "Variability can be introduced in the measurement of the LVOT diameter or the velocity at the outflow tract. In vivo EOA values for bileaflet valves might be underestimated when evaluated by means of echocardiography because of localized high-velocity jets. Poor echocardiographic windows and suboptimal Doppler recordings with improper alignment of the Doppler scan with the direction of flow might also affect the accuracy of the method" (p. 314) [7]. In the same paper, Gillinov also points out the role of patient characteristics: "In vivo EOA might change from moment to moment with patient activity, cardiac output and blood pressure, and dynamics of the LVOT…" (p. 314).

Faced with the variety of available EOA results and the pressure of competition, valve manufacturers tend to select the most flattering EOA data available. In fact, since there is no way of knowing which study is the most valid, the study showing the highest EOAs could be considered as reasonable a choice as any.

Table 1. Sixteen published EOA results for the Edwards size 21 valve range from 1.10 to 1.90 cm^2, demonstrating the poor reliability of EOA measurement

Edwards size 21 only	
A range of published EOAS	
Milano – Annals 2001	1.10
Dellgren – JTCS 2002	1.10
Pelletiert – J Card Surg 1988	1.13
Perier – J Card Surg 1991	1.17
Borger – Annals 2007	1.30
Aupart – Eur J CT Surg 1994	1.30
Aupart – Eur J CT Surg 1996	1.30
Rao – JTCS 1999	1.30
Khan – Annals 2000	1.30
Eichinger – JTCS 2005	1.39
Vitale – Annals 2003	1.48
McDonald – Annals 1997	1.49
Tasca – Annals 2003	1.45
Dalmau – ICTS 2006	1.69
Dalmau – ICTS 2007	1.75
Dalmau – ICTS 2006	1.90

■ Patient-prosthesis mismatch and effective orifice area index

When selecting the best bioprosthetic aortic valve for a patient on the operating table, many cardiac surgeons rely on the concept of patient-prosthesis mismatch (PPM), first introduced by Rahimtoola in 1978 [1] and later quantified by the concept of indexed effective orifice area (often referred to as "effective orifice area index" or "EOAI") by Dumesnil and colleagues in 1990 [2]. PPM refers to a case where the valve is inadequate to perfuse the patient sufficiently. Research by Dumesnil and his frequent collaborator Pibarot demonstrates a higher rate of clinical complications and mortality for patients who are mismatched with their valves [3–6].

EOAI is appealing because the concept quantifies a limit for PPM as the minimum acceptable ratio between the effective orifice area (EOA) of a given valve to the volume of tissue to be perfused. The calculation of EOA has been described above. Measurement of the volume of tissue to be perfused for any given patient is provided in terms of the body surface area (BSA). The body surface area (BSA) expresses a patient's tissue volume or body mass in two-dimensional terms (m^2) according to the function:

$$BSA(m^2) = 0.007184 \times \text{weight (kg)}^{0.425} \times \text{height (cm)}^{0.725}$$

The EOAI ratio is expressed simply as,

EOAI = EOA/BSA

Based on clinical results, Pibarot and Dumesnil [4] have established the minimum EOAI as

$EOAI_{min} = 0.85$

Note that EOAI has no unit designation; this is an attribute of an index. Using a simple algebraic calculation, it is possible to determine the minimum acceptable EOA as

$EOA_{min} = 0.85$ BSA

Valve manufacturers have simplified the process by creating cross-reference charts specifically for their valves (Fig. 3).

Once again, the appeal of basing the valve selection for a patient on a mathematics-based chart is irresistible. However, like any parameter, the reliability of EOAI is only as good as the variables used to calculate it. Thus, the lack of reliability of EOA is passed on to calculated EOAIs. The options for EOAI charts are as numerous as the available EOAs. To remain competitive, manufacturers create the most flattering EOAI charts from the most flattering EOAs, diminishing EOAI charts to little more than marketing brochures.

Valve Size	19 mm	21 mm	23 mm	25 mm	27 mm
EOA (cm²)	*1.16*	*1.37*	*1.66*	*1.63*	*1.81*
1.0	1.16	1.37	1.66	1.63	1.81
1.1	1.06	1.24	1.51	1.48	1.65
1.2	0.97	1.14	1.38	1.36	1.51
1.3	0.89	1.05	1.28	1.25	1.39
1.4	0.83	0.98	1.19	1.16	1.29
1.5	0.77	0.91	1.11	1.09	1.21
1.6	0.73	0.85	1.04	1.02	1.13
1.7	0.68	0.80	0.98	0.96	1.06
1.8	0.65	0.76	0.92	0.91	1.01
1.9	0.61	0.72	0.87	0.86	0.95
2.0	0.58	0.68	0.83	0.82	0.91
2.1	0.55	0.65	0.79	0.78	0.86
2.2	0.53	0.62	0.75	0.74	0.82
2.3	0.51	0.59	0.72	0.71	0.79
2.4	0.48	0.57	0.69	0.68	0.75
2.5	0.46	0.55	0.66	0.65	0.72

Body Surface Area (m²)

■ Acceptable: EOAI ≥ 0.85 cm²/m²
■ Marginal: 0.85 cm²/m² > EOAI ≥ 0.75 cm²/m²
■ Unacceptable: EOAI < 0.75 cm²/m²

Fig. 3. A fabricated example of an EOAI chart. The appropriate fit of a valve can be determined by cross-referencing the patient's BSA to the valve size

Even if EOAI charts were reliable, the very concept of patient-prosthesis mismatch has been challenged by a number of researchers [7–14]. Blackstone et al. [14], in a study of more than 13 000 patients and almost 70 000 patient-years, showed that deviation by as much as 3.0 standard deviations below the normal expected native valve size for a given patient had no effect on moderate to long-term mortality. However, deviations over 2.5 standard deviations did result in a 2% increase in short-term mortality. On this basis, Blackstone and colleagues established 2.5 standard deviations as the cutoff for patient-prosthesis mismatch. This standard places only about 0.6% of patients in the mismatch category making PPM extremely unlikely. The authors suggested that reference to geometric orifice valve areas may be a more valid and reliable method for intraoperative decision making.

Cardiac surgeons who rely on indexed effective orifice area to determine PPM find that, for a large percentage of patients, they are unable to meet the 0.85 EOAI standard established by Pibarot and Dumesnil. For example, among a series of 1823 St. Jude valve patients, Emery and colleagues showed that 65% of the patients experienced moderate to severe mismatch [15].

Confronted with the unreliability and complex issues surrounding the EOAI charts provided by manufacturers and the challenges to the concept of patient-prosthesis mismatch, the cardiac surgeon is left with a simple solution: strive to fit the patient with the valve that provides the largest GOA possible.

Geometric orifice area – a valid alternative

The geometric orifice area (GOA) can be considered a performance measure in the sense that gradients and EOAs are directly based on and correlated to the flow area of a valve. Furthermore, unlike EOA, the GOA is a highly reliable measure because it is determined by direct observation and measurement. The GOA for any given bioprosthetic valve is here defined as the area of the valve at its greatest opening. This is a valid approximation because the GOA of a bioprosthetic heart valve changes little during systole.

But how can a cardiac surgeon know the GOAs of various bioprosthetic heart valves? Bioprosthetic valve manufacturers often provide orifice areas for their valves in their Instructions for Use (IFU) and in brochures. However, these areas are misrepresented because they are based on the area of the inner diameter of the stent. This is invalid; tissue valves do not open like circular tubes that encompass the inner stent (Fig. 4). In fact, the opening configuration of a bioprosthetic valve is always smaller than the inner perimeter of the stent and too complex for calculation by a simple trigonometric function. Fortunately, digital planimetry makes possible the

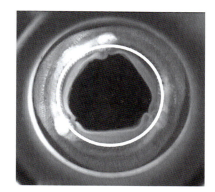

Fig. 4. Maximum opening of a 21 mm pericardial valve at 5 lpm. The actual opening is smaller than the inner stent area whose perimeter is represented by the white circle

calculation of the areas of the most irregular bioprosthetic valve openings. The following analysis illustrates the comparison of bioprosthetic valves using characteristics discernable by direct observation.

Comparison of seven commercially available bioprosthetic valves on the basis of geometric orifice area and space efficiency

▋ Materials and methods

Materials

The observations that follow are not made to compare specific manufacturers but rather the effects of specific designs on the orifice areas and space efficiencies of bioprosthetic valves. To emphasize the design basis for these comparisons, valves are code named with design-related terms. The stented pericardial valves included in this investigation are shown in Fig. 5. *Peri-out Supra* is a supraannular pericardial valve whose leaflets consist of a single ribbon of pericardium secured around the *outside* of the three stent posts. *Peri-in* is composed of three separate leaflets attached *inside* the stent posts. The *Peri-in Supra* is the supraannular version of the Peri-in valve and differs from the Peri-in only by the repositioning and reduction of the sewing ring. A more detailed comparison of the assembly processes for the Peri-out and the Peri-in pericardial valves is shown in Fig. 6.

The stented porcine valves included in this study are shown in Fig. 7. The *Porc-intact* is a stented porcine valve fabricated from a single intact pig valve. It is not known how the porc-intact pig valve is attached to the stent. This valve retains the muscle shelf at the right coronary cusp of the natural pig valve. The *Porc-intact Supra* is the supraannular version of this valve. The *Porc-tricomp* is a stented tricomposite porcine valve assembled

320 ■ J. Sauter

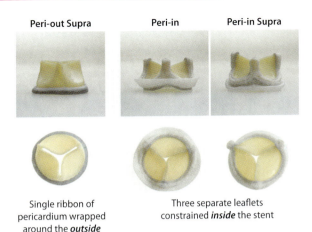

Fig. 5. Shown are three stented pericardial heart valves included in the study. The Peri-out valves are differentiated from the Peri-in valves by the configuration and assembly of the pericardial leaflets

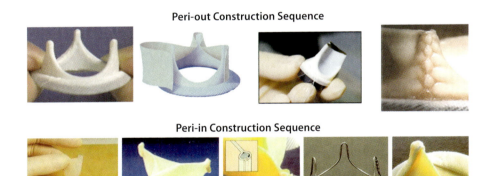

Fig. 6. *Peri-out construction sequence:* The covered stent is completed and is loosely wrapped with a pre-cut ribbon of pericardial tissue. The stent-tissue combination is placed over a plastic frame. The wet leaflets adhere to the frame to create three identical cusps. A special cross-stitch attaches the pericardium to the outside of the covered stent posts and the assembly is attached to the sewing ring. *Peri-in construction sequence:* A cutting die cuts three exact leaflets. The leaflet tabs are joined and are placed over a polyester tab and the fabric-tab-leaflet combination is attached to a frame. The wire stent is then inserted over the leaflets and inside the frame, and the stent is secured to the assembly. Finally, the sewing cuff is attached. The lower five photos reproduced with permission from Edwards Lifesciences, Irvine, CA

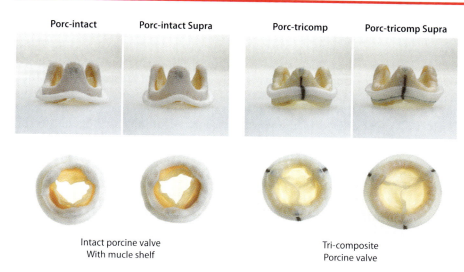

Fig. 7. Four porcine valves were included in the study. Porc-intact valves are fabricated from a single intact pig valve that includes the right coronary muscle shelf. Porc-tricomp is assembled from three leaflets selected from different animals and matched to fit. The muscle shelf is excluded

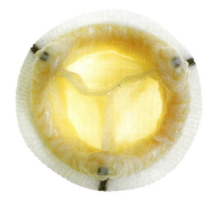

Fig. 8. The Porc-tricomp valve is assembled from three leaflets selected from different animals

from leaflets obtained from different animals (Fig. 8). The muscle shelf is excluded. The *Porc-tricomp Supra* is the supraannular version of this valve.

One each of sizes 19, 21, and 23 were obtained for each of seven valve models manufactured by four different companies. The Porc-tricomp which is not available in size 19 was the sole exception and only two sizes were studied for this valve. Thus, there were a total of 20 valves. Peri-out Supra valves packaged for sale were randomly selected by warehouse staff while the remaining valves were purchased new and in their boxes.

Methods

All the valves were video recorded on the same day using the same setup and flow parameters. Each valve was fitted to a plastic holder and placed in the aortic position of a ViVitro pulse duplicator (ViVitro Systems Inc., Victoria, British Columbia, Canada). An Olympus Encore Mac PCI 2000s digital high-speed video camera (Olympus America Inc., Melville, New York, USA) was affixed to the viewport centered on and orthogonal to the valve holder. Each valve was run at 72 beats per minute at cardiac outputs of 5 lpm and 7 lpm. The camera recorded two cycles for each valve at 500 frames per second and these images were uploaded to the Encore MAC PCI's – High Speed Digital Imaging System (Olympus America Inc., Melville, New York, USA).

Once the dynamic recordings for the valves were complete, the author analyzed each video frame by frame until he identified the largest opening. For pericardial valves the largest opening occurred at mid-systole and differed only slightly from the opening near the beginning and end of systole. For porcine valves, the largest opening occurred at the instant of opening. Thereafter the opening varied minutely and unpredictably throughout systole due to high-frequency fluttering of the leaflets. Once identified, the frame showing the largest opening was captured as a still image. The image was imported into a computer-aided design program (SolidWorks, Dassault Systèmes SolidWorks Corp., Vélizy, France) and digital markers were placed around the perimeter of the opening. The software converted the digital markers into a perimeter and calculated the area inside the perimeter (Fig. 9). The GOAs were recorded and filed with the analyzed image.

In addition to the GOA measurements, observations of the dynamic behavior of each valve were made by repeated examination of its video in both normal and slow motion.

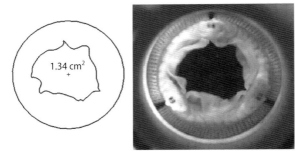

Fig. 9. Planimetric area measurement for a 23 mm porcine valve at 7 lpm

Results

Geometric orifice areas

The geometric orifice areas of the pericardial valves at 5 lpm are shown in Fig. 10. Among these single samples the Peri-out Supra had the largest GOA of the 19 mm valves, the Peri-in Supra had the largest GOA of the 21 mm valves, and the Peri-in had the largest GOA of the 23 mm valves. The single samples of each valve preclude any statistically based comparative conclusions. Furthermore, the largest GOAs were dispersed among the three pericardial valve types. At this point, we can only conclude that there is no significant difference in GOAs among the valves on a size-by-size basis.

On a visual basis, some differences are apparent. The openings of the Peri-out valves are more symmetrical than the openings of the Peri-in valves. At 5 lpm, there was not a single Peri-in or Peri-in Supra valve all of whose leaflets opened to more or less match the inner perimeter of the stent. This limitation appears to have diminished the potential orifice area of the Peri-in valves. Although, as mentioned above, one cannot make statistical comparisons among the valves due to the single samples, the size-by-size variability between the Peri-in and Peri-in Supra valves appears to

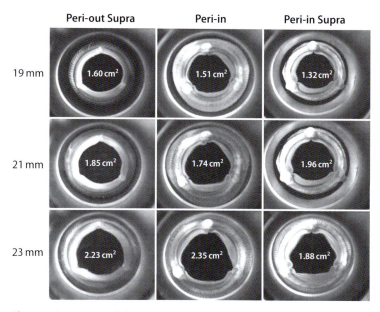

Fig. 10. A summary of the GOAs obtained for stented pericardial valves

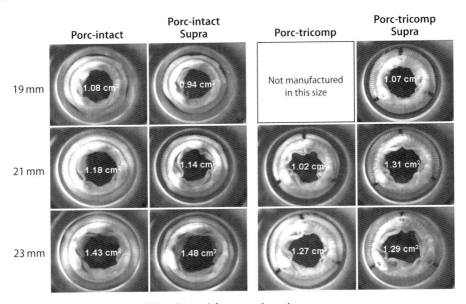

Fig. 11. A summary of the GOAs obtained for stented porcine

correlate with the fit of the leaflets to the inner perimeter of the stent. The most notable case is the 23 mm Peri-in Supra all three of whose leaflets were unable to reach the inner perimeter of the stent, creating an almost triangular opening. As a result, the GOA of the 23 mm Peri-in Supra is actually smaller than that of the 21 mm Peri-in Supra.

The geometric orifice areas for the stented porcine valves at 5 lpm are shown in Fig. 11. Although opening configurations are generally irregular with porcine valves, two of them, 21 mm Porc-tricomp and 21 mm Porc-tricomp Supra, approximate a shield-like symmetry. As was the case with the pericardial valves, the single samples of each valve do not permit a statistical comparison of porcine GOAs on a size-by-size basis. Complicating a size-by-size comparison further, sizing for the Porc-tricomp Supra is unique. In general, a supraannular bioprosthetic valve is given the same size designation and the intraannular valve from which it was derived. For example, the 19 mm Porc-intact Supra is simply a modified version of the 19 mm standard Porc-intact. In the case of the Porc-tricomp the supra version is modified from the original and then designated with the next smaller size. Thus, the 21 mm Porc-tricomp became the 19 mm Porc-tricomp Supra. We should expect then to see the GOA of the 21 mm Porc-tricomp match the GOA of the 19 mm Porc-tricomp and so on in a staggered pattern. Indeed the GOAs were offset as expected with the exception of the 23 mm Porc-tricomp Supra, whose opening was about the same size as the 21 mm Porc-tricomp Supra. The GOAs of the Porc-intact and the Porc-intact Supra valves matched remarkably well on a size-by-size basis.

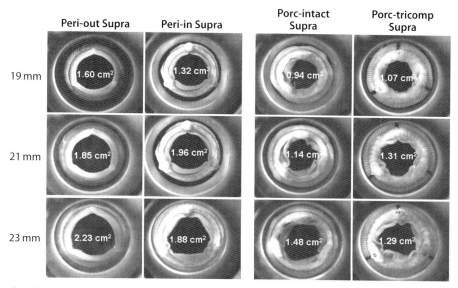

Fig. 12. A comparison among the supraannular models of pericardial and porcine valves at 5 lpm showed a size-by-size advantage for pericardial valves ranging from a minimum of 27% to a maximum of 73%

Examination of Figs. 10 and 11 clearly shows the GOA advantage of pericardial over porcine valves. In Fig. 12, supraannular pericardial and supraannular porcine valves are compared. Size-by-size comparisons among this subset of pericardial valves and porcine valves showed the GOAs of the supraannular pericardial valves to be larger than the GOAs of the supraannular porcine valves by a minimum of 27% to a maximum of 73%. Although not shown, the GOAs of the standard Peri-in pericardial valves obviously dominate the GOAs of the standard porcine valves as well (Figs. 10 and 11).

The effect of cardiac output

Although cardiac outputs vary among individual patients, the discussion thus far has focused on GOAs at a cardiac output of 5 lpm. For research purposes it is common practice to consider 5 lpm as the average resting cardiac output. While this generalization is useful for simple comparisons, a more thorough picture emerges when we analyze the GOAs and opening configurations at both 5 lpm and 7 lpm. Table 2 shows the change in area at 7 lpm with respect to the 5 lpm GOAs. Almost all the valves demonstrated a growth in GOA at the higher cardiac output ranging from 0.5% to 22.5%. The two exceptions were the 23 mm Porc- intact and the 19 mm Porc-intact showing GOA decreases of 4.5% and 2.9%, respectively. The

Table 2. Comparisons of GOAs at 5 lpm and 7 lpm. With two exceptions the GOAs were larger at the higher cardiac output. The most extreme growth in GOA was seen for several of the Peri-in category of valves

	Peri-out supra	Peri-in	Peri-in supra	Porc-intact	Porc-intact supra	Porc tricomp	Porc-tricomp supra
19 mm							
GOA 5 lpm (cm^2)	1.60	1.51	1.32	1.08	0.94	Not available in this size	1.07
GOA 7 lpm (cm^2)	1.69	1.61	1.47	1.13	0.89		1.08
% Growth	6.1	6.8	11.0	4.5	−4.9		1.1
21 mm							
GOA 5 lpm (cm^2)	1.85	1.74	1.96	1.18	1.14	1.31	1.02
GOA 7 lpm (cm^2)	1.97	2.03	2.02	1.21	1.21	1.39	1.02
% Growth	6.3	16.8	3.1	3.2	5.5	6.4	0.5
23 mm							
GOA 5 lpm (cm^2)	2.23	2.35	1.88	1.43	1.48	1.29	1.27
GOA 7 lpm (cm^2)	2.29	2.58	2.30	1.36	1.56	1.34	1.34
% Growth	2.8	9.7	22.5	−4.5	5.4	3.8	5.3

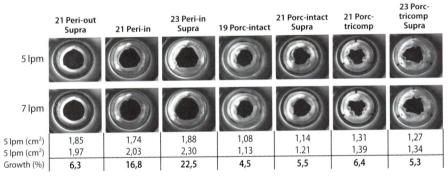

Fig. 13. A graphic depiction of the greatest GOA changes from 5 lpm to 7 lpm for each valve type regardless of size

most remarkable GOA growth was seen in the Peri-in category of valves. The 19 mm Peri-in Supra gained 11.0%, the 21 mm Peri-in gained 16.8%, and 23mm Peri-in Supra gained 22.5%. Relative to the Peri-in valves, the Peri-out valves maintained a more constant GOA, changing by a maximum of 6.3%.

Fig. 13 is a graphic depiction of the greatest GOA increase observed for each of the seven valve models regardless of size. For the pericardial valves, the increased cardiac output forced the valve openings into a more circular configuration. The most dramatic changes from 5 lpm to 7 lpm were observed for the 21 mm Peri-in and the 23 mm Peri-in Supra whose openings were somewhat constricted at 5 lpm but opened to an approximately circular configuration at 7 lpm. These dramatic changes in configuration coincided with the most dramatic GOA changes of 16.8% and 22.5%, respectively, illustrating the effect of incomplete leaflet opening at lower cardiac outputs. For porcine valves, the growth at the higher cardiac output caused little observable change in their opening configurations.

Space efficiency

When choosing the valve that provides the biggest flow area for his or her patient, a surgeon's knowledge of GOAs is insufficient. Valve selection by GOA alone is somewhat like choosing a wheel-tire combination for your car based on the wheel diameter alone (Fig. 14).

Space efficiency determines the capacity of a bioprosthetic valve to fit a greater GOA into the limited space of the aortic root. In general, space efficiency is defined as the ratio of the flow area (GOA) of a valve to an occupied space (Fig. 15).

Two categories of space efficiency will be discussed. *Stent space efficiency* is the ratio of the GOA to the space occupied by the stent or, where SE refers to space efficiency, A refers to area and OD refers to outer diameter:

$$SE_{STENT}(\%) = (GOA/A_{STENT}) \times 100$$

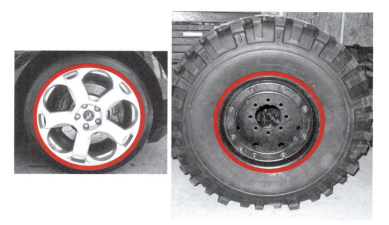

Fig. 14. Knowing the diameter and area of one component alone is not sufficient; one must consider the space efficiency of the entire assembly. Clearly, although the metal wheels of the Lamborghini on the left and the truck on the right are identical in diameter and area (indicated by the red circles), the huge tire of the truck makes it impossible to fit the truck tire-wheel assembly into the wheel well of the Lamborghini

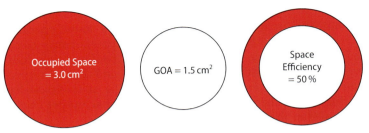

Fig. 15. Definition of space efficiency: occupied space (OS) = 3.0 cm² and GOA = 1.5 cm². Space efficiency (%) = [GOA/OS] × 100 = [1.5 cm²/3.0 cm²] × 100 = 50%

where

$$A_{STENT} = \prod(OD_{STENT}^2/4)$$

Overall space efficiency is the ratio of the GOA to the overall space occupied by the valve. Where SR refers to the sewing ring, the overall space efficiency is calculated by

$$SE_{OVERALL}(\%) = (GOA/A_{SR}) \times 100$$

where

$$A_{SR} = \prod(OD_{SR}^2/4)$$

Stent space efficiency is important because the essence of a bioprosthetic valve's design is contained within the stent. The design that maximizes the GOA contained within the stent would be expected to maximize the performance potential of the valve within the limited space of the aortic root. In Fig. 16, stent configurations of three different 19 mm valves have been normalized to equalize the outer diameters of the stents, shown by the iden-

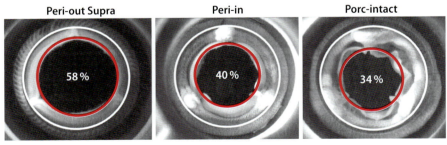

Fig. 16. A normalized comparison of the space efficiencies of three 19-mm valves allows a visual comparison of the ratio of the GOA to the stent areas of the valves. To make this comparison the valves are normalized such that the ODs of the stents, indicated by the white circle, are identical. The red circle approximates the GOA of the valve. Among these three valves, the Peri-out Supra makes the most efficient use of the available stent area for flow

tical white circles. This normalization enables visual comparisons of the stent space efficiency while avoiding the inconsistent sizing schemes of various manufacturers.

In this simplification, GOAs are represented by the areas inside the red circles. At face value, it is clear that the Peri-out Supra makes the most efficient use of the available stent area because the inner red circle occupies most of the stent space indicated by the white circle. By calculating the ratio of the area inside the red circle to the area inside the white circle, one can make approximate percentage comparisons among the stent space efficiencies for the three valves. In this analysis, the Peri-out Supra uses 58% of the stent area for GOA, the Peri-in uses 40%, and the Porc-intact uses 34%.

As mentioned, these normalized graphics do not depict the valves as they actually are. For example, it has been shown that the GOA of the 19 mm Peri-out Supra is similar to that of the 19 mm Peri-in. Fig. 17 shows the three valves at their actual sizes, providing yet another angle on space efficiency. As demonstrated earlier, even at actual size, the porcine valve's GOA is smaller than its pericardial counterparts. However the porcine valve occupies almost as much total area as the Peri-in. On the other hand, while the Peri-out Supra and the Peri-in have similar GOAs, the Peri-out occupies 35% less space than the Peri-in. The Peri-out Supra uses more of its occupied space for flow and is, therefore, the most space-efficient of the three valves.

Figs. 16 and 17 have provided visual examples of space efficiency with respect to both the area of the stent and the overall area of the valve. Table 3 provides a comprehensive table of overall space efficiencies using the equation for $SE_{OVERALL}$ as expressed above. The overall areas were calculated using the equation for A_{SR} as expressed above and sewing ring diameters

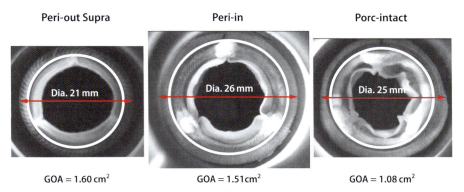

Fig. 17. As expected from our previous analysis of these 19 mm valves, the porcine valve's GOA is smaller than the GOAs of the pericardial valves. However, the porcine valve occupies almost as much space as the Peri-in. Although the Peri-in valve possesses a GOA that is very similar to the GOA of the Peri-out Supra, the Peri-out Supra valve occupies 35% less space

Table 3. A comparison of the overall space efficiencies (the ratio of the GOA to the area occupied by the valve) of the valves examined in this investigation. The Peri-out Supra is the most space efficient of the seven valve types

	Peri-out supra	Peri-in	Peri-in supra	Porc-intact	Porc-intact supra	Porc tricomp	Porc-tricomp supra
19 mm	45.6%	28.4%	29.2%	22.1%	20.8%	n/a	21.8%
21 mm	41.0%	26.3%	36.9%	20.5%	21.5%	16.5%	26.6%
23 mm	42.0%	31.2%	30.5%	20.2%	24.0%	19.3%	22.5%

(OD_{SR}) obtained from each manufacturer's specifications. As expected the pericardial valves exhibit greater overall space efficiencies than the porcine valves. Because of its dominating stent space efficiency, the Peri-out Supra shows a more efficient use of its total occupied space than the Peri-in and Peri-in Supra models.

An additional observation – leaflet flutter

Leaflet flutter is a source of forward flow energy loss. A presentation of the dynamic videos would provide the most meaningful description of relative leaflet stabilities but we are limited to still shots. Fig. 18 depicts the dynamic leaflet stabilities of a 23 mm porcine valve, a 23 mm Peri-in, and a 23 mm Peri-out Supra as a sequence of hi-speed video frames. Leaflet flutter is observed for both the 23 mm porcine valve and the 23 mm Peri-in valve. The Peri-out Supra's leaflets remained stable throughout systole, changing slightly in diameter during opening and closing.

Only one porcine valve was chosen to represent this class because the leaflet instability was consistent across all porcine valve types and sizes. One cannot discern the difference between the leaflet flutter of the porcine valve and that of the Peri-in valve by observing these still sequences. The leaflet flutter for porcine valves was of a very high-frequency, while the leaflet flutter of the Peri-in valve was of only moderate frequency.

Fig. 18. It is difficult to show leaflet flutter without presenting the hi-speed videos. However, by scanning the six sequential frames for the three valves shown the observer can gain an appreciation of the relative leaflet stability. The porcine valve exhibited hi-frequency flutter, the Peri-in valve exhibited moderate frequency flutter, and the Peri-out valve exhibited no flutter

Evaluation of bioprosthetic valve performance | 331

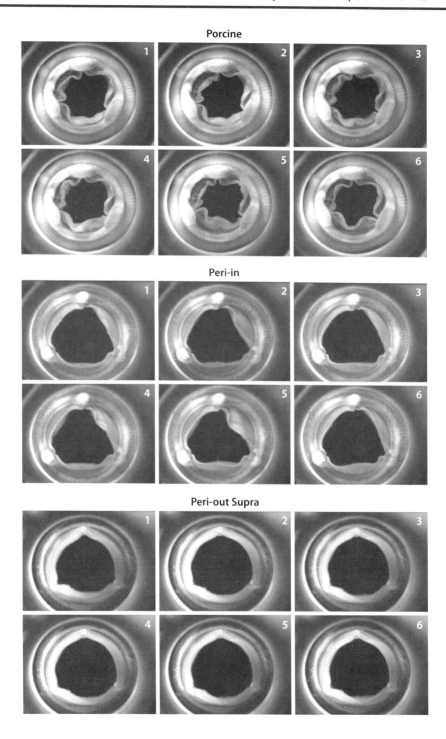

Discussion

When it comes to choosing the best stented bioprosthetic valve for a patient, the surgeon can obtain more information by looking at the valves than by looking at unreliable and perhaps exaggerated performance data in the form of EOAs and EOAIs. To get the valve with the best performance, there are two characteristics to consider: GOA and space efficiency. While each of these variables is important, the best outcome most directly depends on replacing a stenotic valve with the greatest GOA possible. The GOA, a directly measurable feature of a bioprosthetic valve, is the most valid and reliable measure of a valve's expected performance. However, this investigation has shown that a large GOA is insufficient if the size of the device limits its potential fit to the patient's aortic root. The investigation also demonstrated that opening quality and consistency determine the dependability of performance for a valve as well as expose leaflet irregularities that contribute to forward flow energy loss.

An analysis of GOAs for three pericardial models manufactured by two different companies and four porcine valves manufactured by two other companies leads to several observations. Porcine valves provide substantially smaller GOAs and substantially diminished space efficiencies compared to pericardial valves. This fact, combined with a high-frequency flutter exhibited by all of the porcine valves in this study, leads to an expectation of high forward flow energy losses for porcine valves in comparison to pericardial valves.

The selection process then focuses on pericardial valves. Pericardial valves fabricated from a single ribbon of pericardium wrapped around the outside of the stent are more space efficient than pericardial valves fabri-

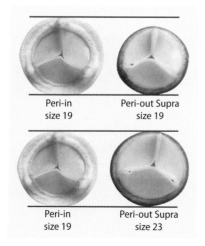

Fig. 19. Size 19 Peri-in and Peri-out Supras have similar GOAs but the Peri-out valve occupies less space. The 23 mm Peri-out Supra occupies the same space as the 19 mm Peri-in

Fig. 20. More space efficient than the Peri-in, the 21 mm Peri-in Supra occupies the same space as the 23 mm Peri-out. Still, the GOA of the Peri-out Supra is larger than the GOA of the Peri-in Supra

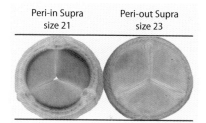

cated from three separate leaflets that are constrained inside the stent. The improved space efficiency of the wrap-around design can be expected to enable the placement of a larger GOA into any given aortic root.

Fig. 19 illustrates the practical value of this improved space efficiency for a patient with a 19 mm annulus. On one hand, if the patient has a narrow aortic root the 19 mm Peri-out Supra is more likely to fit than the 19 mm Peri-in. On the other hand, if the 19 mm root is larger and the surgeon is able to implant a Peri-in 19, the surgeon should also be able to implant a Peri-out Supra 23, which occupies the same space. For the set of valves analyzed in this study, the Peri-out Supra enables a 48% GOA advantage over the Peri-in valve. With respect to the other Peri-in model, the Peri-in Supra is more space efficient than its Peri-in counterpart due to a supraannular design and reduced sewing ring. Thus, for the same patient with a 19 mm annulus, the surgeon can place a 21 mm Peri-in Supra. As mentioned before, the 23 mm Peri-out Supra also fits the 19 mm annulus. For this set of valves, the GOA of the Peri-out Supra gains 14% over the GOA of the Peri-in Supra (Fig. 20).

The Peri-in and Peri-in Supra models can be characterized by irregular opening, inconsistent GOAs within and across sizes and cardiac outputs, and leaflet flutter. These problems seem attributable to the irregular fit of the leaflets to the stent. At 5 lpm, it was observed that for each Peri-in and Peri-in Supra valve two or more leaflets were unable to reach the perimeter of the stent ID. This phenomenon results in lost orifice area and may cause the instability that creates leaflet flutter. While it is easy enough to attribute these inconsistencies to the design of the Peri-in valve, the problems are more likely related to the manufacturing process.

Recall that the Peri-in valves are composed of three separate leaflets. The assembler first attaches the leaflets to one another and ultimately to the stent assembly. The challenge it seems is to fit the correctly sized leaflet to a given stent. In most cases, it appears that the leaflets are too small. As mentioned above, in many cases the inadequate length of the edge of the leaflet creates a chord across the stent posts rather than a curved circumferential opening (Fig. 21).

The mismatches of the leaflets to the stents of the Peri-in category of valves reduce the GOA of the valve, especially at a cardiac output of 5 lpm

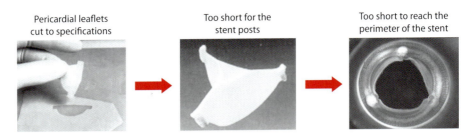

Fig. 21. The pre-cut dimensions of the Peri-in and Peri-in Supra leaflets may not be adequate for the final stent assembly. As a result all of the valves observed in this study had two or more leaflets that were too short to reach the perimeter of the stent ID. The first and second photos reproduced with permission from Edwards Lifesciences, Irvine, CA

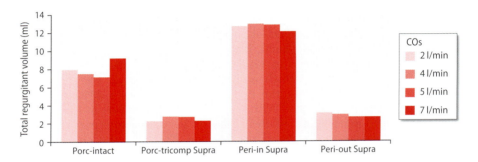

Fig. 22. Total regurgitant volume for four of the valves from the present investigation. Total regurgitant volume is the sum of the closing volume, which is the fluid that escapes back through the valve while it is closing at the end of systole, and leakage volume, which is the volume of fluid that escapes through the valve after it is closed

and presumably lower. But the negative effect on forward flow may also translate into higher regurgitant losses. Simply stated, if the leaflets are unable to reach the perimeter of the ID of the stent, they may also restrict the coaptation at closure. Work by Gerosa and colleagues [16] may support this deduction. Gerosa reported the results of in vitro testing of five different bioprosthetic valves, four of which are included in this study. Fig. 22 shows Gerosa's results for total regurgitant volume at four cardiac outputs and Fig. 23 shows Gerosa's results for total leakage volume at four cardiac outputs. *Total regurgitant volume* is the sum of the closing volume and the leakage volume. The *closing volume* is the fluid that escapes back through the valve while it is closing at the end of systole. The *leakage volume* is the volume of fluid that escapes through the valve after it is closed. The highest total regurgitant volume per cardiac cycle is seen for the Peri-in Supra at around 12 ml followed by the Porc-intact at around 8 ml. The total regurgitant volumes for the Porc-tri-

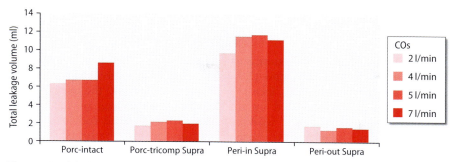

Fig. 23. Total leakage volume for four of the valves from the present investigation. Total leakage volume is the volume of fluid that escapes through the valve after it is closed

comp Supra and the Peri-out Supra are negligible at about 2 ml. By comparing Fig. 22 with Fig. 23 one can determine the percentage of total regurgitation contributed by leakage using the function:

Leakage % = [Leakage volume (ml)/Total Regurg volume (ml)] × 100

Approximating the total regurgitant volumes and the total leakage volumes for a cardiac output of 5 lpm from Gerosa's graph, the function estimates that, for the Porc-intact valve, leakage accounts for about 85% of the total regurgitant volume and for the Peri-in Supra, leakage accounts for about 90% of the total regurgitant volume.

The reason for the high leakage volume for the Porc-intact valve in comparison to the negligible leakage for the Porc-tricomp valve is not known but may be an advantage of the tricomposite valve design of the Porc-tricomp. The high leakage volume of the Peri-in Supra valve may reinforce the author's suspicions about incomplete coaptation due to mismatched leaflets.

Study limitations

This investigation was limited by the single sample for each valve size and type. It is recommended that this analysis be repeated with samples that are large enough to make a statistical comparison among the GOAs of different bioprosthetic valves as well as an analysis of the variance in GOAs within valve types. Such a study would make possible a table of GOAs and space efficiencies for all models and sizes to facilitate the surgeon's prosthesis choice.

Conclusions

Performance comparisons among valves are made difficult and unreliable by the application of EOA and EOAI. Knowing that a valve's opening area is the primary determining factor for these parameters, the surgeon can ignore EOAI charts provided by manufacturers and focus on GOAs. The valve that places the largest GOA into the patient's aortic root can be expected to reduce forward flow energy losses and provide better clinical outcomes.

Porcine valves fall short in this analysis, providing small GOAs in bulky valves and exemplifying very high-frequency leaflet flutter. As a class, pericardial valves provide substantially larger GOAs on a size-for-size basis and better leaflet stability making pericardial valves the better choice of the two biomaterials.

GOAs among the three pericardial models are about the same on a size-for-size basis. However, the space efficiency of the valve constructed from a single ribbon of pericardium secured outside the stent is superior to the space efficiency of the valve composed of three separate pericardial leaflets fastened inside the stent. Space efficiency is not the only difference between the two pericardial valves. The Peri-in valve is also characterized by orifice areas that vary within and across sizes and cardiac outputs, incomplete opening, the possibility of incomplete closing with its associated regurgitation, and leaflet flutter. All of these Peri-in characteristics may be expected to contribute to higher energy losses. It is reasonable to argue that these are not issues of design, but of the manufacturing process.

The outside-the-stent pericardial design provides the greatest GOA in the most space-efficient fashion with leaflets that open uniformly and remain stable throughout systole. This pericardial design is the most likely to provide the greatest available GOA with negligible losses due to leaflet instability.

References

1. Rahimtoola SH (1978) The problem of valve prosthesis-patient mismatch. Circulation 58:20–24
2. Dumesnil JG, Honos GN, Lemieux M, Beauchemin J (1990) Validation and applications of indexed aortic prosthetic valve areas calculated by Doppler echocardiography. J Am Coll Cardiol 16:637–643
3. Pibarot P, Honos GN, Durand LG, Dumesnil JG (1996) The effect of patient-prosthesis mismatch on aortic bioprosthetic valve hemodynamic performance and patient clinical status. Can J Cardiol 12:379–387

4. Pibarot P, Dumesnil J, Lemieux M et al (1998) Impact of Prosthesis-Patient Mismatch on Hemodynamic and Symptomatic Status, Morbidity and Mortality after Aortic Valve Replacement with a Bioprosthetic Heart Valve. J Heart Valve Dis 7(2):211–218
5. Pibarot P, Dumesnil J (2000) Hemodynamic and clinical impact of prosthesis-patient mismatch in the aortic valve position and its prevention. J Am Coll Cardiol 36:1131–1141
6. Dumesnil J, Pibarot P (2006) Prosthesis-patient mismatch and clinical outcomes: The evidence continues to accumulate. J Thorac Cardiovasc Surg 131:952–955
7. Dumesnil J, Pibarot P vs Blackstone E, Gillinov A, Cosgrove D (2004) [Point-Counterpoint] Prosthesis size and prosthesis-patient size are unrelated to prosthesis-patient mismatch. J Thorac Cardiovasc Surg 127:1852–1854
8. Emery R, Emery A, Holter A, Krogh C (2005) Prosthesis-Patient Mismatch: Impact on Patient Survival. 41st Annual Meeting of the Society of Thoracic Surgeons, Tampa, Florida
9. Izzat M, Kadir I, Reeves B, Wilde P, Bryan A, Angelini G (1999) Patient-prosthesis mismatch is negligible with modern small-size aortic valve prostheses. Ann Thorac Surg 68:1657–1660
10. Medalion B, Blackstone E, Lytle B, White J, Arnold J, Cosgrove D (2000) Aortic valve replacement: Is valve size important? J Thorac Cardiovasc Surg 119:963–974
11. Knez I, Rienmuller R, Maier R, Rehak P, Schrottner B, Machler H, Anelli-Monti M, Rigler B (2001) Left ventricular architecture after valve replacement due to critical aortic stenosis: an approach to dis-/qualify the myth of valve prosthesis-patient mismatch? European J Cardio-Thoracic Surg 19:797–805
12. Hanayama N, Christakis G, Mallidi H, Joyner C, Fremes S, Morgan C, Mitoff P, Goldman B (2002) Patient prosthesis mismatch is rare after aortic valve replacement: Valve size may be irrelevant. Ann Thorac Surg 73:1822–1829
13. Gillinov A, Blackstone E, Rodriquez L (2003) Prosthesis-patient size: measurement and clinical implications. J Thorac Cardiovasc Surg 126:313–316
14. Blackstone E, Cosgrove D, Jamieson W, Birkmeyer N, Lemmer J, Miller D, Butchart E, Rizzoli G, Yacoub M, Chai A (2003) Prosthesis size and long term survival after aortic valve replacement. J Thorac Cardiovasc Surg 126:783–796
15. Emery R, Emery A, Holter A, Krogh C (2005) Prosthesis-Patient Mismatch: Impact on Patient Survival. 41st Annual Meeting of the Society of Thoracic Surgeons, Tampa, Florida
16. Gerosa G, Tarzia V, Rizzoli G, Bottio T (2006) Small aortic annulus: The hydrodynamic performances of 5 commercially available tissue valves. J Thorac Cardiovasc Surg 131:1058–1064

Long-term results of biological valves

Stentless bioprostheses

Stented and stentless aortic bioprostheses: competitive or complimentary?

W. R. E. JAMIESON

Aortic valve replacement (AVR) is the established treatment for patients with symptomatic aortic stenosis. Left ventricular hypertrophy, a known manifestation of aortic stenosis, is associated with increased risk of sudden death, congestive heart failure, and stroke. The superior outcome after AVR is achieved with regression of left ventricular hypertrophy, known as left ventricular mass and indexed to body surface area.

The goal of aortic valve replacement is to provide an effective orifice area of the implanted prosthesis equivalent to the left ventricular outflow tract to minimize prosthesis-patient mismatch and provide adequacy of left ventricular mass regression. The stented bioprostheses were considered to have an obstructive nature from the sewing ring and stent or prosthesis-patient mismatch. Stentless bioprostheses were developed without stent and sewing ring with the goal of maximizing the effective orifice area and facilitating left ventricular mass regression. The purpose of this chapter is to consider whether stentless or stented aortic bioprostheses are competitive or complimentary.

To assess the concept of "competitiveness" the results of randomized controlled trials (RCTs) were evaluated [1–15]. Table 1 documents the hemodynamics of studies between stented and stentless bioprostheses that lack differentiation [1–10, 12]. Ten studies have documented lack of differentiation of hemodynamic performance, particularly of left ventricular mass regression (LVMR) expressed as left ventricular mass index (LVMI) at 12 months. These RCTs demonstrated differences in hemodynamics (mean gradients, effective orifice areas, and left ventricular mass regression) favoring stentless bioprostheses in the early months (up to 6 months) following AVR but equivalence of LVMI at the 12-month interval.

Table 1. Chronology of randomized clinical trials (RCTs) showing lack of differentiation

Authors	Prosthesis		Findings
	Stentless	Stented	
Santini et al. (1998) [1]	Toronto SPV/SJM Biocor	HII	LVMR no difference at 12 months
Williams et al. (1999) [2]	Toronto SPV	CE-SAV	No difference in LVMI at 6 months Peak velocity and mean gradients better with SPV at 32 months
Cohen et al. (2002) [3]	Toronto SPV	CE-P	No difference in EOAs, gradients or LVMR at 12 months
Doss et al. (2003) [4]	Edwards PP	CE-P	LVMR no difference at 12 months
Sensky et al. (2003) [5]	MF	MM	LVMR no difference at 6 months
Totaro et al. (2005) [6]	Edwards PP	CE-P/CE-PM	Mean gradients and EOAs no difference. LVMR not assessed
Ali et al. (2006) [7]	Edwards PP	CE-P	No difference in gradients or LVMR at 12 months
ASSERT (2005) [8] (de Arenaza et al.)	MF	MM	MF-EOA and EOAI and peak flow velocity better. LVMR similar at 6 months
Chambers et al. (2006) [9]	Toronto SPV	CE-P	No difference in gradients or LVMR at 12 months
Dunning et al. (2007) [10]	Sorin Freedom	Sorin More	No difference in LVMI at 12 months
Kunadian et al. (2007) [12] (meta-analysis)	Sorin Freedom, Mitroflow, Edwards PP, Toronto SPV, SJM Biocor	CE-P, MM, MI, HII, Sorin More	Differentiation 6 months LVMI, mean gradients and EOAI. No difference LVMI at 12 months

Toronto SPV St. Jude Medical Toronto SPV, *SJM Biocor* St. Jude Medical Biocor, *HII* Hancock II, *LVMR* Left Ventricular Mass Regression, *CE-SAV* Carpentier-Edwards Supra Annular Valve, *LVMI* Left Ventricular Mass Index, *CE-P* Carpentier-Edwards PERIMOUNT, *EOA* Effective Orifice Area, *Edwards PP* Edwards Prima Plus, *MM* Medtronic Mosaic, *CE-PM* Carpentier-Edwards PERIMOUNT Magna, *MF* Medtronic Freestyle, *EOAI* Effective Orifice Area Index, *MI* Medtronic Intact

A meta-analysis of RCTs conducted by Kunadian and colleagues [12], considering the majority of this literature determined that, at 6 months, there was differentiation in favor of stentless bioprostheses for LVMI, mean gradients, and EOAI, but at 12 months, there was no differentiation determined by LVMI.

Table 2. Chronology of randomized clinical trials (RCTs) showing differentiation

Authors	Prosthesis		Findings
	Stentless	Stented	
Maselli et al. (1999) [13]	MF/Toronto SPV	Medtronic Intact	LVMR more complete and faster with MF/Toronto SPV
Szafranek et al. (2006) [14]	MF	MM	LVMI favours MF at 12 months. EOAI undifferentiated
Miraldi et al. (2006) [15]	Sorin Freedom	CE-P	LVMR faster and better with Sorin Freedom at 12 months

MF Medtronic Freestyle, *Toronto SPV* St. Jude Medical Toronto SPV, *LVMR* Left Ventricular Mass Regression, *MM* Medtronic Mosaic, *LVMI* Left Ventricular Mass Index, *CE-P* Carpentier-Edwards PERIMOUNT

Table 2 shows the results of the RCTs that determined there was presence of differentiation between stentless and stented aortic bioprostheses [13–15]. There were only three studies in this group and the findings were LVMR over the initial 12 months, resulting in complete regression of the left ventricular mass for stentless bioprostheses at 12 months, which was superior over stented bioprostheses.

The RCTs compared the hemodynamic performance of stentless bioprostheses to stented bioprostheses of the second generation. The third-generation diameter-enhanced bioprostheses introduced to optimize hemodynamics were not evaluated in the RCTs except for Totaro and investigators [6] who combined the Carpentier-Edwards PERIMOUNT and the Carpentier-Edwards PERIMOUNT Magna in comparison to the Edwards Prima Plus.

The results of the RCTs documenting comparable hemodynamic performance at one year have eliminated the competitiveness of these aortic bioprostheses. There are yet no comparative studies of durability that, if favorable for stentless bioprostheses, could support the prostheses being competitive. The increased implant difficulty and extended ischemic times and cardiopulmonary bypass times may never support these prostheses being competitive. The low proportion of stentless bioprostheses compared to stented bioprostheses since the introduction will likely continue to signal the lack of competitive nature of these prostheses.

The International Society of Minimally Invasive Cardiothoracic Surgery (ISMICS) has developed a consensus statement from an expert panel on stentless and stented bioprostheses for aortic valve replacement [16, 17]. The purpose was to determine whether stentless prostheses improve clinical and resource outcomes. The panel, following evaluation of 17 randomized and 14 nonrandomized trials comprising 1317 and 2485 patients, respectively, outlined the evidence-based recommendations for the use of stentless and stented bioprostheses for adult aortic valve replacement. The consensus document revealed that both stentless and stented bioprostheses provide an excellent valve substitute for aortic valve disease [17]. The consensus panel revealed that the hemodynamic performance of stentless bioprostheses is better than stented bioprostheses over the first 6 to 12 months following aortic valve replacement. However, at the one-year interval, transvalvular gradients and left ventricular mass regression are comparable [17]. There is inadequate knowledge, at this stage, to determine whether durability with stentless bioprostheses is different than stented bioprostheses. The majority of randomized and non-randomized controlled trials between stented and stentless bioprostheses were performed with second-generation prostheses and, in the majority, not with the current, diameter-enhanced stented bioprostheses. The consensus panel recommended that the patient groups in the RCTs and non-RCTs be continually evaluated to obtain 15-year comparative data [17]. This evidence from the ISMICS consensus panel provides further consideration that the two types of bioprostheses are not competitive.

There have been no RCTs comparing subcoronary stentless with root replacement. The consensus document made two recommendations in this regard [17]. In the absence of aortic root disease and with an annulus ≥21 mm, either stented or stentless bioprostheses are acceptable alternatives for the majority of patients when a current (second or third) generation bioprosthesis is indicated. In the presence of an aortic annulus <21 mm, the use of a free-standing bioprosthetic root can be considered as an alternative to diameter-enhanced stented bioprosthesis or a root enlargement procedure.

These circumstances make stented and stentless bioprostheses complimentary. When there is a definite role for the stentless bioprostheses to serve as an aortic root conduit in patients with aortic root disease who qualify for replacement surgery and are in an acceptable age bracket for bioprostheses, then the two types of prostheses can again be considered to be complimentary.

This report provides supporting evidence that stented and stentless aortic bioprostheses are not competitive but are complimentary in the management of aortic valve disease and, in certain circumstances, for aortic root disease.

References

1. Santini F, Bertolini P, Montlbano G, Vecchi B, Pessotto R, Prioli A, Mazzucco A (1998) Hancock versus stentless biopostheses for aortic valve replacement in patients older than 75 year. Ann Thorac Surg 66:S99–S103
2. Williams RJ, Muir DF, Pathi V, MacArthur K, Berg GA (1999) Randomized controlled trial of stented and stentless aortic biopostheses: hemodynamic performance at 3 years. Semin Thorac Cardiovasc Surg 4(Suppl 1):93–97

3. Cohen G, Christakis GT, Joyner CD, Morgan CD, Tamariz M, Hanayama N, Mallidi H, Szalai JP, Katic M, Rao V, Fremes SE, Goldman BS (2002) Are stentless valves hemodynamically superior to stented valves? A prospective randomized trial. Ann Thorac Surg 73:767–778
4. Doss M, Martens S, Wood JP, Aybek T, Kleine P, Wimmer Greinecker G, Moritz A (2003) Performance of stentless versus stented aortic valve bioprostheses in the elderly patients: a prospective randomized trial. Eur J Cardiothoracic Surg 23:299–304
5. Sensky PR, Loubani M, Keal RP, Samani NJ, Sosnowski AW, Galinanes M (2003) Does the type of prosthesis influence early left ventricular mass regression afgter aortic valve replacement? Assessment with magnetic resonance imaging. Am Heart J 146:746
6. Totaro P, Degno N, Zaidi A, Youhana P, Argano V (2005) Carpentier-Edwards PERIMOUNT Magna bioprosthesis: A stented valve with stentless performance? J Thorac Cardiovasc Surg 130:1668–1674
7. Ali A, Halstead JC, Cafferty F, Sharples L, Rose F, Coulden R, Lee E, Dunning J, Argano V, Tsui S (2006) Are stentless valves superior to modern stented valves? A prospective randomized trial. Circulation 114[suppl I]:I-535–I-540
8. Perez de Arenaza D, Lees B, Flather M, Nugara F, Husebye T, Jasinski M, Cisowski M, Khan M, Henein M, Gaer J, Guvendik L, Bochenek A, Wos S, Lie M, Van Nooten G, Pennell D, Pepper J, on behalf of the ASSERT (Aortic Stentless versus Stented valve Assessed by Echocardiography Randomized Trial) (2005) Circulation 112:2696–2702
9. Chambers JB, Rimington HM, Hodson F, Rajani R, Blauth CI (2006) The subcoronary Toronto stentless versus supra-annular Perimount stented replacement aortic valve: early clinical and hemodynamic results of a randomized comparison in 160 patients. J Thorac Cardiovasc Surg 131:878–882
10. Dunning J, Graham RJ, Thambyrajah J, Stewart JM, Kendall SW, Hunter S (2007) Stentless vs stented aortic valve bioprostheses: a prospective randomized controlled trial. Eur Heart J 28:2369–2374
11. Lehman S, Walther T, Kempfert J, Leontjev S, Rastan A, Falk V, Mohr FW (2007) Stentless versus conventional xenograft aortic valve replacement: midterm results of a prospectively randomized trial. Ann Thorac Surg 84:467–472
12. Kunadian B, Vijayalakshmi K, Thornley AR, de Belder MA, Hunter S, Kendall S, Graham R, Stewart M, Thambyrajah J, Dunning J (2007) Meta-analysis of valve hemodynamics and left ventricular mass regression for stentless versus stented aortic valves. Ann Thorac Surg 84:73–79
13. Maselli D, Pizio R, Bruno LP, Di Bella I, De Gasperis C (1999) Left ventricular mass reduction after aortic valve replacement: Homografts, stentless and stented valves. Ann Thorac Surg 67:966–971
14. Szafranek A, Jasinski M, Kolowca M, Gemel M, Wos S (2006) Plasma ANP and rennin-angiotensin-aldosterone system as new parameters describing the hemodynamics of the circulatory system after implantation of stented or stentelss aortic valves. J Heart Valve Dis 15:702–709
15. Miraldi F, Spagnesi L, Tallarico D, Di Matteo G, Brancaccio G (2007) Sorin stentless pericardial valve versus Carpentier-Edwards Perimount pericardial bioprosthesis: is it worthwhile to struggle? Int J Cardiol 118(2):253–255
16. Cheng D, Pepper J, Martin J, Stanbridge RDL, Ferdinand FD, Jamieson WRE, Berg G, Sani G (2009) Stentless versus stented bioprosthetic aortic valves: a systematic review and meta-analysis of controlled trials. Innovations 4:61–73
17. Pepper J, Cheng D, Stanbridge RDL, Ferdinand FD, Jamieson WRE, Stelzer P, Berg G, Sani G, Martin J (2009) Stentless versus stented bioprosthetic aortic valves: a consensus statement of the International Society of Minimally Invasive Cardiothoracic Surgery (ISMICS). Innovations 4:49–60

Edwards Prima Plus Stentless Bioprosthesis: long-term clinical and hemodynamic results

A. Fabbri, A. D'Onofrio, S. Auriemma, G.D. Cresce, C. Piccin, A. Favaro, P. Magagna

Introduction

Stentless aortic xenografts were introduced into clinical practice in order to improve clinical outcomes following aortic valve replacement for their better hemodynamic performance and durability. Edwards Lifesciences Prima Plus stentless xenograft (EPP) (Edwards Lifesciences, Irvine, CA, USA) is a bioprosthesis made of a porcine aortic root reinforced with Dacron fabric.

The aim of this single center, retrospective study was to describe early and late clinical and hemodynamic outcomes after aortic valve replacement with EPP. This paper, written for the "Berlin Heart Valve Symposium 2008", is an update of a previously published article [1].

Materials and methods

Clinical data – patients

Between January 1993 and June 2008, 450 consecutive patients underwent aortic valve replacement with the EPP at our institution. Selection criteria for implantation of the EPP were the following: age older than 65 years; contraindication to oral anticoagulant therapy; request for a biological valve by the patient; small aortic annulus and surgeon's preferences. Furthermore, an EPP was intentionally implanted in patients with pathologies of the aortic root and of the ascending aorta, whenever the aortic valve could not be preserved. There were no absolute contraindications to EPP implantation; relative contraindications mainly due to potential technical problems that could arise were: very low take-off of the coronary arteries, extremely calcified coronary ostia, and abnormal origin of the coronary ostia.

Senile calcific degeneration represented the most common indication to surgery. Associated lesions requiring combined procedures were present in

Table 1. Preoperative patients' characteristics

	No	Mean	Range
Patients	450		
Age (years)		69 ± 9	37–90
Gender (male)	270 (60%)		
NYHA class			
– I	None		
– II	144 (32%)		
– III	230 (51%)		
– IV	76 (17%)		
Aortic stenosis	175 (39%)		
Aortic regurgitation	162 (36%)		
Mixed aortic lesion	58 (13%)		
Type A dissection	63 (14%)		
Aortic root aneurysm	27 (6%)		
Ascending aorta dilatation	198 (44%)		
CAD	133 (29.5%)		
Urgent/Emergency	75 (17%)		

NYHA New York Heart Association, *CAD* coronary artery disease

87% of patients. The most common associated procedure was ascending aorta replacement, performed in 226 patients (58%). The main preoperative clinical features are summarized in Table 1.

Surgical technique and medical management

The EPP was implanted with the "inclusion technique" using 3 polypropylene 4/0 running sutures for the inflow rim [2, 3]. In case of an associated replacement of the ascending aorta, valve inflow rim and coronary ostia sutures were performed first and the proximal vascular anastomosis was performed, after an appropriate trimming of the xenograft, including both the patient's ascending aorta and porcine aortic wall (Fig. 1).

Oral anticoagulation therapy was generally started on the first postoperative day and stopped after two months. Thereafter, antiplatelet agents (acetylsalicylic acid 100 mg daily or ticlopidine 250 mg daily) were administered to all patients.

Follow-up

Direct patient clinical and echocardiographic assessments were planned at 6 and 12 months after surgery and subsequently every 12 months. Patients

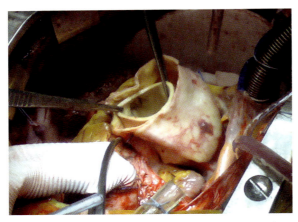

Fig. 1. Aortic valve replacement with the EPP. The prosthesis is implanted with the "miniroot" technique into the native aortic root and the coronary ostia sutures are completed before the proximal vascular anastomosis

unable to attend our outpatient clinic were followed-up by phone interviews or by contacting the referring cardiologists. Follow-up was 100% complete. Mean follow-up was 60 ± 22 months (range: 6 months–14 years), total cumulative follow-up was 1154 patient/years. Echocardiography was performed with an iE 33 cardiac ultrasound scanner (Royal Philips Electronics, Amsterdam, The Netherlands) according to the American Society of Echocardiography guidelines. Mean transvalvular pressure gradients were derived using the modified Bernoulli equation.

Morbidity and fatal valve-related events were categorized as resulting from structural valve deterioration (SVD), nonstructural valve dysfunction (NSVD), thromboembolism, prosthetic valve endocarditis, hemorrhagic complication, reoperation, valve-related mortality or cardiac-related mortality according to the STS and AATS guidelines for reporting morbidity and mortality after cardiac valvular operations [4].

Statistical analysis

Continuous data are expressed as mean ± 1 SD. Categoric data are expressed as percentages. Survival analyses with the Kaplan-Meier method were used to estimate survival and freedom from valve-related adverse events. Incidence of late adverse events is shown using "linearized" rates (events per 100 patient/years). Statistical analysis was performed with the SPSS statistical package (SPSS Inc., Chicago, IL, USA).

Table 2. Operative variables

	Mean ± SD
■ **Stentless valve diameter (mm)** ⌀ 21: 22 (4.8%) ⌀ 23: 155 (34.5%) ⌀ 25: 125 (27.8%) ⌀ 27: 112 (24.9%) ⌀ 29: 36 (8.0%)	
■ **Aortic cross-clamp time (min)** – Isolated AVR – Combined procedures	66 ± 10 124 ± 83
■ **Cardiopulmonary bypass time (min)** – Isolated AVR – Combined procedures	92 ± 15 212 ± 94
■ **Associated procedures** 391 (87%) – CABG 133 (34%) – Ascending aorta replacement 226 (58%) – Other 32 (8%)	

SD standard deviation, *CABG* coronary artery bypass grafting, *AVR* aortic valve replacement

Results

Operative data

Operations were performed by four different surgeons at our institution. Mean cardiopulmonary bypass and cross-clamp times for isolated AVR were 92 ± 15 and 66 ± 10 min, respectively. Operative data are summarized in Table 2.

Survival

Operative mortality was 5.3% (24 pts). There were 50 late deaths (4.3% pt/years). Causes of early deaths are listed in Table 3. Actuarial overall survival at 5 and 10 years was 82 ± 3% and 34 ± 9%, respectively. Actuarial survival of the elective population was 83 ± 4% and 55 ± 13% at 5 and 10 years, respectively (Fig. 2).

Valve-related mortality occurred in 13 patients (1.1% pt/years). Actuarial freedom from valve-related mortality at 5 and 10 years was 94 ± 3% and 76 ± 11%, respectively (Fig. 3).

Table 3. Causes of early death and late adverse events

	No of patients
Early deaths	
– LCO	8
– MOF	6
– Sepsis	3
– Pulmonary insufficiency	5
– Stroke	2
Late adverse events	
– SVD	4 (0.3% pt/years)
– NSD	15 (1.3% pt/years)
– Endocarditis	7 (0.6% pt/years)
– Reoperations	4 (0.3% pt/years)
– Thromboembolic events	11 (1.0% pt/years)

SVD structural valve deterioration, *NSD* nonstructural dysfunction, *LCO* low cardiac output, *MOF* multi-organ failure

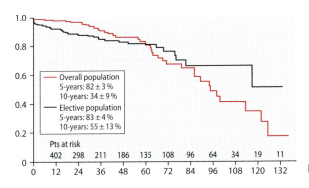

Fig. 2. Actuarial patient survival

Late adverse events (Table 3)

Structural valve deterioration

Structural valve deterioration (SVD) was diagnosed in 4 patients (0.3% pt/years); two died before reoperation, their diagnosis was made at autopsy where one leaflet tear and one leaflet prolapse were found; the others had clinical and echocardiographic assessment showing primary valve failure with significant regurgitation and increase in functional NYHA class and consequently underwent reoperation. Actuarial freedom from SVD was 100% at 5 years and 79 ± 12% at 10 years after the operation (Fig. 4). Calcific degeneration of the implanted xenograft was never observed.

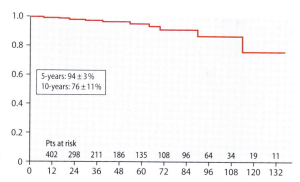

Fig. 3. Freedom from valve-related mortality

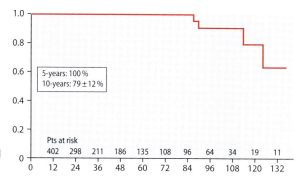

Fig. 4. Freedom from structural valve deterioration

▌ **Embolic events.** Thromboembolic events occurred in 11 patients (1% pt/year), including 7 neuroembolic events and 4 peripheral embolic events.

▌ **Endocarditis.** Bacterial endocarditis occurred in 7 patients (0.6% pt/year). There were 4 deaths from bacterial endocarditis before reoperation, 2 patients were reoperated, and 1 patient with severe aortic regurgitation refused reoperation. Actuarial freedom from bacterial endocarditis at 5 and 10 years was 96 ± 2% and 94 ± 3% respectively.

▌ **Valve reoperation.** Four patients (0.3% pt/years) underwent reoperation. Causes of reoperation were SVD (leaflet prolapse) and endocarditis in 2 patients each. The 2 patients with SVD underwent AVR with a stented xenograft implanted in the porcine root after leaflets removal ("valve in valve"), while those with endocarditis underwent a complete extirpation of the infected prostheses with a subsequent implantation of another EPP.

▌ **Late New York Heart Association functional classification.** In all survivors a significant clinical improvement was observed; 95% of them are currently in NYHA functional class I.

Table 4. Mean transprosthetic gradients

	⌀ 23	⌀ 25	⌀ 27
Hospital discharge (mmHg)	16±4	14±5	13±4
6 months (mmHg)	14±4	12±3	11±3
1 year (mmHg)	11±3	10±6	8±4

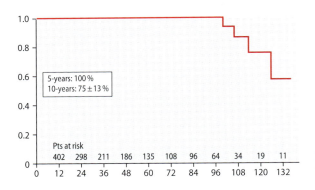

Fig. 5. Freedom from reoperations

■ **Hemodynamic data.** Mean transvalvular gradients before discharge, as well as 6 and 12 months postoperatively are shown in Table 4 for valve sizes 23, 25, and 27.

Discussion

Stentless aortic xenografts have been used in clinical practice for over a decade. The first authors who reported the use of a stentless aortic xenograft were Binet and colleagues [5] in 1965. It has been shown that freehand aortic homografts have better outcomes than stent-mounted homografts [6]; this led to a new interest in stentless porcine xenografts [7, 8]. Furthermore, David and co-workers [9] found stentless valves to have a better hemodynamic performance when compared to stented valves. This improved outcome could be explained by the reduced mechanical stress on the valve leaflets due to the absence of a stent and with a uniform distribution of fluidodynamic forces on the aortic root.

Another important reason of interest is that stentless xenografts could be suitable in the surgical treatment of many complex pathologies like small aortic annulus, ascending aorta aneurysm, aortic root disease, endocarditis with annular abscess and left ventricular dysfunction [10]. In particular, many authors consider aortic root and ascending aorta dilatation a contraindication to stentless valve implantation [11]. The EPP has been available for clinical use since 1991 [12]. In our opinion, the EPP implanted using the "inclusion technique" is a good option in patients suffering from aortic valve pathology associated with dilatation of the aortic root and of the ascending aorta. In fact, in the first case the "inclusion technique" is sufficient to treat both valve and root disease and, in the second case, an associated replacement of the ascending aorta is easily feasible in order to perform a complete surgical treatment. Even for isolated AVR, we have mainly implanted the EPP with the "inclusion technique" for many reasons. First, some authors raised concern about the hemodynamic performance of this prosthesis when implanted in the subcoronary position, since high transaortic gradients were measured early after surgery. This could be at least in part explained by the different anatomy of the porcine root that has a higher right coronary ostium. If the inferior rim of the right coronary ostium is not properly trimmed the Dacron fabric that reinforces the valve at that level could bend inward, thus, causing an obstacle to the left ventricle outflow tract. This mechanism could be exacerbated by the use of an excessively large prosthesis [13, 14]. Different technical alternatives have been suggested in order to avoid this potentially harmful complication: clockwise rotation of the prosthesis so that the polyester cloth corresponds to the noncoronary sinus and the "full root" implantation. The second reason is that the "inclusion technique" significantly reduces the risk of bleeding since the inflow rim as well as the coronary ostia anastomoses are included in the patient's native aortic root. This is particularly true in patients presenting with acute type A aortic dissection. Furthermore, with the "inclusion technique" the coronary arteries are not mobilized but anastomosed in a side to side fashion, this reduces the risk of coronary malpositioning and/or kinking and consequently protects from ischemic complications that are described when using the full root technique. In our experience, we have never had ischemic complications or pseudo-aneurysm of the aortic root [15, 16].

The peculiar design of the EPP makes it particularly useful also in the surgical treatment of bacterial endocarditis with annular abscesses and discontinuity of the aortoventricular junction.

Actuarial overall survival at 10 years is 34%; this could appear low but one has to consider carefully patients' characteristics; mean age was around 70 years and more than 80% of patients underwent combined procedures. Freedom from primary valve failure is 100% and 79% after 5 and 10 years, respectively; looking at the Kaplan-Mayer curve, freedom from SVD falls from 100% to 79% after 7 years, which could be explained by the small number of patients at risk and does not seem to show a critical time point of the prosthesis.

Hemodynamic data show low gradients both early and 12 months postoperatively; gradients tend to progressively decrease over time, which could reflect a kind of adaptation process of the porcine root in the patient's native aorta.

The limitations of this study are those commonly related to all retrospective studies and the fact that there are a small number of patients at risk at 10–14 years; furthermore, echocardiographic data about the effective orifice area and the left ventricular mass regression are not available. In conclusion, our experience shows that the EPP implanted with the "inclusion technique" provides good clinical and hemodynamic results. Thus, we currently consider the EPP as the bioprosthesis of choice when combined AVR and replacement of the ascending aorta is required, especially in elderly patients and if the aortic valve cannot be preserved. Furthermore, we found that the "inclusion technique" was safe, reproducible, and effective.

References

1. Auriemma S, D'Onofrio A, Brunelli M, Magagna P, Paccanaro M, Rulfo F, Fabbri A (2006) Long-term results of aortic valve replacement with Edwards Prima Plus stentless bioprosthesis: eleven years' follow up. J Heart Valve Dis 15(5):691–695, discussion 695
2. Konertz W, Hamann P, Schwammenthal E et al (1992) Aortic valve replacement with stentless xenografts. J Heart Valve Dis 1:249–252
3. Westaby S, Katsumata T, Arifi A et al. (1996) Valve replacement with a stentless biprosthesis: versatility of the porcine aortic root. J Thorac Cardiovasc Surg 112: 708–711
4. Edmunds LH Jr, Clark RE, Cohn LH et al (1996) Guidelines for reporting morbidity and mortality after cardiac valvular operations. Ann Thorac Surg 62:932–935
5. Binet JP, Carpentier A, Langlois J (1965) Heterologous aortic valve transplantation. Lancet 2:1275
6. Angell WW, Angell JD, Oury JH et al (1987) Long-term follow-up of viable frozen aortic homografts: a viable homograft valve bank. J Thorac Cardiovasc Surg 93: 815–822
7. O'Brien MF, Clareborough JK (1967) Heterograft aortic-valve replacement. Lancet 1(7496):929–930
8. Binet JP, Carpentier A, Langlois J (1968) Clinical use of heterografts for replacement of the aortic valve. J Thorac Cardiovasc Surg 55(2):238–242
9. David TE, Bos J, Rakowski H (1988) aortic valve replacement with the Toronto SPV bioprosthesis. J Cardiac Surg 3:501–505
10. Luciani GB (2004) Stentless aortic valve replacement: current status and future trends. Expert Rev Cardiovasc Ther 2(1):127–140
11. Desai ND, Gideon OM, Cohen N et al (2004) Long-term results of aortic valve replacement with the St Jude Toronto Stentless Porcine Valve. Ann Thorac Surg 78:2076–2083
12. Vanermen H, Dossche K, Daenen W et al (1995) Early results of the Edwards Prima stentless aortic bioprosthesis in 200 patients. In: Piwnica A, Westaby S (eds) Stentless bioprosthesis. Eur J Cardiothorac Surg 9:562–567
13. Bortolotti U, Scioti G, Milano A et al (1999) The Edwards Prima stentless valve: Hemodinamic performance at one year. Ann Thorac Surg 68:2147–2151

14. Westaby S, Amarasena N, Long V et al (1995) Time-related hemodinamic changes after aortic replacement with the Freestyle stentless xenograft. Ann Thorac Surg 60:1633–1639
15. D'Onofrio A, Auriemma S, Magagna P, Abbiate N, Fabbri A (2008) The inclusion technique reduces ischemia after stentless aortic root replacement. Ann Thorac Surg 85: 1143–1144
16. Kincaid EH, Cordell AR, Hammon JW, Adair SM, Kon ND (2007) Coronary insufficiency after stentless aortic root replacement: risk factors and solutions Ann Thorac Surg 83:964–968

The Cryo-Life O'Brien stentless valve: 1991–2008

U. Hvass, T. Joudinaud

The hemodynamics of stentless valves are generally recognized as being superior to that of stented devices. Low gradients and large effective orifice areas reflect minimal residual obstruction improving systolic performance, while regression of left ventricular mass diminishes ventricular stiffness improving ventricular filling and diastolic performance.

Physiological advantages conferred by stentless devices must, however, be measured against long-term durability and low complication rates. This report relates the 17-year results of the Cryo-Life O'Brien stentless porcine aortic valve in 1231 consecutive and unselected patients in a single center and by a single surgeon.

The study valve

Cryo-Life International manufactured the Cryo-Life O'Brien stentless porcine aortic bioprosthesis between 1991 and 2004 (Cryo-Life International Inc, 1655 Roberts Blvd, NW Kennesaw, GA 30144, USA). This stentless valve is of a composite design, constructed with noncoronary leaflets obtained from three porcine valves. It is devoid of Dacron reinforcement. Starting in 2004, the valve was manufactured in Brazil by Labcor and then checked and sterilized in Atlanta.

Patients

Demographics are depicted in Table 1. There were no pre-established exclusion criteria. During the study period, only 27 stent-mounted biological valves were used essentially in patients requiring root replacement for annuloaortic ectasia. Patients were predominantly female with a ratio of 4 to 1. The mean age has changed throughout the study, 62 ± 14 during the early years, 78 ± 6 during more recent years, reflecting a general trend of operating on elderly patients.

Table 1. Patient's demographics

■ No. of patients	1231	
■ Age (years)	76 ± 4.2	range 14–90
■ Sex M/F	296/935	(25/75%)
■ Sinus rhythm	837	(68%)
■ NYHA I–II/III–IV	233/998	(19/81%)
■ Calcified aortic stenosis	1194	(97%)
■ Associated lesions		
– Coronary	258	(21%)
– Mitral valve	147	(12%)
– Failed bioprosthesis	98	(8%)

Postoperative anticoagulation was systematic, vitamin K inhibitors replaced by low-dose aspirin or according to the referring cardiologists preference.

Follow-up information was obtained over an 8-month interval through questionnaires addressed to cardiologists, general practitioners, and patients and also telephone contacts. Survivors were followed for an average of 8.6 years, and the total follow-up was 5982 patient-years. Recent echographic information was obtained in 95% of patients living in France where follow-up was 98% complete. Of 35 young patients living abroad, essentially North Africa, 21 were lost to follow-up.

Standard actuarial and linearized statistical techniques were used to describe survival and the incidence of valve-related events. Continuous variables are presented as mean ± standard deviation; actuarial probability and linearized rates are given as mean ± 95% confidence limits of the mean. The STS/AATS/EACTS guidelines were used for reporting morbidity and mortality after cardiac valve operations.

∎ Operative technique

The stentless porcine aortic valve was secured to the patient's aortic root with a single line of three interrupted running sutures. The suture is started at the nadir of each scalloped segment of the aortic annulus and run up to one commissure then to the next, as previously described [1]. With the valve being positioned above the annulus and not inside or below the annulus as with the other stentless valves, the selected valve, to be nonobstructive, must have an inflow diameter that is ideally identical to the diameter of the aortic annulus. This diameter is measured with a cylindrical Hegar probe. Thus, for a measured aortic annulus of 25 mm, one should select a stentless valve that offers an inflow diameter of 25 mm. However, considering that the manufacturing size of the stentless valve as indicated on the prosthesis packaging does not give the inflow diameter we use, but only the exterior diameter of the valve that adds the thickness of the porcine aortic wall to the inflow orifice, we systematically select a valve 2 mm larger than the measured diameter. For example, a 27 mm valve will accept the 25 mm Hegar probe through its inflow orifice. Oversizing a valve is only considered if the Valsalva sinuses are bulging.

Results with the original valve manufactured at the Cryo-Life facility

A total of 1009 patients were followed for 13 years (mean 6.8 years, 4825 patient-years).

Patient survival

The 30-day operative mortality for isolated procedures was 2.7%; the mean age of these patients was 72 ± 4.2 years (Fig. 1). In patients with associated lesions, mean age 77 ± 5.3 years, operative mortality was 14%. The 3-month operative mortality comprises 76 patients (7.7%). Only one of these deaths can be directly related to the valve (traumatic dissection of the left coronary ostia). The other deaths were related to the patient's preoperative status: emergency, severe left ventricular dysfunction, reoperations, prosthetic valve endocarditis and/or respiratory or renal failure.

Late mortality

There were 464 late deaths (Table 2). The causes of these deaths were valve related in 22 (0.42%/year), cardiac related in 57 (0.56%/year), and noncardiac related in 385 (7.8%/year). The actuarial survival rate, including operative mortality was $76\% \pm 6\%$ at 10 years and $46\% \pm 3\%$ at 13 years (Fig. 1).

Nonfatal cardiac events such as myocardial infarction occurred in 18 patients, while 12 had previously undergone coronary bypass procedures. Of the 469 patients alive and with their original stentless porcine aortic valve, 75% are in New York Heart Association functional class I or II.

Table 2. Late mortality (9.6%/year) in 464 of cases

Valve related	22	0.42%/year
Cardiac related	57	0.56%/year
Noncardiac	385	7.8%/year

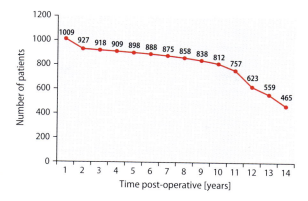

Fig. 1. Actuarial 10-year patient survival rate

Valve-related complications (Table 3)

Nonstructural dysfunction. Six patients showed evidence of nonstructural valve dysfunction (0.33% per patient-year). Three patients had severe aortic regurgitation related to early technical errors, such as slack sutures, prolene rupture, and leaflet perforation leading to reoperations during the first 2 years, mean 12 ± 6 months. Three other cases of progressive aortic insufficiency developed in patients whose initial moderate early regurgitation increased over years leading to reintervention at a mean of 6 ± 2 years. All had successful reoperations with a new stentless valve.

Table 3. Linearized rate of valve-related events (No. events/patient-years × 100)

Patients	1009	
Patient-years	4825	
Mean follow-up	6.6 years	
Mean age	76 ± 4.2 years	
Linearized rate of events (No. events/patient-years × 100)		
Embolism	28	0.5%/year
Bleeding	32	0.6%/year
Endocarditis	15	0.3%/year
Nonstructural deterioration	6	0.12%/year
Structural deterioration		
≥ 65 years	3	0.05%/year
< 65 years	29	0.5%/year
Thrombosis	2	0.04%/year
Reoperations	53	1.1%/year
Total deaths	464	9.6%/year
Death valve related	22	0.4%/year

■ **Valve thrombosis** occurred in a young patient, 36 years old, 3 months postoperatively with a mean transvalvular gradient of 80 mmHg. At reoperation, the valves were thick with layers of thrombus. Another case of valve thrombosis occurred in a 62-year-old patient during the first postoperative year with evidence of thick leaflets, high gradients, and valvular regurgitation that returned to normal after a few months of oral anticoagulation and has remained normal over the following 12 years (0.13% patient-year). The two patients had no evidence of endocarditis.

■ **Hemorrhagic and embolic complications.** All patients received anticoagulants for the first 2 to 3 months. Continuation of anticoagulation was indicated by atrial fibrillation in 252 patients or according to the cardiologist's decision leading to a higher than usual anticoagulant-related bleeding: 32 cases that translate into a linearized rate of 0.32% per patient-year. Correlatively, the incidence of embolic events is relatively low, 28 cases (0.27% per patient-year).

■ **Operated valvular endocarditis.** There were three cases of postoperative early stentless aortic valve endocarditis due to *Staphylococcus aureus*, two of which healed with antibiotics, leaving only mild regurgitation in spite of a sterilized periannular abscess. Two other cases of endocarditis affected only the stented mitral porcine prosthesis with a periannular mitral abscess. The stentless aortic valve was not involved in the septic process at reoperation. Late endocarditis was documented in 12 cases, one died before surgery.

■ **Structural valve deterioration.** The freedom from structural deterioration at 13 years is 98% in patients 65, mean age 76±8 and 53% in 57 patients <65, mean age 35±21 (Fig. 2).

Thirty-two patients showed evidence of structural valve deterioration during the follow-up period and were successfully reoperated. Twenty-nine

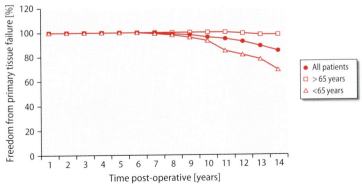

Fig. 2. Actuarial freedom from structural valve deterioration

of the patients were under 65 with a mean age at initial surgery of 27.5 ± 12.2 years and a mean delay of 7 ± 1.41 years. Twenty-one patients received a mechanical valve, six a stent-mounted bioprosthesis and two a stentless pericardium valve (Sorin Solo). Three patients >65 years of age underwent reoperations between 3 and 9 years after the initial operation. They received a new stentless valve.

▌ Reoperations. There were 52 aortic valve reoperations in this series (0.68% per patient-year). Six reoperations were indicated for nonstructural deterioration, 12 for aortic valve endocarditis, 1 for valve thrombosis, and 32 for structural deterioration. Two stentless valves were changed during reoperations for mitral prosthesis endocarditis although there was no apparent involvement of the aortic valve. Three reoperations were necessary for mitral valve repairs; there were no coronary bypass operations during the follow-up period.

▌ Hemodynamic data

The distribution of valve sizes is shown in Fig. 3. Transvalvular gradients at discharge and beyond the first year are depicted in Fig. 4. About 30% of the patients over 70 years of age receive a small size device, size 21 and 23 corresponding, respectively, to a measured aortic annulus of 19 and 21 mm. The gradients are consistently low, with an indexed effective orifice area at discharge over 0.80 cm^2/m^2 and above 0.90 cm^2/m^2 after the first year, reflecting only very mild residual obstruction.

An exercise hemodynamic evaluation was performed between 6 and 12 months in ten patients using echocardiography and Doppler during exertion by cycling in a semisupine position. With a moderate workload of 60 W, the results show that stentless valves exhibit a normal pattern of adaptation, augmenting cardiac output through increased stroke volume, while residual gradients remain low.

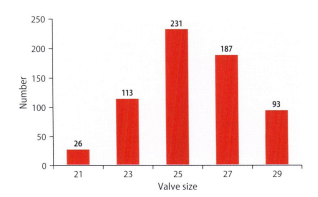

Fig. 3. Distribution of valve sizes in 650 patients. Reprinted with permission from [6]; ICR Publishers

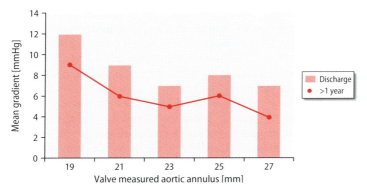

Fig. 4. Transvalvular gradients (mmHg). Reprinted with permission from [6]; ICR Publishers

Results with the second-generation valve manufactured at the Labcor facility in Brazil and sterilized at Cryo-Life

A total of 222 patients received implants and were followed from 2004–2008 (cumulating 1157 patient-years).

Over the last 4 years, valve manufacture has changed. The second-generation valve was mounted and glutaraldehyde fixed at zero pressure by Labcor in Brazil then sterilized in Atlanta. A total of 222 valves were implanted. After a period of 18 to 24 months, there was an abnormally high incidence of endocarditis (8.1%), which resulted in 17 reoperations. All these patients had echographic evidence of periannular abscesses with aortic insufficiency.

At reoperation, cavities were found around the valve, destroying the aortic annulus. The valve was dehiscent, explaining aortic regurgitation. The valve leaflets were normal, without vegetations (except two cases) or perforations. Only two patients had previously been operated on for endocarditis. Explanting the valve from the patient's wall was abnormally easy, as though there had been little healing process between the stentless porcine aortic wall and the patient's aortic wall.

Comment

Initially used in the early 1960s by O'Brien [1], stentless aortic valves came back into practice in the late 1980s pioneered by David with the Toronto SVP stentless valve. Since then, a variety of stentless valves have been introduced, proposing different handling characteristics. Huysmans and Westaby, among others, established the results of the Freestyle Medtronic stentless valve, while O'Brien [2] and Hvass [3] reported results of the Cryo-Life

O'Brien stentless valve. All these stentless devices went through a learning curve that temporarily affected early results, introducing nonstructural deteriorations apparent in all publications.

A 'stentless identity' was soon recognized, consistently being associated with an improved resting hemodynamic profile with low gradients and large effective indexed orifice areas indicating only mild residual obstruction after aortic valve replacement even in the small aortic roots [4], a characteristic rarely contested and further demonstrated by a more efficient regression of left ventricular hypertrophy [5]. These physiological advantages constantly raised a controversial debate centered on whether the stentless device was more than only a surgical tool on which we were focusing our attention and whether the patient would really benefit from it.

The debated question relating functional and survival benefits, intuitively anticipated by improved left ventricular performance, was addressed in several studies and trials in which a pattern that 'stentless' patients experienced fewer cardiac events appeared and that survival advantages perceptible in younger patients tapered off in the elderly groups which are the recognized recipients of biological valves.

Long-term durability of the stentless devices was expected on arguments of dampened mechanical stresses, the flexible and expanding aortic root being the most physiological support for any aortic valve. The long-term results of the Toronto SVP valve show stability of the stentless valve when not affected by subsequent sinotubular dilatation that disturbs the initial geometry of the valve and leads to central regurgitation. The results of the Freestyle valve have been reported by single centers using a variety of techniques and have also reached the 8-year mark with stable results in a multicenter subgroup of 104 root replacements. 'Stentless identity', however, is not sufficient to be able to transfer conclusions from one device to another. The design of the Toronto SVP, the Freestyle and the Cryo-Life O'Brien are specific, leading to implantation rules and possibilities that are not all shared from one device to the other. In particular, the recommended implantation position of the Cryo-Life O'Brien stentless, in opposition to all other stentless designs, is above the annulus, a feature that easily allows the surgeon to oversize when the Valsalva sinuses are large. Patients whose indication for surgery was aortic insufficiency or a calcified bicuspid aortic valve represent a not infrequent subset of patients who more often have a larger than normal Valsalva sinus and sinotubular junction that tend to further enlarge during the follow-up period. The stentless Cryo-Life O'Brien is oversized mainly within this group of patents, and therefore it is not affected to the same extent by an eventual further widening of the sinotubular junction. It is essentially in patients with aortic insufficiency and bicuspid valves that other stentless valves experience late valve insufficiency and dilation of the sinotubular junction leading to noncoaptation of otherwise usually normal leaflets.

The 10-year results of the Cryo-Life O'Brien stentless valve as previously reported [6] equate the 10-year results of the Carpentier-Edwards pericardial valve [7], which stands as a reference for many. This pericardial valve is stable with degenerative changes being infrequent in patients 65+ years old. The results also equate the 10-year mark of the important series published by Jamieson [8] reporting porcine Carpentier-Edwards SAV and Hancock-II bioprostheses.

A question that seems central to the future of stentless devices is the surgeon's ability to use them in all situations. Different lines of investigation have been tested in which one can recognize three tendencies. The most widespread is probably represented by elective indications confirmed or rejected by the surgeon in the operating room on the basis of perceived feasibility giving full latitude to implant or renounce. This flexible approach allows the surgeon to become progressively familiar with the device and with experience eliminate previously resented contraindications. Another tendency is to have at hand a variety of stentless opportunities that suggests that the large spectrum of available devices allows optimizing the fit between a specific valve design, the patient's pathology, and the precise root anatomy. This seems to be a misleading message to young surgeons conveying the impression that commitment towards stentless devices is a highly selective process and very complicated to master. The third position is a systematic approach as we have proposed with our large series of Cryo-Life O'Brien stentless valves from the very beginning. During the 17-year period, only patients with annuloaortic ectasia did not receive a Cryo-Life O'Brien stentless valve. Four patients with coronary anomalies (coronary ostia on each side of a commissure or anomalous circumflex running through the aortic wall) and a case of porcelain aorta, for which we renounced to perform any procedure, represent the only technical impossibilities discovered in the operating room. Implantation time, with experience, is even shorter than conventional devices, and however complex associated procedures may be they never raise even the thought of preferring a stented device.

Conclusion

At 13 years, the initial generation of Cryo-Life O'Brien stentless porcine aortic valve gives excellent results in terms of durability that equates the results of the stent-mounted devices. The stentless valve furthermore displays specific physiological advantages (gradients, orifice areas and mass regression that translate into an appropriately adapted left ventricular exertion profile) that may be related to symptomatic and eventual survival improvements.

However, the second generation of the valve, regardless of the reasons, was associated in our series with an 8% reoperation rate 16 ± 9 months after initial implantation.

References

1. O'Brien MF, Clarebrough JK (1966) Heterograft aortic valve transplantation for human valve disease. Med J Aust 2:228–230
2. O'Brien MF (1995) Composite stentless xenograft for aortic valve replacement. Clinical evaluation of function. Ann Thorac Surg 60:S406–S409
3. Hvass U, Palatianos GM, Frassani R, Puricelli C, O'Brien M (1999) Multi-center study of stentless valve replacement in, the small aortic root. J Thorac Cardiovasc Surg 117:267–272
4. Rao V, Jamieson WR, Ivanov J, Armstrong S, David TE (2000) Prosthesis-patient mismatch affects survival after aortic valve replacement. Circulation 102(Suppl 3): III-5–III-9
5. Jin XY, Zhang Z, Gibson DG, Yacoub MH, Pepper JR (1996) Changes in left ventricular function and hypertrophy following aortic valve replacement using aortic homografts, stentless or stented valves. Ann Thorac Surg 62:683–690
6. Hvass U, Baron F, Elsebaey A, N'Guyen D, Fisher E (2004) The stentless Cryo-Life stentless porcine valve at 10 years. The Journal of Heart Valve disease 13:977–983
7. Aupart MR, Sirinelli AL, Diemont FF, Meurisse YA, Dreyfus XB, Marchand MA (1996) The last generation of pericardial valves in the aortic position: ten-year follow-up in 589 patients. Ann Thorac Surg 61:615–620
8. Jamieson WRE, David TE, Feindel CMS, Miyagishima RT, Germann E (2002) Performance of the Carpentier-Edwards SAV and Hancock-II Bio prostheses in aortic valve replacement. J Heart valve disease 11:424–430

Medtronic stentless Freestyle® porcine aortic valve replacement

J. Ennker, A. Albert, I. Florath

Introduction: stentless biological valves

Biological heart valve prostheses offer the opportunity of avoiding the risk of thromboembolic and hemorrhagic complications due to anticoagulation therapy. Current indications recommend a bioprosthesis for aortic valve replacement in patients of any age, who will not take warfarin or who have major medical contraindications to anticoagulation therapy (Class I), in patients older than 65 years without risk factors for thromboembolism (Class IIa) and in patients under 65 years for lifestyle considerations after detailed discussion of the risks of anticoagulation versus the likelihood of a second valve replacement [1].

Stentless bioprostheses were designed to avoid the obstructive stent and sewing cuff present in a conventional stented biological valve, because the sewing ring and the stent of conventional bioprostheses reduce the blood flow across the artificial valve. This may increase the risk of a valve prosthesis-patient mismatch accompanied by higher transprosthetic gradients and a reduced effective orifice area, which in turn may result in less regression of left ventricular hypertrophy and decreased survival [20]. The design of stentless bioprostheses is assigned to achieve a more physiological flow pattern and superior hemodynamics in comparison to stented valves.

Randomized trials revealed controversial results concerning the superiority of stentless in comparison to stented valves during the last few years [3, 11, 12, 33, 41]. Most of them showed a hemodynamic advantage for stentless valves but several could not reach a significant level. A meta-analysis of ten recent randomized trials comparing stentless and stented bioprostheses including over 500 patients demonstrated a significant advantage of stentless valves concerning transvalvular gradients, effective orifice valve areas and regression of left ventricular mass 6 months after aortic valve replacement [26]. Also, a survival advantage for stentless bioprostheses in comparison to stented ones was reported in a randomized study of 223 patients [27].

The Medtronic Freestyle® aortic root bioprosthesis is composed of a porcine aortic root fixated in glutaraldehyde solution under net zero-differential pressure at the leaflets and treated with the anticalcification AOA® (α-amino oleic acid) agent to maintain the natural leaflet structure and reduce structural valve failure caused by calcification.

The Freestyle® bioprosthesis: surgical technique

Normothermia, intermittent ante- and retrograde cold blood cardioplegia, and a left atrial vent was introduced routinely. Between April 1996 and October 2008, 2033 patients underwent aortic valve replacement with stentless Freestyle® bioprostheses, 343 of them in full root technique. The ascending aorta was concomitant replaced in 203 patients.

Subcoronary technique

In the case of a planned subcoronary implantation technique, the aortic incision was made over at least half to two thirds of the aortic circumference to accommodate good access to the aortic valve. It is recommended to perform the aortic incision 1 cm to 2 cm above the three commissures. This is important because the commissures of the Freestyle prosthesis often go above those of the human aorta. The aortic valve, the position of the left and right coronary ostia as well as the constitution of the aortic wall in the sinus of Valsalva should be carefully examined in order to prevent intraoperative obstacles (see Technical issues of subcoronary implantation technique and the impact of the surgeons on hemodynamic outcome section below). After excision of the native aortic valve, the size of the aortic annulus was measured using standard Medtronic Freestyle® sizers. Generally, the size of the bioprosthesis should be chosen according to the largest sizer that could be passed through the aortic root. Freestyle® bioprostheses should be neither under- nor oversized.

The porcine root was trimmed down to less than 5 mm above the level of the cloth covering, and generally all porcine sinuses were excised.

As the porcine coronary ostia are usually situated at a smaller angle to each other than the human coronary ostia, the Freestyle® bioprosthesis was routinely rotated in a clockwise manner, directing the higher part of the Dacron towards the noncoronary sinus in order to prevent coronary obstruction after implantation. In the case of a marked asymmetry of the human commissures (in comparison to the Freestyle commissures), further rotation of the valve may be necessary and/or the choice of where the new commissures should be placed to avoid interference of the commissures of the Freestyle valve with the coronary ostia.

The bioprosthesis was brought into the annulus and then sutured to the aortic annulus using one or three continuous sutures with 5/0 Prolene. Particular care should be taken to keep the suture line in a level plane through the lowest points of the dense fibrous tissue of the hinge of the native valve. The suture line is below the annulus, which is below the interleaflet triangle, except in the region of the membranous septum, where the suture line follows the annulus directly to protect the conduction system. The second suture line for the outflow tract was started at the top of the left coronary commissure using a 5/0 Prolene suture. The bioprosthesis commissures were cautiously sutured to the aortic wall as high as possible in order to prevent excessive overlapping or folding of the prosthesis valve leaflets. The suture line was then run along the left sinus of Valsalva beneath the left coronary ostium to the acoronary commissure where it was tied at the outside of the aortic wall with the other end of the suture run along the right and acoronary sinus.

After completion of implantation the aortic incision was closed in a standard fashion using a double armed 5/0 Prolene suture.

∎ Total root technique

In the case of a planned full root technique, oversizing was often performed: the size of the prosthesis was chosen one or two valve sizes greater than the size of the aortic annulus, measured using standard Medtronic Freestyle® sizers. Similar to the subcoronary technique, the Freestyle® bioprosthesis was mostly rotated in a clockwise manner directing the higher part of the Dacron towards the noncoronary sinus. Part of the wall of the noncoronary sinus and the left coronary ostia of the Freestyle® prosthesis were excised as buttons. The coronary ostium of the Freestyle® valve directed to the acoronary side was than oversewn. For root replacement, the stentless bioprosthesis was connected to the left ventricular outflow tract using a running 4-0 polypropylene suture. Similar to the subcoronary technique, the sutures are placed below the level of the commissures to create a circle of stitches in a single plane. In the case of fragile tissue, we used a pericardial strip for reinforcement. The coronary ostia were reattached directly to the prosthesis using a running 5-0 polypropylene suture in all patients, reinforced by a pericardial strip in the case of fragile tissue. The Freestyle® prosthesis is then sutured to the patient's aorta (or in the case of a combined replacement of the aorta ascendens to a Hemashield prosthesis) with 4-0 or 5-0 continuous Prolene, occasionally reinforced by a pericardial strip.

The Freestyle® bioprosthesis: hemodynamic outcome

A number of issues concerning hemodynamics after stentless valve implantation are important to study: after implantation of stentless valves, characteristically, a perivalvular hematoma develops between the prosthesis and the natural aortic wall. Resolving the hematoma during the 3 to 6 months postoperatively may contribute towards a marked decrease in transvalvular gradients over time [5, 24]. What is the extent of the decrease in the gradient postoperatively?

Second, if stentless bioprostheses are hemodynamically superior in comparison to stented bioprostheses, could a lower incidence of prosthesis-patient mismatch after aortic valve replacement be expected?

Third, what is the effect of the full root technique in comparison to the subcoronary technique concerning hemodynamic outcome and risks of the procedure?

Fourth, what is the impact of the surgeon's experience and skill on hemodynamic outcome after implantation and what are the consequences? It was already mentioned that the performance of stentless valves may depend to a larger extent on surgical experience [2, 6].

Decrease in gradients postoperatively

Mean and peak transprosthetic gradients were measured at our institute between 5 and 7 days after aortic valve replacement. Late echocardiographic data were obtained from the patients' family cardiologists. In 362 patients, mean transprosthetic gradient obtained before discharge and from the family cardiologist were compared (Fig. 1a, b). During follow-up, the peak transprosthetic gradients decreased in 80% of the patients for the subcoronary implantation technique since the gradients were measured at discharge. The gradients decreased on average even more in patients presenting high gradients at discharge (Fig. 1a). In patients presenting with peak transprosthetic gradients higher than 35 mmHg at discharge, classified as moderate aortic stenosis according to the ACC/AHA 2006 Guidelines [1], the peak gradients decreased on average about 20 mmHg (Fig. 1a). In comparison, the amount of decrease was on average only 4 mmHg during follow-up for patients with peak gradients below 36 mmHg at discharge (Fig. 1b).

Valve prosthesis-patient mismatch

Valve prosthesis-patient mismatch may occur "when the effective prosthetic valve area, after insertion into the patient, is less than that of a normal

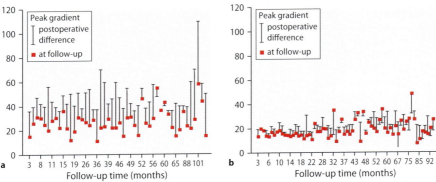

Fig. 1a, b. Comparison of transprosthetic gradients at follow-up to transprosthetic gradients at discharge. Reprinted with permission from Ennker J, et al. (2009) J Card Surg 24:41–48; © Wiley-Blackwell

valve" [35]. In a study population of 533 patients, the effective orifice area was measured by echocardiography 5 to 7 days after aortic valve replacement. Severe mismatch (indexed effective orifice area ≤0.6 cm^2/m^2, Hazard Ratio: 1.9 (1.08–3.21)) was a significant predictor of survival time after adjustment for age, LVEF, atrial fibrillation, NYHA class, serum creatinine and hemoglobin level. The 5- and 7-year survival rates were 71±4% and 54±8% for patients with severe mismatch, 76±3% and 63±6% for patients with moderate mismatch, 83±4% and 80±8% for patients with mild mismatch, respectively. As expected, the incidence of prosthesis-patient mismatch observed after insertion of stentless valves (27% in subcoronary technique) was lower than after the use of stented biological valves (47%) [20].

Technical issues of subcoronary technique and the impact of the surgeons on hemodynamic outcome

In previous studies, suboptimal hemodynamics after stentless valve implantation were reported in a considerable number of patients (20% of the population): these patients showed higher mean transprosthetic gradients than expected (>20 mmHg) at discharge with persistence over 1 year and less complete LV mass regression. They were more often female and had both lower BSA and smaller valve sizes [4]. In our institution, transprosthetic gradients measured at discharge were even higher than reported elsewhere, which may be partly explained by the more frequent use of the subcoronary technique in patients with small aortic roots than in other series. However, it may also be explained by the fact that the valves were frequently implanted by a cumulative number of 25 surgeons and trainees during the last 10 years. We studied the performance over time: Fig. 2 shows the mean transvalvular pressure gradients at discharge by year of implantation for each valve size. The decrease in transprosthetic gradients

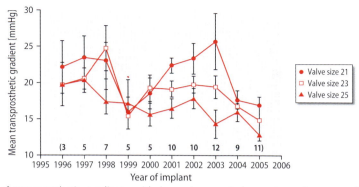

Fig. 2. Decrease of transprosthetic gradients with increasing surgical experience by years of implantation. Reprinted with permission from Ennker J, et al. (2009) J Card Surg 24:41–48; © Wiley-Blackwell

during the first few years until 1999 reflects the learning curve of three surgeons implanting 191 stentless bioprostheses between 1996 and 1998. In the year 2000, the number of surgeons implanting stentless valves increased to ten, whereas only five surgeons implanted stentless valves continuously during all years. The increase in the transprosthetic gradients from year 2000 may be caused by less experience of the surgeons starting to implant the stentless bioprosthesis, whereas the gradients in smaller valve sizes were affected more. These variations seem to reflect the learning effects of the surgeons [19].

Thus, we assessed each individual surgeon's impact on the transvalvular gradient in a multivariate model. We demonstrated that the surgeon's skills and differences in their individual histories of training seem to be more important than experience over time and the number of cases [2].

The goal is to fit the Freestyle® prosthesis properly into the aortic root, so that it adapts smoothly to the aortic wall ("snug fit"), avoiding buckling of the prosthesis into the outflow tract, which affects the hemodynamic outcome. Higher transvalvular gradients through Freestyle bioprosthesis may develop already by slight distortions of the valve, horizontal or vertical folding of valve tissue into the outflow tract, impaired movements of the noncoronary cusp, oversizing, or due to a large paravalvular hematoma. Because these phenomena may neutralize the presumed benefit of stentless valves concerning hemodynamic outcome and impair functional recovery, we stress the importance of proper training of surgeons in stentless valve implantation.

Pioneers in stentless valve implantation have already given advice to prevent buckling of the prosthesis or ostial obstruction and have emphasized: the importance of optimal aortotomy [14, 39], the risk of oversizing [8], the problems of sinus calcifications for the second suture line [25, 40], the problems of low ostia especially the right, with the need for rotation of the

Table 1. Common problems increasing the risk of higher mean pressure gradients

Problem	Consequence	Safeguard
Too low aortotomy	Tendency to bend the commissures into the outflow tract leading to outflow obstruction	A small transverse aortotomy is made initially 1 to 2 cm above the right coronary ostium. Then the aortic commissures should be identified before extending the aortotomy
Deviation from the virtual plane defined by the nadirs when constructing the proximal suture line	Buckling of the Freestyle valve above the commissures into the outflow tract. Impaired opening of the leaflets	In the area of the commissures the needle is passed through the ventricular muscle and the sub-aortic curtain to form a circle of stitches in a single plane
Coronary ostia situated close to the annulus	Implantation requires an element of folding, dictated by the height of the cloth part of the valve	Rotation of the valve directing the higher part of the Dacron towards the noncoronary sinus, or avoidance of subcoronary technique
Coronary ostia (mostly right) situated close to the commissures	Risk of bending the valve trying to avoid obstructing the coronary flow	Further rotation of the Freestyle valve deviating its commissures from the original patient's commissures
Disproportion between intercommissural length of the Freestyle prosthesis and the patients annulus (e.g., larger noncoronary sinus of the patient)	Shortening and folding the patient's annulus leading to bulging the Dacron into the outflow tract	Further rotation of the Freestyle valve deviating its commissures from the original patient's commissures

valve to place the higher cloth towards the acoronary sinus [14, 39, 40], the optimal level plane of the proximal suture line defined by the nadirs of the cusps [40], and need of an radial orientation of the stitches close to the ostia [14]. We have listed below those technical aspects we consider most important to optimize stentless valve implantation (Table 1) and illustrate some important issues of implantation technique using two different examples (see Figs. 3–10). Techniques of Freestyle® implantation reported often in the literature differ somewhat from the techniques used normally in our institute: interrupted instead of continuous sutures for the proximal suture line [40], the start of the second suture line below the ostia instead of starting at the commissures [14, 39, 40], rotation of the Freestyle® valve with position of the prosthesis right coronary sinus towards the human acoronary only in selected patients instead of routine rotation [14, 25, 40]. Nevertheless, we consider these techniques to have minor importance regarding hemodynamic outcome.

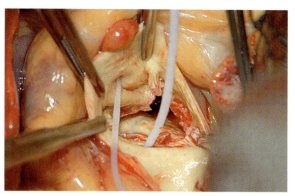

Fig. 3. Favorable anatomy of the aortic root for implantation of Freestyle bioprosthesis. Both coronary ostia are situated in the middle of the sinus with sufficient distance to the commissures as well as to the annulus. The intercommissural distances are of equal size. Note: the aortotomy was made with sufficient distance to the commissures (>2 cm) (Patient 1)

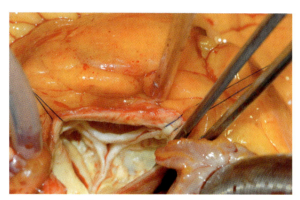

Fig. 4. Special anatomy of the aortic root with left coronary ostia situated close to the commissure between the left and acoronary sinuses. The acoronary inter-commissural distance is significantly longer than the right and left coronary. In this case it is recommendable to place the new left/acoronary commissure about 1 cm toward the acoronary sinus (Patient 2)

In our experience, it is helpful, at least for the surgeon who is not specialized in stentless valve surgery, to follow the implantation rules stepwise. For example it is mandatory to check four conditions *before starting with the first suture line*:
- optimal placement of aortotomy with sufficient distance to the human commissures,
- observation of the aortic sinus for severe calcification,
- assessment of distance of coronary ostia to the annulus, and
- comparison of the angles of the Freestyle's commissures with the human commissures and subsequent choice of where to place the Freestyle commissures: in an anatomic or extra-anatomic position.

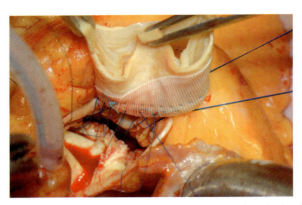

Fig. 5. The freestyle bioprosthesis was orientated with the higher Dacron part towards the acoronary sinus. Due to the special anatomy of this aortic root (see Fig. 4), the commissures of the prosthesis (see markers on the Freestyle Dacron) are placed towards the acoronary sinus; thereby obstruction of the left coronary ostia is avoided and symmetry of length between the commissural distances between the (relatively longer) human acoronary sinus and prosthesis is achieved. Note: all sinuses of the Freestyle bioprosthesis are completely removed (Patient 2)

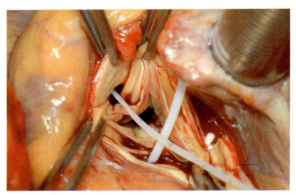

Fig. 6. After the first suture line has been finished, the relationship between the prosthesis and the coronary ostia is fixed. A bending of the commissures to avoid interference with coronary ostia would usually result in buckling of the prosthesis into the outflow tract (Patient 1)

We suggest gaining experience with larger valve sizes because the transvalvular gradients are correlated to some extent with the indexed effective orifice area [34]. Second, we recommend active participation in the operating room (expert cognitive modeling), prolonged assistance and correction by an expert and interactive discussions.

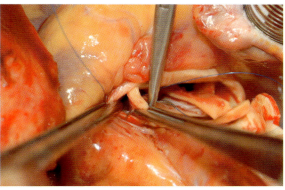

Fig. 7. We start with the second suture line at one commissure. The assistant has to pull on the patient's commissures to achieve congruence between the prosthesis and the aortic wall (Patient 1)

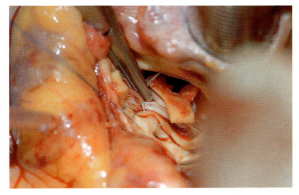

Fig. 8. It is important to place radial stitches around the coronary ostia to avoid obstruction or distortion of the coronary (Patient 1)

∎ Subcoronary versus total root implantation technique *

The Freestyle® aortic root bioprosthesis can be implanted by several surgical techniques similar to the use of different implant techniques with human tissue valves: complete or modified subcoronary, root inclusion, and full root. Using human tissue valves, aortic root replacement was associated with a lower incidence of early reoperation, greater effective orifice area and with less prominent aortic regurgitation on Doppler echocardiography in comparison to the subcoronary technique [24, 30]. However, contradictory results exist neglecting the superiority of root replacement technique with regard to aortic regurgitation [9, 42]. A comparison of dif-

---

* The study was supported by Medtronic Inc., Düsseldorf (Germany)

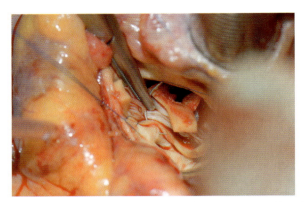

Fig. 9. Check of the valve opening after implantation. Here the prosthesis smoothly fits with the aortic wall (Patient 2)

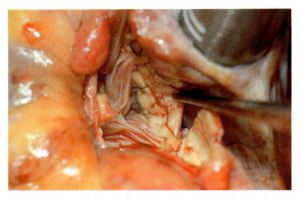

Fig. 10. Check of the leaflet closure, leaflet heights and symmetry (Patient 2)

ferent implantation techniques for porcine stentless bioprostheses reported higher operative mortality, better hemodynamics, functional class and freedom from regurgitation with the full root in comparison to subcoronary implantation technique [6]. We reported our experience with the full root technique recently: between 1996 and 2005, 1014 patients underwent AVR with stentless Freestyle® bioprostheses, 169 of them using the full root technique. The full root technique was more often performed in female patients, in patients of smaller body height, and in patients requiring concomitant replacement of the ascending aorta. We compared early and late outcomes for the subcoronary versus full root implantation technique using a propensity score-based matching analysis. Thus, 148 matched pairs were created with a mean age of 73 years, 64% being women. We found that the mean transprosthetic gradients were on average 7 mmHg less for the full root technique than for the subcoronary technique, but early and late outcomes were equal: overall survival was 71±33% and 78±29% after 5 years and 33±20% and 34±24% after 9 years, respectively, for the subcoronary

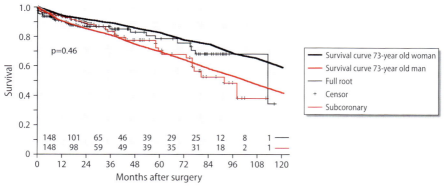

Fig. 11. Comparison of survival curves after implantation of Freestyle bioprosthesis to the German population. Reprinted with permission from Ennker J, et al. (2008) Ann Thorac Surg 85: 445–453; © The Society of Thoracic Surgeons

and full root group (p = 0.46) and was similar to men and women of the German general population with the mean age of the study population (Fig. 11) [18]. However, despite proper training and the development of routines, many surgeons are reluctant to perform the total root technique routinely due to the known difficulties of this technique and the fear of bleeding and coronary complication, especially in the elderly [6]. We use the total root technique mainly in patients with small aortic roots, in cases of annuloaortic ectasia and replacement of ascending aorta, and in cases where a prosthesis-patient mismatch would be expected.

Another drawback of the full root implantation technique is the demanding surgery in case of re-replacement of the aortic valve due to prosthetic valve endocarditis or structural valve deterioration. Excellent midterm freedom from reoperation because of structural valve deterioration was reported to be 95% at 10 years [7, 28]. Long-term studies showed similar results with stented bioprostheses, whereas the reoperation rate increased more profoundly after 10 to 15 years especially for patients younger than 60 years [22, 23]. As the maximum follow-up in the most recent studies about stentless valves is 10 years, no recommendation concerning total root replacement with stentless bioprosthesis can be given at the moment for younger patients ([18], Society of Thoracic Surgeons (2008)).

The Freestyle® bioprosthesis: operative risk in isolated and combined procedures

As simultaneous myocardial revascularization is a more complex surgical technique than isolated aortic valve replacement, longer operation times and as a result an increased operative risk may be expected. In a study population of 1014 patients undergoing Freestyle valve replacement with a mean age of 73±21 years and a mean EuroSCORE of 8.1±2.4, we observed a significantly prolonged cardiopulmonary bypass time for simultaneous myocardial revascularization (130±47 min) in comparison to isolated valve replacement (106±39 min, p<0.001). However, no increased operative risk (p=0.16) was observed for patients undergoing Freestyle® valve replacement and simultaneous myocardial revascularization after adjustment by the following risk factors diabetes mellitus, congestive heart failure, concomitant mitral valve replacement, smaller body height and body mass index less than 24.

Compared with isolated valve replacement and despite more extensive surgery and prolonged bypass time, simultaneous myocardial revascularization can be performed without an increased operative risk in patients with stentless valve implantation [16].

The Freestyle® bioprosthesis: valve related morbidity and mortality *

We have studied valve-related morbidity and mortality in 1014 consecutive patients who received a Freestyle bioprosthesis. Mean age was 73 years, 50% were female. According to the EuroScore, 81.9% of the patients were in the high-risk group, 16.8% in the medium-risk group and 1.4% in the low-risk group. The actuarial survival rate was 71±3% and 46±9% at 5 and 9 years, respectively, and was between the survival rates of men and women of the general German population of age 73 years.

The actuarial freedom from aortic valve reoperation and structural valve deterioration were 97.0±1.2% and 92.4±7.4% at 5 years and 99.9±0.2%, 97.0±4.9% at 9 years, respectively. Twenty-eight patients required reoperations. The causes for reoperations are given in Table 2. Structural valve deterioration occurred in two patients. In one patient the deteriorated valve was re-replaced after 100 months because of cusp rupture. Another patient was reoperated after 3 months due to pericarditis after a postmyocardial infarction syndrome. The valve was replaced because of a mean gradient of 30 mmHg. Intraoperatively, only a stiffening of the cusps was observed. The histological examination described a low-grade inflammation with some leukocytes in the cusps, some mucoid swelling and edema, connective tissue with some fibrosis, and no calcification. Of the 28 patients undergoing reoperation, in 21 (75%) patients, the Freestyle® valve was explanted and 11 (39%) patients died within 30 days. The linearized rates of late adverse events (later 30 days) were 0.57% per patient-year and 0.07% per patient-year for reoperation and structural valve deterioration, respectively.

---

* The study was supported by Medtronic Inc., Düsseldorf (Germany)

Table 2. Causes of reoperation. Reprinted with permission from Ennker J, et al. (2009) J Card Surg 24:41–48; © Wiley-Blackwell

Reoperation (N = 28)	N	Implant duration (months)	Type of replaced valve
▍ Subcoronary technique			
Structural valve deterioration	2	3, 100	NA, Freestyle
Nonstructural dysfunction	18		
– paravalvular leak	7	0, 0.1, 0.1, 1.4, 4, 6, 10	SJM Regent, 2 Medtronic Hall
– entrapment by pannus	2	within 1st month	3 Freestyle FR, 3 SJM Regent
– hemodynamic	6	5 within 1st	SJM HP, Carbomedics
– intraoperative replaced	2	month, 24	
– incompetent valve because of dilation of sinotubular junction	1	69	no
Valve thrombosis	1	3	Carbomedics
Operated valvular endocarditis	5	1, 2, 5, 46, 80	Mosaic, Supra, Freestyle, no, Hancock
▍ Full root technique			
Operated valvular endocarditis	2	6, 12	Tissuemed AR, Freestyle FR

AR aortic root, *FR* full root, *NA* not available, *no* no valve replaced, *SJM* St. Jude Medical

The 5- and 9-year actuarial freedom from endocarditis was 98.3 ± 0.9% and 96.6 ± 5.9%, respectively. The linearized rate was 0.43% per patient-year. There were 12 endocarditis episodes. The mean interval of occurrence was 2.1 ± 2.3 years. Seven patients required reoperation (Table 2).

Actuarial freedom from neurological events at 5 and 9 years was 88.3 ± 2.3% and 69.5 ± 15.7%, respectively. Neurological events were observed in 72 patients. The linearized rate was 2.69% per patient-year.

Actuarial freedom from major bleeding events at 5 and 9 years was 95.8 ± 1.0% and 94.8 ± 1.4%, respectively. Major bleeding occurred in 19 patients with a linearized rate of 0.69% per patient-year. 21% of the patients required anticoagulation therapy due to generalized atherosclerotic disease or chronic atrial fibrillation presenting pre- or postoperatively.

Linearized rates of valve-related morbidity were almost equal to a previous report about the Freestyle® bioprostheses (Table 3). Also, similar results were obtained in comparison to other stentless valves, whereas we observed higher rates for thromboembolic events (Table 3). In comparison to stented bioprostheses, linearized rates of adverse events were also almost similar with apparently little increased rates of structural valve deterioration and reoperation for stented valves.

A wide variation in the thromboembolic rate from 0.52 to 2.66 events per patient-year (Table 3) was observed between the different biological prostheses. Because the complication rates depend significantly on patient-related factors [36], comparing the outcome from different studies may be

Table 3. Linearized rates of late adverse events in % per patient-year. Reprinted with permission from Ennker J, et al. (2009) J Card Surg 24:41–48; © Wiley-Blackwell

Valve	N	Age	Follow-up	PVE	Re-OP	SVD	MBE	NE
▪ Freestyle [present]	1014	73	9 years	0.43	0.57	0.07	0.69	2.69
▪ Freestyle [7]	725	72	10 years	0.43	0.7	0.27	NA	2.66
▪ Freestyle [29]	608	68	10 years	NA	0.25	0.11	NA	NA
▪ Cryolife-O'Brien [30]	402	73	8 years	0.35	0.35	0.04	NA	1.56
▪ Cryolife-O'Brien [31]	185	73[a]	10 years	0.22	0.91	1.04	NA	NA
▪ Toronto SPV [13]	200	64	10 years	0.43	1.12	0.32	NA	0.52
▪ CE-porcine [23]	1823	68	20 years	0.36	1.12	0.91	NA	2.33
▪ Mosaic [37]	255	67	10 years	0.5	1.4	0.3	0.31	0.8
▪ Hancock II [38]	809	68	15 years	0.44	0.73	0.4	0.5	1.29
▪ Mitroflow, pericardial [43]	1513	73	21 years	0.28	1.4	0.9	0.065	0.79

[a] Median age, otherwise mean age
MBE major bleeding events, *NA* not available, *NE* neurological events, *PVE* prosthetic valve endocarditis, *Re-OP* reoperation

quite difficult due to the different baseline characteristics. For instance, the prevalence of risk factors for stroke (e.g., advanced age, diabetes mellitus, hypertension, atrial fibrillation, left ventricular hypertrophy, cardiovascular disease) may differ in the various studies.

The incidence of first clinical strokes reported from the Framingham study was 0.87%/patient-year in persons older than the 65 years [10]. In the presented study cohort, additional risk factors were more prevalent in comparison to the Framingham cohort: Hypertension (66% vs. 56%), diabetes mellitus (25% vs. 7%), cardiovascular disease (38% vs. 19%) and atrial fibrillation (19% vs. 5%), which may account for the higher rates of strokes observed in our study [18]. In conclusion, our results compare favorably with those of other biological valve studies. The Freestyle® bioprosthesis showed encouraging durability up to 9 years with low rates of valve-related morbidity and can be safely implanted without an increased operative risk even during the learning phase.

The Freestyle® bioprosthesis: special indications

▪ Concomitant replacement of the ascending aorta

Between 2000 and 2007, the aortic valve and the ascending aorta were replaced in 304 patients. A total of 64 patients received separate replacement of the aortic valve and the ascending aorta (52 biological); 144 patients received a mechanical composite graft and 96 patients received a stentless bioprostheses using the full root technique and replacement of the ascending aorta (biological composite graft). From this patient population 56 matched-pairs, receiving either a mechanical (M) or a biological composite graft (B), were created based on a saturated propensity score. The matched study population was predominantly male (n=90; 79%) and the mean age was 65±8 years (range: 43-83 years). No significant differences within 6 months after valve replacement were observed between the two groups with respect to mortality (M: N=1 (1.8%) vs. B: N=2 (3.6%)), bleeding (M: N=3 (5.8%) vs. B: N=3 (5.8%)), and neurological events (M: N=1 (1.8%) vs. B: N=3 (5.8%)). One patient with a biological composite graft required re-replacement due to prosthetic valve endocarditis 72 days after initial surgery.

The low 6-month mortality and good clinical outcome in comparison to mechanical composite graft replacement suggests that concomitant replacement of the total aortic root and the ascending aorta with stentless Freestyle® valves is a perfectly acceptable operation for elderly patients with aortic valve disease, normal or mildly dilated aortic sinuses, and a dilated ascending aorta to avoid anticoagulation therapy.

Octogenarians

The steadily increasing life expectancy of the population in the Western World, together with the progress in noninvasive diagnostic methods and operating techniques are leading to an increase in aortic valve surgery in elderly people. Between 1996 and 2002, 503 patients older than 60 years underwent aortic valve replacement with a stentless Freestyle bioprosthesis, with 76 of them being older than 80 years. In general, risk-adjusted analyses did not reveal an increased risk of operative mortality (p=0.4), postoperative atrial fibrillation (p=0.2), prolonged ventilation (p=0.5), prolonged stay in intensive care unit (p=0.3), or mid-term valve-related morbidity as prosthetic valve endocarditis (p=0.2), reoperation (p=0.4), bleeding events (p=0.1) and stroke (p=0.8), for octogenarians. Continuously increasing age was an independent risk factor for postoperative neurological complications (OR=1.8 per 10 years, p=0.04). Quality of life was equal to the general population of the same age. Median survival time of octogenarians was 5.2±0.5 years. Except for postoperative neurological complications, octogenarians receiving stentless bioprostheses had no increased risk of adverse perioperative and mid-term outcome in comparison to younger patients. As quality of life and life expectancy after AVR with stentless valves were equal to the general population, AVR with stentless bioprostheses should not be withheld from octogenarians [17].

Young patients

Current guidelines recommend a bioprosthesis for aortic valve replacement in patients under 65 years for lifestyle considerations after detailed discussion of the risks of anticoagulation versus the likelihood of a second valve replacement [1]. A recent review pointed out that for a 50-year-old man the mortality risk is not different after mechanical or after biological valve replacement, whereas the valve-related morbidity is more than 6 times higher after mechanical valve replacement. But after bioprosthetic replacement a 50-year-old man should anticipate at least one reoperation. The authors argue that if the patient wants no anticoagulation, minimal changes to lifestyle, and accepts the risk of at least one reoperation, then a biological valve is recommended. In contrast, if the patient wants to minimize the risk of reoperation and accepts significant lifestyle changes due to anticoagulation therapy, then a mechanical valve is recommended [15].

A multicenter study population of 127 patients under 60 years underwent aortic valve replacement with the Medtronic Freestyle® stentless bioprosthesis between 1993 and 2001. Median age was 48 years (range 10–59). The 30-day mortality was 1.6% (2/127). Mean follow-up was 7.4 ± 3.1 years. There were 11 late deaths (9.9%). Overall survival at 5 and 10 years was 95.2% and 89.3%, respectively. Freedom from reoperation for structural valve deterioration was 99.0% at 5 years and 76.4% at 10 years.

References

1. American College of Cardiology; American Heart Association Task Force on Practice Guidelines (Writing Committee to revise the 1998 guidelines for the management of patients with valvular heart disease), Society of Cardiovascular Anesthesiologists, Bonow RO, Carabello BA, Chatterjee K, de Leon AC Jr, Faxon DP, Freed MD et al (2006) ACC/AHA 2006 guidelines for the management of patients with valvular heart disease: Circulation 114(5):e84–e231
2. Albert A, Florath I, Rosendahl U, Hassanein W, Hodenberg EV, Bauer S et al (2007) Effect of surgeon on transprosthetic gradients after aortic valve replacement with Freestyle stentless bioprosthesis and its consequences: A follow-up study in 587 patients. J Cardiothorac Surg 2:40
3. Ali A, Halstead JC, Cafferty F, Sharples L, Rose F, Goulden R et al (2006) Are stentless valves superior to modern stented valves? A prospective randomized trial. Circulation 114(1 Suppl):I535–I540
4. Bach DS, Lemire MS, Eberhart D, Armstrong WF, Deeb GM (2000) Impact of high transvalvular velocities early after implantation of Freestyle stentless aortic bioprosthesis. J Heart Valve Dis 9:536–543
5. Bach DS, Cartier PA, Kon N, Johnson KG, Dumesnil JG, Doty DB (2001) Impact of high transvalvular to subvalvular velocity ratio early after aortic valve replacement with Freestyle stentless aortic bioprosthesis. Sem Thorac Cardiovasc Surg 13(4):75–81

6. Bach DS, Cartier PC, Kon ND, Johnson KG, Deeb GM, Doty DB et al (2002) Impact of implant technique following Freestyle stentless aortic valve replacement. Ann Thorac Surg 74:1107–1114
7. Bach DS, Kon ND, Dumesnil JG, Sintek CF, Doty DB (2005) Ten-year outcome after aortic valve replacement with the Freestyle stentless bioprosthesis. Ann Thorac Surg 80:480–487
8. Barratt-Boyes BG, Christie GW, Raudkivi PJ (1992) The stentless bioprosthesis: surgical challenges and implications for long-term durability. Eur J Cardiothorac Surg 6 [Suppl 1]:S39–S43
9. Böhm JO, Botha CA, Hemmer W, Schmidtke C, Bechtel JFM, Stierle U et al (2004) Hemodynamic performance following the ross operation: comparison of two different techniques. J Heart Valve Dis 13:174–181
10. Caradang R, Seshadri S, Beiser A, Kelly-Hayes M, Kase CS, Kannel WB et al (2006) Trends in incidence, lifetime risk severity, and 30-day mortality of stroke over the past 50 years. JAMA 296:2939–2946
11. Chambers JB, Rimington HM, Hodson F, Rajani R and Blauth CI (2006) The subcoronary Toronto stentless versus supra-annular Perimount stented replacement aortic valve: early clinical and hemodynamic results of a randomized comparison in 160 patients. J Thorac Cardiovasc Surg 131(4):878–872
12. Cohen G, Christakis GT, Joyner CD, Morgan CD, Tamariz M, Hanayama N et al (2002) Are stentless valves hemodynamically superior to stented valves? A prospective randomized trial. Ann Thorac Surg 73(3):767–775
13. Desai ND, Merin O, Cohen GD, Herman J, Mobilos S, Sever JY et al (2004) Long-term results of aortic valve replacement with the St. Jude Toronto Stentless Porcine Valve. Ann Thorac Surg 78:2076–2083
14. Doty JR, Flores JH, Millar RC, Doty DB (1998) Aortic valve replacement with medtronic freestyle bioprosthesis: operative technique and results. J Card Surg 13(3):208–217
15. El Oakley R, Kleine P and Bach DS (2008) Choice of prosthetic heart valve in today's practice. Circulation 117:253–256
16. Ennker J, Bauer S, Rosendahl U, Lehmann A, Mortasawi A, Schröder T et al (1999) Simultaneous myocardial revascularization and aortic valve replacmenent: Stentless versus stented Bioprostheses. Sem Thorac Cardiovasc Surg 11:83–87
17. Ennker J, Dalladaku F, Rosendahl U, Ennker IC, Mauser M, Florath I (2006) The stentless Freestyle Bioprosthesis: Impact of age over 80 years on quality of life, preoperative and mid-term outcome. J Card Surg 21:1–7
18. Ennker J, Albert A, Rosendahl U, Ennker IC, Dalladaku F, Florath I (2008) Ten-year experience with stentless aortic valves: Full-root versusu subcoronary implantation. Ann Thorac Surg 85:445–453
19. Ennker J, Ennker I, Albert A, Rosendahl U, Bauer S, Florath I (2009) The Freestyle stentless bioprosthesis in more than 1000 patients: a single-center experience over 10 years. J Card Surg 24:41–48
20. Florath I, Albert A, Rosendahl U, Ennker IC, Ennker J (2008) Impact of valve prosthesis-patient mismatch estimated by echocardiographic-determined effective orifice area on long-term outcome after aortic valve replacement. Am Heart J 155(6):1135–1142
21. German Federal Statistical Office (Statistisches Bundesamt der BRD, Abgekürzte Sterbetafel, 1996/98), Wiesbaden
22. Hammermeister K, Sethi GK, Henderson WG, Grover FL, Oprian C, Rahimtoola SH (2000) Outcomes 15 years after valve replacement with a mechanical versus a bioprosthetic valve: Final report of the veterans affairs randomized trial. J Am Coll Cardiol 36:1152–1158

23. Jamieson WRE, Burr LH, Miyagishima RT, Germann E, MacNab JS, Stanford E et al (2005) Carpentier-Edwards supra-annular aortic porcine bioprosthesis: Clinical performance over 20 years. J Thorac Cardiovasc Surg 130:994–1000
24. Kilian E, Oberhoffer M, Gulbins H, Uhlig A, Kreuzer E, Reichardt B (2004) Ten years' experience in aortic valve replacement with homografts in 389 cases. J Heart Valve Dis 13:554–559
25. Kon ND, Westaby S, Amarasena N, Pillai R, Cordell AR (1995) Comparison of implant techniques using the freestyle stentless porcine aortic valve. Ann Thorac Surg 59:857–862
26. Kunadian B, Vijayalakshmi K, Thornley AR, der Belder MA, Hunter S, Kendall S et al (2007) Meta-analysis of valve hemodynamics and left ventricular mass regression for stentless versus stented aortic valves. Ann Thorac Surg 84:73–79
27. Lehmann S, Walther T, Kempfert J, Leontyev S, Holzhey D, Rastan AJ et al (2007) Stentless versus conventional xenograft aortic valve replacement: Midterm results of a prospectively randomized trial. Ann Thorac Surg 84:467–472
28. Matsue H, Sawa Y, Takahashi T, Matsumiya G, Ohtake S, Hamada S et al (2001) Three-dimensional flow velocity quantification of freestyle aortic stentless bioprosthesis by magnetic resonance imaging: Surgical considerations. Sem Thorac Cardiovasc Surg 13:60–66
29. Mohammadi S, Baillot R, Voisine P, Mathieu P, Dagenais F (2006) Structural deterioration of the Freestyle aortic valve: Mode of presentation and mechanisms. J Thorac Cardiovasc Surg 132:401–406
30. O'Brien MF, Harrocks S, Stafford EG, Gardner MA, Pohlner PG, Tesar PJ, Stephens F (2001) The homograft aortic valve: a 29-year, 99.3% follow up of 1022 valve replacements. J Heart Valve Dis 10:334–344
31. O'Brien MF, Gardner MAH, Gralick B, Jalali H, Gordon JA, Whitehouse SL et al (2005) CryoLife-O'Brien stentless valve: 10-year results of 402 implants. Ann Thoracic Surg 79:757–766
32. Pavoni D, Badano LP, Ius F, Mazzero E, Frassini R, Gelsomino S et al (2007) Limited long-term durability of the Cryolife O'Brien stentless procine xenograft valve. Circulation 116:I-307–I-313
33. Perez de Arenaza D, Lees B, Flather M, Nuagara F, Husebye T, Jasinsky M et al (2005) Randomized comparison of stentless versus stented valves for aortic stenosis: effects on left ventricular mass. Circulation 112(17):2696–2702
34. Pibarot P, Dumesnil JG (2000) Hemodynamic and Clinical impact of prosthesis-patient mismatch in the aortic valve position and its prevention. J Am Coll Cardiol 36:1131–1141
35. Rahimtoola SH (1978) The problem of valve prosthesis-patient mismatch. Circulation 58:20–24
36. Rahimtoola SH (2003) Choice of prosthetic heart valve for adult patients. JACC 41:893–904
37. Riess F-C, Bader R, Cramer E, Hansen L, Kleijnen B, Wahl G et al (2007) Hemodynamic performance of the Medtronic Mosaic porcine bioprosthesis up to ten years. Ann Thorac Surg 83:1310–1318
38. Rizzoli G, Mirone S, Ius P, Polesel E, Bottio T, Salvador L et al (2006) Fifteen-year results with the Hancock II valve: A multicenter experience. J Thorac Cardiovasc Surg 132:602–609
39 Sintek CF, Pfeffer TA, Kochamba GS, Yun KL, Fletcher AD, Khonsari S (1998) Freestyle valve experience: technical considerations and mid-term results. J Card Surg 13(5):360–368
40. Stelzer P (2008) Stentless aortic valve replacement: porcine and pericardial. In: Cohn LH (ed) Cardiac surgery in the adult. 3 ed. CTSNet, pp 915–934

41. Walther T, Falk V, Langebartels G, Krüger M, Bernhardt U, Diegeler A et al (1999) Prospectively randomized evaluation of stentless versus conventional biological aortic valves: impact on early regression of left ventricular hypertrophy. Circulation 100(19 Suppl):II6–II10
42. Willems TP, van Herwerden LA, Steyerberg EW, Taams MA, Kleyburg VE, Hokken RB et al (1995) Subcoronary implantation or aortic root replacement for human tissue valves: sufficient data to prefer either technique? Ann Thorac Surg 60:S83–S86
43. Yankah CA, Pasic M, Musci M, Stein J, Detschades C, Siniawski H, Hetzer R (2008) Aortic valve replacement with the Mitroflow pericardial bioprosthesis: durability results up to 21 years. J Thorac Cardiovasc Surg 136(3):688–696

The ATS 3f Aortic Bioprosthesis

J. L. Cox

Introduction

Artificial tissue valves are less durable than artificial mechanical valves but they require less anticoagulation than mechanical valves and, thus, are associated with fewer bleeding complications. The past 40 years have witnessed persistent efforts to manufacture either a mechanical valve that does not require warfarin therapy or a tissue valve with greater long-term durability. The ATS 3f Aortic Bioprosthesis was developed specifically to address the durability problem with previously designed artificial tissue valves.

There are a variety of reasons why artificial tissue valves fail prematurely, including inherent deficiencies in the tissue chosen for the valve, failure to abolish its antigenicity during the fixation process, and detrimental alterations in its structural matrix due to the fixation process. While recognizing the potential importance of these factors, we believe that the major cause for the suboptimal durability of artificial tissue valves is improper valve *design*. In the past, artificial tissue valves were largely based on the erroneous concept that if an artificial valve *looks* like the native aortic valve it will probably *function* like the native aortic valve. This notion that "function follows form" is a faulty engineering concept and one that invariably results in the maldistribution of stress on the valve leaflets and in excessive turbulence of blood flow across the valves, both of which doom the valves to failure. The design of the ATS 3f valve is based on the proven engineering concept that "form follows function", i.e., it was designed not to *look* like the native aortic valve but rather to *function* like the native aortic valve. The fact that once implanted, it is difficult for even experienced echocardiographers to tell the difference between the ATS 3f Bioprosthesis and a normal native aortic valve (Fig. 1) simply confirms that we have accurately determined how heart valves *function* and that the *form* of the ATS 3f valve simply conforms to that function.

We believe that native heart valves function as if they were simple tubes whose sides collapse passively in response to external pressure [1]. The specific form that an individual native valve takes upon closure is determined by the anatomic constraints placed on the movements of that native

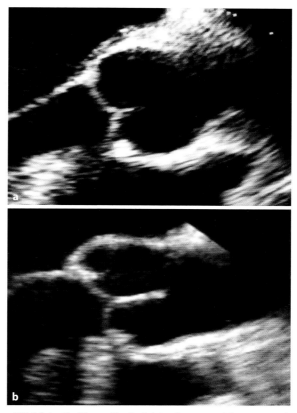

Fig. 1. Anatomic similarity of the ATS 3f Aortic Bioprosthesis (**a**) to the normal human aortic valve (**b**). (Courtesy of Dr. X.Y. Jin)

tubular valve. Indeed, if any one of the four native valves is completely excised and replaced by a simple tube and constrained in the same manner as the excised native valve, the replacement tube will assume the form of the native valve upon closure ... form follows function. Furthermore, both the distribution of stress on the "leaflets" of the replacement tubular valve when "closed" and the flow characteristics across the tubular valve when "open" are virtually superimposable on those of the native valve. The ATS 3f Aortic Bioprosthesis is a tubular valve that intentionally mimics the function of the native aortic valve. Because its design is based on the concept that "form follows function", it should be more durable than previously less well-designed artificial tissue valves.

Development and preclinical evaluation of the ATS 3f Aortic Bioprosthesis

The concept that native heart valves function as simple tubes whose sides collapse in response to external pressures evolved over many years of experimentation. Pilot experiments evaluating our hypothesis extended from 1987–1999 during which time we used small intentine submucosa (SIS) as the replacement valve tissue because it came naturally in tubular form and was close enough in diameter to those of the mitral, tricuspid and aortic valves that it could be used rather easily to replace all three of these native valves. When the "preliminary" studies over a dozen years proved promising, 3f Therapeutics, Inc. was founded and the development of a commercially viable product was initiated.

The choice of equine pericardium

Early studies demonstrated that SIS was simply not strong enough to withstand the rigors of the in vitro durability evaluations required by the USFDA. Multiple types of tissue, including bovine pericardium, were subsequently subjected to extensive tensile strength tests. Equine pericardium proved to be the strongest of all materials *in the areas of the valve where the stress was known to be greatest*, i.e., in the "belly" of the valve leaflets and it was at least as strong as bovine pericardium in all other areas of the newly constructed valve. Moreover, equine pericardium is thinner and more pliant than bovine pericardium and unlike bovine pericardium, there is little variation in the natural thickness of equine pericardium. The combination of equal or superior tensile strength in all planes and uniform thickness in a thinner, more pliant material in comparison to bovine pericardium and all other tissues evaluated, led to the selection of equine pericardium as the tissue of choice. However, any number of other tissues could have been chosen because the important characteristic of this valve is its *design*, not its tissue type.

Transvalvular flow dynamics

As the design of the commercial product necessarily evolved from a simple tube of tissue to its ultimate form, we were careful to maintain its tubular structure (Fig. 2). Prototype valves were then given to Dr. Mory Gharib, Professor and Chairman of the Department of Biomedical Engineering at the California Institute of Technology who voluntarily performed all transvalvular flow studies that were completely independent of 3f Therapeutics, Inc. Dr. Garib, a world-renowned expert in flow dynamics, summarized his findings by noting that the flow pattern across this new valve were "... vir-

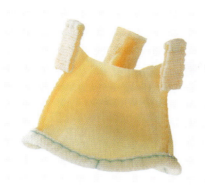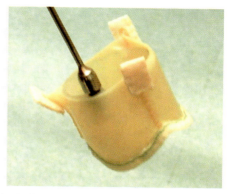

Fig. 2. Final design of the ATS 3f Aortic Bioprosthesis demonstrating that the tubular structure is maintained. Reproduced with permission from [1]; © American Association for Thoracic Surgery

tually superimposable on that of a normal human aortic valve ..." and that there was "... virtually no turbulence across the valve, again mimicking the normal human aortic valve ..." [1].

▌ Stress distribution on the valve leaflets

Finite-element analysis (FEA) had been performed in 1991 on simple tubes using a CAD-CAM system borrowed from the McDonnel-Douglas Aircraft Company in St. Louis, MO that was modified to measure the stress distribution in the heart and its valves rather than the distribution of stress on the F-15 Eagle and F-18 Hornet fighter planes that McDonnel-Douglas manufactured. After the commercial 3f valve was designed and constructed, it was subjected to a new series of FEA studies beginning in 1999 with more advanced dynamic capabilities. All of these studies revealed a remarkable and absolutely critical finding ... the site of lowest stress on the 3f valve occurred at the commissural posts (Fig. 3). This is precisely the distribution of stress in a normal human aortic valve and differs distinctly from the stress distribution of every other artificial tissue valve ever constructed in that the latter all have the highest stress at their commissural posts! This is generally thought to be why the common failure mode of artificial tissue valves is leaflet tear at or near their commissural post attachments. Similarly, it is a major reason why we expect the ATS 3f valve to last longer than previously designed artificial tissue valves.

▌ In vitro hemodynamic performance

All in vitro hemodynamic and durability tests of the 3f valve were performed using the St. Jude Medical Toronto SPV valve as a control. That valve was chosen as our control because at the time, it was considered to be the state-of-the-art tissue valve with the best hemodynamics of any tis-

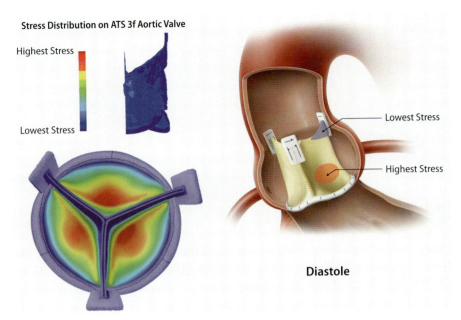

Fig. 3. Results of Finite Element Analysis of the distribution of stress on the leaflets of the ATS 3f Aortic Bioprosthesis during ventricular diastole. Note the highest stress in the "belly" of the leaflets and the LOWEST stress at the commissural posts. This stress distribution pattern is common to the ATS 3f Aortic Bioprosthesis and the normal human aortic valve. Other artificial tissue aortic valves have the *highest* level of stress at their commissural posts, their most common site of failure

sue valve yet designed. Prior to initiating those studies, we sought the advice of the USFDA with a testing problem unique to the 3f valve. Unlike other stentless valves, including the SPV valve, the 3f valve actually has no stent. Therefore, whatever material was used to mount the valve for study purposes had the potential to alter the function of the valve. We had designed a latex aorta with sinuses of Valsalva (aortic sinuses) and the USFDA directed us to use it to mount the 3f valve during our hemodynamic studies. However, the USFDA stipulated that we use two groups of latex aortas, one engineered to have a compliance of 16% (mimicking a normal aorta) and another engineered to a compliance of 4% (mimicking a "stiff" aorta). All valve sizes from 19 mm to 29 mm were then subjected to both groups of latex aortas at varying cardiac outputs. The results clearly demonstrated the superior flow characteristics of the 3f valve in comparison to the SPV valve at all flow rates in both normal and "stiff" latex aortas (Fig. 4). Subsequent experimental studies in calves by Mueller and von Segesser confirmed the hemodynamic superiority of the ATS 3f valve over other stentless prostheses in the immediate postimplant period [2].

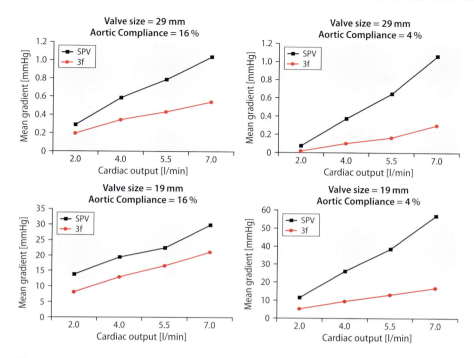

Fig. 4. In vitro comparison of the gradients across the ATS 3f Aortic Bioprosthesis and the Toronto SPV valve. The two top panels compare size 29 mm valves and the two lower panels compare size 19 mm valves. The two left panels compare valves implanted inside latex aortas with a compliance of 16% and the two right panels compare valves implanted inside latex aortas with a compliance of 4%. The ATS 3f valve outperforms the Toronto SPV valve at both sizes, at both degrees of aortic "stiffness" and across all cardiac outputs measured. Reproduced by permission from [1]; © American Association for Thoracic Surgery

■ In vitro durability tests

Accelerated wear tests were performed using six standard accelerated wear testers each of which housed 10 individual valves, nine 3f valves and one SPV valve. The testers were set to open and close the valves at physiologic transvalvular pressures 700 times per minute. At this rate, 200 million cycles was "equivalent" to 5 years clinically, far more than the USFDA required of any tissue valve for approval. Again, the 3f valve outperformed the SPV valve at all sizes in both normal and "stiff" aortas (Fig. 5). Subsequent studies that have been allowed to extend nearly three times as long continue to show that the ATS 3f valve outperforms other valves, including the Edwards Perimount valve, in terms of its durability (Fig. 6).

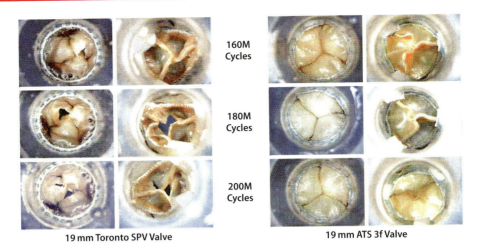

Fig. 5. In vitro comparison of the durability of the ATS 3f Aortic Bioprosthesis and the Toronto SPV valve as determined by their relative degrees of destruction in accelerated wear testers. Each of six testers held 9 ATS 3f valves and 1 Toronto SPV valve. The valves were opened and closed 700 times per minute for the designated number of cycles. This figure shows the typical results for 19 mm valves but similar results were attained at all valve sizes up to 29 mm. 200 million cycles is equivalent to the average number of heartbeats in 5 years but to more than 5 years of actual clinical durability. Reproduced by permission from [1]; © American Association for Thoracic Surgery

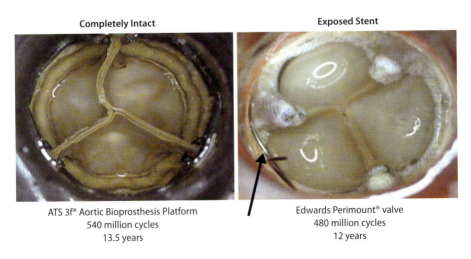

Fig. 6. In vitro comparison of the durability of the ATS 3f Aortic Bioprosthesis and the Edwards Perimount valve as determined by their relative degrees of destruction in accelerated wear testers. The valves were opened and closed 700 times per minute for the designated number of cycles

Clinical performance and results

The first 3f valve was implanted clinically by Drs. Hugo Vanermann and Philippe Castleman in Aalst, Belgium on October 3, 2001. The initial clinical trial included 405 patients. The European CE Mark was issued for the 3f valve in September 2004 and the company was subsequently purchased by ATS Medical, Inc. in 2007. The valve, subsequently known as the ATS 3f Aortic Bioprosthesis, received final USFDA approval on October 31, 2008.

Clinical hemodynamic performance

Approximately 2500 ATS 3f valves have now been implanted world-wide and there has been only one reported instance of what had to be classified technically as a "structural valve failure". Early clinical implants during the European Clinical Trial which ended in March 2004 demonstrated that when properly sized, the valves had extremely small gradients and excellent hemodynamics. However, because the valve is devoid of any type of stent, it can be folded, collapsed or "crimped" so that almost any size valve can be physically inserted into almost any size aortic root. This led to problems early in the trial in which some surgeons implanted valves that were too large for the aortic root, often by two full sizes, resulting in unacceptable transvalvular gradients. Once the oversizing problem was recognized, the low transvalvular gradients across the ATS 3f valve proved to be one of its strongest attributes [3–7].

Clinical flow dynamics and aortic root preservation

One day in 2004, we received a surprising and unsolicited note from Dr. X.Y. Jin, an echocardiographer at the Radcliffe Infirmary, Oxford University stating that as a part of his on-going evaluation of all commercial stentless tissue valves, he had performed an extensive study of the 3f valves that had been implanted by his surgical colleague, Mr. Ravi Pillai as a part of our European Clinical Trial. His note stated that "The 3f valve represents a major milestone towards achieving native aortic valve structure and function" [8]. In addition to *looking* almost exactly like a normal human aortic valve on Echo (form follows function), Jin's studies showed remarkably similar flow characteristics in the aortic root, especially during ventricular systole when the valve leaflets are open. As blood passes out the distal end of the valve, a portion of it "wraps around" over the ends of the leaflets and swirls downward into the aortic sinuses to initiate the actual closure of the leaflets during end-systole. The flow patterns in the normal aortic valve and in the ATS 3f valve are virtually indistinguishable at this critical point in the cardiac cycle (Fig. 7). This flow characteristic results in both

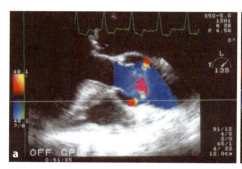 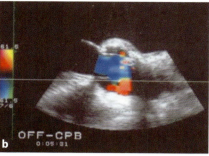

Fig. 7. Color Doppler-flow studies of the trans-valvular flow dynamics of the normal human aortic valve (left panel) and the ATS 3f Aortic Bioprosthesis (right panel). Note that as the blood is ejected from the left ventricle through the open aortic valve during systole, it is already beginning to flow over the edges of the open leaflets to enter the aortic sinuses. This characteristic, which is unique to the ATS 3f valve among artificial prostheses, not only enhances coronary artery flow during ventricular systole but also augments the optimal distribution of stress on the aortic valve leaflets during diastole [8, 9]. (Courtesy of Dr. X.Y. Jin)

the normal human aortic valve and the ATS 3f valve closing *from the belly of the leaflets upward* towards the commissural posts, a major factor that further reduces the stress on the commissural posts and adjacent leaflet edges (see Fig. 3).

Dr. Jin also has unpublished data that cannot be disclosed in any detail here but which demonstrate that unlike all other artificial valves of any type, mechanical or tissue, the ATS 3f valve allows the normal anatomy and hemodynamic function of the aortic root to be preserved following implantation [9]. This is true partly because of the implantation technique that is unique to the ATS 3f valve in which the continuity of the left ventricular outflow tract (LVOT) and the sinotubular junction (STJ) are maintained but without any intervening sutures between the two that traverse the aortic sinuses and destroy their ability to reduce, regulate, and properly distribute stress on the aortic valve leaflets throughout the cardiac cycle.

Summary

The ATS 3f Aortic Bioprosthesis is the vanguard of a new generation of artificial tissue valves that diverge markedly from previous generations in its design characteristics. Every in vitro study and every controlled clinical evaluation performed to date indicates that this valve design is superior to previous tissue valve design and, therefore, should result in enhanced long-term durability. The two major goals of the original radical design change were the following: (1) superior flow characteristics with a minimum of transvalvular flow turbulence, and (2) improved distribution of stress on the valve leaflets. It was believed that these two goals would result in improved durability of artificial tissue valves. To those two goals has been added the observation that normal aortic root anatomy and function are essential to the long-term durability of any artificial tissue valve. The ATS 3f valve accomplishes all three of these goals and is unique in doing so, thus, offering the greatest promise of a truly long-term artificial tissue heart valve.

References

1. Cox JL, Ad N, Myers K, Gharib M, Quijano RC (2005) Tubular heart valves: a new tissue prosthesis design – preclinical evaluation of the 3F aortic bioprosthesis. J Thorac Cardiovasc Surg 130(2):520–527
2. Mueller XM, von Segesser LK (2003) A new equine pericardial stentless valve. J Thorac Cardiovasc Surg 125(6):1405–1411
3. Sadowski J, Kapelak B, Bartu K, My J, Drwita R (2004) Stentless 3F Therapeutics Aortic Bioprosthesis – a new alternative to aortic valve replacement. Acta Cardiol 59(2):231–232
4. Doss M, Martens S, Wood JP, Miskovic A, Christodoulou T, Wimmer-Greinecker G, Moritz A (2005) Aortic leaflet replacement with the new 3F stentless aortic bioprosthesis. Ann Thorac Surg 79(2):682–685
5. Eckstein FS, Tevaearai H, Keller D, Schmidli J, Immer FF, Seiler C, Saner H, Carrel TP (2004) Early clinical experience with a new tubular equine pericardial stentless aortic valve. Heart Surg Forum 7(5):E498–502
6. Grubitzsch H, Linneweber J, Kossagk C, Sanli E, Beholz S, Konertz WF (2005) Aortic valve replacement with new-generation stentless pericardial valves: short-term clinical and hemodynamic results. J Heart Valve Dis 14(5):623–629
7. Linneweber J, Kossagk C, Rogge ML, Dushe S, Dohmen P, Konertz W (2006) Clinical experience with the 3F stentless aortic bioprosthesis: one-year follow up. J Heart Valve Dis 15(4):545–548
8. Jin XY: Personal Communication
9. Jin XY, Du X, Kattach H, Ratnatunga C, Pillai R (2009) Effects of prosthetic valve substitute on aortic root geometry and dynamics. Submitted to Annals of Thoracic Surgery

The Vascutek Elan stentless porcine prosthesis – the Glasgow experience

G. A. Berg, P. Sonecki, R. B. S. Berg, K. J. D. MacArthur

Introduction

The ideal aortic valve implant will provide maximum restoration of aortic valve dynamics, a low transvalvular gradient, minimal long-term structural valvular degeneration, a low infection rate and will be relatively easy to implant. Stentless bioprosthetic valves have been shown to provide excellent hemodynamics in comparison to first and second generation stented bioprostheses, with corresponding early greater regression in left ventricular mass [14]. We assessed the medium term outcome of implantation of the Vascutek Elan aortic stentless bioprosthesis (Vascutek, Newmains Avenue, Inchinnan, Renfrewshire PA4 9RR, Scotland, UK) in a single center (Fig. 1).

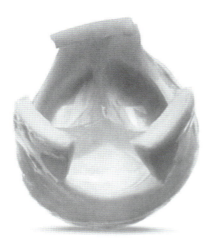

Fig. 1. Vascutek Elan stentless bioprosthesis

Materials and methods

This study was approved by the local hospital research ethics committee. All patients underwent an aortic valve replacement in the Western Infirmary, Glasgow between September 1999 and January 2008. Patients had follow-up echocardiographic examination as clinically indicated. Clinical follow-up of all survivors was carried out in October 2007. Data was prospectively entered into a clinical database Late deaths were correlated with the Information Services Division of the Scottish NHS. All surviving patients underwent clinical follow-up. Echocardiographic data was analyzed where available.

Study population

From August 1999 to February 2008, 363 Elan stentless valves were inserted into 361 consecutive patients in a single institution. The patient mean age (± standard deviation was 71.7 ± 8.4 (range 27 to 88 years). Age groupings are shown in Fig. 2. Preoperative clinical characteristics are presented in Table 1 and operative procedures in Table 2.

Echocardiography

Echocardiographic studies were analyzed at 2 ± 0.6 and 6 ± 1.4 years after valve replacement. Data collected included fractional shortening and left ventricular mass, left ventricular systolic and diastolic dimensions. Data on aortic valve and root morphology and the mechanism of valve failure, where relevant, were also collected. Structural and nonstructural valve deterioration was defined according to guidelines published by Edmunds [7].

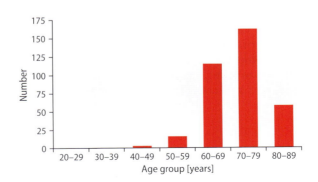

Fig. 2. Patient age range

Table 1. Patient characteristics

Recipient number	361
Mean age	71.7 ± 8.4 yrs Range 27–88
Male	168 (46.5%)
Coronary artery disease (%)	145 (40.2%)
Mitral valve disease (%)	25 (6.9%)
NYHA I	32 (8.9%)
NYHA II	134 (37.1%)
NYHA III	165 (45.7%)
NYHA IV	30 (8.3%)
Emergency	5 (1.4%)
Urgent	26 (7.2%)
Previous open heart surgery	16 (4.4%)
Cerebrovascular disease	46 (12.7%)

NYHA New York Heart Association class

Table 2. Operative procedures

	All	Isolated AVR	AVR + CABG	AVR + Other
Patients	361	185	145	31
Mean age (yrs)	71.7	70.6	74.0	68.2
Male	46.5%	42.2%	51.7%	48.4%
Logistic EuroSCORE	8.9%	8.1%	7.7%	18.8%
Redo	16 (4.4%)	2	1	13

Surgical technique

The indications for surgery are shown in Table 3. All prostheses were inserted using a similar subcoronary technique. The aorta was opened using a horizontal aortotomy. After excision of the aortic valve and decalcification, the annulus and sinotubular junction were measured separately. A stentless valve was not deemed suitable for insertion if there was a discrepancy between the measurements of more than 2 mm. The larger of the measurement was used as the appropriate prosthesis size. Prostheses were inserted to using a two layer technique, with interrupted 2/0 Tycron for the first layer and continuous 4/0 Prolene for the second.

Table 3. Indications for surgery

Patients	361
Aortic stenosis (%)	281 (77.8%)
Aortic incompetence (%)	47 (13.0%)
Mixed	33 (9.2%)
Calcific degeneration	284 (77.8%)
Rheumatic	31 (8.6%)
Myxomatous degeneration	10 (2.8%)
Congenital	14 (3.9%)
Infection	17 (4.7%)
Native endocarditis (%)	12
Prosthetic valve endocarditis	5
Aortic/atrial fistula	1
Thrombosed prosthesis	1

Statistical analysis

Survival analyses using the Kaplan-Meier method were used to estimate survival and freedom from valve-related adverse events.

Results

From August 1999 until January 2008, 363 Elan stentless bioprostheses were implanted into 361 consecutive patients at our institution. The range of valve sizes inserted are shown in Fig. 3. An isolated first time aortic valve replacement was performed in 185 (51.2%) patients. Coronary artery bypass grafts were performed in 145 (40.2%) patients. Overall hospital mortality was 4.2% (Logistic EuroSCORE 8.9%). The Elan valve was inserted in 17 (4.7%) patients with native or prosthetic valve endocarditis. Two of these patients presented with aortic root abscesses secondary to native aortic valve infectious endocarditis and subsequently had repeat aortic valve replacements with Elan bioprostheses for continuing infection. Both have competent valves at long-term follow-up. The hospital mortality for isolated first time aortic valve replacement was 2.2% (Logistic EuroSCORE 8.1%). The operative and postoperative outcomes are shown in Table 4. Two patients sustained a postoperative cerebrovascular injury with a severe residual defect (0.6%).

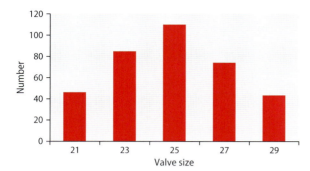

Fig. 3. Size of Elan valve inserted

Table 4. Operative and postoperative outcomes

	All	Isolated AVR	AVR + CABG	AVR + Other
Patients	361	185	145	31
Ischemic time (min)	79	71	82	114
Cardiopulmonary bypass time (min)	103	90	109	149
Ventilation	17 h	12 h	18 h	4 d 4 h
Hospital stay	9 d 6 h	8 d 3 h	9 d 19 h	13 d 10 h
Logistic EuroSCORE	8.90%	8.10%	7.70%	18.80%
Hospital mortality	15 (4.2%)	4 (2.2%)	8 (5.5%)	3 (9.7%)

Total follow-up was 1251 patient years. Late deaths occurred in 65 patients, and six of them were valve related (1.8% patient/years). Overall patient survival was 74.3 ± 2.8% and 54.9 ± 5.9% at 5 and 8 years, respectively (Fig. 4). Seven valves (1.9%) required reoperation. Five were due to endocarditis (three late prosthetic valve endocarditis and two for continuing infection following aortic valve replacement for native valve endocarditis), one for a paravalve leak and one due to a leaflet tear associated with calcification. Freedom from structural and nonstructural valve deterioration (Fig. 5) and reoperation (Fig. 6) was 91% ± 4% with 94% ± 4%, respectively, at 8 years.

Early hemodynamic data measured at echocardiography are shown in Table 5. All valve sizes had a mean gradient of less than 6 mm. Surviving patients who were fit enough to travel to hospital for review had echocardiography carried out at a mean of 75 months following operation. These data are shown in Table 6.

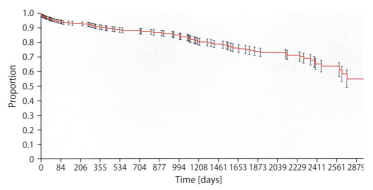

Fig. 4. Kaplan Meier freedom from all cause death after aortic valve replacement with the Elan stentless valve

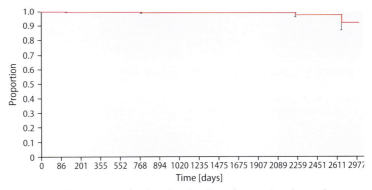

Fig. 5. Kaplan-Meier freedom from structural valve deterioration after aortic valve replacement with the Elan stentless valve

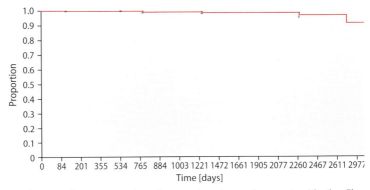

Fig. 6. Kaplan-Meier freedom from reoperation after aortic valve replacement with the Elan stentless valve

Table 5. Early echocardiographic hemodynamic data

Valve size (mmHg)	Mean gradient (mmHg)	Peak gradient (mmHg)	Peak flow velocity (m/s)	EOAI (cm^2/m^2)
21	5.1±0.9	11.0±0.2	1.66±0.18	0.94
23	4.4±0.3	13.5±0.4	1.82±0.1	0.93
25	5.5±0.6	13.4±0.4	1.78±0.1	1.00
27	4.2±0.7	10.2±1.7	1.69±0.1	1.11
29	4.3±0.6	9.6±1.2	1.53±0.1	1.20

Table 6. Medium term echocardiographic hemodynamic data

Valve size (mmHg)	Mean gradient (mmHg)	Peak gradient (mmHg)	Peak flow velocity (m/s)
21	12.0±3.9	27.0±5.2	2.57±1.3
23	10.2±2.3	21.0±3.74	2.26±0.9
25	8.0±1.7	17.0±2.9	2.0±0.3
27	6.3±1.4	6.3±2.2	1.24±0.2
29	3.2±0.9	7.0±2.3	1.3±0.2

Discussion

The Vascutek Elan stentless valve is made from a single piece of porcine tissue component to ensure retention of the proper anatomical shape. It is zero pressure fixated and fresh mounted to minimize bending stresses on the valve during manufacture. The muscle bar of the porcine aortic root is covered with a double layer of porcine pericardium. The valve therefore has a minimal amount of prosthetic material inserted during its manufacture. We found its handling characteristics were similar to a human homograft.

The human homograft is considered to be the best valve to be inserted in the presence of infection [15, 18], because of its handling characteristics and the ability to use the anterior leaflet of the mitral valve to patch defects associated with abscess formation. It also has low reinfection rate, excellent function and longevity [9]. However, human homografts of the appropriate size are not always available. The Shelhigh SuperStentless valve when used with a tissue conduit has been reported to have similar hemodynamic results, ease of implantation and low rates of recurrent endocarditis compared with homografts. Siniawski et al. concluded that these stentless valves were preferable to homografts in cases of aortic endocarditis [17]. The same author also concluded that valves that do not contain artificial fabric material offer resistance to bacterial infection [16].

Table 7. Causes of late death

Total late deaths	65 (18%)
Accidental overdose	1
Cancer	6
Cardiac failure	7
Cerebral infarction	4
Head injury	1
Liver failure	1
Multi-organ failure	1
Myocardial infarction	7
Perforated bowel	1
Pneumonia	6
Renal failure	1
Respiratory failure	3
Septicemia	2
Shock	1
Unknown	23

We inserted the Elan valve in 17 patients with infective endocarditis. In two patients the procedures were done as a salvage procedure in association with end-stage heart failure and gross aortic incompetence with multiple root abscesses. Stentless valves were inserted to achieve aortic valve competence and improve hemodynamics in a situation where insertion of a stented bioprosthesis may not have been possible. Both patients survived but required early re-replacement of the stentless valves with a following full recovery. Other workers have used subcoronary stentless bioprostheses for the treatment of endocarditis [8, 13, 17].

Stentless aortic bioprostheses were reintroduced in order to overcome problems associated with durability of stented bioprostheses at that time and to improve valve hemodynamics. Studies have shown that early hemodynamics of stentless valves are superior to stented valves particularly in the first 12 months following implantation [2, 18]. Although there is a quicker improvement in reduction of left ventricular mass, it has not been translated into a significantly different clinical improvement. Studies show that the medium term results of stentless porcine prostheses are excellent [1, 5, 10, 12] but there are concerns regarding late structural valve deterioration [6]. In addition, when compared to third generation stented bioprostheses the hemodynamic advantage may not be as great across the range of valve sizes [3, 4, 11], although comparison with a stentless valve with a potentially obstructive cloth covering may not be appropriate. We found that the medium term (8 year follow-up) results of the Elan stentless valve were excellent; however, further follow-up to assess the long-term results is required.

Table 8. Freedom from death

At risk	286	122	34
Freedom from	1 year	5 years	7 years
Cardiac-related death	94.5 ± 1.2	91.1 ± 1.8	89.6 ± 2.3
Valve-related death	98.4 ± 0.7	91.9 ± 2.0	84.3 ± 3.8
All death	90.2 ± 1.6	74.7 ± 2.7	64.5 ± 3.9

Limitations of the study

This study has limitations due to the retrospective design. Clinical and echocardiographic examination of all surviving patients was not possible due to travel restrictions of elderly patients in the west of Scotland. There were a relatively small number of patients who had their valves inserted more than five years ago.

Conclusions

The Elan stentless valve, implanted in an elderly population, is associated with excellent clinical outcomes at eight years of follow-up. This study has shown that the valve is durable in the medium term and appears to be a good option for patients with native or prosthetic valve endocarditis in an elderly age group.

References

1. Akar AR, Szafranek A, Alexiou C, Janas R, Jasinski MJ, Swanevelder J, Sosnowski AW (2002) Use of stentless xenografts in the aortic position: determinants of early and late outcome. Ann Thorac Surg 74:1450–1457, discussion 1457–1458
2. Borger MA, Carson SM, Ivanov J, Rao V, Scully HE, Feindel CM, David TE (2005) Stentless aortic valves are hemodynamically superior to stented valves during mid-term follow-up: a large retrospective study. Ann Thorac Surg 80:2180–2185
3. Chambers J, Rimington H, Rajani R, Hodson F, Blauth C (2004) Hemodynamic performance on exercise: comparison of a stentless and stented biological aortic valve replacement. J Heart Valve Dis 13:729–733
4. Chambers JB, Rimington HM, Hodson F, Rajani R, Blauth CI (2006) The subcoronary Toronto stentless versus supra-annular Perimount stented replacement aortic valve: early clinical and hemodynamic results of a randomized comparison in 160 patients. J Thorac Cardiovasc Surg 131:878–872

5. Dellgren G, Eriksson MJ, Brodin LA, Radegran K (2002) Eleven years' experience with the Biocor stentless aortic bioprosthesis: clinical and hemodynamic follow-up with long-term relative survival rate. Eur J Cardiothorac Surg 22:912–921
6. Desai ND, Merin O, Cohen GN, Herman J, Mobilos S, Sever JY, Fremes SE, Goldman BS, Christakis GT (2004) Long-term results of aortic valve replacement with the St. Jude Toronto stentless porcine valve. Ann Thorac Surg 78:2076–2083; discussion 2076–2083
7. Edmunds LHJ, Clark RE, Cohn LH, Grunkemeier GL, Miller DC, Weisel RD (1996) Guidelines for reporting morbidity and mortality after cardiac valvular operations. Eur J Cardiothorac Surg 10:812–816
8. Ennker JA, Albert AA, Rosendahl UP, Ennker IC, Dalladaku F, Florath I (2008) Ten-year experience with stentless aortic valves: full-root versus subcoronary implantation. Ann Thorac Surg 85:445–452; discussion 452–453
9. Knosalla C, Weng Y, Yankah CA, Siniawski H, Hofmeister J, Hammerschmidt R, Loebe M, Hetzer R (2000) Surgical treatment of active infective aortic valve endocarditis with associated periannular abscess – 11 year results. Eur Heart J 21:490–497
10. Martinovic I, Everlien M, Farah I, Wittlinger T, Knez I, Greve H, Vogt P (2005) Midterm results after aortic valve replacement with a stentless bioprosthesis aortic valve. Ann Thorac Surg 80:198–203
11. Nagy ZL, Bodi A, Len A, Balogh I, Peterffy A (2005) Three years' experience with the sorin pericarbon stentless prosthesis: mid-term results with three different implantation techniques. J Heart Valve Dis. 14:72–77
12. O'Brien MF, Gardner MA, Garlick B, Jalali H, Gordon JA, Whitehouse SL, Strugnell WE, Slaughter R (2005) CryoLife-O'Brien stentless valve: 10-year results of 402 implants. Ann Thorac Surg 79:757–766
13. Okada K, Tanaka H, Takahashi H, Morimoto N, Munakata H, Asano M, Matsumori M, Kawanishi Y, Nakagiri K, Okita Y (2008) Aortic root replacement for destructive aortic valve endocarditis with left ventricular-aortic discontinuity. Ann Thorac Surg 85:940–945
14. Raja SG, Macarthur KJ, Pollock JC (2006) Impact of stentless aortic valves on left ventricular function and hypertrophy: current best available evidence. J Card Surg 21:313–319
15. Sabik JF, Lytle BW, Blackstone EH, Marullo AG, Pettersson GB, Cosgrove DM (2002) Aortic root replacement with cryopreserved allograft for prosthetic valve endocarditis. Ann Thorac Surg 74:650–659, discussion 659
16. Siniawski H, Grauhan O, Hofmann M, Pasic M, Weng Y, Yankah C, Lehmkuhl H, Hetzer R (2004) Factors influencing the results of double-valve surgery in patients with fulminant endocarditis: the importance of valve selection. Heart Surg Forum 7:E405–410
17. Siniawski H, Lehmkuhl H, Weng Y, Pasic M, Yankah C, Hoffmann M, Behnke I, Hetzer R (2003) Stentless aortic valves as an alternative to homografts for valve replacement in active infective endocarditis complicated by ring abscess. Ann Thorac Surg 75:803–808, discussion 808
18. Yankah CA, Pasic M, Klose H, Siniawski H, Weng Y, Hetzer R (2005) Homograft reconstruction of the aortic root for endocarditis with periannular abscess: a 17-year study. Eur J Cardiothorac Surg 28:69–75

Sorin pericardial valves

Operative technique and early results of biological valves

S. Beholz, S. Meyer, N. von Wasielewski, W. F. Konertz

Introduction

Porcine stentless valves have proven excellent long-term results in aortic valve replacement [8] with improved left ventricular reverse remodeling as compared to stented biological valves [21]. The Sorin Pericarbon Freedom[TM] stentless valve (Sorin Group, Saluggia, Italy) is a truly stentless valve formed from two sheets of bovine pericardium (Fig. 1) which has been available since 1994 [20]. To overcome the adverse effects of glutaraldehyde as used in most bioprostheses on freedom from structural valve deterioration and reoperation, the pericardium is treated by homocystic acid which has proven to reduce mineralization in vitro and in vivo [19]. The valve is designed for subcoronary implantation [3, 22] using interrupted or continuous suture techniques at the inflow side without differences in early postoperative hemodynamics [2]. As a further improvement of the already excellent hemodynamics of the valve even as compared to other pericardial stentless valves [11], in 2004 a modification of the Sorin Pericarbon Free-

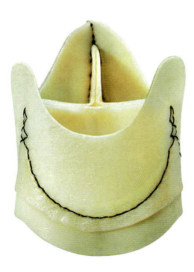

Fig. 1. Sorin Pericarbon Freedom[TM] stentless valve

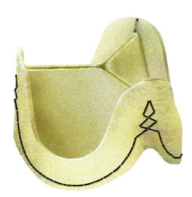

Fig. 2. Freedom™ Solo stentless valve

dom™ stentless valve was introduced. The Freedom™ Solo stentless valve (Fig. 2) (Sorin Group, Saluggia, Italy) uses the same pericardial material but is designed for supraannular implantation [1, 17] using one single running suture line in the sinuses of valsalva.

The paper describes the operative experience and the early clinical and hemodynamic results of both valves.

Material and methods

All patients receiving bovine pericardial stentless valves in our institution were included in the study. From November 2001 to January 2009 the Sorin Pericarbon Freedom™ stentless valve (group Freedom) and from June 2004 to January 2009 the Freedom™ Solo stentless valve (group Solo) were implanted.

The patients were operated on in general anesthesia, median sternotomy, and using normothermic cardiopulmonary bypass. Concomitant procedures were performed prior to the valve replacement except proximal anastomoses of saphenous vein grafts, which were performed immediately prior to declamping the aorta. Intermittent warm antegrade cardioplegia [5] was applied to the aortic root and after transverse aortotomy directly to the coronary ostia. After transverse aortotomy (Fig. 3), thorough resection of the leaflets and, in case of calcification, of all calcified structures (Fig. 4) was performed.

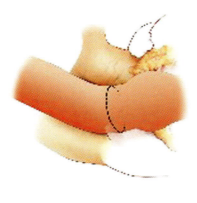

Fig. 3. Transverse aortotomy

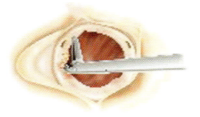

Fig. 4. Thorough resection of calcification

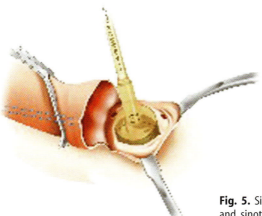

Fig. 5. Sizing of annulus and sinotubular junction

Operative technique Freedom

Sizing was performed according to the diameter of the annulus (Fig. 5) and the sinotubular junction (STJ): if the size of the STJ did not exceed 20% of the diameter of the annulus, the latter was chosen as the valve size. In case of a larger discrepancy between the STJ and annulus, the valve was chosen

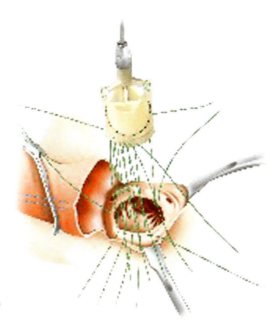

Fig. 6. Interrupted inflow suture line of Freedom valve

one size larger than the annulus and proper aortoraphy was performed with the closure of the aortotomy. The intraoperatively found pathology did not affect the preoperative choice of implantation technique for the inflow suture line: either 18 to 30 single 2-0 braided polyester sutures without reinforcement were used (Fig. 6); before tying the sutures, the valve was inverted into the LVOT according to the instructions for use (Fig. 7). Alternatively one single running 3-0 polypropylene suture was used for fixation in the LVOT (Fig. 8). After eversion of the valve, the outflow site of the valve was fixed to the aortic root using a running 4-0 polypropylene suture in a subcoronary fashion (Fig. 9).

Operative technique Solo

During decalcification, special care was taken not to affect the annulus (Fig. 4). In case of defects, these were closed using 4-0 polypropylene sutures prior to sizing. Then sizing, using intraoperative testing by obturators (Fig. 5), was performed according to the diameter of the STJ in case of the absence of ectasia of the aortic root. If the size of STJ exceeded 20% of the diameter of the annulus, patients were excluded from the implantation. No reinforcement of the sinotubular junction or enlargement of annulus was performed in any patient.

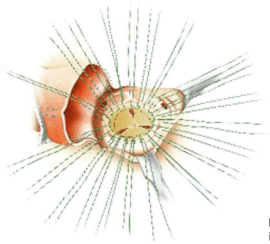

Fig. 7. Inverting the Freedom valve into the LVOT

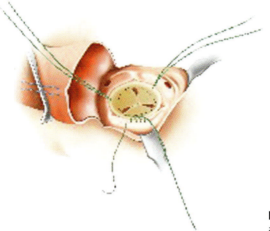

Fig. 8. Continuous suture line at inflow of the Freedom valve

The Freedom™ Solo valve was implanted using a single continuous suture line in supraannular technique similar to the technique described for the CryoLife-O'Brien valve [15] as recommended by the manufacturer: beginning from the deepest point of each sinus of Valsalva (Fig. 10), the pericardial skirt of the outer layer was sewn to the sinus of Valsalva using three 4-0 polypropylene sutures 3–4 mm apart from the annulus (Fig. 11). At the top of the commissures, the sutures were tied outside the aorta without the need for any reinforcement (Fig. 12).

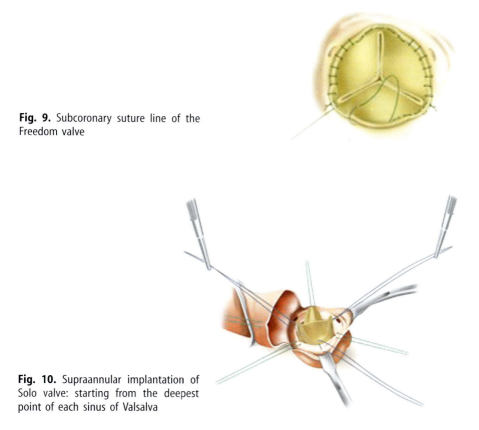

Fig. 9. Subcoronary suture line of the Freedom valve

Fig. 10. Supraannular implantation of Solo valve: starting from the deepest point of each sinus of Valsalva

In both valves after closure of the aortotomy and release of the cross clamp, intraoperative transesophageal echocardiography was performed to monitor deairing of the heart as well as to investigate the proper function of the valve. Special attention was brought to a symmetric opening of the three leaflets and the absence of any paravalvular leakage or transvalvular regurgitation more than trivial. Patients were then weaned from bypass and transmitted to the ICU. No routine anticoagulation was performed after removal of the chest tubes. Warfarin was given only in those patients after left atrial ablation for 3 months. In every patient, 100 mg acetylsalicylic acid was prescribed.

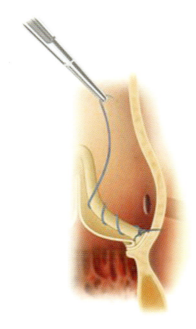

Fig. 11. Supraannular implantation technique of the Solo valve

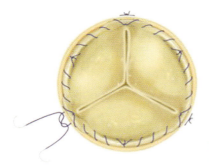

Fig. 12. Completing implantation of the Solo valve

Results

In total 709 patients were included in the study: 430 patients received a Freedom valve and 279 a Solo valve, respectively (Table 1). Due to the restriction in case of enlargement of the ascending aorta including STJ, fewer patients receiving a Solo valve suffered from isolated regurgitation. Comparable rates of associated procedures were performed in both valves; in case of endocarditis the Freedom valve was first choice due to its property to cover any defects after debridement (Table 2).

Table 1. Included patients

	Freedom (n=430)	Solo (n=279)	p
Age (yrs)	72.6 ± 9.0	75.1 ± 8.0	n.s.
Male/female (%)	46/54	53/47	n.s
Weight (kg)	74.9 ± 13.7	76.1 ± 16.5	n.s.
Height (cm)	167.0 ± 8.4	167.0 ± 9.1	n.s.
Stenosis/regurgitation/mixed (%)	64/10/26	72/4/24	p<0.05
LV-EF (%)	55.0 ± 14.0	54.6 ± 12.3	n.s.
Peak gradient (mmHg)	72.6 ± 29.7	72.9 ± 28.7	n.s.
Mean gradient (mmHg)	45.7 ± 20.1	45.4 ± 18.0	n.s.
Regurgitation (°)	1.01 ± 1.07	0.73 ± 0.68	n.s.

Table 2. Operative spectrum

	Freedom (n=430)	Solo (n=279)	p
Isolated procedures (%)	52	55	n.s.
Combined procedures (%)	48	45	n.s.
– CABGx1-5 (%)	66.8	75.9	n.s.
– mitral procedures (%)	19.3	12.5	n.s.
– ablations	17.1	13.4	n.s.
– myectomies	3.9	4.5	n.s.
– others	7.2	7.1	n.s.
Endocarditis (%)	9.6	2.4	<0.01
Reoperations (%)	10.6	9.2	n.s.

Mean valve size was comparable in both groups (Table 3). Due to the lack of a second suture line, overall cross-clamp time and cross-clamp time for isolated cases were significantly shorter in case of implanting a Solo valve. There was no difference in expected and observed mortality in either group.

Postoperative hemodynamics were excellent in both groups (Fig. 13); however, mean gradients were significantly lower in all valve size groups. There was no relevant regurgitation or any paravalvular leakages at discharge (Table 3).

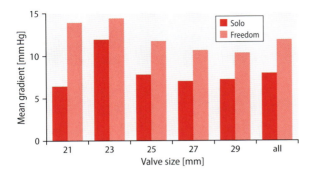

Fig. 13. Hemodynamics at discharge

Table 3. Operative data and expected and observed mortality

	Freedom (n = 430)	Solo (n = 279)	p
■ Mean valve size (mm)	25.7 ± 2.2	26.4 ± 2.1	n.s.
■ Cross-clamp time overall (min)	81.2 ± 32.1	50.1 ± 18.2	< 0.01
■ Cross-clamp time isolated (min)	65.5 ± 25.2	37.9 ± 5.8	< 0.01
■ log. EuroSCORE	11.5 ± 7.1	15.1 ± 13.7	n.s.
■ 30-day mortality (%)	5,3	6,4	n.s.
■ Postop mean gradient (mmHg)	11.2 ± 5.9	8.4 ± 4.5	< 0.05
■ Postop regurgitation (°)	0.07 ± 0.27	0.10 ± 0.31	n.s.

Discussion

Aortic valve replacement has shown excellent results over the last 40 years. Substantial improvements in terms of prosthesis design, preservation of biological materials and postoperative treatment have lead to an increased use of tissue valves in the elderly. Stentless valves compared to stented valves have shown superior results with respect to postoperative effective orifice area and gradients at rest [4, 7, 10, 12–14, 16, 18, 21, 23], at exercise [10, 16], improvement in left ventricular mass reduction [4, 12–14, 16, 18, 21, 23], and recovery of left ventricular function [4, 18, 21]. In addition, improved overall survival could be demonstrated in various retrospective studies [4, 6].

Stented pericardial valves by different manufacturers have been available for decades for aortic as well as for other valve replacement procedures. Folliguet et al. reported excellent long-term results of up to 10 years with respect to structural deterioration in echocardiography of the glutaraldehyde-based fixation process of the bovine pericardium [9]. The detoxification process used in the Sorin Pericarbon Freedom^{TM} stentless valve, which uses homocystic acid for covering remaining aldehyde residues in the tissue, has proven mechanical stability [19] and improved biocompatibility as well as decreased calcification in animal models.

As demonstrated in this study, the implantation of both the Sorin Pericarbon Freedom™ stentless valve and the Freedom™ Solo stentless valve is safe and reliable. Perioperative mortality was low compared to the expected mortality as estimated by the logistic EuroSCORE. Hemodynamics were excellent at discharge.

In conclusion, pericardial stentless valves proved their suitability for aortic valve replacement in combined and isolated aortic valve replacement. However, long-term follow-up is necessary to show the stability of these promising prostheses over time.

References

1. Beholz S, Claus B, Dushe S, Konertz W (2006) Operative technique and early hemodynamic results with the Freedom Solo valve. J Heart Valv Dis 15:429–432
2. Beholz S, Grubitzsch H, Dushe S, Liu J, Dohmen PM, Konertz W (2005) Hemodynamic Results of the Pericarbon Freedom Stentless™ Valve. Thorac Cardiovasc Surg 53:212–216
3. Beholz S, Hunter S, Infantes CA, Zussa C (2005) Recommendations for the implantation of the Pericarbon Freedom stentless valve. Heart Surgery For 8:E409–E411
4. Borger MA, Carson SM, Ivanov J, Rao V, Scully HE, Feindel CM, David TE (2005) Stentless aortic valves are hemodynamically superior to stented valves during mid-term follow-up: a large retrospective study. Ann Thorac Surg 80:2180–2185
5. Calafiore AM, Teodori G, Mezzetti A, Bosco G, Verna AM, Di Giammarco G, Lapenna D (1995) Intermittent antegrade warm blood cardioplegia. Ann Thorac Surg 59:398–402
6. Casali G, Auriemma S, Santini F, Mazzucco A, Luciani GB (2004) Survival after stentless and stented xenograft aortic valve replacement: a concurrent, case-match trial. Ital Heart J 5:282–289
7. De Paulis R, Sommariva L, Colagrande L, De Matteis GM, Fratini S, Tomai F, Bassano C, Penta de Peppo A, Chiariello L (1998) Regression of left ventricular hypertrophy after aortic valve replacement for aortic stenosis with different valve substitutes. J Thorac Cardiovasc Surg 116:590–598
8. Desai ND, Merin O, Cohen GN, Herman J, Mobilos S, Sever JY, Fremes SE, Goldman BS, Christakis GT (2004) Long-term results of aortic valve replacement with the St. Jude Toronto stentless porcine valve. Ann Thorac Surg 78:2076–2083
9. Folliguet TA, Le Bret E, Bachet J, Laborde F (2001) Pericarbon pericardial bioprosthesis: an experience based on the lessons of the past. Ann Thorac Surg 71(Suppl):S289–S292
10. Fries R, Wendler O, Schieffer H, Schafers HJ (2000) Comparative rest and exercise hemodynamics of 23-mm stentless versus 23-mm stented aortic bioprostheses. Ann Thorac Surg 69:817–822
11. Grubitzsch H, Linneweber J, Kossagk C, Sanli E, Beholz S, Konertz W (2005) Aortic valve replacement with new-generation stentless pericardial valves: Short-term clinical and hemodynamic results. J Heart Valv Dis 14:623–629

12. Jin XY, Zhang ZM, Gibson DG, Yacoub MH, Pepper JR (1996) Effects of valve substitute on changes in left ventricular function and hypertrophy after aortic valve replacement. Ann Thorac Surg 62:683–690
13. Maselli D, Pizio R, Bruno LP, Di Bella I, De Gasperis C (1999) Left ventricular mass reduction after aortic valve replacement: homografts, stentless and stented valves. Ann Thorac Surg 67:966–971
14. Milano AD, Blanzola C, Mecozzi G, D'Alfonso A, De Carlo M, Nardi C, Bortolotti U (2001) Hemodynamic performance of stented and stentless aortic bioprostheses. Ann Thorac Surg 72:33–38
15. O'Brien MF (1995) The Cryolife-O'Brien composite aortic stentless xenograft: surgical technique of implantation. Ann Thorac Surg 60:S410–S413
16. Pibarot P, Dumesnil JG, Leblanc MH, Cartier P, Metras J (1999) Changes in left ventricular mass and function after aortic valve replacement: a comparison between stentless and stented bioprosthetic valves. J Am Soc Echocardiogr 12:981–987
17. Repossini A, Kotelnikov I, Bouchikhi R, Torre T, Passaretti B, Parodi O, Arena V (2005) Single-suture line placement of a pericardial stentless valve. J Thorac Cardiovasc Surg 130:1265–1269
18. Santini F, Bertolini P, Montalbano G, Vecchi B, Pessotto R, Prioli A, Mazzucco A (1998) Hancock versus stentless bioprosthesis for aortic valve replacement in patients older than 75 years. Ann Thorac Surg 66:S99–S103
19. Stacchino C, Bona G, Bonetti F, Rinaldi S, Della Ciana L, Grignani A (1998) Detoxification process for glutaraldehyde-treated bovine pericardium: biological, chemical and mechanical characterization. J Heart Valve Dis 7:190–194
20. Stacchino C, Bona G, Rinaldi S, Vallana F (1995) Design and performance characteristics of the Pericarbon stentless valve. J Heart Valve Dis 4:S102–105
21. Walther T, Falk V, Langebartels G, Kruger M, Bernhardt U, Diegeler A, Gummert J, Autschbach R, Mohr FW (1999) Prospectively randomized evaluation of stentless versus conventional biological aortic valves: impact on early regression of left ventricular hypertrophy. Circulation 100(19 Suppl):II6–II10
22. Westaby S (2001) Implant technique for the Sorin stentless pericardial valve. Operat Tech Thorac Cardiovasc Surg 6:101–105
23. Williams RJ, Muir DF, Pathi V, MacArthur K, Berg GA (1999) Randomized controlled trial of stented and stentless aortic bioprotheses: hemodynamic performance at 3 years. Semin Thorac Cardiovasc Surg 11(Suppl 1):93–97

Stented bioprostheses

The changing role of pericardial tissue in biological valve surgery:
22 years' experience with the Sorin Mitroflow stented pericardial valve

C. A. Yankah, M. Pasic, J. Stein, C. Detschades, H. Siniawski, R. Hetzer

Background

The bovine pericardial tissue valve, once prohibited for clinical use, has demonstrated the longest durability (22 years) [1, 15]. With the increase in life expectancy up to 83 years in men and 85 years in women, there is a trend towards the use of non-thrombogenic biological tissue which requires no long-term anticoagulation [1–14]. Because of the natural history of the aortic valve and root diseases, the majority of patients have small aortic roots which require implantation of small and hemodynamically effective valves without the need for an extended procedure of aortic root enlargement [1, 17–25]. On the other hand, there is a group of younger patients, especially women of child-bearing age or persons who are active in sports or because of professional reasons, who prefer biological valves and trade long-term anticoagulation for a second operation in their lifetime [1, 3, 13–16].

The study was designed to evaluate the long-term (21 years) results in patients <65 and >65 years old with Mitroflow pericardial bioprostheses (Sorin Group Canada, Inc. Mitroflow Division, Vancouver) for aortic valve replacement (AVR) since its introduction at our institution. The study further evaluated the hemodynamic performance (transvalvular gradients, effective orifice area) and patient-related factors for defining the age threshold for the use of pericardial valves.

Patients and methods

Between 3/1986 and 4/2007, 1513 patients who received isolated Mitroflow pericardial bioprostheses (1071 females, 442 males) at a mean age of 73.2 ± 0.22 years (SEM), range 22–95 years, were followed up to 9/2007. A total of 1031 patients (mean age 74.6 ± 0.3 years) received model 12 Mitroflow valves.

The clinical characteristics of the patients are summarized in Table 1. Distribution of patients by age group is shown in Fig. 1. A total of 759 (50.2%) patients underwent concomitant coronary artery bypass. The etiology of the aortic valve disease is summarized in Fig. 2.

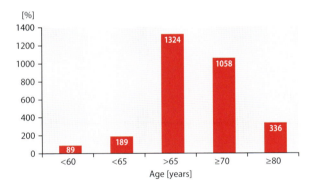

Fig. 1. Age-group distribution of 1513 patients who underwent aortic valve replacement with the Mitroflow pericardial aortic bioprosthesis

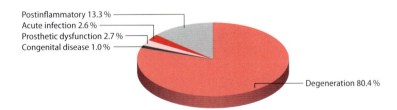

Fig. 2. Etiology of the aortic valve and root diseases of 1513 patients who underwent aortic valve replacement with the Mitroflow pericardial aortic bioprosthesis

Table 1. Characteristics of patients. Reprinted with permission from [1] © American Association for Thoracic Surgery

No. of patients:	1513
Mean:	73.2 ± 0.22 years (SEM)
Range:	22–95
Female:	1071 (70.8%)
Male:	442 (29.2%)

Distribution of patients by age group

Age (years)	n	%
< 60	89	5.8
60–69	366	24.2
70–79	722	47.7
≥ 65	1324	87.5
≥ 70	1058	69.9
≥ 80	336	22.2

NYHA

II:	620 (41%)
III:	633 (41.8%)
IV:	210 (13.9%)
Unknown:	50 (3.3%)

Body mass index

Mean:	25.74 ± 0.12 kg/m^2 (SEM)
Range:	12.98–47.5 kg/m^2
Renal failure:	159 (10.5%)
Pulmonary disease (COPD):	152 (10%)
Carotis stenosis:	104 (6.9%)

Implanted valve size | Explanted valve size

Implanted valve size		Explanted valve size	
N = 1513		N = 86	
19 mm	204 (13.5%)	10 (0.7%)	
21 mm	869 (57.4%)	35 (2.3%)	
23 mm	347 (22.9%)	30 (2.0%)	
25 mm	76 (5.0%)	6 (0.4%)	
27 mm	17 (1.1%)	1 (0.06%)	
Unknown:		4 (0.3%)	

Table 2. Three-center hemodynamic study of pericardial aortic valve replacement [1, 3, 12]

Size (mm)	Berlin MF	Canadian CE-P	French CE-Magna	French CE-P
19	1.4	1.1	1.0	1.1
21	1.6	1.3	1.3	1.4
23	1.85	1.5	1.96	1.7

MF Mitroflow, *CE* Carpentier-Edwards, *P* Perimount

Aortic root disease and morphology

Natural history of aortic stenosis: 54.6% (n=827) of 1513 patients presented with aortic stenosis. The patients were distributed into the following age groups: 53.4% of patients were aged >60 years and 1.2% of patients were aged <60 years (p=0.001). In the age group ≥65 and <65 years, the figure was 50.8% and 3.8%, respectively (p=0.001); 42.3% of patients ≥70 years had aortic stenosis.

Design and characteristics of the Mitroflow pericardial bioprosthesis

The Mitroflow pericardial bioprosthesis has been in clinical use since 1982 (Model 11) and it was redesigned (Model 12) for further clinical use in 1991 [8, 12]. It is a single sheet of pericardial tissue fixed with 0.5% glutaraldehyde at zero pressure mounted outside the low profile stent and has a smaller sewing ring than other bioprostheses.

This offers a wide opening and synchronous opening and closure of the leaflets with a maximum unimpeded laminar blood flow. It reduces the risk of interference with the sinotubular junction and of squeezing in a small aortic root.

Its small, soft, and pliable sewing cuff facilitates implantation into the smallest aortic annulus (19 mm, 21 mm) without the need for annular enlargement. Therefore, it reduces the risk of patient-prosthesis mismatch and high transvalvular gradients. The hemodynamics, transvalvular gradients, and effective orifice area compete with those of stentless bioprostheses (stented Mitroflow bovine pericardial valve 19 mm: 1.9 mmHg/ 1.4 cm^2; 21 mm: 7.1 mmHg/1.6 cm^2; 23 mm: 4.7 mmHg, 1.9 cm^2 [1]; stentless Freestyle porcine valve: 19 mm: not available; 21 mm: 8.2 mmHg/ 1.4 cm^2; 23 mm: 5.0 mmHg/1.9 cm^2 [26]).

The following indications are recommended for valve replacement with a biological prosthesis by the American College of Cardiology/American Heart Association task force report:
- patients who cannot or will not take warfarin therapy (class I),
- patients >65 years old needing aortic valve replacement who do not have risk factors (atrial fibrillation, left ventricular dysfunction, previous thromboembolism, and hypercoagulable situation (class II),
- patients considered to have possible compliance problems with warfarin (class IIa).

Surgical procedure

The standard surgical procedure was performed as described previously [9]. The objectives and principles of implantation of the Mitroflow pericardial bioprosthesis and techniques of aortic root enlargement are described in Tables 3 and 4. The percentage distribution of valve sizes implanted in 1513 patients is shown in Fig. 3.

Table 3. Objectives and surgical principles of AVR with a low profile stented Mitroflow pericardial bioprosthesis

- Due to its external pericardial sheet covering meticulous decalcification of the aortic annulus is warranted to obtain soft annulus tissue for suturing and avoid leaflet abrasion
- Sizing: Use the appropriate obturator to measure the native annulus for selection of proper valve size
- Avoid oversizing to create valve deformation
- Relief of subaortic obstructive septal hypertrophy, preferably by resection (myectomy)
- Supraannular implantation: clinical judgement of the aortic root space for supraannular positioning
- Pledgeted fixation sutures (LV-aortic fashion)
- Supraannular implantation provides 100% geometric orifice – aortic annulus match, good coaptation of leaflets and minimum hemodynamic stress
- Valve struts should correspond to native commissures and tall tied knots should be reduced to avoid coronary ostial impingement
- Concomitant replacement of aortic valve and ascending aorta: When using the MF pericardial bioprosthesis for concomitant replacement of the ascending aorta, the conduit size should be equivalent to the external diameter of the bioprosthesis (i.e., one size larger than the labeled size) to avoid leaflet impingement and abrasion

Table 4. Techniques of aortic root enlargement in adults with small aortic root

▮ Nicks 1970 [19]
Posterior annuloplasty. Extension of aortic incision posteriorly
To the noncoronary sinus across the aortic annulus to the mitral annulus

▮ Manougian: 1979 [20]
Aortic-mitral annuloplasty. Extension of the aortic incision posteriorly into the noncoronary sinus across the aortic annulus to the anterior mitral leaflet

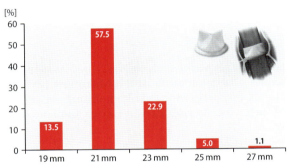

Fig. 3. Percentage distribution of Mitroflow pericardial aortic bioprostheses by sizes (19–27 mm) in the supraannular position which were implanted in 1513 patients

Follow-up

Follow-up was complete in 99.3% patients (11 patients were lost to follow-up) with a mean of 7.23 ± 0.287 years (3482 pt-years) for Model 11 and 2.6 ± 0.08 years (2682 pt-years) for Model 12; thus, the data from a total of 6163.5 patient-years were available for analysis. There was no implantation of Mitroflow valves between 1992 and 1996. A total of 1297 (85.7%) of the hospital survivors underwent routine echocardiographic studies at 3 and 9 months after operation and thereafter annually. Transthoracic Doppler echocardiography was performed at different institutions in a uniform manner and the evaluations were comparable. If a patient had undergone more than one echocardiographic or clinical evaluation, the result of the most recent investigation was reported.

Follow-up information was obtained from the state registry of births and deaths, and from our institutional department for clinical studies. In some cases, it was documented by questionnaire or telephone interview, or from the records of the patients' family physicians or cardiologists. The primary endpoint of the clinical follow-up was described as mutually time-related outcomes such as event-free survival, valve-related morbid events (structural valve deterioration, bleeding, thromboembolism, prosthetic valve endocarditis), or death from other causes before explants. The maximal follow-up of the 86 explanted valves was 14.9 years and 642.65 patient-years at a mean of 7.39 ± 0.4 years, whereas for the 64 valves explanted for structural valve deterioration (SVD) it was 552.1 patient-years at a mean of 8.76 years [1]. We evaluated 189 measurements of mean gradients in 120 patients. Measurements of mean gradients and time intervals between serial echocardiographic studies were not uniform in some patients. Therefore, we did not apply the mixed model longitudinal regression analysis as described by Banbury et al. [4]. Evolution of mean transvalvular gradients of valve sizes 19–25 mm and their median values over time are shown in Fig. 7.

Structural and nonstructural deterioration of the Mitroflow valves, diagnosed preoperatively by echocardiographic studies, was confirmed at the time of explantation.

At the time of the last follow-up study, 150 patients (29%) were in New York Heart Association class I, 232 (45%) in class II, and 120 (23%) in class III; 14 patients (3%) could not be classified because of advanced age.

NYHA functional classification of the patients was inconsistent and unreliable to reproduce due to a high proportion of patients in advanced age (mean age at operation 73 years). Many follow-up patients discontinued or irregularly took their medication partly because of the risk and fear of bleeding and stroke. Therefore, a statistical approach to estimate a time-related proportion of patients in NYHA functional class and on anticoagulants did not yield meaningful, reproducible clinical information.

Postoperative anticoagulation

During the first 6 weeks after surgery AVR patients received coumarol/Coumadin or antiplatelet drugs. Those in atrial fibrillation continued to take their anticoagulation. A total of 97 (7.6%) patients were under anticoagulation treatment with Coumadin and 260 (20.5%) with antiplatelet drugs. There were 995 patients enrolled for follow-up at 1 year, 493 at 5 years, 156 at 10 years, and 58 at 15 years (Fig. 5). At 1 year 13.9%, at 5 years 23.5%, and at 10 years 33.3% were on anticoagulants (antiplatelet or Coumadin, Fig. 4). 7.6% were on Coumadin, 20.5% on antiplatelet therapy [1]. There were 315 (24.8%) patients ≥65 years using anticoagulants as compared to 42 (3.3%) patients <65 years (Table 5).

Table 5. Distribution of patients on anticoagulant therapy and thromboembolic complication by age group

Age group	Anticoagulants late Antiplatelet	Coumadin	Total	TE Early	Late	Total
<65 years	32	10	42 (3.3%)	2 (0.15%)	4 (0.3%)	6 (0.45%)
>65 years	228	87	315 (24.8%)	24 (1.8%)	19 (1.6%)	43 (1.6%)
Total	260	97	357 (28.1%)	26 (2.0%)	23 (1.8%)	49 (3.8%)

TE thromboembolism, *early* <6 weeks postop, *late* >6 weeks postop
Linearized rate (%/pts-year): <65 years 0.50; ≥65 years 0.93

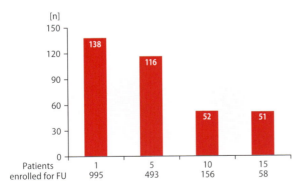

Fig. 4. Distribution of follow-up patients on anticoagulant therapy (figures in red columns) in relation to the entire cohort of follow-patients enrolled in year periods, 1, 5, 10, and 15 years after aortic valve replacement with the Mitroflow pericardial aortic bioprosthesis

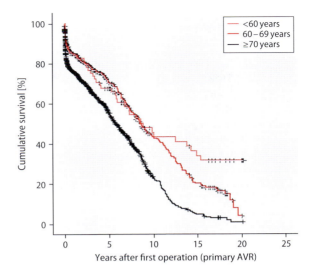

Fig. 5. Kaplan-Meier estimates of survival by age group of the 1513 patients who received aortic valve replacement with the Mitroflow pericardial aortic bioprosthesis at a mean age of 73 years

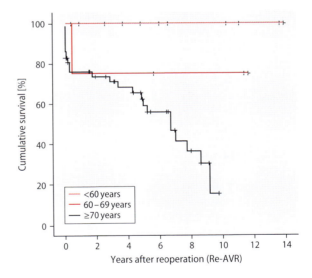

Fig. 6. Kaplan-Meier estimates of survival by age group of the 64 patients who underwent re-operation and replacement of the Mitroflow pericardial aortic bioprosthesis after structural valve deterioration

Statistical analysis

The guidelines for reporting morbidity and mortality after cardiac valvular operations, approved by the Society of Thoracic Surgeons were used to analyze postoperative complications [32]. All continuous variables were expressed as mean ±SEM. Actuarial curves were calculated by the Kaplan-Meier method.

Linearized occurrence rate of events and confidence limits were calculated according to the Poisson distribution. Actual competing risk analysis (cumulative incidence) was performed. A p value of <0.05 was considered as evidence of statistical significance. Predictors of events during follow-up were identified by means of Cox's proportional hazards regression.

Results

Early mortality

Early survival was 97.5% for elective and 90.6% for emergency surgery and was defined as mortality within 30 days or during the same hospitalization. There was no significant difference between patients with and without concomitant coronary artery surgery (p=0.118). The causes of early death were cardiac related in 96 (61%) patients and noncardiac in 61 (39%) patients.

Significant predictive factors for early mortality were emergency operation (OR: 1.53, CI (95% CL) 1.33–1.75, p value<0.001) and preoperative renal failure (OR: 2.76, CI (95% CL) 0.98–7.76, p value 0.054).

Long-term survival

The number of late deaths during the 20-year follow-up was 615 (40.6%). Actuarial freedom from valve-related death at 20 years was 82.9±4.0%.

Survival after primary aortic valve replacement at 1, 5, 10, 15, and 20 years was 78.9±1.1%, 60.6±1.5%, 31.9±1.8%, 12.7±1.4%, and 6.1±1.5%, respectively. Survival by age group is demonstrated in Fig. 8. There was a striking difference in overall late survival for patients with and without coronary bypass or coronary artery disease (p=0.0002). The most common cause of cardiac, nonvalve-related death was congestive heart failure, while sudden death and unexplained death were the most common cause of cardiac, valve-related death. If sudden death was excluded from the data, the most frequent cause of valve-related death was stroke.

The actuarial survival rate including operative death in our cohort at 10, 15, and 20 years was 31.9±1.8%, 12.7±1.4%, and 6.1±1.5%, respectively. Univariate and multivariate analysis showed that NYHA III–IV, (OR: 1.37, CI (95% CL) 1.18–1.59, p value <0.001), renal insufficiency (OR: 1.74, CI (95% CL) 1.40–2.17, p value <0.001), chronic obstructive pulmonary disease (COPD), (OR: 1.54, CI (95% CL) 1.22–1.95, p value 0.001), body mass index <20 kg/m^2 (OR: 1.46, CI (95% CL) 1.13–1.88, p value 0.001), and advanced age (OR: 1.82, CI: 1.56–2.16, p value: <0.001) were predictive factors for late death. On the other hand, small valve size (19 mm, OR: 1.09, CI: 0.86–1.38, p value: 0.458; 21 mm, OR: 1.68, CI: 0.65–4.38: 1.38, p value: 0.286) and gender (OR: 1.11, CI: 0.96–1.29, p value: 0.158) were not independent risk factors. When the body mass index (BMI) and valve size are regarded as functions of survival BMI>30 vs. 21 mm Mitroflow valve the p value was p=0.630, BMI<30 vs 21 mm it was p=0.615. There was better survival in those patients who underwent reoperation during the follow-up period than in those without (Fig. 5 and 6). Survival at 1, 5, and 10 years after reoperation for SVD was 80.3±5.1%, 67.2±6.5%, and 40.6±4.5%, respectively.

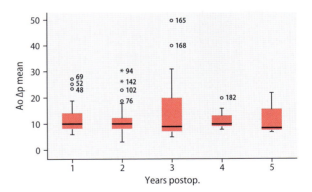

Fig. 7. Transvalvular mean gradients (mmHg) of Mitroflow pericardial aortic bioprostheses measured over time (1, 5, 10, 15, and >15 years) in relation to labeled valve sizes, 19–25 mm. Solid lines represent time-related estimates of median values for the prostheses 19–25 mm

Years postop	1	5	10	15	>15
■ Range [mmHg]	6–27	5–30	5–50	8–20	7–22
■ Median [mmHg]	10.0	10.0	9.0	10.0	8.5

Postoperative hemodynamic profile

The postoperative transvalvular gradients (mmHg), effective orifice area (cm^2) and regression of left ventricular hypertrophy are shown in Figs. 7 and 8, and Table 2. Valves with size 19 mm and 21 mm showed a higher transvalvular gradient than those with 23 mm and 25 mm, and this decreased during the first postoperative year (Fig. 7). The mean gradients at 5 years in patients over 65 with valve sizes 19–25 mm ranged from 12 to 6 mmHg, and at 10 years, from 18 to 8 mmHg. At 15–20 years the gradients remained stable. In contrast to the gradients in patients under 65 years with valve sizes 21 and 23 mm, the mean gradients ranged from 40 to 19 mmHg (p = 0.004). The mean transvalvular gradients over time in relation to prosthesis sizes 19 mm–25 mm are shown in Fig. 8. Regression of the LV hypertrophy of 32% was measured by echocardiography at a mean follow-up time of 2.9 years (Fig. 9).

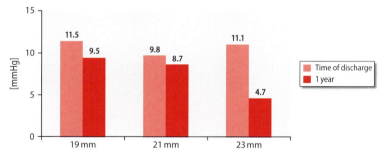

Fig. 8. Transvalvular mean gradients (mmHg) of Mitroflow pericardial aortic bioprostheses, sizes 19–23 mm measured at the time of discharge and 1 year after aortic valve replacement

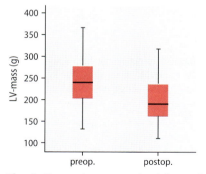

Fig. 9. Pre- and postoperative left ventricular mass (g) measured by echocardiography as an expression of the left ventricular hypertrophy (LV) showing 32% regression of the LV hypertrophy at a mean follow-up time of 2.9 years after aortic valve replacement with the Mitroflow pericardial aortic bioprostheses
The solid lines in the boxes express the mean LV mass (g)

Reoperation

In total, 86 (5.7%) patients (53 females and 33 males) with a median age of 66.0 years (range 27–84 years) underwent reoperation after 20 years. The mean follow-up to the time of reoperation was 7.39±years, maximum 14.95±years at 552.09 patient-years. There were 64 (4.2%) valves explanted for primary SVD including one leaflet tear, 17 for infective endocarditis and 1 for paravalvular leakage including one leaflet tear (linearized rate: 0.016%/pts-year).

Structural valve deterioration

Bioprosthetic valve dysfunction due to primary SVD occurred in 64 patients (4.2%). Distribution of explantations in age groups is shown in Figs. 10–12.

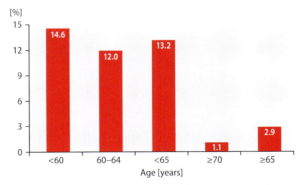

Fig. 10. Percentage explantation of Mitroflow pericardial aortic bioprosthesis for structural valve deterioration (SVD) after aortic valve replacement in the different age groups

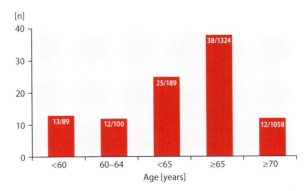

Fig. 11. Distribution of explantations for structural valve deterioration (SVD) after aortic valve replacement with the Mitroflow pericardial aortic bioprosthesis by age group in relation to the patient population

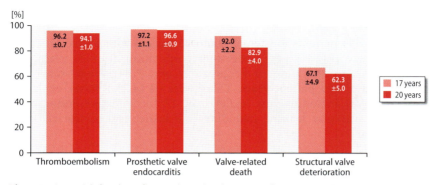

Fig. 12. Actuarial freedom from valve-related events after aortic valve replacement with the Mitroflow pericardial aortic bioprosthesis at 17 and 20 years [1, 9]

Table 6. Incidence of and actuarial freedom from structural valve deterioration and linearized rate of events

Age (years)	Incidence of SVD (%)	Linearized rate (%/pt./year)	Actuarial freedom from SVD (%) (18–20 year)
>65	2.9	0.76	71.8
>70	1.1	0.34	84.6
<65	13.2	2.1	48.2

The mean follow-up to the time of reoperation was 8.76±years, maximum 14.95±years at 642.15 patient-years. The actuarial freedom from explantation due to SVD was 62.3±5.0 (female: 67.12±7.8%, male: 64.8±7.8) (actual 88.6±4.1%). In Table 7 results of other authors are listed for comparison. Statistical differences in the incidence of SVD were found between the age groups ≥65 and <65 years (Fig. 13, p=0.004). Linearized rate of SVD in patients over 65 years was 0.76%/pt-year (CI, 0.6–1.3), under 65 years was 2.3%/pt-year (CI, 1.5–3.5) (Table 6). At 20 years, the actuarial freedom from SVD in the age groups ≥65 and ≥70 years was 72% and 84.8%, respectively (Fig. 13). In patients under 65 years and those under 60 years, at 10 and 18 years the actuarial freedom from SVD was 78.8±5.2% and 48.2±8.1% and 71.4±9.0% and 42±12.0%, respectively (Figs. 13, 14). In Table 8 the results of similar age group of patients are presented.

The linearized rate of SVD within 5 years in the age group ≥65 years was 0.2%/pt-year (CI, 0.002–0.7). Subsequently, it was observed in 18 patients ≥60 years with aortic stenosis, 62% of whom were free from SVD at 18 years; however, this finding is not highly conclusive because of the low number of patients. In patients aged 60–64 years freedom from SVD at 18 years was 53±10.9% (actual 76.1±6.2%).

Table 7. Structural valve deterioration of porcine and pericardial bioprostheses [1–4, 7, 12]

Author	Prosthesis	Mean age	Age group	Freedom from SVD Actuarial (%)	Actual (%)	Time (yrs.)
Eichinger et al. 2008	SJM Biocor	72.5±9	–	86.5±4.5	–	20
			>75	95.1±2.7	–	15
			66–74	59.9±18	–	20
			<65	56.5±15	–	20
Borger et al. 2008	Hc II	67±11	>65	73±16	–	20
			<65	39±9	–	20
Myken et al. 2009	SJM Biocor	70.8±10.9	–	61.1±8.5	85.6±2.2	20
			71–80	97.8±1.2	–	20
			61–70	81.0±5.1	–	20
			>65	92.1±2.5	–	20
			<65	44.5±9.2	–	20
Aupart et al. 2006	CE-P	72.6	–	68±12	–	18
			>70	99±1	–	18
			60–70	77±12	–	18
			<60	45±15	–	18
Jamieson et al. 2005	CE-SAP	68.9±10.9	–	64±3.6	88.9±1	18
			>70	94.6±2.3	98.2±0.6	18
			61–70	77.6±4.9	–	18
			<60	51±7	70.6±4	18
Yankah et al. 2005/08	MF	72.4±8.4	–	67±4.9	95.3±0.7	17
		73.2±0.22	–	62.3±5.02	88.6±0.9	20
			<70	84.8±0.7	96.6±0.8	20
			>65	72±6	92.6±4.6	20

Table 8. Actuarial freedom from SVD after pericardial and porcine AVR in patients <65 years [1–4, 7, 12]

Author	Year	Prosthesis	Age group	Actuarial freedom from SVD (%) (years)	Time (years)
Myken et al.	2009	SJM-BioCor	<65	44.5±9.2	20
Eichinger et al.	2008	SJM-BioCor	<65	56.5±15	17
Borger et al.	2005	Hc II	<65	39±9	20
Aupart et al.	2006	Ce-P	<60	45±15	18
Jamieson et al.	2005	CE-SAP	<60	51±7	18
Yankah et al.	2008	Mitroflow	<60*	62±12	18

* Aortic stenosis

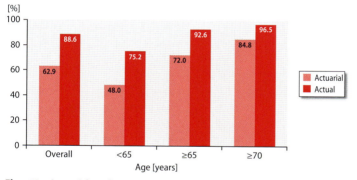

Fig. 13. Actuarial and actual (cumulative incidence) freedom from reoperation for structural valve deterioration (SVD) by age group after aortic valve replacement with the Mitroflow pericardial aortic bioprosthesis

Nonstructural valve deterioration

There were four explantations due to nonstructural valve deterioration (NSVD). One patient presented with paravalvular leak (0.07%), without clinical signs or histological/bacteriological findings of concomitant infection; one case was due to intraoperative patient-prosthesis mismatch. The two other cases were related to technical problems. Actuarial freedom from NSVD at 20 years was 98.6±0.7%.

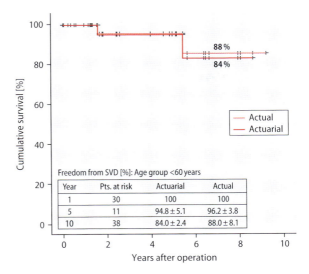

Fig. 14. Actuarial and actual (cumulative incidence) freedom from reoperation for structural valve deterioration (SVD) in the age group <60 years after aortic valve replacement with the Mitroflow pericardial aortic bioprosthesis (Model 12)

Prosthetic valve endocarditis

Prosthetic valve endocarditis (PVE) developed in 17 (1.1%) patients; none of them had native valve endocarditis before surgery. Reinfection developed within the first 60 days in one patient and late in 16 patients at between 0.29 and 9.83 years (mean: 3.44 years, SEM). Eleven reoperations for PVE were carried out electively and 6 urgently. Linearized rate of prosthetic infection was 0.08%/pt-year (CI:0.03–0.17). At 15 and 18 years, actuarial freedom from PVE was 96.8 ± 0.9% after AVR (Fig. 12).

Hemorrhage

Anticoagulant induced hemorrhage was significantly low (n = 4, 0.3%) with a linearized rate of 0.06%/pt-year (CI: 0.02–0.15). There was no incidence of hemorrhage-related death or recurrent bleeding. At 20 years, the actuarial freedom from hemorrhage was 97.4%.

Thromboebolism

Valve thrombosis was seen in one patient. There were 49 embolic episodes. A total of 40 patients suffered a single episode, while 9 suffered two episodes which were fatal. Among the 49 episodes, 4 resulted in permanent neurological consequences. Six patients had a cerebral transient ischemic attack (TIA) at a linearized rate of 0.09%/pt-year. At 20 years after AVR, the actuarial freedom from thromboembolism was 94.1% (Fig. 12).

Discussion

The indication for implantation of tissue valves in elderly patients is evidently based on the fact that there is a relation between age and bleeding complications during anticoagulant therapy. The rate of major hemorrhagic complication is highest above the age of 60 years: 6.8 per 100 treatment years, compared with 2.9 per 100 treatment years below 60 years. However the complications can be minimized by the current self-management of anticoagulation [42]. Incidences of postoperative thromboembolic episodes (transient ischemic attack and stroke) after technically advanced heart surgery are not well understood, although they are frequently observed in advanced age [1, 4, 11, 27]. Anticoagulant-induced hemorrhage was significantly low in our series with a linearized rate of 0.06%/pt-year (CI: 0.02–0.15). Primary SVD is the critical valve-related complication with pericardial bioprostheses, and it was the reason for their limited use in the past [33–35]. The study was aimed at evaluating age- and valve-related clinical performance of the Mitroflow pericardial aortic bioprosthesis and comparing the results with those of the current bioprostheses. Age at implantation was regarded as a determinant of long-term durability of both porcine and pericardial valves. Magilligan et al. first reported a high incidence of SVD in young patients, while Jamieson et al. subsequently showed SVD to be less frequent with advancing age [36, 37]. Patients who are currently undergoing AVR are elderly and would therefore benefit more from tissue valves. In our series with a mean age of 73 years, the overall actuarial freedom from SVD at 20 years was 62.3±5.0%; in the age groups >65 and >70 years it was 72% and 84%, respectively. Similar results have been reported by others [1–14].

Improved design of pericardial bioprostheses has contributed significantly to the durability of the pericardial valves which was evidenced by several clinical trials and large follow-up studies [3–9, 14, 16]. Age- and valve-related factors have influenced and determined the long-term performance of pericardial tissue valves and this has influenced the decision-making processes during selection of bioprostheses in aortic valve surgery in the last 20 years. Other critical issues on decision-making for device selection for patients relate to the underlying etiology and the natural history of the aortic valve disease, patients' comorbidity, hemodynamic performance, and durability of the device [1, 9–15, 17, 18, 21–23]. Patients with small aortic roots could benefit from small size bioprostheses with a large effective orifice area and low transvalvular gradient which are similar to those of a stentless bioprosthesis. These hemodynamic factors are determinants for postoperative regression of the left ventricular hypertrophy, and functional recovery and subsequently the life-expectancy of the patients [21–26, 29–31, 38]. The possibility of patient-prosthesis size mismatch with the Mitroflow pericardial bioprosthesis is reduced, which is associated with rapid regression of left ventricular hypertrophy.

The excellent hemodynamic profile of the Mitroflow valve of size 19 and 21 mm is attributed to its design with the pericardial sheet outside the struts in addition to its small sewing ring which provides a wider orifice and allows matching of the annulus to the orifice at implantation without the need for aortic root enlargement. Subsequently, the Mitroflow prosthesis provides a low mean transvalvular gradient between 7 and 13 mmHg and a large effective orifice area (EOA) of 1.4 and 1.6 cm^2. The impact of patient-prosthesis mismatch of various types of bioprostheses on regression of left ventricular hypertrophy and function is reported by several authors [1, 23–26, 29–31]. In the present series, valve size was not found to be a risk factor for early or late deterioration of New York Heart Association functional class as judged by echocardiographic studies [1, 21].

Myken & Bech-Hansen and Eichinger et al. recently reported data on the St Jude Medical Biocor porcine bioprosthesis (St Jude Medical, St Paul, MN, USA) with identical low incidence of SVD within a 20-year term with the only discrepancy in the age group <65 years. The results of Eichinger et al. on freedom from SVD were superior, 71.8±9.2% at 20 years vs. 44.5% found by Myken & Bech-Hansen [2, 7]. In the series of Borger et al. with the Hancock II porcine valve in a similar age group, freedom from SVD was 39±9% at 20 years [4].

It has been reported by several authors that an age of <65 years carries higher risk for primary tissue failure as compared with the older age group [4, 12–16, 36, 37]. The incidence of SVD in our series was lower than that of the recently reported series by others [2, 4, 7]. The actuarial freedom from SVD at 10 and 18 years in the age groups <65 years and <60 years was 78.8±5.2%, 48.2±8.1% and 71.4±9.0% and 42±12%, respectively. Some patients below the age of 60 years in our series even demonstrated lower incidence of explantation with freedom from SVD of 62% at 18 years. However, the findings are not highly conclusive because of the low number of patients in this group.

Leaflet tears or disruption are rare complications but occur in all types of bioprosthesis even in allograft valves usually at the commissures or body cusp [1, 4, 7, 16, 33–35]. The etiology is variable; therefore, unless it is an acute or subacute spontaneous leaflet tear, it is not easy to distinguish and to interpret the morphology. The Carpentier-Edwards Perimount (Edwards

Lifesciences, Irvine, CA) and Mitroflow pericardial valves have confirmed improved 20- and 21-year clinical performance with reports on a low incidence of leaflet tear in both, a complication which is seen in porcine valves as well [3, 4, 16]. Two cases observed in our series of 1513 implants and patients were due to
- primary tissue failure and
- sequelae of infection [1].

There are a few underlying causes which are not well appreciated in the literature: the primary tissue failure and inflammatory processes such as bacterial infection or immune reaction. For a better understanding of the etiology, Simionescu and Thiene suggested evaluation of valve matrix changes by electron microscopic techniques to verify collagen breakdown and of macrophagic infiltration which could cause collagen disruption through metalloproteinase release by histochemistry [40, 41].

Previous reports have indicated that most late deaths after valve surgery are due to cardiac or valvular problems, sudden death, myocardial infarction and congestive heart failure [24, 39]. In our series with a mean age of 73 years, congestive heart failure, COPD, and stroke were the most frequent causes of late death. Other factors such as valve size 19/21 mm vs. >23 mm were not shown to be a significant cause of early or late death (p=0.549) [1, 9].

In search of an ideal tissue valve, tissue engineering could be a positive step towards solving the biological factors such as graft-related and host-related factors which accelerate SVD in young patients. Decellularization of xenografts and allografts is a technique that allows host cells to repopulate the implant, thus, producing a biocompatible heart valve. The two concepts could dictate the future direction for the production of tissue-engineered heart valves. The stentless pericardial tissue valve at its tenth year has shown satisfactory clinical performance and, therefore, could compete well with the porcine and allograft valves because of its unique anatomic structure. The pericardial covered sewing ring of a stented valve as a total biological tissue can resist local infection and minimize the incidence of prosthetic valve endocarditis. The innovative technology in valve replacement, such as percutaneous and transapical catheter-based aortic valve replacements (Edwards Sapien, Corvalve or Sadra Lotus devices) which are currently used to treat high-risk patients, would change the role of traditional valve surgery and even make a reentry sternotomy unnecessary for re-re-placement of biologic tissue valves. The device needs further improvement in the design to enable it to achieve this aim and also to ensure long-term durability.

Inferences

The Mitroflow pericardial bioprosthesis is very easy to handle and to implant in the supraannular position without the need for aortic root enlargement. It has excellent hemodynamics (larger effective orifice area, low postoperative transvalvular gradient), especially in small sizes 19 and 21 mm. Therefore, it promotes rapid regression of left ventricular hypertrophy and functional recovery

It has demonstrated a low incidence of SVD in patients ≥65 years which suggests and supports a reduction of the age threshold from 70 to 65 years. Thus, patients under 65 years could be offered the pericardial bioprosthesis for a specified indication with a low risk of re-replacement in their life time.

Conclusion

Our data suggest that the Mitroflow pericardial bioprosthesis provides excellent long-term results especially in patients over 65 years and a satisfactory lower incidence of SVD in younger patients under 65 years and even under 60 years with aortic stenosis. It is, thus, an option for those patients <65 years who prefer a second operation for various reasons to long-term anticoagulation.

Acknowledgments. The authors are grateful to Anne M. Gale, ELS, for editorial assistance, Astrid Benhennour for bibliographic support, and Carla Weber for providing the graphics.

References

1. Yankah CA, Pasic M, Musci M, Stein J, Detschades C, Siniawski H, Hetzer R (2008) Aortic valve replacement with the Mitroflow pericardial bioprosthesis: durability results up to 21 years. J Thorac Cardiovasc Surg 136(3):688–696
2. Myken PSU, Bech-Hansen O (2009) A 20-year experience of 1712 patients with the Biocor porcine bioprosthesis. J Thorac Cardiovasc Surg 137(1):76–81
3. Jamieson WR, Burr LH, Miyagishima RT, Germann E, MacNab JS, Stanford E, Chan F, Janusz MT, Ling H (2005) Carpentier-Edwards supra-annular aortic porcine bioprosthesis: clinical performance over 20 years. J Thorac Cardiovasc Surg 130(4):994–1000
4. Borger MA, Ivanov J, Armstrong S, Christie-Hrybinsky D, Feindel CM, David TE (2006) Twenty-year results of the Hancock II bioprosthesis. J Heart Valve Dis 15(1):49–56

5. Khan SS, Trento A, DeRobertis M, Kass RM, Sandhu M, Czer LS, Blanche C, Raissi S, Fontana GP, Cheng W, Chaux A, Matloff JM (2001) Twenty-year comparison of tissue and mechanical valve replacement. J Thorac Cardiovasc Surg 122(2):257–269
6. Legarra JJ, Llorens R, Catalan M, Segura I, Trenor AM, de Buruaga JS, Rabago G, Sarralde A (1999) Eighteen-year follow up after Hancock II bioprosthesis insertion. J Heart Valve Dis 8(1):16–24
7. Eichinger WB, Hettich I, Ruzicka D, Holper K, Schricker C, Bleiziffer S, Lange R (2008) Twenty-year experience with the St.-Jude medical biocor prosthesis in the aortic position. Ann Thorac Surg 86(4):1204–1211
8. Pomar JL, Jamieson WR, Pelletier LC, Gerein AN, Castella M, Brownlee RT (1995) Mitroflow pericardial bioprosthesis: clinical performance to ten years. Ann Thorac Surg 60(2 Suppl):S305–S310
9. Yankah CA, Schubel J, Buz S, Siniawski H, Hetzer R (2005) Seventeen-year clinical results of 1,037 Mitroflow pericardial heart valve prostheses in the aortic position. J Heart Valve Dis 14(2):172–180
10. Moggio RA, Pooley RW, Sarabu MR, Christiana J, Ho AW, Reed GE (1994) Experience with the Mitroflow aortic bioprosthesis. J Thorac Cardiovasc Surg 108(2):215–220
11. Sjögren J, Gudbjartsson T, Thulin LI (2006) Long-term outcome of the MitroFlow pericardial bioprosthesis in the elderly after aortic valve replacement. J Heart Valve Dis 15(2):197–202
12. Aupart MR, Mirza A, Muerisse YA, Sirinelli AL, Neville PH, Marchand MA (2006) Perimount pericardial bioprosthesis for aortic calcified stenosis: 18-year experience with 1133 patients. J Heart Valve Dis 15(6):768–776
13. Smedira NG, Blackstone EH, Roselli EE, Laffey CC, Cosgrove DM (2006) Are allografts the biologic valve of choice for aortic valve replacement in nonelderly patients? Comparison of explantation for structural valve deterioration of allograft and pericardial prostheses. J Thorac Cardiovasc Surg 131(3):558–564
14. Hammermeister K, Sethi GK, Henderson WG, Grover FL, Oprian C, Rahimtoola SH (2000) Outcomes 15 years after valve replacement with a mechanical versus a bioprosthetic valve: final report of the Veterans Affairs randomized trial. J Am Coll Cardiol 36(4):1152–1158
15. Yankah CA, Weng Y, Meyer R, Siniawski H, Hetzer R (2006) Twenty-two-year durability of Ionescu-Shiley pericardial aortic bioprosthesis implanted in a 49-year-old woman: a valuable insight into the performance of current pericardial bioprostheses. J Thorac Cardiovasc Surg 132(2):427–428
16. Jamieson WR, David TE, Feindel CM, Miyagishima RT, Germann E (2002) Performance of the Carpentier-Edwards SAV and Hancock-II porcine bioprostheses in aortic valve replacement. J Heart Valve Dis 11(3):424–430
17. Passik CS, Ackermann DM, Pluth JR, Edwards WD (1987) Temporal changes in the causes of aortic stenosis: a surgical pathologic study of 646 cases. Mayo Clin Proc 62(2):119–123
18. Wood P (1958) Aortic stenosis. Am J Cardiol 1(5):553–571
19. Nicks R, Cartmill T, Bernstein L (1970) Hypoplasia of the aortic root. The problem of aortic valve replacement. Thorax 25(3):339–346
20. Manouguian S, Seybold-Epting W (1979) Patch enlargement of the aortic valve ring by extending the aortic incision into the anterior mitral leaflet. New operative technique. J Thorac Cardiovasc Surg 78(3):402–412
21. Banbury MK, Cosgrove DM 3rd, Thomas JD, Blackstone EH, Rajeswaran J, Okies JE, Frater RM (2002) Hemodynamic stability during 17 years of the Carpentier-Edwards aortic pericardial bioprosthesis. Ann Thorac Surg 73(5):1460–1465

22. Cosgrove DM, Lytle BW, Williams GW (1985) Hemodynamic performance of the Carpentier-Edwards pericardial valve in the aortic position in vivo. Circulation 72(3 Pt 2):II146–II152
23. Garcia-Bengochea J, Sierra J, Gonzalez-Juanatey JR, Rubio J, Vega M, Fernandez AL, Sanchez D (2006) Left ventricular mass regression after aortic valve replacement with the new Mitroflow 12A pericardial bioprosthesis. J Heart Valve Dis 5(3):446–452
24. David TE, Puschmann R, Ivanov J, Bos J, Armstrong S, Feindel CM, Scully HE (1998) Aortic valve replacement with stentless and stented porcine valves: a case-match study. J Thorac Cardiovasc Surg 116(2):236–241
25. Sintek CF, Fletcher AD, Khonsari S (1996) Small aortic root in the elderly: use of stentless bioprosthesis. J Heart Valve Dis 5(Suppl 3):S308–S313
26. Westaby S, Jin XY, Katsumata T, Arifi A, Braidley P (1998) Valve replacement with a stentless bioprosthesis: versatility of the porcine aortic root. J Thorac Cardiovasc Surg 116(3):477–484
27. Butchart EG, Moreno de la Santa P, Rooney SJ, Lewis PA (1995) Arterial risk factors and ischemic cerebrovascular events after aortic valve replacement. J Heart Valve Dis 4(1):1–8
28. Nollert G, Miksch J, Kreuzer E, Reichart B (2003) Risk factors for atherosclerosis and the degeneration of pericardial valves after aortic valve replacement. J Thorac Cardiovasc Surg 126(4):965–968
29. Frater RW, Furlong P, Cosgrove DM, Okies JE, Colburn LQ, Katz AS, Lowe NL, Ryba EA (1998) Long-term durability and patient functional status of the Carpentier-Edwards Perimount pericardial bioprosthesis in the aortic position. J Heart Valve Dis 7(1):48–53
30. Minami K, Schereika S, Kortke H, Gleichmann U, Koerfer R (1993) Long term follow-up of Mitroflow pericardial valve prostheses in the small aortic annulus. J Cardiovasc Surg (Torino) 34(3):189–193
31. Rao V, Jamieson WR, Ivanov J, Armstrong S, David TE (2000) Prosthesis-patient mismatch affects survival after aortic valve replacement. Circulation 102(19 Suppl 3):III5–III9
32. Edmunds LH, Jr., Clark RE, Cohn LH, Grunkemeier GL, Miller DC, Weisel RD (1996) Guidelines for reporting morbidity and mortality after cardiac valvular operations. J Thorac Cardiovasc Surg 112(3):708–711
33. Roselli EE, Smedira NG, Blackstone EH (2006) Failure modes of the Carpentier-Edwards pericardial bioprosthesis in the aortic position. J Heart Valve Dis 15(3):421–428
34. Scully H, Goldman B, Fulop J, Butany J, Tong C, Azuma J, Schwartz L (1988) Five-year follow-up of Hancock pericardial valves: management of premature failure. J Card Surg 3(3 Suppl):397–403
35. Leandri J, Bertrand P, Mazzucotelli JP, Loisance D (1992) Mode of failure of the Mitroflow pericardial valve. J Heart Valve Dis 1(2):225–231
36. Magilligan DJ, Lewis JW, Stein P, Alan M (1989) The porcine bioprosthetic heart valve: Experience at 15 years. Ann Thorac Surg 48(3):324–330
37. Jamieson WR, Burr LH, Tyers GF, Miyagishima RT, Janusz MT, Ling H, Fradet GJ, MacNab J, Chan F, Henderson C (1995) Carpentier-Edwards supraannular porcine bioprosthesis: Clinical performance to twelve years. Ann Thorac Surg 60(2 Suppl): S235–S240
38. Puvimanasinghe JP, Takkenberg JJ, Edwards MB, Eijkemans MJ, Steyerberg EW, Van Herwerden LA, Taylor KM, Grunkemeier GL, Habbema JD, Bogers AJ (2004) Comparison of outcomes after aortic valve replacement with a mechanical valve or a bioprosthesis using microsimulation. Heart 90(10):1172–1178

39. Blackstone EH, Kirklin JW (1985) Death and other time-related events after valve replacement. Circulation 72(4):753–767
40. Thiene G, Bortolotti U, Valente M (1998) The Hancock II xenograft: a step forward in bioprosthetic valve longevity? J Heart Valve Dis 8(1):1–3
41. Simionescu A, Simionescu D, Deac R (1996) Biochemical pathways of tissue degeneration in bioprosthetic cardiac valves. The role of matrix metalloproteinases. ASAIO J 42(5):M561–M567
42. Körtke H, Körfer R (2001) International normalized ratio self-management after mechanical heart valve replacement: is an early start advantageous? Ann Thorac Surg 72(1):44–48

20 years' durability of Carpentier-Edwards Perimount stented pericardial aortic valve

E. Bergoënd, M.R. Aupart, A. Mirza, Y.A. Meurisse, A.L. Sirinelli, P.H. Neville, M.A. Marchand

Aortic valve disease is the most common cardiac valve condition in developed countries, and its prevalence increases with patient age, especially due to calcified aortic stenosis [24]. Although aortic valve replacement (AVR) remains the most effective treatment in the majority of cases for significant aortic stenosis as well as aortic regurgitation, few data are available for long-term surgical outcome. Perimount pericardial valves offer excellent hemodynamic function, and the present authors' 10 year experience proved to be satisfactory when these valves were implanted in both the aortic and mitral positions [2, 3]. However, the long-term durability and performance of the valve remained questionable. The study aim was to evaluate long-term results of valve replacement for significant aortic valve disease, and long-term behavior of the aortic Perimount pericardial bioprosthesis, which the present authors have been implanting since 1984.

Clinical material and methods

Patients

Between July 1984 and December 2003, a total of 1600 consecutive patients aged >60 years, and 257 selected patients aged <60 years, underwent AVR for isolated aortic valve disease with a Perimount pericardial bioprosthesis at the authors' institution. The 257 selected patients presented with contraindications to anticoagulation treatment, mental inability, poor life expectancy with comorbidities, and a few had refused anticoagulation treatment due to lifestyle (women wishing to become pregnant, young people participating in sporting activities, or traveling). Indications for surgery followed international guidelines [6] as well as the European Association of Cardiology report [15] for asymptomatic patients. The indication was calcified aortic stenosis in 1133 (61%) cases, regurgitation in 468 (25%) and mixed in 256 (14%). The patient cohort comprised 1279 males (69%). Mean age was 69.8 years (range: 19 to 91 years). Mean NYHA functional status was

2.4, with 780 patients (42%) in NYHA classes III or IV. Chronic atrial fibrillation was observed in 166 patients (8.9%), and a pacemaker was present in 61 (3.3%).

Surgical technique

Patients were operated using a standard procedure via a median sternotomy with cardiopulmonary bypass, hemodilution, and general body hypothermia. Myocardial protection was achieved with crystalloid or blood cardioplegia and topical cooling. Valves implanted in each patient were as large as possible. As the aortic annulus was not enlarged in patients aged >60 years, 19 and 21 mm valves were used, despite their reputation for mild stenosis. Concomitant surgical procedures were required in 606 patients (32%); these included aortocoronary bypass in 335 patients (18%).

Anticoagulation

The postoperative anticoagulant protocol included heparin administration for two days, followed by one month treatment with calcium heparin (activated partial thromboplastin time >1.5 times normal) or acenocoumarol (International Normalized Ratio 2.5–3). After one month, anticoagulation treatment was discontinued at the cardiologist's discretion, except in patients with atrial fibrillation. Since 1998, postoperative treatment has been modified with prophylactic doses of low molecular weight heparin for one month.

Follow-up

The population was followed up in alternate years, using a consistent procedure. The latest data were obtained during a 6-month interval (April–September, 2004) through questionnaires sent to the cardiologist, family physician and patients, and completed by telephone contacts. The questionnaire included an echocardiographic study by the cardiologist and a survey on the patient's health condition. If a questionnaire was not returned or was unclear, repeated mailing and telephone contact were undertaken. Any patient with a discrepancy or with an abnormal echocardiographic examination was directly followed up at the authors' institution by one of the consultant cardiologists. Guidelines for reporting mortality and morbidity after cardiac valvular operation [10] were observed in these studies. An echocardiographic definition of structural failure was indicated by a mean gradient >40 mmHg or aortic insufficiency of grade 3 or 4 (based on a scale of 1 to 4).

Data analysis

All data were analyzed with Sedistat (SEDIA SA, Paris, France). Standard actuarial and linearized statistical techniques were used to describe survival and the incidence of valve-related complications. Only the first event for each patient was considered in the actuarial analysis, whereas all events for each patient were considered in the linearized rate. Data were presented as mean and 95% confidence limits of the mean. The log rank test was used to compare actuarial data. Comparisons between continuous variables were made using t-tests or analysis of variance, as appropriate. Comparisons between categorical variables were made with the chi-square test. Because of the small number of events in the subgroups, multivariable analysis was not performed.

Results

Follow-up

A total of 20 patients (1.1%) were lost to follow-up. Average duration of follow-up was 5.9 years, and cumulative follow-up was 10 828 patient-years. A total of 36 patients remained at risk at 18 years. Among the patient cohort, 1130 were alive during the follow-up period, while 74 living patients had incomplete cardiologic status (patient in institution for neurological disorders, especially Alzheimer's disease; at end of life; not wishing to reply). Enquiries concerning the echocardiography of each patient were asked of the respective cardiologists. The questionnaire included mainly prosthesis parameters: peak and mean gradients, effective orifice area, permeability index, insufficiency if any. Echocardiographic study was obtained for 1102 patients. For 28 patients, no echocardiographic data were available.

Patient survival

There were 52 early deaths (30-day mortality 2.8%), the main cause of early death being cardiac failure (n = 32); none was valve-related. Overall, the mortality rate among patients remained consistent during the entire study period (1984–2004). There were 581 late deaths, causes being valve-related in 36 patients (6%), cardiac but not valve-related in 103 (18%), and noncardiac in 381 (66%). Sixty-one patients (10%) died of unknown cause, while 75 required reoperation and were excluded (still alive except one) from the study on discharge from the rehabilitation center. The actuarial survival rate at 18 years (including operative mortality) was 22 ± 4% (Fig.

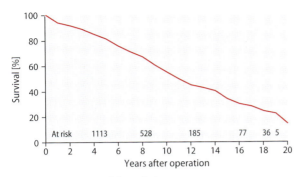

Fig. 1. Patient actuarial survival

1). Although survival was significantly influenced by age and preoperative atrial fibrillation, other factors (e.g., gender, preoperative NYHA status, size of prosthesis, coronary artery bypass grafting (CABG)) did not significantly influence survival. No patient with preoperative atrial fibrillation was alive after 12 years, and none of them required reoperation for structural valve deterioration.

Clinical status

At the time of follow-up, mean NYHA clinical status was 1.3. There were 896 patients (79%) in sinus rhythm, 95 in atrial fibrillation (8%), and 108 had a pacemaker (10%). 192 patients (17%) were being treated with warfarin, and 700 (62%) with antiplatelet drugs, among whom were patients who underwent CABG. Health condition was considered as 'satisfactory' by 1040 patients (92%), and 80% of patients estimated that valve replacement had improved their clinical state.

Valve-related complications

A total of 273 valve-related complications were observed, and there were 62 unexplained deaths. Hence, the actuarial rate of freedom from all valve-related complications was 42 ± 5%, with a linearized rate of 2.7% patient per year (%/yr).

Valve-related death

Thirty-five patients died from valve-related causes (22 thromboembolisms, 4 endocarditis, 5 bleeding events, 4 structural failures). At 18 years, actuarial rate of freedom from valve-related death was 94 ± 2%, with a linearized rate of 0.3%/yr. Sixty-two patients died of unknown cause; at the time of follow-up, the cause of death could not be determined from either the family or physician/cardiologist. Additionally in France, there is no reliable register of cause of death. According to the guidelines utilized, the actuarial rate of freedom from valve-related death including unexplained death was $78 \pm 4\%$ at 18 years, with a linearized rate of 0.9%/yr.

Thromboembolism

Sixty-five patients presented with thromboembolic events, with 22 deaths. Freedom from thromboembolism at 18 years was $93 \pm 1\%$, with a linearized rate of 0.6%/yr. No thrombosis of the bioprosthesis was observed.

Bleeding events

There were 37 cases of hemorrhagic complications meeting the definition of the guidelines and accounting for a linearized rate of 0.3%/yr. Freedom from bleeding at 18 years was $96 \pm 1\%$.

Endocarditis

Endocarditis was reported in 45 patients. Fourteen of these patients were reoperated, two died without reoperation at another institution, and 29 were medically treated with success. Three of the medically treated patients were reoperated for structural failure a few years later. At 18 years, the actuarial rate of freedom from endocarditis was $95 \pm 2\%$, with a linearized rate of 0.4%/yr.

Hemolysis

No hemolytic episodes were reported among this patient group.

Reoperation

Seventy-five patients required reoperation: 45 for structural failure, 14 for endocarditis, and 4 for perivalvular leak, while 12 valves were prophylactically explanted due to other diseases (4 CABG, 4 mitral valve replacement and 4 aortic aneurism treatment). The actuarial rate of freedom from reoperation was $57 \pm 9\%$ at 18 years. Only one perioperative death, due to cardiac failure, was observed for reoperation, and no emergency reoperation was necessary. Two patients older than 80 years required reoperation.

Structural valve deterioration

There were 48 patients with structural valve deterioration (SVD), with an actuarial freedom from structural valve failure of 67±8% at 18 years. Among those patients, 45 were reoperated; three patients died without reoperation (one patient had Alzheimer's disease and the two others had severe associated conditions that prevented reoperation). Age was an important factor that influenced durability (Table 1). Actuarial freedom from structural failure (Fig. 2) varied from 99±1% in patients aged >70 years to 80±5% in those aged 60–70 years, and to 48±7% in those aged <60 years. SVD was observed in no patients older than 75 years, and in 2 patients aged 70–75 years. In the present study, age did not represent a contraindication to reoperation. Only one perioperative death occurred during reoperation for structural valve deterioration. Explanted valves showed calcifications leading to valve stenosis in 28 patients, and late fatigue-induced leaflet tear without calcification in 18 cases. In 2 cases, there were both leaflet tear and calcifications. Calcifications occurred mainly between 5 to 11 years after implantation, whereas leaflet tears occurred in older prosthesis (usually between 9 to 15 years after operation). The mean period before valves explantation was 10 years.

Table 1. Relationship between structural valve deterioration and age

Age	<60	60–70	>70
■ No. of patients	257	480	1120
■ 18-year survival	55%	50%	4%
■ SVD (n)	28	18	2

SVD structural valve deterioration

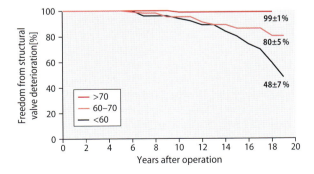

Fig. 2. Actuarial freedom from structural failure according to age at implantation

Table 2. Follow-up echocardiographic data*

	No. of patients	Mean gradient (mmHg)	Peak gradient (mmHg)	EOA (cm^2)
19 mm	136	17.1	29.2	1.1
21 mm	374	14.9	25.8	1.4
23 mm	360	13.1	23.4	1.7
25 mm	232	12.6	22.4	1.9

* Values are mean ± standard deviation.
EOA effective orifice area

Hemodynamics

The echocardiography results detailed in Table 2 comprised 1102 examinations. In addition, among those patients, insufficiency of grade 2 was found in 67 patients, and of grade 1 in 422 patients.

Discussion

The main treatment of significant aortic valve stenosis or regurgitation is aortic valve replacement (AVR). The decision to perform valve surgery requires knowledge of the long-term results of surgical therapy. Despite the well-known finite durability of tissue valves that limits their use, the long-term outcome has been satisfactory, particularly in older patients, in those with a limited life expectancy, and in those undergoing valve replacement in the aortic position. Herein are presented details of the authors' long-term experience with the aortic Perimount pericardial valve. These 18-year data showed good long-term survival for patients who underwent AVR with a Perimount bioprosthesis, with a mean follow-up of 5.9 years and the evolution of patients at risk with time corresponding to the inclusion rate.

Between 1984 and 1994, the authors' team undertook increasing numbers of valve implantations each year and currently implants approximately 200 bioprostheses each year. The cardiologic status of patients was satisfactory, with clear improvements in clinical status and almost all patients being either asymptomatic or pauci-symptomatic. The follow-up echocardiographic studies (Table 2) showed the mean ventricular parameters to be within standard limits; the distribution of data was due mainly to the echocardiographic investigations having been conducted by a variety of operators as the study population was too large to be followed solely at the authors' institution. Late mortality was mainly related to noncardiac rather than valve-related causes though, as in the general population, mortality due to cancer was also significant. Unfortunately, an increasing rate of neurological disorders according to age was observed in the followed population. Sixty-one deaths were of unknown cause, despite aggressive follow-up, though this appeared also to be related to age. Preoperative atrial fibrillation appeared to be a risk factor for poor survival. Indeed, in a recent study, Chaput et al. [8] concluded that patients with preoperative atrial fibrillation had a poorer survival than those without. However, in the present authors' experience this did not contraindicate the use of a biological valve, as no patient with preoperative atrial fibrillation was alive after 12 years and none required reoperation for structural valve failure. The risk of structural valve failure decreased with age; none was observed in patients aged >75 years, and in only two patients aged 70–75 years. Thus, in this population the valve durability exceeded life expectancy. In the present study, an echocardiographic definition was used to reduce the risk of underevaluating the rate of SVD. For those patients who died inexplicably, it was possible to know the echocardiographic status before death, as all patients were followed up every two years. None of the patients who died had signs of SVD at their last follow-up, though the only way to underestimate SVD would be to miss an echocardiography study or to lose the patient to follow-up, and in the present study this risk was low. Although the rate of SVD remained acceptable in patients aged <60 years, the proportion of the present patients aged <60 was low and these were selected; hence, it was impossible to draw any firm conclusion among this population. The indications for tissue valves in the aortic position, according to age, are increasingly better defined in line with advances in valve design, preservation, and the management of reoperations. Although some patients requiring cardiac valve replacement clearly benefit more from one type of valve than from another, some are in the 'gray zone', where optimal choice is difficult. Biological valves tended to be implanted in older patients and mechanical ones in younger patients, but the cut-off level remains controversial [13]. A Veterans' trial [12] and other recent publications with the Perimount pericardial valve [4] suggested the use of a bioprosthesis in patients aged >65 years, and the results of the present study supported this suggestion. During the present study, all patients aged >60 years were implanted with a Perimount valve, there being no selection bias. Moreover, this choice was reinforced by an increasing rate of bleeding among patients with a mechanical prosthesis and age >60 years [5]. Although the risk of reoperation increased with time, the operative risk of reoperation remained low. Few reports have shown an increasing risk of reoperation in elderly patients [21]; in the present study only two patients aged >80 years required reoperation. Many other reports have shown a low risk of mortality [18, 25], with mortality being linked to clinical status or to a need for emergency reoperation. Hence, it was concluded that the trends toward reducing the age at which tissue valve implantation is performed may be justified [9]. Only one death following reoperation for SVD was observed in the present study. All reoperations were performed in an elective situation, and no emergency reoperation was necessary. Patients were reoperated on in case of structural valve failure, before cardiac failure. In this situation, close echocardiographic follow-up is mandatory, and an aggressive reoperation policy offers the best route to good results. The risk of other complications was comparable to those published elsewhere with regard to the use of mechanical and biological valves, and no change has been observed during the past 20 years. In the present study, thromboembolic and hemorrhagic complications rates were low; although as the study was retrospective in nature the rates may have been minimized by the fact that patients do not always report minor events that have no sequel and tend to be forgotten. On the other hand, the guideline definition may have overestimated the real risk of embolism, with some neurological events not being related to the prosthesis. The rate should be compared to neurological events in a normal population. The risk of hemorrhage compared favorably to that seen with mechanical valves (most studies have also been retrospective). Age, associated diseases, and the rate of cancer in the followed population encouraged us to include as short as possible a postoperative period of anticoagulation, as this increases the risk of cerebral hemorrhage [29] and is difficult to manage in case of associated disease, especially for neurological disorders, cancer, and trauma [19, 27]. The present rates of valve-related morbidity and mortality were comparable to those reported recently for the long-term implantation of mechanical valves [14, 22]. Indications for the use of mechanical or biological valves are based on long-term comparisons of valve-related complication rates [12, 20, 28], but these randomized studies were carried out with first-generation bioprostheses and during the study period the reoperation mortality was high. With time, the risk of reoperation has decreased to a point that, today, it is similar to that for primary AVR [18, 25]. In addition, the durability of bioprostheses has increased. Despite their long-term durability, the use of mechanical valves is handicapped by the drawbacks of lifelong anticoagulation, and the choice between mechanical and biological valve implantation in the aortic position remains controversial. The risk of complications and especially of valve failure may be favorably compared with long-term results observed in patients with stented porcine valves [16, 26]. The present 20-year data confirmed an intermediate comparison between stented porcine and pericardial valves [11, 17]. A comparison between pericardial and stentless valves cannot be made as no 20-year data are available. Nonetheless, two points should be highlighted from the present investigation, namely the absence of premature leaflet failure [7] and the absence of valve thrombosis. An even longer-term follow-up of the population will be necessary in order to evaluate the impact of any new valve treatment or other treatment on pericardial tissue calcification processes [1, 23].

In conclusion, the long-term results of AVR with the Perimount pericardial valve were satisfactory, and the long-term behavior of this prosthesis confirmed the findings of previous reports, with a low rate of valve-related complications and an especially low rate of structural valve failure. The present data support the clinical use of this prosthesis in patients aged >60 years and in those with atrial fibrillation.

References

1. Antonini Canterin F, Zuppiroli A, Bogdan A et al (2003) Effect of statins on the progression of bioprosthetic aortic valve degeneration. Am J Cardiol 92:1479–1482
2. Aupart MR, Sirinelli AL, Diemont FF, Meurisse YA, Dreyfus XB, Marchand MA (1996) The last generation of pericardial valves in the aortic position: ten-year follow-up in 589 patients. Ann Thorac Surg 61:615–620
3. Aupart MR, Neville PH, Hammami S, Sirinelli AL, Meurisse YA, Marchand MA (1997) Carpentier-Edwards pericardial valves in the mitral position: ten-year follow-up. J Thorac Cardiovasc Surg 113:492–498
4. Banbury MK, Cosgrove DM, White JA, Blackstone EH, Frater RW, Okies JE (2001) Age and valve size effect on the long-term durability of the Carpentier-Edwards aortic pericardial bioprosthesis. Ann Thorac Surg 72:753–757
5. Bergoend E, Aupart M, Kendja F, Sirinelli A, Neville P, Marchand M (2004) Twelve years' experience with Carbomedics bileaflet valves. Arch Mal Coeur Vaiss 97: 214–220
6. Bonow RO, Carabello B, Chatterjee K et al (1998) Guidelines for the management of patient with valvular heart disease. Circulation 98:1949–1984
7. Bortolotti U, Milano A, Thiene G et al (1987) Early mechanical failures of the Hancock pericardial xenograft. J Thorac Cardiovasc Surg 94:200–207
8. Chaput M, Bouchard D, Demers P et al (2005) Conversion to sinus rhythm do not improve long term survival after valve surgery: insight from a 20 year follow up study. Eur J Cardiothorac Surg 28:206–210
9. Dalrymple-Hay MJ, Crook T, Bannon PG et al (2002) Risk of reoperation for structural failure of aortic and mitral tissue valves. J Heart Valve Dis 11:419–423
10. Edmunds LH Jr., Clark RE, Cohn LH, Grunkemeier GL, Miller DC, Weisel RD (1996) Guidelines for reporting morbidity and mortality after cardiac valvular operations. Ad Hoc Liaison Committee for Standardizing Definitions of Prosthetic Heart Valve Morbidity of The American Association for Thoracic Surgery and The Society of Thoracic Surgeons. J Thorac Cardiovasc Surg 112:708–711
11. Gao G, Wu Y, Grunkemeier GL, Furnary AP, Starr A (2004) Durability of pericardial versus porcine aortic valves. J Am Coll Cardiol 44:384–388
12. Hammermeister K, Sethi GK, Henderson WG, Grover FL, Oprian C, Rahimtoola SH (2000) Outcomes 15 years after valve replacement with a mechanical versus a bioprosthetic valve: final report of the Veterans Affairs randomized trial. J Am Coll Cardiol 36:1152–1158
13. Hanania G, Michel PL, Montely JM et al (2004) The long term (15 years) evolution after valvular replacement with mechanical prosthesis or bioprosthesis between the age of 60 and 70 years. Arch Mal Coeur Vaiss 97:7–14

14. Ikonomidis JS, Kratz JM, Crumbley AJ et al (2003) Twenty year experience with the St. Jude Medical mechanical prosthesis. J Thorac Cardiovasc Surg 126:2022–2031
15. Iung B, Gohlke-Barwolf C, Tornos P et al (2002) Recommendations on the management of the asymptomatic patients with valvular heart disease. Eur Heart J 23: 1253–1266
16. Jamieson WR, Burr LH, Munro AI, Miyagishima RT (1998) Carpentier-Edwards standard porcine bioprosthesis: a 21-year experience. Ann Thorac Surg 66(6 Suppl): S40–S43
17. Jamieson WR, Marchand MA, Pelletier CL et al (1999) Structural valve deterioration in mitral replacement surgery: comparison of Carpentier-Edwards supra-annular porcine and Perimount pericardial bioprostheses. J Thorac Cardiovasc Surg 118:297–304
18. Jamieson WR, Burr LH, Miyagishima RT et al (2003) Reoperation for bioprosthetic aortic structural failure: risk assessment. Eur J Cardiothorac Surg 24:873–878
19. Karni A, Holtzman R, Bass T et al (2001) Traumatic head injury in the anticoagulated patient: a lethal combination. Am Surg 67:1098–1100
20. Khan SS, Trento A, DeRobertis M et al (2001) Twenty year comparison of tissue and mechanical valve replacement. J Thorac Cardiovasc Surg 122:257–269
21. Kirsh M, Nakashima K, Kubota S, Houel R, Hillion ML, Loisance D (2004) The risk of reoperative heart valve procedures in octogenarian patients. J Heart Valve Dis 13:991–996
22. Lund O, Nielsen SL, Arildsen H, Ilkjaer LB, Pilegaaard HK (2000) Standard aortic St. Jude at 18 years: performance profile and determinants of outcome. Ann Thorac Surg 69:1459–1465
23. O'Brien KD (2005) Converting enzyme inhibitor and aortic calcification. Arch Intern Med 165:858–862
24. Otto CM (1998) Aortic stenosis. Clinical evaluation and optimal timing of surgery. Cardiol Clin 16:353–373
25. Potter DD, Sundt TM, Zehr KJ et al (2005) Operative risk of reoperative aortic valve replacement. J Thorac Cardiovasc Surg 129:94–103
26. Rizzoli G, Bottio T, Thiene G, Toscano G, Casarotto D (2003) Long-term durability of the Hancock II porcine bioprosthesis. J Thorac Cardiovasc Surg 126:66–74
27. Rosand J, Eckman MH, Knudsen KA, Singer DE, Greesberg SM (2004) The effect of warfarin and intensity of anticoagulation on outcome of intracerebral haemorrhage. Arch Intern Med 164:880–884
28. Sidhu P, O'Kane H, Ali N et al (2001) Mechanical or bioprosthetic valves in the elderly: a 20-year comparison. Ann Thorac Surg 71(5 Suppl.):S257–S260
29. Sjalander A, Engstrom G, Berntrop E, Svensson P (2003) Risk of hemorrhagic stroke in patient with oral anticoagulation compared with the general population. J Intern Med 254:434–438

Twenty-year experience with the St. Jude Medical Biocor bioprosthesis in the aortic position

W. Eichinger

Bioprostheses are prone to continuous degeneration, which over time may lead to structural valve deterioration (SVD). In turn, SVD may require reoperation [1–3]. Improvements in valve design and conservation methods have extended the lifetime of bioprotheses [4, 5]. Thus, data on valve dysfunction and the risk of reoperation over the long term are of particular interest.

Over a 12-year period, from January 1985 through December 1996, the St. Jude Medical Biocor prosthesis was implanted in a series of 455 consecutive patients at the German Heart Center Munich. This study was designed to provide 21-year outcome data in patients who received a St. Jude Medical Biocor valve in the aortic position. The Biocor valve (St. Jude Medical, Inc., St. Paul, MN, USA) is a triple-composite, porcine bioprosthesis, first introduced in 1982 in Brazil [5].

Material and methods

Patients

Data on all 455 patients who received a St. Jude Medical Biocor bioprosthesis in the aortic position between January 1985 and December 1996 are included in the study.

Follow-up

Follow-up was conducted with the patients in 2003 and 2006 via questionnaires and telephone contact. The latest follow-up occurred from January 2006 to July 2006. The follow-up questionnaire was designed to answer questions regarding clinical outcome according to the criteria of Edmunds [6]. All possible valve-related complications were checked. In addition, all available medical reports were obtained from the patients' cardiologists or home physicians. Causes of death were determined from hospital records and the government registration office.

Valve selection

Patients older than 65 years received a bioprosthesis. The decision to implant a Biocor valve was made by the surgeon according to his or her preference.

Operative techniques

Operations were performed using standard cardiopulmonary bypass with moderate hypothermia. The valves were secured to the annulus with interrupted pledgeted mattress sutures.

Anticoagulation management

Except in patients with atrial fibrillation or other indications for continuous anticoagulant therapy, there was no routine postoperative anticoagulation. The target international normalized ratio (INR) for patients who received anticoagulant therapy was 2.0 to 2.5. (INR analysis had been available since the end of the 1990s.)

Outcomes

Predefined study outcomes included survival and adverse events (bleeding, endocarditis, embolism, leak, tear, valve degeneration, and reoperation). All adverse events related to the heart valve prosthesis were assessed. Valve-related death was defined as death caused by structural valvular deterioration, nonstructural dysfunction, valve thrombosis, embolism, bleeding events, valvular endocarditis, or death related to operative replacement of a dysfunctional prosthesis. Sudden, unexplained deaths were counted as valve-related deaths [6].

Adverse events data were collected in accordance with the standards described by Edmunds and colleagues and the U.S. Food and Drug Administration document, "Replacement of Heart Valve Guidance" 1996 [6, 7].

Statistical analysis

Statistical evaluation was performed with the Statistical Package for Social Sciences, version 13 (SPSS, Inc., Chicago, IL).

Categorical variables were reported using the number and percent of observations. Continuous variables were reported as mean ± standard deviations. Complication rates and survival rates were calculated using a nonparametric actuarial Kaplan-Meier product-limit estimator [8]. To compare survival and complications, patients were grouped into the following age classes: 65 years or younger; 66 to 74 years; and 75 years or older. A p value of < 0.05 was considered statistically significant.

Results

Patient population

Over a 12-year period, 455 patients who underwent aortic valve replacement with the Biocor valve at the German Heart Center Munich were included. The follow-up covered up to 21 years. It was 99.6% complete for the endpoint "death." Cumulative follow-up time was 3, 321 patient years. Mean follow-up time was 8.2 years.

Patient survival

The overall 30-day mortality was 5.3% (24/455). Twelve patients who died had concomitant coronary artery bypass grafting (CABG); one patient had concomitant CABG and replacement of the ascending aorta; and one patient had concomitant repair of the ascending aorta. All other patients who died within 30 days had isolated aortic valve replacement. The most frequent cause of death was congestive heart failure (2.8%: 13/455). Two of the early deaths were valve related: one patient with defect of one cusp in combination with a hemorrhagic pericarditis and one patient with unclear cause of death, which was classified as valve-related in accordance with the guidelines [6].

Actuarial survival rates at 5, 10, 15, and 20 years were 74.7% ± 2.0%, 44.9% ± 2.4%, 20.9% ± 2.5%, and 9.4% ± 2.8%, respectively.

Survival was significantly superior in younger patients (i.e., younger than 65 years).

Freedom from valve-related death at 5, 10, 15, and 20 years was 94.3% ± 1.2%, 90.9% ± 1.5%, 87.8% ± 2.6% and 87.8% ± 2.6%, respectively. It was comparable in all age groups.

Hemorrhage

Major bleeding occurred in 28 patients. Of those with a major bleeding event, seven patients had atrial fibrillation, each of whom was under permanent anticoagulation with Coumadin with a target INR between 2–2.5. Exact INR values at the time of the bleeding events were unknown. Three other patients died of an intracerebral hemorrhagic event; the anticoagulation status of those patients at the time of the events was also unknown. The remaining 18 patients had major bleeding events without further sequelae.

The actuarial freedom from hemorrhagic complications at 5, 10, 15, and 20 years was 96.6% ± 1.0%, 93.0% ± 1.6%, 92.2% ± 1.8% and 76.8% ± 14.1%, respectively. Freedom from hemorrhage was comparable in all age groups.

Endocarditis

A total of 18 patients suffered from prosthetic valve endocarditis (PVE): 3 patients received antibiotic treatment without reoperation; 8 patients required reoperation due to PVE; 7 patients died. Actuarial freedom from PVE after 5, 10, 15, and 20 years was 96.1% ± 1.0%, 95.0% ± 1.2%, 95.0% ± 1.2% and 95.0 ± 1.2%, respectively.

The risk of postoperative PVE was significantly ($p < 0.005$) higher in patients younger than 65 years than in patients 65 or older. In those younger than 65 years, the incidence of preoperative endocarditis was higher (3 of 49 patients: 6.1%) than in patients 65 to 74 years (4 of 221 patients: 1.8%) and patients 75 years or older (1 of 184: 0.5%).

Structural valve deterioration

Structural valve deterioration (SVD) was defined as a decrease of one New York Heart Association (NYHA) functional class resulting from an intrinsic abnormality of the valve that causes stenosis or regurgitation [6]. In addition, a mean pressure gradient exceeding 40 mmHg was defined as structural valve deterioration.

In total, 23 patients suffered from SVD. Of those, 16 required reoperation. Four patients were not referred for or they refused reoperation and were treated conservatively (NYHA I, III – one patient each; NYHA II – two patients). Two patients were too old for reoperation (NYHA I and II). One patient was mentally retarded and the custodian refused reoperation (NYHA IV).

Overall mortality of the reoperated patients was 37.5% (6/16) and 28.6% (2/7) for non-reoperated patients. There was no early death in the group of the reoperated patients (mean days to death: 995 d ± 964.4 d; range: 71 d ± 2141 d). Causes for deaths in the reoperated group were chronic heart failure (2), acute nonvalve-related death (2), valve-related death (1), and death due to other causes (1). In the group of patients who did not undergo reoperation, both deaths were due to unknown causes. The actuarial freedom from SVD after 5, 10, 15, and 20 years was 98.4% ± 0.6%, 93.1% ± 1.7%, 88.4% ± 3.5%, and 70.3% ± 10.9%.

The risk for SVD was significantly different ($p < 0.05$) for the different age groups. In patients under 65 years of age, the risk of SVD began to increase 7 years postoperatively.

Nonstructural valve dysfunction

The actuarial freedom from nonstructural valve dysfunction (NSVD) at 5, 10, 15, and 20 years was 97.5% ± 0.8%, 97.5% ± 0.8%, 97.5% ± 0.8%, and 97.5% ± 0.8%, respectively. It was similar in all age groups.

Reoperation

Reoperation was defined as any operation that repaired, altered or replaced a previously operated valve [6]. During the 20-year follow-up period, 32 patients required reoperation. Reasons for reoperation were SVD in 16 patients, PVE in seven patients, and paravalvular leakage in four patients. (A further group of six patients exhibited paravalvular leakage without the need for reoperation; all 10 patients with paravalvular leakage survived.) One patient suffered from valve dysfunction due to thrombotic material on the leaflets, two patients were reoperated due to an aneurysm of the ascending aorta, and one patient had a coronary artery bypass operation. One patient had reoperation without the cause being known. Actuarial freedom from reoperation after 5, 10, 15, and 20 years was 95.4% ± 1.1%, 90.6% ± 1.8%, 88.2% ± 2.4%, and 84.0% ± 4.7%.

The actuarial freedom from reoperation due to SVD at 5, 10, 15, and 20 years was 95.9% ± 1%, 91.9% ± 1.6%, 90.6% ± 2.1%, and 86.5% ± 4.5% (Fig. 1).

Thromboembolism

Thromboembolism occurred in 70 patients. Of those, 41 suffered from major cerebral thromboembolism, 1 patient suffered from minor cerebral thromboembolism and 19 patients suffered from a reversible ischemic neurologic deficit. In 9 patients, thromboembolism of the extremities occurred. Of the 41 patients with major stroke, 8 had atrial fibrillation and were under anticoagulation. Sixteen patients died after the acute event and 25 patients had residual neurological deficits. Coagulation status of the patients with sinus rhythm was unknown. Overall freedom from thromboembolism after 5, 10, 15, and 20 years was 90.3% ± 1.5%, 80.7% ± 2.3%, 76.0% ± 2.9%, and 71.2% ± 5.3%. Older patients had an increased risk of thromboembolism.

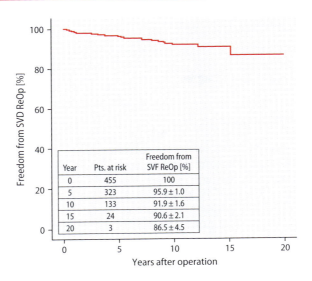

Fig. 1. Freedom from reoperation due to SVD

Comment

From 1999 to 2002, the implantation of bioprostheses increased from 50% to 65% [2]. Thus, as a majority of patients have begun to request biological valve prostheses, complete long-term follow-up studies have become increasingly important in helping to advise patients of their risks following valve replacement. The main focus of long-term biological valve studies lies in the incidence of SVD, thromboembolism, and major bleeding events, compared with their incidence in association with mechanical prostheses.

This is one of the longest and largest follow-up studies of a bioprosthetic heart valve. It does not evaluate the valve's hemodynamic performance: several papers on the Biocor valve's hemodynamic function [9, 10] have been published.

Survival

Until now, the longest follow-up study for the Biocor valve is a 17-year follow-up of around 1,500 patients, published by Myken et al. The study reported an actuarial survival of 28.2% ± 3.7% at 17 years for patients (mean age 70 ± 11 years) receiving the valve in the aortic position [11]. The study observed a survival rate of 9.4% ± 2.8% at 20 years. Freedom from death after 17 years was calculated to be 17.4% ± 2.7%.

Valve-related mortality

The incidence of valve-related mortality in the patient group was 7.9% (36/455 patients) and was higher than in the Gothenburg population after 17 years (2.7%: 35/1283) [11].

Reoperation

Freedom from reoperation in the study population was 84.0% ± 4.7% after 20 years. These results are comparable with published outcomes describing other bioprosthetic valves. Recipients of the Biocor prosthesis (n = 254) at the Karolinska Institute, Stockholm, were reported to have about 87% freedom from reoperation after 11 years (mean age 78.5 ± 5 years)[12]. For the Carpentier-Edwards pericardial valve, Jamieson published freedom from valve-related reoperation of 62.3 ± 3.5% at 18 years (mean age 68.9 ± 10.9 years) [13].

Structural valve deterioration

Overall freedom from SVD was 70.3% ± 10.9% after 20 years in the study population, but patients up to age 65 were at a significantly ($p < 0.05$) higher risk of SVD than patients over 65. Kaplan-Meyer calculations also showed significant differences regarding the time of occurrence of SVD for patients younger than 65 years, starting about 7 years postoperatively. After 20 years, freedom from SVD was 56.5% ± 15.3%, 59.9% ± 18.5%, and 95.1% ± 2.7% for patients younger than 65 years, 66 to 74 years, and 75 and over, respectively. Similar age-related differences in valve degeneration for the Biocor prosthesis in both the aortic and mitral positions have been reported previously [10, 14].

Results from the current study compare favorably with published data on the Carpentier-Edwards porcine valve, which showed a freedom from SVD of 64.0% after 18 years (compared to 70.3% after 20 years in the current study) [13]. Subdivided into age groups, freedom from SVD was reported in 77.6% of patients from 61 to 70 years and in 94.6% of patients older than 70 [13]. The age groups (65 years or younger, 66 to 74, and 75 or older) are not fully comparable, but results are slightly superior for patients older than 75 years (95.1% ± 2.7%). Nevertheless, the results seem to be worse for younger patients (56.5% ± 15.3% for patients 65 years or younger and 59.9% ± 18.5% for patients aged 66 to 74 years).

SVD is an age dependent phenomenon, demonstrated for all biological prostheses. However, younger patients request such implants, mostly for lifestyle considerations. Although the speed of SVD may be significantly different for specific biological valves, patients younger than 65 years should be advised that, even with the most durable biological valve today, they take an approximate 50% chance of having a reoperation for replacement within 20 years.

Reoperations due to SVD

Structural valve deterioration (SVD) is a major cause of reoperation. It is generally due to either major calcification or to primary cusp deterioration without significant dystrophic calcification [3, 15, 16], both of which can lead to a partial or total valve dysfunction. The study by Myken at al. of Biocor valves in the aortic position reported a freedom from reoperation due to SVD of 73.9% after 17 years [11], which was lower than was found in the current study (86.5% after 20 years).

The mortality of patients who underwent reoperations due to SVD seems to be considerably higher than that of patients with SVD and no reoperation (37.5% vs. 28.6%). Because the groups were small, these results must be interpreted carefully. They do not justify any general statement concerning the indication for reoperation.

Hemorrhage

In the current study, the overall freedom from anticoagulant-related hemorrhage (ARH) was 76.8% ± 14.1% after 20 years. It was similar for all age groups. This result seemed surprisingly low – and comparable to results when mechanical valves are implanted, followed by an aggressive anticoagulant regime. With the St. Jude Medical mechanical valve, freedom from ARH at 20-year follow-up was 77.9% (mean age 62 ± 14.1 years) compared to 76.8% in the current study [17]. In the current study group, no routine anticoagulation was applied postoperatively except in patients with atrial fibrillation or other indications for continuous anticoagulant therapy. It is possible, however, that in the current study, bleeding was related to age rather than to the anticoagulation regime. The population's mean age was higher than in some other studies [11, 13]. The risk of hemorrhagic events, such as gastrointestinal and cerebral bleeding, rises in the general population with increasing age and is further increased by medication, such as low-dose aspirin [18].

In this study, a single hemorrhagic event led to a drop in the freedom from ARH at 17 years from 92.2% to 76.8%. This was a nonpermanent, nonlethal cerebral event in an 89-year-old man. At that time, only five patients were at risk, so this had a large impact on the overall result.

At 17 years (before the occurrence of the single hemorrhagic event described above), results of the current study (92.2% ± 1.8%) were comparable to Myken's data using the Biocor valve (91.4% ± 2.2% freedom from ARH at 17 years), and Minami's experience with the Mitroflow prosthesis at 15 years (94.4% freedom from bleeding: mean age 75.6 years) [11, 19].

Other complications

Freedom from thromboembolism also decreased with increasing age. This may be due to the general observation that the incidence of transient ischemic attacks, ischemic stroke, and hemorrhagic stroke rises with advanced age by more than 1% in people over 65 years [20]. Myken et al. published very similar results with the Biocor valve after 17 years of follow-up; freedom from thromboembolic events was 98.8% in patients up to 50 years, but it fell with increasing age to 73.7% in patients over 80 years of age [11].

Younger patients seemed to have an increased risk of developing PVE postoperatively. This is also consistent with other studies. Minami et al. reported a significant reduction in the frequency of PVE with increasing age in their study population of Mitroflow valve recipients [19].

Influence of patient age on outcome

Younger patients had a higher valve degeneration rate (leading to an increased risk of reoperation) and an increased risk of PVE compared with older patients. The opposite was true, however, for hemorrhagic and thromboembolic events [18, 20]. With a trend toward the selection of bioprostheses for younger patients, the risk of reoperation due to SVD should be carefully discussed. However, results for the Biocor valve showed extremely low reoperation rates compared with other bioprostheses in the aortic position [13, 21–23].

Limitations of the study

It is difficult to collect data and maintain follow-up over a long timeframe. In this study, systematic echocardiographic data was not obtained, a fact that could result in an underestimation of SVD rates. The large numbers of variables that influence outcome make it difficult to compare results from different studies, and few data are available to guide interpretation of individual factors. In this study, effort was made to select the most appropriate comparators and to avoid potentially misleading 'actual' data analyses.

Conclusion

Compared with other bioprostheses for which long-term results are available, the St. Jude Medical Biocor porcine bioprosthesis in the aortic position demonstrated very satisfying outcomes at 20-year follow-up. Results indicate an age-dependent risk for SVD beginning as soon as 7 years postoperatively for patients younger than 65 years of age. But the results also showed a lower overall incidence of valve-related complications, indicating excellent durability, especially when used in patients older than 65 years.

Study results, thus, support the recent changes in the "Guidelines for the Management of Patients with Valvular Heart Disease" from 2006 [2], which recommend bioprostheses for patients older than 65 years (Class IIa). In addition, for the first time, bioprostheses are recommended for patients younger than 65 years for lifestyle considerations (Class IIa). It needs to be stressed that the choice of using a bioprosthesis is driven by logic and discussion with the patient since second-generation tissue valves – porcine and pericardial – provide patients with similar outcomes to mechanical valves [24].

Acknowledgments. The study was financially supported by St. Jude Medical, Inc.

References

1. Oxenham H, Bloomfield P, Wheatley DJ et al (2003) Twenty-year comparison of a Bjork-Shiley mechanical heart valve with porcine bioprostheses. Heart 89(7):715–721
2. Bonow RO, Carabello BA, Kanu C et al (2006) ACC/AHA 2006 guidelines for the management of patients with valvular heart disease: a report of the American College of Cardiology/American Heart Association Task Force on Practice Guidelines (writing committee to revise the 1998 Guidelines for the Management of Patients with Valvular Heart Disease): developed in collaboration with the Society of Cardiovascular Anesthesiologists: endorsed by the Society for Cardiovascular Angiography and Interventions and the Society of Thoracic Surgeons. Circulation 114(5):e84–e231
3. Bortolotti U, Milano A, Mossuto E, Mazzaro E, Thiene G, Cassorotto D (1995) Porcine valve durability: a comparison between Hancock standard and Hancock II bioprostheses. AnnThorac Surg 60(2 Suppl):S216–S220
4. Vesely I (1991) Analysis of the Medtronic Intact bioprosthetic valve. Effects of "zero-pressure" fixation. J Thorac Cardiovasc Surg 101(1):90–99
5. Vrandecic MO, Gontijo Filho B, Paula e Silva JA et al (1991) Clinical results with the Biocor porcine bioprosthesis. J Cardiovasc Surg (Torino) 32(6):807–813
6. Edmunds Jr LH, Clark RE, Cohn LH, Grunkemeier GL, Miller DC, Weisel RD (1996) Guidelines for reporting morbidity and mortality after cardiac valvular operations. The American Association for Thoracic Surgery, Ad Hoc Liaison Committee for Standardizing Definitions of Prosthetic Heart Valve Morbidity. Ann Thorac Surg 62(3):932–935
7. Johnson DM, Sapirstein W (1994) FDA's requirements for in-vivo performance data for prosthetic heart valves. J Heart Valve Dis 3(4):350–355
8. Grunkemeier GL, Jin R, Eijkemans JM, Takkenberg JJ (2007) Actual and actuarial probabilities of competing risks: apples and lemons. Ann Thorac Surg 83(5):1586–1592
9. Bech-Hanssen O, Wallentin I, Larsson S, Caidahl K. (1998) Reference Doppler echocardiographic values for St. Jude Medical, Omnicarbon and Biocor prosthetic valves in the aortic position. J Am Soc Echocardiogr 11(5):466–477
10. Bottio T, Rizzoli G, Thiene G, Nesseris G, Casarotto D, Gerosa G (2004) Hemodynamic and clinical outcomes with the Biocor valve in the aortic position: an eight-year experience. J Thorac Cardiovasc Surg 127(6):1616–1623

11. Myken PS (2005) Seventeen-year experience with the St. Jude Medical Biocor porcine bioprosthesis. J Heart Valve Dis (14(4):486–492
12. Dellgren G, Eriksson, MJ, Brodin, LA, Radegran K (2002) Eleven years' experience with the Biocor stentless aortic bioprosthesis: clinical and hemodynamic follow-up with long-term relative survival rate. Eur J Cardiothorac Surg 22(6):912–921
13. Jamieson WR, Burr, LH, Miyagishima RT et al (2005) Carpentier-Edwards supra-annular aortic porcine bioprosthesis: clinical performance over 20 years. J Thorac Cardiovasc Surg 130(4):994–1000
14. Kirali K, Guler M, Tuncer A et al (2001) Fifteen-year clinical experience with the Biocor porcine bioprosthesis in the mitral position. Ann Thorac Surg 71(3):811–815
15. Fann, JI, Miller DC, Moore KA et al (1996) Twenty-year clinical experience with porcine bioprostheses. Ann Thorac Surg 62(5):1301–1311, discussion 1311–1312
16. Jamieson, WR, Burr LH, Munro AI, Miyagishima RT (1998) Carpentier-Edwards standard porcine bioprosthesis: a 21-year experience. Ann Thorac Surg 66(6 Suppl):S40–S43
17. Emery RW, Krogh CC, Arom KV et al (2005) The St. Jude Medical Cardiac Valve Prosthesis: A 25-year experience with single valve replacement. Ann Thorac Surg 79(3):776–782
18. Nelson MR, Liew D, Bertram M, Vos T (2005) Epidemiological modeling of routine use of low-dose aspirin for the primary prevention of coronary heart disease and stroke in those aged > or =70. BMJ 330(7503):1306
19. Minami KA, Zitterman S, Schulte-Eistrup S, Koertle H, Korfer R (2005) Mitroflow synergy prostheses for aortic valve replacement: 19 years' experience with 1516 patients. Ann Thorac Surg 80(5):1699–1705
20. Kolominsky-Rabas PL, Sarti C, Heuschmann PU et al (1998) A prospective community-based study of stroke in Germany – the Erlangen Stroke Project (ESPro): incidence and case fatality at 1, 3 and 12 months. Stroke 29(12):2501–2506
21. Aupart, MR, Mirza A, Meurisse Y.A., Sirinelli AL, Neville PH, Marchand MA (2006) Perimount pericardial bioprosthesis for aortic calcified stenosis: 18-year experience with 1, 133 patients. J Heart Valve Dis 15(6):768–775, discussion 775–776
22. Borger MA, Ivanov J, Armstrong S, Christie-Hrybinsky D, Feindel CM, David TE (2006) Twenty-year results of the Hancock II bioprosthesis. J Heart Valve Dis 15(1):49–55, discussion 55–56
23. Yankah CA, Schubel J, Buz S, Siniawski H, Hetzer R (2005) Seventeen-year clinical results of 1037 Mitroflow pericardial heart valve prostheses in the aortic position. J Heart Valve Dis 14(2):172–179, discussion 179–180
24. Hammermeister KE, Sethi GK, Henderson WG, Oprian C, Kim T, Rahimtoola S (1993) A comparison of outcomes in men 11 years after heart-valve replacement with a mechanical valve or bioprosthesis. Veterans Affairs Cooperative Study on Valvular Heart Disease. N Engl J Med 328(18):1289–1296

20-Year durability of bioprostheses in the aortic position

W. R. E. Jamieson

Bioprostheses have become the predominant diseased aortic valve substitute for aortic valve replacement. The experience of the Society of Thoracic Surgeons was published in 2009 by Brown and colleagues [1] documenting that the use of bioprostheses increased from 42% in 1996 to 78.4% in 2006. The mechanical prostheses use declined to 20.5%. The use of bioprostheses for aortic valve replacement has increased in Western Europe but not to the same extent. The current contemporary bioprostheses utilized worldwide were, in some cases, delayed by regulatory market approval in the United States. There is considerate opinion in the United States that current bioprostheses have the opportunity for advanced durability. Patients have had a renewed concern of anticoagulation management and complications. The knowledge of durability of the contemporary bioprostheses is of extreme importance in determining the risk of reoperation for SVD.

There are a number of contemporary bioprostheses that have or nearing to have published reports of 20-year durability results. Some publications have reported 20-year experiences but without having adequate numbers at risk to have a valid 20-year durability experience. The contemporary bioprostheses evaluated in this chapter are detailed in Table 1 [2–11]. The formulation of these bioprostheses has been stable since their introduction, with the majority dating back to the early 1980s. The Medtronic Mosaic porcine bioprosthesis was introduced as an investigational prosthesis in 1994 and has the shortest documented experience. The prostheses are all formulated with glutaraldehyde collagen cross-linking for tissue preservation.

Glutaraldehyde-treated tissue is subject to degenerative collagen changes and calcification due to residual aldehydes and/or phospholipids. Calcium-mitigation therapy attempts to control or retard mineralization by altering these two mechanisms of calcification. The compounds most commonly utilized are surfactants, alpha oleic acid, and ethanol. Thermafix heat treatment of the Carpentier-Edwards PERIMOUNT pericardial bioprosthesis is the only new biological tissue treatment since the introduction of these contemporary bioprostheses on the worldwide market. The improvements to bioprostheses have incorporated improved tissue procurement and processing, as well as tissue formulation to reduce tissue stress, a contributing factor to altered durability. Several manufacturers have come forward with

Table 1. Summary of reported freedom from structural valve deterioration of predominant marketed porcine and pericardial bioprostheses (aortic valve replacement)

Author	Prosthesis	Mean age	Age group	Freedom from SVD (%) Actuarial	Actual	Time interval (years)
Jamieson et al. (2005) [2]	CE-SAV	68.9 ± 10.4		74.9 ± 2.3	88.9 ± 1.0	15
			>70	94.6 ± 2.3	98.2 ± 0.6	15
			61–70	85.7 ± 3.2	92.8 ± 1.5	15
			51–60	62.6 ± 5.4	75.4 ± 3.6	15
			≤50	44.0 ± 5.8	56.5 ± 4.9	15
				64.0 ± 3.6	86.4 ± 1.2	18
			>70	94.6 ± 2.3	98.2 ± 0.6	18
			61–70	77.6 ± 4.9	90.5 ± 1.8	18
			51–60	51.0 ± 7.0	70.6 ± 4.0	18
			≤50	31.9 ± 6.3	48.4 ± 5.3	18
Borger, David et al. (2006) [3]	Hancock II	67.0 ± 11.0		64.0 ± 3.0		20
			<65	39.0 ± 9.0	72.0 ± 7.0	20
			≥65	73.0 ± 16.0	97.0 ± 2.0	20
			<65	72.0 ± 5.0		15
			≥65	99.0 ± 1.0		15
Eichinger et al. (2008) [4]	SJM Biocor	72.5 ± 9.0		88.4 ± 3.5		15
				70.3 ± 10.9		20
			≤65	56.5 ± 15.3		15
			>65–<75	93.2 ± 2.1		15
			≥75	95.1 ± 2.7		15
				90.6 ± 2.1*		15
				86.5 ± 4.5*		20
			≤65	71.8 ± 9.2*		15
			>65–>75	92.8 ± 2.0*		15
			≥75	95.7 ± 1.8*		15
Myken, Bech-Hansen (2009) [5]	SJM Biocor	70.8 ± 10.9		61.1 ± 8.5*	85.6 ± 2.2*	20
			51–60	60.7 ± 10.3*		20
			61–70	81.0 ± 5.1*		20
			71–80	97.8 ± 1.2*		20
			>80	100*		20
			≤65	44.5*		20
			>65	92.1*		20
Aupart et al. (2006) [6]	CE-P	72.6		68.0 ± 12.0		18
			>60	45.0 ± 15.0		18
			60–70	77.0 ± 12.0		18
			>70	99.0 ± 1.0		18

Table 1 (continued)

Author	Prosthesis	Mean age	Age group	Freedom from SVD (%)		Time interval (years)
				Actuarial	Actual	
Cosgrove, Frater (2003) [7]	CE-P		≥60	77.1*	92.6*	20
			≥65	81.5*	96.3*	20
Clinical Communique			61–70	77.9*	90.5*	20
			>70	69.9*	96.0*	18
Prasongsukarn et al. (2005) [8]	CE-SAV	68.9±10.9				
			61–70	86.1±3.1	93.0±1.5	15
			>70	94.5±2.3	98.2±0.6	15
Jamieson et al. (2006) [9]	CE-P	69.5±10.4				
			61–70	88.9±4.0	92.7±2.5	15
			>70	99.4±0.6	99.6±0.4	15
Jamieson et al. (2009) [10]	Mitroflow		≥60	85.2±3.9*	93.3±1.8*	12
			≥65	85.0±4.0*	94.2±1.8*	12
			61–70	95.7±4.3*	97.4±2.6*	10
			>70	83.2±4.6*	94.0±1.9*	12
Yankah et al. (2008) [11]	Mitroflow	73.2±0.22				
			≥65	71.8±6.0*	92.6±4.6*	20
			≥70	84.8±0.7*	96.6±0.8*	20

*SVD diagnosed by reoperation

SVD Structural valve deterioration, *CE-SAV* Carpentier-Edwards supra annular valve, *SJM* St. Jude Medical, *CE-P* Carpentier-Edwards PERIMOUNT

diameter-enhanced designs to facilitate optimal hemodynamics, namely the Carpentier-Edwards PERIMOUNT Magna, Medtronic Mosaic Ultra, St. Jude Medical Epic Supra, and the Medtronic Hancock II Ultra. These formulations are designed to facilitate implantation upsizing.

The pathological features of structural valve deterioration differ for porcine and pericardial bioprostheses. Jamieson and colleagues [2] reported on the Carpentier-Edwards SAV porcine aortic bioprosthesis in 2005 – calcification with leaflet tear 61%, primary tears 15%, calcification without accompanying leaflet tear 23%, and stent dehiscence 1%. Aupart and coauthors [6] reported on the Carpentier-Edwards PERIMOUNT aortic bioprosthesis and reported that, of explanted prostheses, dystrophic calcification and valvular stenosis was present in 79% and late fatigue induced leaflet tear without calcification in 21%. These findings confirmed the porcine bioprostheses fail with insufficiency (usually acute) in approximately 80% of cases, while pericardial bioprostheses fail by dystrophic calcification (usually chronic) in approximately 80% of cases.

The durability of the predominant marketed porcine and pericardial bioprostheses are documented in Table 1 as actuarial and actual freedom from structural valve deterioration [2–11]. Table 1 shows the prostheses by reporting authors, by mean age, by age groups, and time intervals. The 20-year experience is often reported but patients-at-risk only allow for robustness of data to 15 and 18 years. Actuarial freedom denotes the prostheses durability, while actual freedom denotes freedom from structural valve deterioration as clinical performance in specific populations, such as the elderly where the risk of mortality is more multifactorial during the anticipated failure-free period of the prostheses.

This chapter is not formulated to compare the durability of specific porcine and pericardial bioprostheses or to compare porcine to pericardial bioprostheses. Several series are reported as SVD at reoperation, while others attempt to report by a composite of reoperation, autopsy, and echocardiography. Table 1 designates the reporting method for designated series.

The major reported studies of porcine aortic bioprostheses comprise of 4595 patients – CE-SAV 1847 (Jamieson et al. [2]) (Figs. 1 and 2), Hancock II 1010 (Borger and David et al. [3]) (Figs. 3 and 4), St. Jude Medical Biocor 1283 (Myken and Bech-Hansen [5]) and St. Jude Medical Biocor 455 (Echinger et al. [4]) (Figs. 5 and 6). For pericardial aortic bioprostheses of 2646 patients – CE-PERIMOUNT 1133 (Aupart et al. [6]) and Sorin-Mitroflow 1513 (Yankah et al. [11]). Figures 1–6 document the actuarial and actual freedom from structural valve deterioration demonstrating known durability of these biorpostheses.

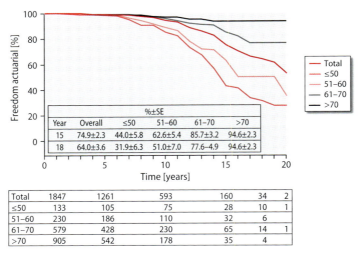

Fig. 1. Aortic valve replacement Carpentier-Edwards supra-annular valve – actuarial freedom from structural valve deterioration overall and by age groups. Reprinted with permission from [2]; © American Association of Thoracic Surgery

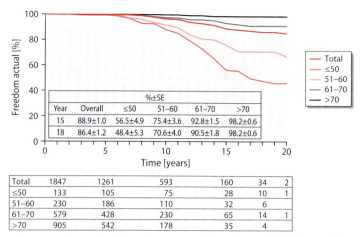

Fig. 2. Aortic valve replacement Carpentier-Edwards supra-annular valve – actual freedom from structural valve deterioration overall and by age groups. Reprinted with permission from [2]; © American Association of Thoracic Surgery

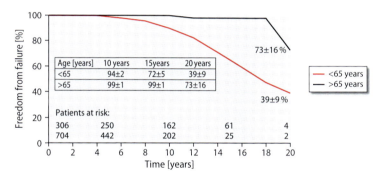

Fig. 3. Aortic valve replacement: Hancock II actuarial freedom from failure by age. Reprinted with permission from [3] and David (2009); © ICR Publishers, Ltd.

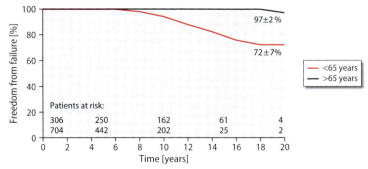

Fig. 4. Aortic valve replacement: Hancock II actual freedom from failure. (Personal communication with Tirone David (2009))

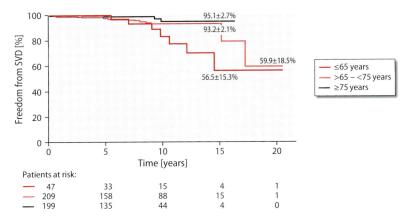

Fig. 5. Aortic valve replacement St. Jude Medical Biocor – freedom from structural valve deterioration for patients divided by age groups. Reprinted with permission from [4]; © The Society of Thoracic Surgeons

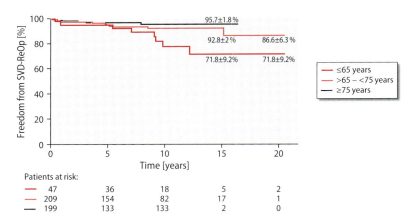

Fig. 6. Aortic valve replacement St. Jude Medical Biocor – freedom from reoperation due to structural valve deterioration for patients divided by age groups. Reprinted with permission from [4]; © The Society of Thoracic Surgeons

The 20-year durability knowledge of aortic porcine and pericardial bioprostheses requires further documentation from the reporting centers with adequate patients at risk at 20 years to provide robust data for comparative evaluation.

References

1. Brown JM, O'Brien SM, Wu C, Sikora JA, Griffith BP, Gammie JS (2009) Isolated aortic valve replacement in North America comprising 108,687 patients in 10 years: changes in risks, valve types, and outcomes in the Society of Thoracic Surgeons National Database. J Thorac Cardiovasc Surg 137(1):82–90
2. Jamieson WRE, Burr LH, Miyagishima RT, Germann E, Macnab JS, Stanford E et al (2005) Carpentier-Edwards supra-annular aortic porcine bioprosthesis: Clinical performance over 20 years. J Thorac Cardiovasc Surg 130(4):994–1000
3. Borger MA, Ivanov J, Armstrong S, Christie-Hrybinsky D, Feindel CM, David TE (2006) Twentyyear results of the Hancock II bioprosthesis. J Heart Valve Dis 15(1):49–55, discussion 55–56
4. Eichinger WB, Hettich IM, Ruzicka DJ, Holper K, Schricker C, Bleiziffer S, Lange R (2008) Twenty-year experience with the St. Jude medical Biocor bioprosthesis in the aortic position. Ann Thorac Surg 86(4):1204–1210
5. Myken PS, Bech-Hansen O (2009) A 20-year experience of 1712 patients with the Biocor porcine bioprosthesis. J Thorac Cardiovasc Surg 137(1):76–81
6. Aupart MR, Mirza A, Meurisse YA, Sirinelli AL, Neville PH, Marchand MA (2006) Perimount pericardial bioprosthesis for aortic calcified stenosis: 18-year experience with 1133 patients. J Heart Valve Dis 15(6):768, 775, discussion 775–776
7. Edwards Lifesciences LLC (2003) Carpentier-Edwards PERIMOUNT aortic pericardial bioprosthesis: 20-year results. Clinical Communique, Edwards Lifesciences
8. Prasongsukarn K, Jamieson WRE, Lichtenstein SV (2005) Performance of bioprostheses and mechanical prostheses in age group 61–70 years. J Heart Valve Dis 14(4):501–508, 510–511, discussion 509
9. Jamieson WRE, Germann E, Aupart MR, Neville PH, Marchand MA, Fradet GJ (2006) 15-year comparison of supra-annular porcine and PERIMOUNT aortic bioprostheses. Asian Cardiovasc Thorac Ann 14(3):200–205
10. Jamieson WRE, Koerfer R, Yankah CA, Zittermann A, Hayden RI, Ling H, Hetzer R, Dolman WB (2009) Mitroflow aortic pericardial bioprosthesis – clinical performance. Eur J Cardio-Thorac Surg (in press)
11. Yankah CA, Pasic M, Musci M, Stein J, Detschades C, Siniawski H, Hetzer R (2008) Aortic valve replacement with the Mitroflow pericardial bioprosthesis: durability results up to 21 years. J Thorac Cardiovasc Surg 136(3):688–696

Clinical results including hemodynamic performance of the Medtronic Mosaic porcine bioprosthesis up to ten years*

F.-C. Riess, R. Bader, E. Cramer, L. Hansen, B. Kleijnen, G. Wahl, J. Wallrath, S. Winkel, N. Bleese

The main advantage of bioprosthetic cardiac valves in comparison to mechanical prosthesis is the lower incidence of antithromboembolic-related hemorrhages. However, bioprostheses have limited durability due to progressive tissue degeneration and calcification resulting in structural valve deterioration (SVD) and suboptimal hemodynamic performances. The Medtronic Mosaic bioprosthesis is a supraannular third-generation stented porcine bioprosthesis which was introduced in 1994. It is built upon the historical durability of the Hancock II valve [1] and technical innovations were incorporated into the design in an attempt to improve hemodynamic performance and durability [2]. Tissue fixation with the Medtronic Physiologic Fixation^{TM} process is performed with glutaraldehyde in order to minimize the consequences of antigenicity after porcine valve implantation [3]. Furthermore, the valve design includes predilatation of the porcine aortic root and using zero net pressure across the leaflets (Fig. 1a) [4]. By this treatment, natural leaflet morphology is generally preserved. The tissue is mounted on a low-profile flexible polymer stent (Fig. 1b) to minimize hemodynamic disturbance and to make it suitable for patients with small aortic root diameters. The bioprosthesis is treated with the long-chain fatty acid alpha-amino oleic acid (AOA) which binds to the aldehyde fractions of the glutaraldehyde-preserved porcine tissue by forming Schiff base covalent linkages with the aldehydes which remain after fixation with glutaraldehyde (Fig. 1c). The AOA process has been shown in several animal studies to reduce porcine valve mineralization of both leaflets and aortic wall, while improving valve gradients [5–7].

Our hospital was a contributing center to the US Food and Drug Administration (FDA) multicenter, prospective, nonrandomized trial which completed actuarial data in late 2000. This is a report of our data obtained from the ongoing post-FDA approval long-term clinical evaluation study of

---

* This article is a modified version of an article published in 2007 in The Annals of Thoracic Surgery, Vol 83, pp 1310–1318, Riess et al., "Hemodynamic Performance of the Medtronic Mosaic Porcine Bioprosthesis Up to Ten Years". Additional figures were incorporated with permission of the Medtronic Company.

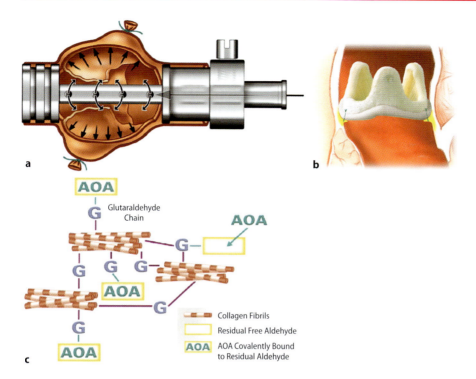

Fig. 1. Supraannular valve implantation technique

the Medtronic Mosaic valve. Efficacy, safety, and clinical performance including hemodynamic data from a total of 302 contributed patients are provided, collected by prospective, serial, standarized echocardiographic follow-up for up to 10 years.

Patients and methods

Patient population and study design

Patients diagnosed with valvular heart disease and requiring isolated replacement of either the aortic or mitral valves were eligible to enter the study. Concomitant procedures in addition to valve replacement were permitted. Patients requiring a concomitant valve replacement, or who had a preexisting prosthetic valve in another position, were excluded. Between 02/1994 and 10/1999, we enrolled a total of 302 patients into this prospective and nonrandomized study. Aortic valve replacement (AVR) was per-

Table 1. Characteristics of patients undergoing aortic valve replacement (AVR) or mitral valve replacement (MVR) with the Mosaic bioprosthesis

Variable	AVR n=255	MVR n=47
Gender		
Male	150 (58.8%)	14 (29.8%)
Female	105 (41.2%)	33 (70.2%)
Concomitant procedures		
Coronary artery bypass	95 (37.3%)	8 (17.0%)
Ascending aorta replacement/repair	31 (12.2%)	0
Aortic root enlargement	20 (7.8%)	0
Myotomy/myectomy	11 (4.3%)	0
Age at Implant (years)		
23–50	9 (3.6%)	1 (2.1%)
51–65	70 (27.5%)	12 (19.4%)
66–70	59 (23.1%)	15 (31.9%)
71–75	79 (31.0%)	12 (25.5%)
>75	38 (14.0%)	7 (14.9%)
Cardiac rhythm		
Sinus rhythm	229 (89.8%)	25 (53.2%)
Atrial fibrillation	13 (5.1%)	20 (42.6%)
Heart block	6 (0.6%)	0
Paced rhythm	7 (2.8%)	2 (4.2%)
NYHA classification		
Class I	4 (1.6%)	0
Class II	74 (29.0%)	17 (36.2%)
Class III	150 (58.8%)	28 (59.6%)
Class IV	27 (10.6%)	2 (4.3%)
Valvular lesion		
Stenosis	43 (16.9%)	2 (4.3%)
Insufficiency	38 (14.9%)	30 (63.8%)
Mixed	174 (68.2%)	15 (31.9%)

formed in 255 patients (mean age 67±8.5 years, range: 23 to 82 years) and mitral valve replacement (MVR) in 47 patients (mean age 67±8.2 years, range: 41 to 84 years). Coronary artery bypass surgery was performed as a concomitant procedure in 95 patients (37.3%) during AVR and 8 patients (17%) during MVR. Further demographic data are summarized in Table 1. The study was approved by the respective institutional ethics committee and all patients provided their informed consent to participate.

Surgical technique

Patients were operated using standard cardioplegia, cardiac arrest, and crystalloid or modified blood cardioplegia. Prosthetic valves were implanted using the supraannular technique with felt-armed single stitches (Fig. 1b). In case of mitral valve implantation, posterior chordae were preserved, if possible.

Postoperative anticoagulation

Postoperatively all patients received unfractionated heparin intravenously and subcutaneously until complete mobilization. A total of 95 patients (37.1%) received phenprocoumon for three months postoperatively with an INR target range of 2.5 to 3 in the AVR group and 38 patients (80.9%) with an INR target range of 3 to 4 in MVR group. Indications for phenprocoumon treatment were chronic atrial fibrillation or severely impaired left ventricular ejection fraction (LVEF < 30%).

Follow-up

Data of the clinical and hemodynamic follow-up were collected at the early evaluation (prior to discharge or within 30 days after implantation), late evaluation (at 3–6 months postimplantation), at one year (11–14 months postimplantation), and annually thereafter. The examination included a patient interview, the registration of valve-related adverse events, ECG, and a laboratory check for hemolysis. Furthermore, hemodynamic assessments were made using transthoracic echocardiography to assess the structure and hemodynamics of the Mosaic valve. The mean transvalvular gradient for the aortic bioprosthesis was calculated using the long form of the Bernoulli equation, and effective orifice area (EOA) was calculated using the continuity equation. The valve-related complications, composites of complications, and deaths were classified and reported according to the guidelines of the Society of Thoracic Surgeons, of the American Association of Thoracic Surgery and of the European Association of Cardio-Thoracic Surgery [8]. A total of 57 patients from the AVR group and 14 patients from the MVR group were lost to follow-up. This provided for a cumulative follow-up of 1540 patient-years (pt-years) for AVR (mean 6.1 maximum 10 years) and 250 pt-years for MVR (mean 5.4, maximum 10 years).

Statistical analysis

Statistical analysis was performed using the SAS® statistical software. Descriptive statistics were used to characterize the patient population data, operative and follow-up clinical data. For continuous variables, the number of patients, mean (±SD), minimum, and maximum were provided. For categorical variables, the number and percentage of patients were provided. Early event rates were calculated as the number of patients having the event divided by the total number of patients, expressed as a percentage. Linearized rates (% per pt-year) were used to summarize late events, and calculated by dividing the number of late events by the sum of the late pt-year of experience, expressed as a percentage. Survival analyses using the actuarial Kaplan-Meier method were used to estimate survival and the freedom from valve-related adverse events. Peto's formula [9] was used to calculate standard errors of these estimates. Events that occurred during the early and late postoperative periods were included in the analysis.

Results

Echocadiography

Echocardiographically obtained mean systolic valve gradients (SVG) and effective orifice area (EOA) 1, 5, 9 and 10 years after Mosaic bioprosthesis implantation in the aortic position are presented in Table 2. Corresponding data for the mitral valve group are summarized in Table 3. Postoperative NYHA class recorded after AVR or MVR are presented in Table 4. The number of patients with transvalvular regurgitation and degree of regurgitation are presented in Table 7.

Table 2. Echocardiographic results after aortic valve replacement (AVR)

Variable/ follow-up	Valve size (mm)					
	19 (n)	21 (n)	23 (n)	25 (n)	27 (n)	29 (n)
Mean SVG (mmHg)						
1 year	16.0±4.0 (7)	13.6±4.7 (59)	12.5±4.9 (86)	12.0±5.5 (72)	10.3±3.2 (12)	13.0±3.6 (2)
5 years	18.3±4.6 (2)	14.3±5.1 (39)	13.4±6.2 (56)	12.3±5.3 (52)	11.0±3.5 (10)	15.0±10.5 (2)
9 years	–	18.6±7.0 (6)	12.8±5.5 (16)	13.0±5.9 (17)	9.4±2.2 (3)	8.1 (1)
10 years	–	13.9 (1)	11.6±3.4 (5)	32±22.5 (3)	12.8±1.4 (2)	–
EOA (cm^2)						
1 year	1.2±0.2 (7)	1.5±0.3 (59)	1.8±0.4 (86)	2.1±0.5 (72)	2.5±0.4 (12)	2.3±0.6 (2)
5 years	1.3±0.1 (2)	1.5±0.3 (39)	1.8±0.5 (54)	2.1±0.5 (52)	2.6±0.3 (10)	2.5±0.8 (2)
9 years	–	1.3±0.3 (6)	1.7±0.2 (17)	2.0±0.4 (17)	2.4±0.2 (3)	3.2 (1)
10 years	–	1.5 (1)	1.6±0.3 (5)	1.5±0.5 (3)	2.3±0.6 (2)	–

EOA effective orifice area, *SVG* systolic valve gradient

Table 3. Echocardiographic results after mitral valve replacement (MVR)

Variable/ follow-up	Valve size (mm)			
	25 (n)	27 (n)	29 (n)	31 (n)
Mean SVG (mmHg)				
1 year	6.7 ± 1.7 (7)	4.9 ± 1.3 (12)	4.4 ± 1.4 (16)	3.7 ± 0.9 (6)
5 years	6.1 ± 3.2 (2)	5.0 ± 1.4 (7)	4.6 ± 1.9 (11)	3.3 ± 1.1 (5)
9 years	–	6.2 (1)	4.8 (1)	–
10 years	–	3.9 (1)	3.0 (1)	4.0 (1)
EOA (cm^2)				
1 year	1.9 ± 0.3 (7)	1.9 ± 0.4 (12)	2.0 ± 0.5 (16)	2.3 ± 0.6 (6)
5 years	1.9 ± 0.4 (2)	2.3 ± 1.0 (6)	2.4 ± 0.6 (11)	2.3 ± 0.7 (5)
9 years	–	1.7 (1)	2.2 (1)	–
10 years	–	3.3 (1)	2.5 (1)	3.4 (1)

SVG systolic valve gradient, *EOA* effective orifice area

Table 4. NYHA classification of patients after Mosaic valve replacement in the aortic (AVR) or mitral (MVR) position

NYHA class	AVR			MVR		
	after 1 year	5 years	10 years	after 1 year	5 years	10 years
I	118 (52.2%)	73 (45.3%)	1 (9.1%)	10 (24.4%)	2 (8.0%)	0 (0.0%)
II	99 (43.8%)	79 (49.1%)	10 (90.9%)	31 (75.6%)	23 (92.0%)	3 (100.0%)
III	5 (2.2%)	3 (1.9%)	0 (0.0%)	0 (0.0%)	0 (0.0%)	0 (0.0%)
IV	0 (0.0%)	0 (0.0%)	0 (0.0%)	0 (0.0%)	0 (0.0%)	0 (0.0%)

Cardiac rhythm

In the AVR group, 5 years after prosthetic valve implantation, 138 patients (85.7%) stayed in sinus rhythm, 15 (9.3%) in atrial fibrillation/flutter, and 8 patients (5.0%) were paced. At the same time point, 97 patients (61.0%) received aspirin, 10 patients (5.7%) were on phenprocoumon, and 52 patients (33.1%) had no anticoagulation therapy. In the MVR group, 5 years after prosthetic valve implantation 14 patients (56.0%) stayed in sinus rhythm, 9 (36.0%) in atrial fibrillation/flutter, and 2 patients (8.0%) were paced. At the same time, 9 patients (36.0%) received phenprocoumon, 8 patients (32%) aspirin, and 6 patients (24.0%) had no anticoagulation therapy.

Ten years after AVR, 9 patients (81.8%) stayed in sinus rhythm, 1 (9.1%) in atrial fibrillation/flutter, and 1 patients (9.1%) were paced. At the same

Table 5. Frequency of adverse events and actuarial freedom from valve-related adverse events, 5, 9, and 10 years after aortic valve replacement (AVR)

Adverse event	Late events N	%/pt-year	Actuarial freedom from event (% ± SD) 5 years	9 years	10 years
▋ Thromboembolism	13	0.8	95.1 ± 1.5	93.3 ± 1.8	86.6 ± 6.6
– Permanent neurological event	4	0.3	98.2 ± 0.9	98.2 ± 0.9	91.2 ± 6.8
– Transient neurological event	4	0.3	98.1 ± 0.9	97.5 ± 1.1	97.5 ± 1.1
– Acute myocardial infarction	1	0.1	100.0 ± 0.0	99.4 ± 0.7	99.4 ± 0.7
– Valve thrombosis	4	0.3	99.1 ± 1.6	98.6 ± 0.8	98.2 ± 0.8
– Peripheral embolic event	0	0.0	100.0 ± 0.0	100.0 ± 0.0	100.0 ± 0.0
– Infarction of spleen	1	0.1	99.6 ± 0.5	99.6 ± 0.5	99.6 ± 0.5
▋ Structural valve deterioration	4	0.3	100.0 ± 0.0	96.2 ± 2.7	87.1 ± 6.7
▋ Endocarditis	7	0.5	98.3 ± 0.9	95.4 ± 4.6	95.4 ± 4.6
▋ Paravalvular leak	6	0.4	97.1 ± 1.1	97.1 ± 1.1	97.1 ± 1.1
▋ Mismatch	3	0.2	99.1 ± 0.6	98.6 ± 0.8	98.6 ± 0.8
▋ Hemolysis	0	0.0	100.0 ± 0.0	100.0 ± 0.0	100.0 ± 0.0
▋ Major hemorrhage	5	0.3	98.7 ± 0.8	96.8 ± 1.3	96.8 ± 1.3
▋ Reoperation	22	1.4	94.8 ± 1.5	84.9 ± 3.9	72.5 ± 8.1
▋ Explant	20	1.3	96.0 ± 1.3	86.0 ± 3.9	73.4 ± 8.2

N number of patients, *%/pt-year* percent per patient year; data are presented as mean ± standard deviation

time 5 patients (45.5%) received aspirin and 3 patients (27.3%) had no anticoagulation therapy. In the MVR group, 10 years after prosthetic valve implantation 1 patient (33.3%) stayed in sinus rhythm and 2 (66.6%) in atrial fibrillation/flutter. At the same time 2 patients (66.6%) received phenprocoumon and 1 patient (33.3%) aspirin.

▋ Adverse events

Late valve-related adverse events and actuarial freedoms from valve-related adverse events 5 year, 9 years, and 10 years after AVR are summarized in Table 5. Corresponding data of the MVR group are presented in Table 6.

Table 6. Frequency of adverse events and actuarial freedom from valve-related adverse events 5, 9, and 10 years after mitral valve replacement (MVR)

Adverse event	Late events N	%/pt-year	Actuarial freedom from event (% ± SD) 5 years	9 years	10 years
■ Thromboembolism	2	0.8	100.0 ± 0.0	86.3 ± 9.8	86.3 ± 9.8
– Permanent neurological event	1	0.4	100.0 ± 0.0	90.9 ± 8.7	90.9 ± 8.7
– Transient neurological event	0	0.0	100.0 ± 0.0	100 ± 0.0	100.0 ± 0.0
– Acute myocardial infarction	0	0.0	100.0 ± 0.0	100 ± 0.0	100.0 ± 0.0
– Valve thrombosis	0	0.0	100.0 ± 0.0	100 ± 0.0	100.0 ± 0.0
– Peripheral embolic event	1	0.4	100.0 ± 0.0	95.8 ± 4.1	95.8 ± 4.1
■ Structural valve deterioration	0	0.0	100.0 ± 0.0	100 ± 0.0	100.0 ± 0.0
■ Paravalvular leak	0	0.0	100.0 ± 0.0	100 ± 0.0	100.0 ± 0.0
■ Mismatch	0	0.0	100.0 ± 0.0	100 ± 0.0	100.0 ± 0.0
■ Endocarditis	2	0.8	95.0 ± 3.5	95.0 ± 3.5	95.0 ± 3.5
■ Paravalvular leak	0	0.0	100.0 ± 0.0	100.0 ± 0.0	100.0 ± 0.0
■ Hemolysis	0	0.0	100.0 ± 0.0	100.0 ± 0.0	100.0 ± 0.0
■ Major hemorrhage	2	0.8	93.5 ± 3.6	93.5 ± 3.6	93.5 ± 3.6
■ Reoperation	3	1.2	92.4 ± 4.3	92.3 ± 4.3	92.3 ± 4.3
■ Explant	2	0.8	95.0 ± 3.5	95.0 ± 3.5	95.0 ± 3.5

N number of patients, *%/pt-year* percent per patient year; data are presented as mean ± standard deviation

Table 7. Patients with transvalvular regurgitation after Mosaic valve replacement in the aortic (AVR) or mitral (MVR) position

Regurgitation	AVR after 1 year (n = 238)	5 years (n = 161)	10 years (n = 11)	MVR after 1 year (n = 41)	5 years (n = 25)	10 years (n = 3)
I	7	13	3	2	–	–
II	4	6	1	–	2	–
III	2	1	–	–	–	–
IV	–	–	–	–	–	–

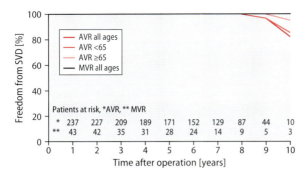

Fig. 2. Freedom from SVD 10 years after Mosaic valve replacement in the aortic (AVR) or mitral (MVR) position

Structural valve deterioration (SVD)

In the AVR group, 4 cases of SVD were observed during the 10-year follow-up with combined aortic valve regurgitation and stenosis in 3 cases and isolated stenosis or regurgitation in 1 case, each. No SVD at all was observed in the MVR group (Fig. 2). In all 4 SVD cases of the AVR group, the explanted valves were studied for calcium content microscopically and confirmed by radiological and histological investigations of all valve prosthesis.

Thrombosed valves

Four cases of aortic valve prosthesis thrombosis were observed. One 73-year-old female showed valve thrombosis at postoperative day 87 with a mean systolic valve gradient (SVG) of 70 mmHg. Phenprocoumon had been administered during the early postoperative course but was discontinued due to severe nasal angiodysplasia with recurrent hemorrhage. The valve prosthesis was replaced with a Hancock II prosthesis, which also developed thrombosis with a mean SVG of 110 mmHg during the early postoperative course. Thrombophilic investigations revealed a congenital antithrombin deficiency (AT III activity 20%). The thrombosed valve prosthesis was replaced with a mechanical valve. Analysis of the explanted valves showed bland thrombotic occlusion without infection or calcification. The second case was a 53-year-old female with aortic valve prosthesis thrombosis at postoperative day 891 under aspirin treatment with mean SVG of 42 mmHg and effective orifice area (EOA) of 0.68 cm^2. The valve was replaced with a mechanical valve. Analysis of the explanted valve showed extensive thrombosis and no signs for cuspal degeneration, calcification, or infection. The third case was a 67-year-old male patient, who developed thrombosis under aspirin treatment 1827 days after surgery aortic valve prosthesis. In the early postoperative course, this patient had suffered from acquired antithrombin (AT) III deficiency and acute heparin-induced thrombocytopenia (HIT) type II had to be treated with AT III concentrates and recombinant hirudin, respectively. The valve was replaced with a second Mosaic valve. The fourth case was an 81-year-old man suffering from aortic stenosis with a mean SVG of 32 mmHg leading to reoperation on day 3304 and replacement with a Hancock II valve. Analysis of ten explanted valve revealed brown thrombotic appearing material on two cusps.

Thromboembolism

Two early cases of thromboembolism occurred in the AVR group and no one in the MVR group. In one 76-year-old female with paroxysmal atrial fibrillation a hemiparesis occurred 7 days after aortic valve implantation, while the patient was on heparin treatment. The second patient (age 72, female) with chronic atrial fibrillation developed a transient neurological event with nausea, vertigo, and amnesia 13 days after aortic valve replacement. A total of 13 late thromboembolisms occurred after aortic valve replacement during the 10-year follow-up. Four of these patients developed permanent neurological dysfunction (stroke), while one of these patients suffered from chronic atrial fibrillation and had no anticoagulation. In the mitral group, two late thromboemblic events occurred. One patient with sinus rhythm and no anticoagulation suffered from a left renal infarction due to renal artery thrombus revealed by CT scan. The patient was heparinized and then treated with phenprocoumon. Several weeks later, the renal artery was shown to be patent. One 64-year-old female patient with atrial fibrillation and aspirin treatment developed 2650 days after mitral valve implantation a stroke with problems of speaking which resolved completely after several days.

Bleeding

One 73-year-old female patient developed 24 days after aortic valve implantation under phenprocoumon treatment severe epistaxis requiring balloon tamponade to stop bleeding. Furthermore, five late hemorrhagic complications were observed after aortic valve replacement including cerebral hematoma (n=2), gastrointestinal bleeding (n=2), and hematoma of the thigh after an accident (n=1). In the mitral group, one patient (75 years, female) suffered from diffuse oral bleeding which occurred under phenprocoumon treatment 8 days after surgery. Two cases of late hemorrhage complication occurred after prosthetic mitral valve implantation. First, a 73-year-old male patient developed under phenprocoumon treatment massive intestinal hemorrhage from the colon (colitis and diverticulitis) 73 days after surgery requiring transfusion. Second, a 67-year-old male patient developed under phenprocoumon treatment subdural hematoma at postoperative day 127 requiring surgical intervention.

Paravalvular leak

Two paravalvular leaks were observed 3 days and 6 days after AVR, respectively. Degree of aortic regurgitation was II to III in both cases. In one patient, valve replacement with a Mosaic prosthesis was performed at postoperative day 102. Six late paravalvular leaks (all degree II) were observed with NYHA class I to II. No surgical intervention was performed in these patients. No paravalvular leaks were observed in the mitral valve group.

Prosthesis mismatch

In three patients of the AVR group, late patient-prosthesis mismatch between the size of the bioprothesis and body surface area was found resulting in aortic stenosis. In two patients prosthesis replacement was necessary due to the increased mean systolic valve gradient. Both valves were replaced with a Mosaic prosthesis of larger size and additional patch enlargement of the ascending aorta.

Endocarditis

No early endocarditis was observed in the AVR and MVR groups. However, 7 cases of late endocarditis were observed after aortic valve replacement (Table 5). In 4 cases a streptococcus was isolated, in one case an enterococcus. In two cases, no bacterium could be cultured. Six patients were treated with valve replacement, while one patient was treated successfully with antibiotics. In the MVR group, two cases of late endocarditis occurred induced by enterococcus and streptococcus, respectively (Table 6). Both patients were treated with mitral prosthesis replacement.

Explants

No valve was explanted during the early (< 30 days) follow-up in both groups. Twenty aortic valve prostheses (1.3%/pt-years) were explanted until the 10-year follow-up. Reasons for explant were endocarditis (n = 7), SVD (n = 4), valve thrombosis (n = 4), incidental replacement due to aneurysm of the ascending aorta (n = 3), mismatch (n = 1), and paravalvular leak (n = 1). In the MVR group, 2 patients (0.8%/pt-years) were explanted both due to prosthetic endocarditis.

Mortality

In the AVR group, the early mortality rate was 0.8% (2 patients). In one patient pulmonary hypertonus due to hypertrophy obstructive cardiomyopathy with left ventricular outlet obstruction occurred (postoperative day 3) and in the other one acute pericardial tamponade due to aortic dissection and perforation (postoperative day 13). The linearized rate for late mortality was 3.5% per pt-year. Out of 54 late deaths, 3 were valve related (0.2%/pt-year), 11 were cardiac (0.7%/pt-year), 26 were noncardiac (1.8%/pt-year), and 14 were unexplained (1.0%/pt-year). The cases of valve-related death after AVR consisted of a 66-year-old man who suffered from a cerebral hemorrhage with phenprocoumon treatment due to chronic atrial fibrillation (INR 2) and developed septicemia after a relieving operation (postoperative day 2119). The second patient was a 49-year-old man with prosthetic valve endocarditis requiring valve replacement the day of operation from low output syndrome (postoperative day 3098). The third patient was a 68-year-old man who died from heart failure after a cerebrovascular accident (postoperative day 983). No autopsy was performed in any of these patients. The 11 cardiac deaths until 10-year follow-up included myocardial infarction (n=5), heart failure (n=5), and cor pulmonale (n=1).

In the MVR group, there was no early mortality. The linearized rate for late mortality (7 deaths) was 2.8% per pt-year. Of these 7 deaths, 1 was cardiac (0.4%/pt-year), 3 were noncardiac (1.2%/pt-year), and 3 were unexplained (1.2%/pt-year) (Fig. 3). Survival at 10 years was 65.5±4.4% for AVR and 84.1±6.0% for MVR (Fig. 4). Freedom from valve-related or unexplained death at 10 years was 88.0±3.2% (SE) for the AVR group, and 94.5.6±3.8% for the MVR group (Fig. 2). There was no case of valve-related death during the total follow-up and only one case of cardiac death after mitral valve replacement in a 75-year-old female with cor pulmonale at postoperative day 1117 due to heart failure.

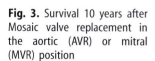

Fig. 3. Survival 10 years after Mosaic valve replacement in the aortic (AVR) or mitral (MVR) position

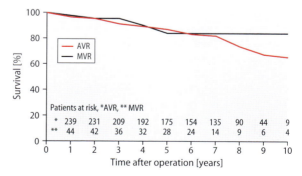

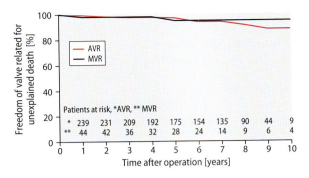

Fig. 4. Freedom from valve-related or unexplained death after Mosaic valve replacement in the aortic (AVR) or mitral (MVR) position

Discussion

These are data from an ongoing post-FDA approval trial investigating the hemodynamic performance and the clinical outcome of patients after implantation of the Medtronic Mosaic porcine prosthesis in the aortic or mitral position. The design of an annual prospective serial standardized echocardiographic follow-up allowing assessment of functionally and hemodynamic data was generally not performed in earlier generation bioprostheses. The serial echocardiographic follow-up here is unique to this study cohort. The intermediate 10-year results demonstrate excellent hemodynamic and clinical performance of this new third generation porcine valve prosthesis in the aortic and mitral positions. Results are comparable with those of other frequently implanted tissue valves [10–13]. Thus, there is no statistically significant difference between the second generation Carpentier-Edwards supraanular porcine valve, the Carpentier-Edwards Perimount pericardial prosthesis, and the third generation Medtronic Mosaic porcine valve with respect to mean transvalvular gradients and effective orifice area [14]. The present echocardiographic data demonstrate stable transvalvular gradients and transvalvular effective orifice area during the 10-year follow-up. Data are comparable with data obtained in earlier Mosaic series which reported up to 7 years echocardiographic findings [2, 14, 15]. Relatively low gradients were found in small valve sizes. It is assumed that these low transvalvular gradients are a direct benefit of this new valve design and tissue processing preserving the normal architecture of the collagen tissue [4]. In contrast to the previous Intact Medtronic valve prosthesis, where fixation in a nondilated root was associated with overcrowding of the leaflets, the Mosaic valve includes dilatation of the aortic root at the time of preservation resulting in normal plane closure of leaflets without restriction. Nevertheless, freedom from structural valve deterioration (SVD) was low in the intact valve at 10-year follow-up [16, 17]. It was expected that improvement in tissue fixation and additional antimineralization treatment with alpha-amino oleic acid (AOA) [17–19] will provide longer durability than current bioprostheses, especially in younger populations [2]. In our study population, a total of 4 cases (age at implant 31, 55, 55, 63 years) out of 255 aortic implants occurred during the 10-year follow-up resulting in a freedom from SVD of 87.1±6.7% (Fig. 2). Since hazards are not constant, the presentation of linearized rates is not really quantitative. None of these documented cases of SVD in the AVR group occurred in a patient older than 65 years at implant. Thus, freedom from SVD in patients >65 years was 100%. Jamieson and colleagues [20] and Malligan and coworkers [21] found that even though SVD occurred at all ages, the freedom was greater with advancing of age. These results suggest that the evolution in valve design allow for performance superior to that reported for earlier generation bioprostheses. Sarris reported Hancock standard 10-year SVD freedom rates of 59±9% and 72±2%, respectively, for aortic and mitral replacement [22]. Jamieson et al. [23] reported 10-year freedom rates of 79% and 72% with the Carpentier-Edwards aortic and mitral replacements, respectively. Jones et al. [24] documented 10-year freedom from SVD with standard prosthesis of 79% for AVR and 63% for MVR. Pelletier reported 87% freedom from SVD at 10 years for the Carpentier-Edwards Perimount pericardial valve in the aortic position [25].

Most remarkable in our study is that not a single case of SVD was observed in a total of 47 patients having undergone mitral valve replacement during the 10-year follow-up and no case of moderate or severe transvalvular regurgitation was observed. This observation is in contrast to other authors, who reported tissue valves to be more durable in the aortic than in the mitral position [1, 16, 24, 26–28]. It was suggested [23] that the difference in durability may be due to elevated closing pressures and, thus, increased hemodynamic stress in the mitral position. This suggests that the Mosaic valve seems to withstand the high stress in the mitral position.

Valve thrombosis occurred in four cases of the AVR group and none of the MVR group. In one patient with prosthesis thrombosis a congenital antithrombin defect with residual activation of only 20% was detected, which can be considered to be the reason for this adverse event. This theory is supported by the reoccurrence of thrombosis after implant of a Hancock II prosthesis. Another patient developed valve thrombosis of the Mosaic prosthesis 1827 days after implant. This special patient had suffered from heparin-induced thrombocytopenia (HIT) type II as well as AT III deficiency during the early postoperative course and was treated with recombinant hirudin (lepiriudin, Pharmion, Great Britain) as an alternative anticoagulant instead of heparin. The overlapping treatment with phenprocoumon had to be stopped early after initiation due to a gastrointestinal hemorrhage. The intraoperative findings and histological investigation supported the theory of HIT, because a thin layer of white clot formation was found in all three cusps of the Mosaic valve resulting in prosthetic stenosis with a transvalvular peak gradient of 55 mmHg.

Seven patients of the AVR group and two patients of the MVR group developed endocarditis during the postoperative course resulting in freedom from endocarditis rates of 95.4 ± 4.6% for the AVR group and 95.0 ± 3.5% for the MVR group. Thus, the rates of infective endocarditis after AVR and MVR with the Mosaic valve prosthesis are similar to those reported for other stented porcine and pericardial valves, such as Hancock II [1], Carpentier-Edwards Perimount [26, 29, 30], Biocor [31, 32], Medtronic Intact [16], and the Carpentier-Edwards porcine prostheses [33].

The risk of endocarditis was reported by David et al. [1] to be highest during the first year after the operation. In contrast to this, in our cohort, 7 cases of endocarditis in the AVR group occurred 261, 615, 782, 833, 1886, 1909 and 3015 days after implant, and in 2 cases mitral position endocarditis was observed 133 and 1265 days, respectively, after implant. A major benefit of a bioprosthesis in comparison to a mechanical valve is the low incidence of thromboembolic and major anti-thromboembolic-related hemorrhage. In the present trial, late thrombotic rates of 0.8% per patient year (pt-year) were observed in the AVR and MVR groups, respectively, which is favorable to other studies. In this context, it seems to be important that all patients without the need for phenprocoumon (e.g., chronic atrial fibrillation) were treated with aspirin.

A comparable low rate of major hemorrhages was observed for both groups with only 0.3%/pt-year after AVR and 0.8%/pt-year after MVR. The freedom from hemorrhage rates at 10 years were 96.8 ± 1.3% (AVR) and 93.5 ± 3.6% (MVR), respectively. The number of major hemorrhages was lower than in other series [34]. The reason might be the relatively low percentage of patients of our study under continuous anticoagulation therapy at 6 months after surgery in comparison to other studies (52.5%/pt-year [34]).

Conclusion

The long-term performance of the Mosaic valve is encouraging, as this third-generation porcine bioprosthesis continues to provide excellent hemodynamic data, a small number of valve-related adverse events, and a low incidence from structural valve deterioration. Continued clinical follow-up and monitoring of this patient population should demonstrate if indeed this valve will provide patients with increased durability and low morbidity, when compared with bioprosthetic valves of an earlier design and generation.

References

1. David TE, Ivanov J, Armstrong S, Feindel CM, Cohen G (2001) Late results of heart valve replacement with the Hancock II bioprosthesis. J Thorac Cardiovasc Surg 121:268–278
2. Fradet G, Bleese N, Busse E, Jamieson E, Raudkivi P, Goldstein J, Metras M (2004) The Mosaic valve clinical performance at seven years:results from a multicenter prospective clinical trial. J Heart Valve Dis 13(2):239–247
3. Carpentier A, Lemaigre G, Robert L, Carpentier S, Dubost C (1969) Biological factors affecting long-term results of valvular heterografts. J Thorac Cardiovas Surg 58:467
4. Vesley I (1991) Analysis of the Medtronic Intact bioprosthesis valve. Effects of zero-pressure fixation. J Thorac Cardiovasc Surg 101:90–99
5. Duarte IG, MacDonald MJ, Cooper WA et al (2001) In vivo hemodynamic, histologic, and antimineralization charateristics of the Mosaic Bioprosthesis. Ann Thorac Surg 71:92–99
6. Girardot MN, Girardot JM, Schoen FJ (1991) Alpha amino oleic acid, a new compound, prevents calcification of bioprosthetic heart valves. Trans Soc Biomater 14:114–116
7. Walther T, Falk V, Diegeler A et al (1999) Effectiveness of different anticalcification treatments for stentless aortic bioprosthesis. Thorac Cardiovasc Surg 47:23–25
8. Edmunds LH, Clark RE, Cohn LH, Grunkemeier GL, Miller DC, Wiesel RD (1996) Guidelines for reporting morbidity and mortality after cardiac valvular operations. Ann Thorac Surg 62:932–935
9. Peto R, Pike MC, Armitage P et al (1977) Design and analysis of randomized clinical trials requiring prolonged observation of each patient. Br J Cancer 35:1–39
10. Salomon NW, Okies JE, Krause AH, Page US, Bigelow JC, Colburn LQ (1991) Serial follow-up of an experimental bovine pericardial aortic bioprosthesis. Circulation 84:140–144
11. David TE, Armstrong S, Sun Z (1992) Clinical and hemodynamic assessment of the Hancock II bioprosthesis. Ann Thorac Surg 54:661–667
12. McDonald ML, Daly RC, Schaff HV et al (1997) Hemodynamic performance of small aortic valve bioprostheses: Is there a difference? Ann Thorac Surg 63:362–366
13. Jamieson WR, Janusz MT, Burr LH, Ling H, Miyagishima RT, Germann E (2001) Carpentier-Edwards supraannular porcine bioprosthesis: Second-generation prosthesis in aortic valve replacement. Ann Thorac Surg 71:224–227
14. Jamieson WRE, Janusz Mt, MacNab J, Henderson C (2001) Hemodynamic comparison of second and third generation stented bioprostheses in aortic valve replacement. Ann Thorac Surg 71:282–284
15. Wong SP, Legget ME, Greaves SC, Barratt-Boyes BG, Milsom FP, Raudkivi PJ (2000) Early experience with the mosaic bioprosthesis: A new generation porcine valve. Ann Thorac Surg 69:1846–1850
16. Barratt-Boyes BG, Jaffe WM, Whitlock RM (1998) The Medtronic intact porcine valve: Ten-year clinical review. J Thorac Cardiovasc Surg 116:1005–1014
17. Jones M, Eidbo EE, Hilbert SL, Ferrans VJ, Clark RE (1989) Anticalcification treatments of bioprosthetic heart valves: In vivo studies in sheep. J Card Surg 4:69–73
18. Gott JP, Pan-Chih, Dorsey LMA et al (1992) Calcification of porcine valves: A successful new method of antimineralization. Ann Thorac Surg 53:207–216

19. Melina G, Rubens MB, Birks EJ, Bizzarri F, Khaghani A, Yacoub MH (2000) A quantitative study of calcium deposition in the aortic wall following Medtronic freestyle compared with homograft aortic root replacement. A prospedive randomized lrial. J Heart Valve Dis 9:97–103
20. Jamieson WRE, Janusz MT, Miyagishima RT et al (1988) Carpentier-Edwards standard porcine bioprostheses – primary tissue failure (structural valve deterioration) by age groups. Ann Thorac Surg 46:155–162
21. Magilligan DJ, Lewis JW, Stein P, Alam M (1989) The porcine bioprosthetic heart valve: experiences at 15 years. Ann Thorac Surg 48:324–330
22. Sarris GE, Robbins RC, Miller DC, Mitchell RS, Moore KA, Stinson EB, Oyer PE, Reitz BA, Shumway NE (1993) Randomized, prospective assessment of bioprosthetic valve durability. Hancock versus Carpentier-Edwards valves. Circulation 88(5 Pt 2):II55–II64
23. Jamieson WRE, Allen P, Miyagishima RT, Gerein AN Munro AI, Burr LH et al (1990) The Carpentier-Edwards standard porcine bioprosthesis: a first-generation tissue valve with excellent longterm clinical performance. J Thorac Cardiovasc Surg 99:543–561
24. Jones EL, Weintraub WS, Craver JM, Guyton RA, Cohen CL, Corrigan VE, Hatcher CR (1990) Ten-year experience with the porcine bioprosthetic valve: interrelationship of valve survival and patient survival in 1050 valve replacements. Ann Thorac Surg 49:370–384
25. Pelletier LC, Carrier M, Leclerc Y, Dyrda I (1995) The Carpentier-Edwards pericardial bioprosthesis: clinical experience with 600 patients. Ann Thorac Surg 60 (2 Suppl):297–302
26. Poirier NC, Pelletier LC, Pellerin M, Carrier M (1998) 15 year experience willi the Carpentier-Edwards pericardial bioprosthesis. Ann Thorac Surg 66:57–61
27. Jamieson WR, Munro AI, Miyagishima RT, Allen P, Burr LH, Tyers GF (1995) Carpentier-Edwards standard porcine bioprosthesis: Clinical performance to seventeen years. Ann Thorac Surg 60:999–1006
28. Akins CW, Carroll DL, Buckley MJ, Daggett WM, Hilgenberg AD, Austen WG (1990) Late results with Carpentier-Edwards porcine bioprosthesis. Circulation 82(Suppl IV):65–74
29. Banbury MK, Cosgrove DM, III, Lytle BW, Smedira NG, Sabik JF, Saunders CR (1998) Long-term results of the Carpentier-Edwards pericardial aortic valve: a 12 year follow-up. Ann Thorac Surg 66:S73–S76
30. Frater RW, Furlong P, Cosgrove DM et al (1998) Longterm durability and patient functional status of die Carpentier-Edwards perimount pericardial bioprosthesis in the aortic position. J Heart Valve Dis 7:48–53
31. Myken PS, Caidahl K, Larsson S, Berggren HE (1994) 10-year experience with the Biocor porcine bioprosthesis in the aortic position. J Heart Valve Dis 3:648–656
32. Dellgren G, Eriksson MJ, Brodin LA, Radegran K (2002) Eleven years' experience with the Biocor stentless aortic bioprosthesis: Clinical and hemodynamic follow-up with long-term relative survival rate. Eur J Cardiothorac Surg 22:912–921
33. Bernal JM, Rabasa JM, Lopez R, Nistal JF, Muniz R, Revuelta JM (1995) Durability of the Carpentier-Edwards porcine bioprosthesis: Role of age and valve position. Ann Thorac Surg 60:S248–S252
34. Gansera B, Botzenhardt F, Grünzinger R, Spiliopoulos K, Angelis I, Kemkes BM (2003) The Mosaic bioprosthesis in aortic position: seven years' results. J Heart Valve Disease 12:354–361

Aortic root replacement with the BioValsalva prosthesis

D. Pacini, R. Di Bartolomeo

Introduction

Aortic root replacement with a composite valve graft, according to the Bentall technique and its following modifications [1, 3, 13], represents the treatment of choice for pathologies affecting the aortic root and the aortic valve. The increasing number of elderly patients with complex diseases of the aortic valve and ascending aorta, and the disadvantages of anticoagulation and thromboembolism associated with mechanical valves are stimulating the search for an ideal substitute [9, 16, 17]. Homografts, composite conduits with a biological stented or stentless valve prosthesis intraoperatively assembled and stentless xenografts are currently available, each with its advantages and disadvantages [9, 11, 12, 15, 18]. A new prepacked biological conduit, the BioValsalva porcine aortic valved conduit, has been developed offering the surgeon a new treatment option for elderly patients with combined disease of the aortic valve and root or for patients in whom anticoagulation should be avoided or is contraindicated.

The BioValsalva conduit

The Bio-Valsalva™ conduit is a biological valved conduit composed of a Vascutek Triplex Valsalva™ vascular graft and Vascutek Elan™ stentless heart valve.

The Triplex™ vascular graft consists of three layers or membranes (Fig. 1). The inner layer that is in contact with blood is a standard, non-coated Dacron graft; the central layer is composed of a self-sealing elastomeric membrane; and the outer layer is a standard expanded polytetrafluoroethylene (ePTFE) graft. Thanks to the three-layer structure, blood impermeability is maintained without any need of coating; in vitro tests show that the Triplex graft has a water leakage value of 0.68 ml/cm^2/min, which is significantly lower than a standard Gealweave-coated graft, which

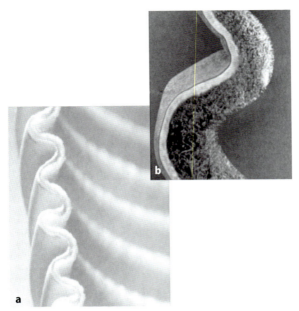

Fig. 1. a Magnification and **b** microscopic view of the three-layer structure of the Triplex™ graft. The inner layer is composed by standard noncoated woven Dacron and the outer layer by standard ePTFE. These two layers are fused together by a central layer of self-sealing elastomeric membrane

is rated at 15 ml/cm^2/min [7]. Such a conduit can, therefore, be easily stored in glutaraldehyde along with a biological valve.

The new Triplex conduit was then manufactured in the Valsalva configuration to determine whether a valved conduit could combine the advantages of the Triplex fabric with the potential of the Valsalva graft for the Bentall application (i.e., facilitation of coronary ostia anastomoses, reduction of the tension on the sutures, and potential improvement of coronary blood flow). The Valsalva configuration consists of three segments joined together:

- the collar with horizontal corrugation,
- the skirt with radially expandable corrugation, and
- the body with horizontal corrugation as extensively described and shown previously by De Paulis [4–6].

The Elan™ valve (Vascutek Terumo, UK), a porcine stentless bioprosthesis that has been shown to afford excellent hemodynamics with performance [10], is inserted into the expandable portion of a 1-mm larger Triplex Valsalva graft.

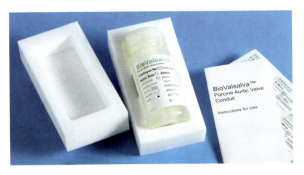

Fig. 2. The BioValsalva conduit is a combination of a Triplex™ Valsalva graft and an Elan porcine stentless heart valve. The composite graft is stored, as other biological valves, in glutaraldehyde solution. It is ready for implantation after a careful washing (three times in 500 ml of sterile saline for 2 min each)

The new biological valved conduit is manufactured in various sizes, is stored in glutaraldehyde, and, as with other biological valves, it is ready-to-use after washing for 6 min in 1500 ml of sterile saline solution (Fig. 2).

Clinical experience

Patients' characteristics

A total of 35 patients (9 females and 26 males, mean age 69 ± 5.4 years) underwent combined replacement of the aortic valve and aortic root with the BioValsalva prosthesis at our institution between April 2007 and September 2008. Aortic root pathologies were degenerative aneurysm in 19 patients, atherosclerotic in 14 and inflammatory in 2. Four patients had type A aortic dissection (2 acute and 2 chronic). A bicuspid aortic valve was detected in 9 patients. Concomitant aortic valve diseases were detected by transthoracic echocardiography and consisted of aortic stenosis, stenoinsufficiency, and severe regurgitation in 12, 15, and 8 patients, respectively. Atrial fibrillation (AF) was detected in three cases while an associated coronary artery disease was found in 2 patients. The preoperative details of the patients are shown in Table 1.

Operative technique

Median sternotomy was performed in all patients. Cardiopulmonary bypass with mild systemic hypothermia (32 °C) was usually instituted through cannulation of the right atrium and the distal ascending aorta or aortic

Table 1. Patient characteristics

■ Age (years) ± SD	69 ± 5.4
■ Gender (male/female)	26 (73.3)/9 (25.7)
■ NYHA classification	
– I–II	7 (20)
– III–IV	28 (80)
■ ASA class ± SD	3.2 ± 1.1
■ Presentation	
– Acute	2 (5.7)
– Chronic	33 (94.3)
■ Hypertension	23 (65.7)
■ COPD	5 (14.3)
■ Smokers	16 (45.7)
■ Diabetes	2 (5.7)
■ Dislipidemy	14 (40)
■ Bicuspid valve	9 (25.7)
■ Previous cardiac/aortic surgery	5 (14.3)
■ Aortic valve disease	
– Stenosis	11 (31.4)
– Stenoinsufficiency	15 (42.9)
– Insufficiency	9 (25.7)
■ Mean ejection fraction	60.4 ± 6.3
■ Disease of the aorta	
– Root aneurysm	17 (81)
– Acute type A dissection	2 (5.8)
– Chronic type A dissection	2 (5.8)

Values are expressed as mean ± standard deviation (SD) or number of patients experiencing the event followed by the corresponding percentage in parentheses, unless otherwise noted. *NYHA* New York Heart Association functional class, *ASA* American Society of Anesthesiologists, *COPD* chronic obstructive pulmonary disease

arch. In patients with aortic arch involvement, a peripheral cannulation (right femoral or axillary artery) was preferred. In these cases, moderate systemic hypothermia (26 °C of nasopharingeal temperature) and antegrade selective cerebral perfusion were used during the period of circulatory arrest. Myocardial protection was achieved by antegrade infusion of cold (5–10 °C) crystalloid cardioplegia (Custodiol; Koehler Chemie, Alsbach-Haenlein, Germany). The left ventricle was vented by inserting a cannula through the superior right pulmonary vein. The aortic root was excised leaving only buttons of aortic tissue surrounding each of the coronary ar-

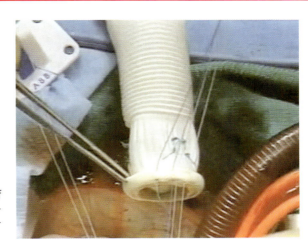

Fig. 3. The soft sewing ring of the graft is sutured to the annulus with 2-0 everting pledgeted mattress sutures

teries. The coronary arteries were mobilized to prevent tension during reimplantation. The size of the graft was selected according to the size of the aortic annulus. The soft sewing ring of the graft was sutured to the annulus with 2-0 pledgeted polyester mattress sutures (Fig. 3). A second suture line with a 4-0 running polypropylene suture was carried out to aid hemostasis. Openings for coronary reimplantation were made with a sharp blade, and not with the cautery, in the appropriate position of the graft skirt. A 5 mm punch was used to create a circular hole, taking care to avoid valve leaflets (Fig. 4a). Coronary ostia were reattached with a continuous 5-0 polypropylene suture (Fig. 4b, c). After the distal anastomosis was performed, the graft was vented with a needle and the heart chambers were deaired. The distribution of the graft sizes chosen is illustrated in Fig. 5.

Results

Inhospital outcomes

Two patients had emergency surgery and 33 were operated on electively. Aortic replacement was extended to the arch or to the hemiarch in 4 cases. Total arch replacement using the frozen elephant trunk procedure was performed in 2 dissected patients (1 acute and 1 chronic type A dissection). Coronary artery bypass grafting and bipolar radiofrequency ablation of the AF were performed, as associated procedures, in 2 and 3 patients, respectively. The mean cross-clamping time was 109.2 ± 31.1 min, while the overall cardiopulmonary bypass time was 147 ± 60.8 min (mean). The mean

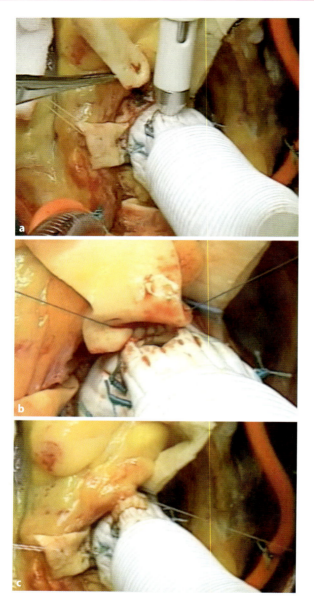

Fig. 4. a Holes for coronary buttons are made with a 5 mm punch. **b, c** The coronary arteries are reattached with continuous 5-0 polypropylene sutures

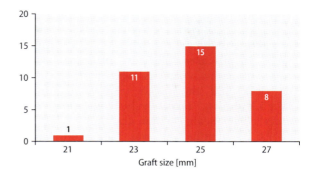

Fig. 5. Graft size distribution

Table 2. Operative data

■ Extension of aortic replacement	
– Ascending aorta	29 (82.9)
– Hemiarch or arch	4 (11.4)
– Frozen elephant trunk	2 (5.7)
■ Associated procedures	
– CABG	2 (5.5)
– Bipolar radiofrequency ablation	3 (8.6)
■ CPB time ± SD	147 ± 0.8
■ Cross-clamp time (min) ± SD	109.2 ± 31.1

Values are expressed as mean ± standard deviation (SD) or number of patients experiencing the event followed by the corresponding percentage in parentheses, unless otherwise noted. *CABG* coronary artery bypass grafting, *CPB* cardiopulmonary bypass

ASCP time was 53.8 ± 30.6 min. All patients were transferred to the ICU after surgery. The median VAM time was 6.7 h (range, 5–37 h), while the median ICU stay was 2.8 ± 5.3 d (range, 1–28 d). Surgical procedures and operative data are reported in Table 2.

Inhospital mortality was 2.8% (1 patient). The cause of death was irreversible arrhythmia. Two patients required rethoracotomy for bleeding, two patients needed prolonged mechanical ventilation (>48 h) and one patient suffered from acute renal failure requiring temporary dialysis. Blood transfusions were necessary in three patients. The mean blood loss from thoracic drains was 271 ± 156.3, 436.2 ± 252.9, 595.7 ± 260.3 ml at 12, 24 and 48 h from ICU admission, respectively. The median inhospital stay was 10.4 d (range, 7–83 d). No others complications were observed.

Hemodynamic characteristics and follow-up

All patients underwent transthoracic echocardiography before hospital discharge. In all cases, the valve prostheses were functioning normally. No images of paravalvular leakage or structural degeneration were detected. The peak and the mean transvalvular gradients were 25.1±8.5 and 13.5±5.1 mmHg, respectively. The mean aortic valve area was 1.72± 0.3 cm^2. The mean ejection fraction was 62.5±9.7%. The mean follow-up was 7.6±4 months and was 100% complete. Clinical examination, ECG, and thorax X-rays, which were performed at 1, 3 or 6 months after discharge and then yearly, always revealed patients in good general condition.

Discussion

A variety of pathological conditions involving the ascending aorta and aortic valve often require concomitant ascending aorta and aortic valve replacement. Since the first successful report of the Bentall-De Bono technique [1], the mechanical valved conduit has traditionally been implanted with excellent results [20]. Throughout the years, many improvements in the materials and surgical techniques have contributed to facilitating the procedure and ameliorating the results. Precoated Dacron grafts have reduced blood loss, while the open-button technique, reducing the tension on the ostial anastomoses, has decreased the risk of bleeding and late pseudoaneurysm formation [13]. However, the use of mechanical valves is limited by their need for anticoagulation and suboptimal hemodynamics. With improved durability of bioprosthetic valves coupled with the aging of the general population, the use of the biological valve has increased enormously, for example, the use of the biological valved conduit [2, 4, 9, 18].

Composite conduits with a biological stented or stentless valve prosthesis have been used with satisfactory results but they need to be assembled intraoperatively, thus, increasing bypass, cross-clamp and procedural times [9]. Stentless xenograft roots offer good outcomes but their length is limited; they are often not long enough to replace the entire ascending aorta, thus, requiring a Dacron graft extension resulting in an additional suture line [2]. However, the xenograft aortic wall is prone to calcification and, if reoperation were required, then their entire replacement would be necessary, compounding the risk of surgery [8].

Preassembled biological valved conduits were unavailable, because conventional protein sealed grafts cannot be sterilized using valve sterilant and storage solutions, i.e., formaldehyde and glutaraldehyde. Graft sterilization by this method would result in the crosslinking of the protein sealant and make it completely nonresorbable. Likewise, biological valves cannot be

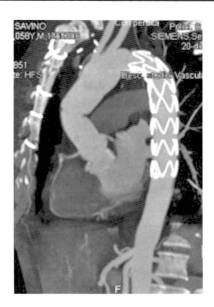

Fig. 6. Multidetector CT scan of a patient underwent Bentall procedure and frozen elephant trunk procedure for diffuse disease of the thoracic aorta. The pseudosinuses of the BioValsalva graft are clearly detectable

sterilized by ethylene oxide or radiation, the two recognized methods for conventional protein sealed grafts.

Unique elastomeric membrane technology, pioneered by The Terumo Corporation, led to the development of Triplex^{TM} a new zero porosity, non-protein sealed vascular thoracic graft. However, Triplex^{TM} when combined with the Vascutek Elan^{TM} stentless porcine biological valve can withstand formaldehyde and glutaraldehyde. This has resulted in the development of a novel biological valved conduit, the BioValsalva^{TM}.

The Valsalva Triplex graft, which better reconstructs the anatomy of the aortic root, facilitates coronary ostia anastomoses and reduces tension on the sutures, with the potential for improved coronary blood flow [4, 6] (Fig. 6). Moreover it may play a role in enhancing durability of the valve improving the movement of the aortic prosthetic cusps [5]. The use of the Elan^{TM} porcine stentless heart valve seems to be supported by the excellent results obtained by Flynn and colleagues [10]. Our own experience with this valve was very encouraging. We performed 128 isolated or combined aortic valve replacements with the Elan valve (series not published) in a 5-year period with a mortality rate of 4.7% (6 patients). The mean aortic gradient was 15.1 mmHg at a mean follow-up time of 14 months.

Another important advantage of the BioValsalva graft is that, if reoperation is needed, the stentless valve can be easily replaced cutting out the valve cusps and implanting a new stentless or stented valve into the suitable position.

Conclusions

In conclusion, the BioValsalva represents a new biological conduit that incorporates the practical advantages of a ready-to-use valved conduit and offers the hemodynamic advantages of a stentless valve prosthesis. It demonstrates ease of implantation and offers rapid hemostasis due to the trilaminate material of the vascular prosthesis. However, more patients, longer follow-up and randomized controlled studies are necessary to validate our early results and to confirm the efficacy of this new biological valved conduit.

Disclosures and freedom of investigation. The authors do not have any personal conflicts of interest.

References

1. Bentall H, De Bono A (1968) A technique for complete replacement of the ascending aorta. Thorax 23:338–339
2. Byrne JG, Mihaljevic T, Lipson WE, Smith B, Fox JA, Aranki SF (2001) Composite stentless valve with graft extension for combined replacement of the aortic valve, root and ascending aorta. Eur J Cardiothorac Surg 20:252–256
3. Cabrol C, Pavie A, Mesnildrey P, et al (1986) Long-term results with total replacement of the ascending aorta and reimplantation of the coronary arteries. J Thorac Cardiovasc Surg 91:17–25
4. De Paulis R, Nardi P, De Matteis GM, Polisca P, Chiariello L (2001) Bentall procedure with a stentless valve and a new aortic root prosthesis. Ann Thorac Surg 71:1375–1376
5. De Paulis R, De Matteis GM, Nardi P et al (2002) Analysis of valve motion after the reimplantation type of valve-sparing procedure (David I) with a new aortic root conduit. Ann Thorac Surg 74:53–57
6. De Paulis R, Tomai F, Bertoldo F et al (2004) Coronary flow characteristics after a Bentall procedure with or without sinuses of Valsalva. Eur J Cardiothorac Surg 26:66–72
7. De Paulis R, Scaffa R, Maselli D et al (2008) A third generation of Dacron vascular grafts for the ascending aorta. Preliminary experience. Ann Thorac Surg 85:305–309
8. Dossche KM, Schepens MA, Morshuis WJ, de la Riviere AB, Knaepen PJ, Vermeulen FE (1999) A 23-year experience with composite valve graft replacement of the aortic root. Ann Thorac Surg 67:1070–1077
9. Etz CD, Homann TM, Rane N, Bodian CA, Di Luozzo G, Plestis KA, Spielvogel D, Griepp RB (2007) Aortic root reconstruction with a bioprosthetic valved conduit: A consecutive series of 275 procedures. J Thorac Cardiovasc Surg 133:1455–1463
10. Flynn M, Iaccovoni A, Pathi V, Butler J, Macarthur KJ, Berg GA (2001) The aortic Elan stentless aortic valve: excellent hemodynamics and ease of implantation. Semin Thorac Cardiovasc Surg. 13:48–54

11. Gulbins H, Kreuzer E, Reichart B (2003) Homografts: a review Expert Rev Cardiovasc Ther 1(4):533–539
12. Hemmer WB, Botha CA, Bohm JO, Herrmann T, Starck C, Rein JG (2004) Replacement of the aortic valve and ascending aorta with an extended root stentless xenograft. Ann Thorac Surg 78:2150–2153
13. Kouchoukos NT, Karp RB (1981) Resection of ascending aortic aneurysm and replacement of aortic valve. J Thorac Cardiovasc Surg 81:142–143
14. Lehmann S, Walther T, Kempfert J, Leontjev S, Rastan A, Falk V, Mohr FW (2007) Stentless versus conventional xenograft aortic valve replacement: midterm results of a prospectively randomized trial. Ann Thorac Surg 84:467–472
15. Musci M, Siniawski H, Knosalla C, Grauhan O, Weng Y, Pasic M, Meyer R, Hetzer R (2006) Early and mid-term results of the Shelhigh stentless bioprosthesis in patients with active infective endocarditis. Clin Res Cardiol 95:247–253
16. Pacini D, Ranocchi F, Angeli E, et al (2003) Aortic root replacement with composite valve graft. Ann Thorac Surg 76:90–98
17. Slaughter MS, Jweied E (2007) Managing mechanical valves with reduced anticoagulation. Expert Rev Cardiovasc Ther 5:1073–1085
18. Urbanski PP, Diegeler A, Siebel A, Zacher M, and Hacker RW (2003) Valved stentless composite graft: clinical outcomes and hemodynamic characteristics. Ann Thorac Surg 75:467–471
19. Westaby S, Katsumata T, Vaccari G (1999) Coronary reimplantation in aortic root replacement: a method to avoid tension. Ann Thorac Surg 67:1176–1177
20. Zehr KJ, Orszulak TA, Mullany CJ et al (2004) Surgery for aneurysms of aortic root. A 30-year experience. Circulation 110:1364–1371

Valve replacement in renal dialysis patients: bioprostheses versus mechanical prostheses

W. R. E. Jamieson, V. Chan

The incidence of end-stage chronic renal failure is increasing. In 1999, Schaubel and colleagues [1] reported on prevalence projections to 2005 in Canada, which can be considered representative of western countries. In 1981, the rate was 49.5 per million population, 2000 projected at 154 per million, and, in 2005, projected at 214.5 per million with a significant increase in nondiabetics 65 years and diabetics both in age categories 45–64 years and ≥65 years [1].

The purpose of this chapter is to review the evidence for prosthesis-type for management of valvular disease in end-stage renal disease (ESRD). The choice of prosthesis remains the subject of debate. In 1998, the Guidelines for the Management of Patients with Valvular Heart Disease (American College of Cardiology and American Heart Association) recommended that mechanical prosthesis were indicated in "patients in renal failure, on hemodialysis, or with hypercalcemia" (class II evidence) [2]. The traditional teaching recommended by the ACC/AHA was that bioprostheses would undergo accelerated calcification in patients with ESRD; therefore, mechanical valves had been the mainstay of treatment for many years.

Following the publication of the ACC/AHA guidelines evidence continued to be presented to alter the prosthesis-type recommendation for ESRD.

In 1997, Lucke and co-authors [3] reported the Duke University experience in 19 patients (9 bioprostheses and 10 mechanical prostheses). The overall survival at 5 years was 42%. Mechanical prostheses were complicated by cerebrovascular accidents or bleeding complications, while no reoperations were required for bioprostheses. Because of the poor survival, these authors recommended that preference be given to bioprostheses over mechanical prostheses for ESRD. In 2002, Brinkman and colleagues [4] documented experience of Emory University. The overall survival of 72 patients was 15.9% at 6 years (Fig. 1). The survival was undifferentiated for mechanical prostheses and bioprostheses (Fig. 2). Mechanical prosthesis patients had a six-fold higher incidence of late bleeding or stroke. Their conclusion was that bioprostheses should be the substitute of choice in ESRD.

The major thrust for reconsideration of the ACC/AHA guidelines occurred when Herzog and colleagues [5], in 2002, reported from the US Renal Data System on 5858 dialysis patients, 881 having had bioprostheses.

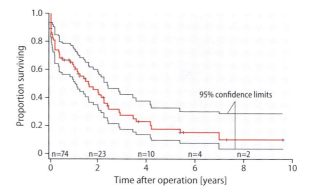

Fig. 1. Kaplan-Meier survival after operation (solid line) with 95% confidence limits (dotted lines) above and below. Reprinted with permission from [4]; © Annals of Thoracic Surgery

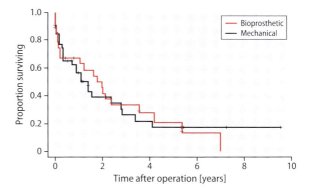

Fig. 2. Survival after valve replacement, stratified by type of valve implanted. No influence of valve type on survival was demonstrated in this review. Reprinted with permission from [4]; © Annals of Thoracic Surgery

There was no difference in survival between the two prosthesis types, at two years, 39.7% for each of bioprostheses and mechanical prostheses (Fig. 3). Of the predictors of death, bioprostheses were not predictive. These authors recommended that bioprostheses should not be excluded in a substitute choice for valve replacement in ESRD (Class II).

Further reports have come forward addressing the prosthesis-choice for valve replacement in ESRD. Gultekin et al. [6] reported on a Turkish experience in 2005 that survival at 5 years was 46.7%. Of this experience, 29 of 30 had mechanical prostheses. These authors provided consideration that life expectancy is extended in valve disease patients with ESRD after valve replacement and provides the opportunity for renal transplantation. The Cleveland Clinic experience was reported in 2000 with a 5-year survival for mechanical prosthesis of 33% and for bioprostheses of 27%, not significantly different [7]. This report documented that prosthesis-related complications were similar for bioprostheses and mechanical prostheses. The report by Filsoufi et al. [8] confirmed that the 5-year survival rates were equivalent for bioprostheses and mechanical prostheses in a patient

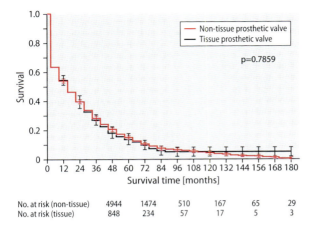

Fig. 3. Estimated all-cause survival of dialysis patients after heart valve replacement surgery with tissue and nontissue prosthetic valves. Bars indicate standard errors. Reprinted with permission from [5]; © Circulation

population combining renal failure/dialysis and nondialysis-dependent renal failure. Consensus recommendations were brought forward in 2004 and 2006 in Canada and the United States, respectively [9, 10]. The Canadian Cardiovascular Society 2004 Consensus on Surgical Management of Valvular Heart Disease recommended bioprostheses for valve replacement in patients in renal failure, on hemodialysis or with hypercalcemia (Class IIb C) [9]. The revision of the ACC/AHA Guidelines for the Management of Patients with Valvular Heart Disease, in 2006, made no specific recommendations for prosthesis selection in dialysis patients but noted difficulties in maintaining anticoagulation in these patients [10].

The University of British Columbia experience was published jointly with Westchester Medical Center, New York, by Chan and co-investigators [11] in 2006. The series comprised 69 patients, 47 with bioprostheses and 22 with mechanical prostheses. The overall survival was 31.4% at 5 years, not different by prosthesis type. There was one case of structural valve deterioration in the bioprosthesis group at 95 months after surgery. The freedom from valve-related complications, at 5 years, for thromboembolism plus thrombosis plus hemorrhage was 93.0% for bioprostheses and 76.4% for mechanical prostheses (Fig. 4). The five-year freedom from all valve-related complications was 82.8% for bioprostheses and 76.4% for mechanical prostheses (Fig. 5).

The conclusions of the manuscript documented that overall survival was poor [11]. Differences between populations were related to age at operation and coronary artery disease. Structural valve deterioration was not accentuated with bioprostheses. Considering lack of homogeneity between prostheses groups there was no superiority of mechanical prostheses over bio-

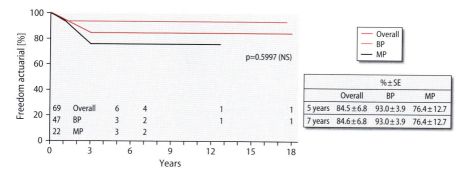

Fig. 4. Actuarial freedom from valve-related thromboembolism, thrombosis, and hemorrhage, overall (solid line) and for bioprostheses (*BP* long-dash line) and mechanical prostheses (*MP* short-dash line) (*NS* not significant). Reprinted with permission from [11]; © Annals of Thoracic Surgery

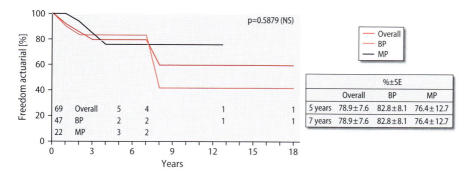

Fig. 5. Actuarial freedom from all valve-related complications, overall (solid line) and for bioprostheses (*BP* long-dash line) and mechanical prostheses (*MP* short-dash line) (*NS* not significant). Reprinted with permission from [11]; © Annals of Thoracic Surgery

prostheses in terms of freedom from composites of complications. Bioprostheses should be considered in the management of valvular disease in end-stage renal disease patients.

This review of the literature, including the authors' contribution, reveal that bioprostheses should not be contraindicated in end-stage renal disease, for valve replacement, given the observed rarity of accelerated calcification and poor intermediate term survival. Bioprostheses offer distinct advantage to circumvent long-term anticoagulation, important given issues of chronic care related to routine dose adjustments and nonmorbid bleeding events.

References

1. Schaubel DE, Morrison HI, Desmeules M, Parsons DA, Fenton SSA (1999) End-stage renal disease in Canada: prevalence projections to 2005. Can Med Assoc J 160:1557–1563
2. Bonow RO, Carabello B, deLeon AC Jr et al (1998) Guidelines for the management of patients with valvular heart disease: executive summary. A report of the American College of Cardiology/American Heart Association Task Force on Practice Guidelines. Circulation 98:1949–1984
3. Lucke JC, Samy RN, Atkins BZ et al (1997) Results of valve replacement with mechanical and biological prostheses in chronic renal dialysis patients. Ann Thorac Surg 64:129–133
4. Brinkman WT, Williams WH, Guyton RA et al (2002) Valve replacement in patients on chronic renal dialysis: implications for valve prosthesis selection. Ann Thorac Surg 74:37–42
5. Herzog CA, Ma JZ, Collins AJ (2002) Long-term survival of dialysis patients in the United States with prosthetic heart valves: should the ACC/AHA practice guidelines on valve selection be modified? Circulation 105:1336–1341
6. Gultekin B, Ozkan S, Uguz E et al (2005) Valve replacement surgery in patients with end-stage renal disease: long-term results. Artificial Organs 29(12):972–975
7. Horst M, Mehlhorn U, Hoerstrup SP, Suedkamp M, de Vivie R (2000) Cardiac surgery in patients with end-stage renal disease: 10-year experience. Ann Thorac Surg 69:96–101
8. Filsoufi F, Chikwe J, Castillo JG, Rahmanian PB, Vassalotti J, Adams DH (2008) Prosthesis type has minimal impact on survival after valve surgery in patients with moderate to end-stage renal failure. Nephrol Dial Transplant 23(11):3613–3621
9. Jamieson WRE, Cartier PC, Burwash IG et al (2004) Canadian Cardiovascular Society. Surgical management of valvular heart disease. Can J Cardiol 20E:1–120
10. Bonow RO, Carabello BA, Chatterjee K, de Leon AC Jr et al (2006) ACC/AHA 2006 guidelines for the management of patients with valvular heart disease: a report of the American College of Cardiology/American Heart Association Task Force on Practice Guidelines. J Amer Col Card 48(3):e1–e148
11. Chan V, Jamieson WRE, Fleisher AG et al (2006) Valve replacement surgery in end-stage renal failure: mechanical prostheses versus bioprostheses. Ann Thorac Surg 81:857–862

Replacement of bioprostheses after structural valve deterioration

C. A. Yankah, M. Pasic, H. Siniawski, J. Stein,
C. Detschades, A. Unbehaun, N. Solowjowa, S. Buz,
Y. Weng, R. Hetzer

Introduction

Xenografts, allografts, and pulmonary autografts have complimentary roles in the treatment of valvular heart diseases. Because the recipients require no long-term anticoagulant therapy, the incidence of thromboembolic events is low in contrast to that in mechanical valve recipients [1–14]. Furthermore, among the biological valves, the allograft has an additional advantage over xenografts and mechanical valves for aortic valve replacement in the setting of endocarditis, with a lower probability of recurrent infections [15–20]. Another purported advantage of biological prostheses (BP) is their anticipated subtle mode of failure in contrast to the catastrophic mechanism of failure anticipated for mechanical prostheses. Despite the obvious advantage of bioprostheses over the mechanical valves some surgeons still favor the mechanical prosthesis (MP) because of its high structural durability and lower reoperation rate for younger patients [21, 22]. The mechanical prosthesis, however, poses a contraindication in elderly and noncompliant patients because of the valve-related hemorrhagic and thromboembolic complications.

The current debate addresses whether anticoagulant-free bioprostheses will outlast the life expectancy of elderly and comorbid patients, so that they will not develop structural valve deterioration (SVD) which would require reoperation in their lifetime. The debate continues with the question of whether a second bioprosthesis after SVD poses a higher risk for early structural deterioration and, thus, a reoperative risk, especially in elderly patients who at younger age preferred the bioprosthesis.

The contemporary risk of reoperative aortic valve replacement, therefore, has implications for the selection of prosthesis type – mechanical or biological – or other procedures such as reconstruction among patients with limited or longer life expectancy.

The purpose of this publication, therefore, is to determine the prosthesis of choice for the replacement of failed implanted bioprostheses after SVD in patients of different age groups and the current reoperative risks, morbidity, and mortality. Our recommendations may serve to guide the surgeons in their decision-making process for the selection of BP for particular patients.

Methods

In the first half of our aortic valve replacement (AVR) program, from 1986–1997, more mechanical prostheses were implanted than bioprostheses. The trend changed in the latter half of the study period (1998–2007) towards the use of more bioprostheses (Fig. 1). Between May, 1986, and December, 2007, 5027 patients underwent primary AVR with and without concomitant coronary artery bypass grafting (CABG). In the same period, 330 patients underwent replacement of biprostheses (BP) for various reasons. Major causes for explantation were the following: structural valve deterioration (53.9%), prosthetic valve endocarditis (29.4%), paravalvular leakage (5.2%), leaflet tear (2.4%), and valve thrombosis (0.9%) (Table 1).

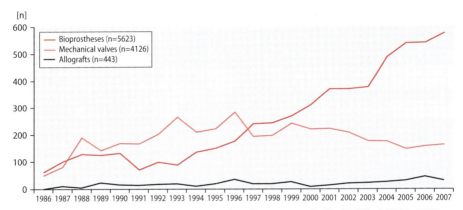

Fig. 1. Trends in aortic valve surgery at Deutsches Herzzentrum Berlin (DHZB), 3/1986–2007

Table 1. Causes of bioprosthetic replacement of bioprostheses at the Deutsches Herzzentrum Berlin (DHZB), No = 330; 5/1986–2007

Diagnoses			
PVE acute	97	Anterior mitral leaflet	1
Healed PVE	29	Leaflet damage distortion by radiation	1
SVD	178	Coronary ostial obstruction	1
Paravalvular leak	17	VSD	2
Prosthetic valve thrombosis	3	Aneurysm of sinus of Valsalva	2
Leaflet tear	7	Pseudoaneurysm asc. aorta	1
Leaflet perforation	1	Type A aortic dissection	1
Patient-prosthesis mismatch	1	LV aneurysm	1

PVE prosthetic valve endocarditis, *SVD* structural valve deterioration, *VSD* ventricular septal defect

A total of 178 patients (93 males and 85 females) aged 14-89, median 67 years had repeat AVR after structural valve deterioration (SVD). A total of 96 patients received the primary AVR at our institution and 82 externally since 1975. Median follow-up after primary AVR was 13.7 (range: 1.8–32.2) years at 2587 patient-years and after re-replacement it was 3.87 (range: 0–20.99) years at 1059.2 patient-years. The age groups were distributed as follows: < 60 years (n = 52), 60–69 years (n = 53) and > 70 years (n = 73) (Table 2). Replacement of bioprostheses with concomitant CABG (1st CABG/re-CABG or hybrid procedure: PTCA with stent implantation) was performed in 41 patients (Fig. 2).

In 2007, 12 265 isolated aortic valve procedures (with 42 allografts, 2814 mechanical prostheses, 9260 xenografts and 149 reconstructions) and 8473

Table 2. Re-AVR with bioprostheses for SVD with concomitant CABG/re-CABG Deutsches Herzzentrum Berlin (DHZB), 5/1986–2007

Patient demographics	
No. of patients	178
Median age (years)	70.7
Range (years)	16.4–91.2
Male/female	88/83
Age groups (years)	n
< 65	47 (26.4%)
≥ 65	131 (73.6%)
≥ 70	104 (58.4%)

AVR aortic valve replacement, *SVD* structural valve deterioration, *CABG* coronary artery bypass grafting

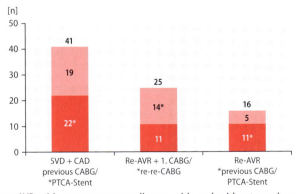

Fig. 2. Patients undergoing repeat AVR with coronary artery disease with and without previous CABG and coronary artery stenting. Red box represnts represents patients undergoing repeat aortic valve replacement with concomitant coronary artery bypass grafting or stenting

procedures combined with coronary bypass grafting (CABG) and 295 Ross procedures were reported by 79 German institutions to the German Society of Cardiothoracic and Vascular Surgery database [23]. The operative risk for isolated aortic valve procedures according to the database was 3.9% and for combined CABG it was 6.3%. The report confirmed further an increased implantation of bioprostheses over the years in Germany because of the aging population. In Table 3, a summary of considerations for prosthesis selection and in Table 4 relevant population statistics are presented.

Table 3. Considerations for prosthesis selection for valve re-replacement for structural valve deterioration (SVD)

- Does a previous structural valve deterioration (SVD) of a bioprosthesis pose a risk for accelerated SVD, and is it, therefore, a contraindication for another bioprosthesis?
- Is a young age a risk factor for accelerated SVD for second bioprosthesis (a second-set reaction)?
- Is the risk of reoperation higher than that of primary operation?
- Is the cumulative patient morbidity (reoperative mortality) for two bioprostheses comparable with that of patients with a single mechanical valve?
- A second bioprosthesis will outlast the life expectancy of which patients?
- Which patients will not experience reoperation for SVD of bioprosthesis before death?
- Do the risks of long-term anticoagulation outweigh those of SVD?
- Does the incidence of PVE differentiate bioprostheses from mechanical prostheses?

Table 4. Life expectancy of German population and patients after aortic valve replacement

Life expectancy (LE) of German population by age groups[a]					
Age groups	60 years	65 years	70 years	75 year	80 years
LE of women (years)	24.61	20.31	16.15	12.31	8.92
LE of men (years)	20.75	16.93	13.3	10.23	7.56
Life expectancy of men after bioprosthetic (BAVR) and mechanical (MAVR) aortic valve replacement by age groups[b]					
Age groups	60 years	65 years	70 years	75 years	80 years
LE after BAVR (years)	13	11	10	8	–
LE after MAVR (years)	13	10.5	8	7	–

[a] Federal Bureau of Population Statistics, Wiesbaden, Germany, [b] Puvimanasinghe et al. 2004 [24]

Operation technique

Preoperative imaging

Chest X-ray in two views and thoracic computer tomography (CT scan) are performed to assess
- the space between the sternum and the epicardium and
- the relationship between the substernal structures (CABG, internal mammary artery (IMA), ascending aorta) and the sternum (Fig. 3).

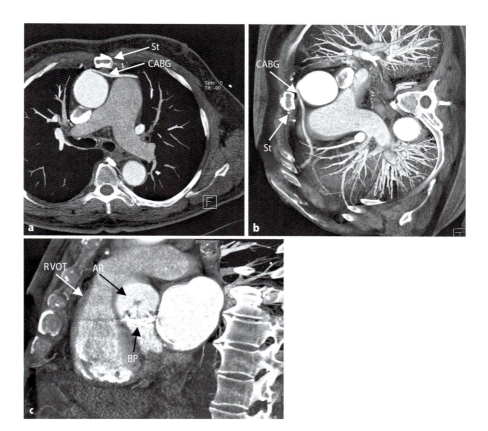

Fig. 3. Preoperative electrocardiographic triggered thoracic computed tomography (64-slice, Siemens Somatron Definition) for assessing the relationship between the sternum (St) and the substernal cardiovascular structures. **a** A transverse cross-sectional view at the level of pulmonary artery bifurcation showing the coronary artery bypass graft (CABG) below the sternum, **b** a sagittal cross-sectional view showing the coronary artery bypass graft below the sternum, **c** a sagittal cross-sectional view showing the right ventricular outflow tract (RVOT) and the aortic root (AR) with a bioprosthesis (BP)

Reentry sternotomy

The groins are prepared as for all sterile operations. The lines for the extracorporeal circulation are primed as the skin incision is performed. After midline skin incision, the sternal wires are cut and removed. Gentle dissection is made of the suprasternal jugulum soft tissue structures, partly bluntly, with absolute care taken not to damage the innominate vein. At the distal sternum around the xyphoid, the linea alba is divided and with a gentle dissection the substernal soft tissue is exposed in line with the midline sternum incision. Using the manually controlled, electrically driven oscillating saw along the midline sternum incision guided by high-pressure suction the two sternal blades (layers) are gently sawed beginning from the manubrium distally towards the distal sternum until the substernal soft tissue site is felt. We classify reentry sternotomy into four grades according to severity of substernal epimyocardial and vascular injury, blood loss, and circulatory situation of the patient:

- Grade 1: Uneventful sternotomy; no epimyocardial damage; easy dissection of adhesions to expose the heart, great arteries, and veins.
- Grade 2: Accomplished sternotomy with minor epicardial/superficial myocardial, atrial or vascular injury with minor controlled bleeding at dissection.
- Grade 3: Epimyocardial injury with significant blood loss; blood transfusion from the cell-saver and hypotension necessitating urgent institution of cardiopulmonary bypass.
- Grade 4: Severe cardiac chamber injury with severe blood loss and cardiac arrest before institution of cardiopulmonary bypass.

Statistical analysis

The guidelines approved by the Society of Thoracic Surgeons for reporting morbidity and mortality after cardiac valvular operations were used to analyze postoperative complications [32]. All continuous variables were expressed as mean ± SEM. Actuarial curves were calculated by the Kaplan-Meier method. Linearized occurrence rate of events and confidence limits were calculated according to Poisson distribution. Actual competing risk analysis (cumulative incidence) was performed. A p value of <0.05 was considered as evidence of statistical significance. Predictors of events during follow-up were identified by means of Cox's proportional hazards regression.

Results

▌ Valve re-replacement with a second bioprosthesis after structural valve deterioration

A total of 92 patients received a bioprosthesis. Frequency of implantation of bioprostheses in age groups is shown in Table 5. Of patients ≥70 years, 81.9% received bioprostheses. One patient under 60 years received allograft aortic valve replacement. Experience gained from transapical valve implantation in native stenotic aorta has allowed an extension of the indication for patients with degenerated bioprosthesis in many cetres (Table 5b, Fig. 4).

▌ Valve re-replacement with mechanical prosthesis after bioprosthetic structural valve deterioration

Eighty-two patients received mechanical prostheses. Frequency of implantation of mechanical prosthesis in the age groups is shown in Table 5a. Seventyfive percent of patients <60 years received mechanical prostheses. In Table 6, types of re-replacement at different institutions are shown.

Table 5a. Types of prosthesis for re-aortic valve replacement in age groups, n=171

Age groups (years)	Total 171	Prosthesis of choice		
		Bioprosthesis n=92 (%)	Allograft n=1 (%)	Mechanical valve n=78 (%)
<60	49	22.4	2.1	75.5
<65	75	26.7	1.3	72
≥65	69	75	–	25
≥70	72	81.9	–	18.1
≥80	16	87.5	–	12.5

Table 5b. Transapical off-pump valve-in-valve implantation in degenerated bioprosthesis. Series at German Heart Centres (6/2009)

Institution	TAVR n	V-i-V n
▌ Leipzig	250	7 (2.8%)
▌ Karlsruhe	130	4 (3.1%)
▌ Berlin	114	9 (7.9%)
▌ Munich	63	1 (1.6%)
▌ Hamburg	55	4 (7.3%)

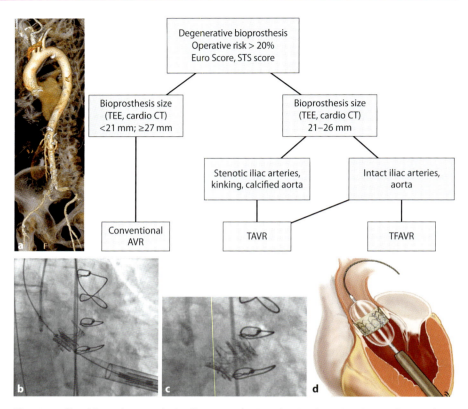

Fig. 4. a Algorithm of transapical off-pump valve-in-valve implantation into a bioprosthesis after structural valve deterioration. **b–d** Implantation of Edwards Sapien valve into a CE-Perimount pericardial bioprosthesis after structural valve deterioration. (From [41])

Hospital survival

Patient survival in the overall period 1986–2007 and in the subperiod 2002–2007 was 90.1±5.4% and 93.3±3.7%, respectively (p=0.580).

Hospital mortality by period: 2002–2007. Hospital mortality for re-AVR was 1.3% (2/151), and for re-AVR and concomitant CABG it was 5.8% (1/17) (Table 7).

Hospital mortality by period: 1986–2007. Hospital mortality for re-AVR was 8.4% (10/118), for re-AVR and concomitant CABG 12.2% (5/41), and for re-AVR + concomitant CABG and re-CABG 12% (3/25) (Table 6). A summary of reoperative hospital mortality with and without CABG at different institutions is shown in Table 8.

Table 6. Types of prosthesis for valve re-replacement at different institutions [11, 27]

Institution	Explanted	Type of re-replacement		
	Bioprosthesis n	Bioprosthesis n (%)	Allograft n (%)	Mechanical n (%)
The Cleveland Clinic	95	50 (53)	2 (2)	43 (45)
The Cleveland Clinic	46[a]	15 (32)	7 (16)	24 (52)
DHZB	171	92 (53.4)	1 (0.5)	78 (46.1)
Mayo Clinic	77	40 (52)	7 (9.1)	30 (39)

DHZB Deutsches Herzzentrum Berlin
[a] Allografts

Table 7. Mortality after valve re-replacement with bioprostheses for SVD and concomitant CABG/re-re-CABG in 2002–2007 compared with the total study period at Deutsches Herzzentrum Berlin (DHZB): 30-day mortality

Period	Primary AVR	Re-AVR	Re-AVR + CABG
1986–2007	10.9%	8.4%	12.2%
	549/5027	10/118	5/41
2002–2007	5.9%	1.3%	5.8%
	119/2020	2/151	1/17

SVD structural valve deterioration, *CABG* coronary artery bypass grafting, *AVR* aortic valve replacement

Table 8. Published data on hospital mortality after reaortic valve replacement ± CABG [3, 27, 29]

Author	Re-AVR ± CABG	Hospital mortality (%)	Mean age (years)
Potter et al. 2005	–	4.9	64
Jamieson et al. 2003	±	6.5	na
Jamieson et al. 2003	+	5	na
Byrne et al. 2002	+	6	na
Yankah et al. 2008	+	5.8	67

AVR aortic valve replacement, *CABG* coronary artery bypass grafting

Long-term survival

Survival primary and after reoperative AVR in patients with SVD and nonstructural valve deterioraton, in different age groups and with and without concomitant CABG, are shown in Figs. 5–8. In Fig. 7 patient survival after primary AVR is presented. The low survival is related to the advanced age at the primary AVR (73 years versus 67 years) and comorbidity. Summaries of long-term survival from the literature are shown in Tables 8 and 9.

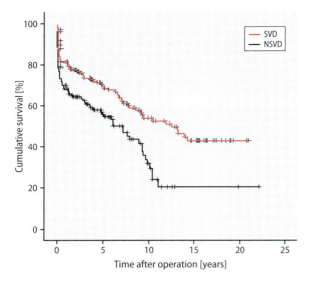

Fig. 5. Survival after replacement of bioprostheses after structural (SVD) and nonstructural (NSVD) valve deterioration (Kaplan-Meier)

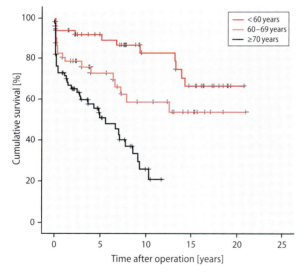

Fig. 6. Survival after replacement of bioprostheses for structural valve deterioration in age groups (Kaplan-Meier)

Comments

The heart valve database at the Deutsches Herzzentrum Berlin (DHZB) started with allografts and bioprostheses and now covers 22 years followup time [1, 18, 20]. Although the average age of AVR patients was greater than 70 years, more mechanical prostheses were implanted in the first half of our program, from 1986–1997, than bioprostheses. The trend changed in

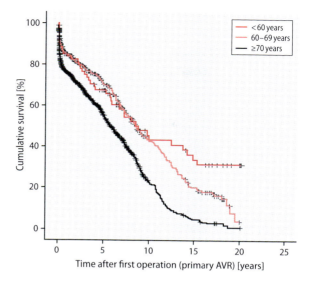

Fig. 7. Survival after primary aortic valve replacement in age groups (Kaplan-Meier)

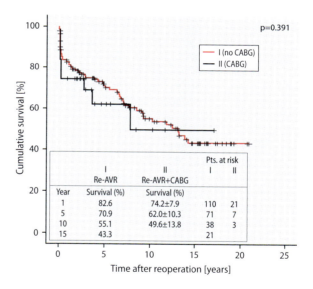

Fig. 8. Survival after replacement of bioprostheses for structural valve deterioration with concomitant primary and repeat coronary artery bypass grafting (Kaplan-Meier)

the latter half of the study period (1998–2007) towards the use of more bioprostheses, primarily for patients aged over 65 years. The reason for this trend was associated with the anticipated durability of bioprostheses and the increased life expectancy of the German population.

According to the German Federal Bureau of Population Statistics (2005–2007) 11 194 720 (13.6%) and 3 927 136 (4.8%) of the population are over 70 and 80 years old, respectively. The life expectancy in Germany for 60, 65,

Table 9. Patient survival (overall) after re-replacement of bioprostheses for structural valve deterioration [6, 26]

Author	Year	Prosthesis	Actuarial freedom SVD (%)		
			5 years	10 years	15 years
Lau et al.	2006	CE-P	62	56	28
Eichinger et al.	2008	SJM-Biocor	51.6	25.1	–
Yankah et al.	2008	Mitroflow	69.5	54	–
Yankah et al.	2009	Bioprostheses	72	59	50

SVD structural valve deterioration, *CE-P* Carpentier Edwards Perimount, *SJM* St. Jude Medical

70, 75, and 80-year-olds is 20.75, 16.93, 13.3, 10.23, 7.56 years for men and 24.61, 20.31, 16.15, 12.31, 8.92 years for women, respectively.

These life expectancy statistics indicate that patients who could have normal life expectancy are those who could achieve functional recovery of their organs after aortic valve replacement. The conditions for maintaining normal life expectancy are early indication for elective surgery without gross functional impairment of the left ventricular and other organs, using prostheses which do not cause patient-prosthesis mismatch and fatal valve-related complications [1–8]. The current technology in cardiac surgery offers low operative risk for aortic valve replacement even in the elderly with symptomatic aortic valve stenosis or failed bioprosthesis [1–8, 23, 24, 40].

It is well appreciated that the operative risk is confounded by several factors. Close follow-up of patients with echocardiographic monitoring and indication for early reoperation prior to development of gross left ventricular failure and advanced functional class (NYHA III and IV) can reduce the operative risks which are predictive of early and late mortality [1, 25, 27]. It is noteworthy that high postoperative morbidity is inversely related to intraoperative reentry sternotomy complications and preoperative left ventricular failure [32–34]. With tutoring and guidance, technical skills can be developed during the learning curve for reentry sternotomy, thus, avoiding catastrophic intraoperative cardiovascular injuries and postoperative morbidity. Re-sternotomy cardiac injury is a predictive factor for prolonged surgery, bleeding, cardiogenic shock, postoperative low cardiac output syndrome, and cardiac mortality [27, 29, 32–34].

The reported reoperative mortality rate after AVR varies between 1.3 and 10.6% [21–27]. Lau et al. reported 95.0±2.2% and 96.6±2.0% actuarial freedom from valve-related mortality with mechanical and bioprosthesis valves and 98.0±1.9% and 85.7±9.4% for patients older than 70 years, respectively [26]. In the period 1986–2007, the overall hospital mortality for primary AVR was 10.9%, and for primary AVR and concomitant coronary artery bypass grafting (CABG) it was 11.8%. Elective and urgent operative mortality was 8.1%. The Vancouver group reported in their early series

10.7% mortality without and 6.7% with concomitant CABG, which has decreased to 6.9% without and 5.0% with concomitant CABG [25–27]. Likewise, in our series for the last 5 years (2002–2007), the operative risk has improved with a decrease to 5.9% for primary elective AVR and 1.3% for re-AVR. The current operative risk for re-AVR and re-AVR with concomitant CABG is as low as that of the primary operations.

In our series 10- and 20-year survival after re-replacement for SVD in patients aged 60–69 years was 60% and 58%, respectively. Survival at 10 years for patients with Mitroflow pericardial prosthesis was 100%. Survival after bioprosthesis replacement with a second bioprosthesis for SVD in patients who received primary AVR under 65 years of age was 59% as compared to 56% in the recent data of Lau et al. and others [26, 28, 30]. The median age at reoperation was 67 years as compared to 73 years in the series with primary AVR [1].

The prosthesis of choice, whether bioprosthesis or mechanical, for different age groups and patients with special wishes remains a controversial issue. Structural valve deterioration (SVD) and subsequent risks of reoperation are the major morbid events with bioprostheses, while thrombosis, and thromboembolic and hemorrhagic episodes are the major events in patients with mechanical valves. Of reoperations in our series, 54% were associated with SVD of bioprostheses as compared to 87% and 74% in other series [11, 35]. Allograft explantation for SVD was 59% in the series of Smedira et al. [11]. The low rate of valve-related complications of the latest bioprostheses has, therefore, changed the strategy for bioprosthesis selection for patients <65 years [1]. Bioprostheses can be used in patients <60 years of age in the aortic position when the patient refuses long-term anticoagulant therapy, desires pregnancy, has a small aortic annulus or has comorbidity with limited life expectancy [1, 11, 21, 22]. The general debate addresses the question of whether a second bioprosthesis poses a higher risk of accelerated structural degeneration which might occur before the expected lifespan of the patient and, therefore, represent a contraindication.

Among the biological valves, the allograft has an additional advantage over xenograft valves for aortic valve replacement in the setting of endocarditis with a lower probability of recurrent infections [10–13, 16–20]. Reoperative risk was 8.1% excluding reinfection of allografts. Another purported advantage of biological valves is their anticipated subtle mode of failure in contrast to the catastrophic mechanism of failure that can occur with a mechanical prosthesis.

At the selection of prosthesis for primary AVR in young patients, the reoperative risk should be weighed against the benefits of anticoagulation and other valve-related events of mechanical valves. The general debate concerns the age cutoff that should be recommended for implanting a bioprosthesis at the primary operation [1, 11, 21, 22, 24].

With reference to other reports, patients between 65 and 69 years show actual freedom from major complications for mechanical and bioprosthesis of 84.7 ± 8.4% and 60.8 ± 13.4%; for patients over 70 years it was 79.0 ± 10.8% and 90.8 ± 3.9% respectively [26]. The relationship between age and SVD of bioprostheses demands general guidelines for selection of prosthesis, mechanical or bioprosthesis, for individual age groups with or without comorbidity and for special indications. Many studies have indicated that durability of mechanical as compared to that of bioprosthetic valves was not beneficial for patients over 65 years and 70 years in view of morbidity and survival [5, 24, 26]. The observation confirms the criteria used for prosthesis selection by age group in our cohort undergoing valve re-replacement for SVD. This observation was reported in the early studies of Jamieson et al. and McGilligan et al. on age and SVD of bioprostheses [36, 37].

Spampinato et al. found in their study that 20-year cumulative survival after implantation of two bioprostheses (primary AVR + re-replacement and reoperative mortality) was favorable to the 20-year survival of patients with a single mechanical valve [21, 22, 31, 38]. This recommendation can be individualized according to age and comorbidity and ultimately, after counseling about the risks, the patient would be able to decide on which risks he or she would accept even in the era of self-monitoring of anticoagulation [39].

Advanced age and NYHA class III–IV at reoperation for a bioprosthesis with SVD are risk factors for re-AVR The reoperative mortality for NYHA class III was 4.2%, for class IV 16%, and for patients 60–70 years and >70 years 5.6% and 11.8%, respectively, in the series of Jamieson et al. [25]. There was a striking difference in the 10-year survival for the age group 60–69 and ≥70 years, which was 60% and 23%, respectively, in our cohort. However, the 58% survival at 20 years for the age group 60–69 years in our cohort was very encouraging. In view of the high reoperative risk for the age group greater than 70 years, the recent innovative catheter-based aortic valve replacement, which is a minimally invasive procedure, offers a lower reoperative risk and better survival for the higher risk patients [40, 41].

Conclusions

Important technical steps at re-entry sternotomy should be strictly observed.

Re-replacement risk and reoperative mortality at elective/urgent surgery are as low as those of primary AVR without catastrophic reentry sternotomy cardiac injury.

Our data support the strategy of the use of bioprostheses in patients <65 years who prefer reoperation to long-term anticoagulation.

Routine regular echocardiographic follow-up after implantation of bioprostheses could contribute to establishing early indications for elective re-replacement which is associated with low hospital mortality.

Patients >70 years would benefit from valve re-replacement with a bioprosthesis, whereas such an indication is appropriate for patients <70 years with comorbidity.

High-risk patients should be offered catheter-based aortic valve-in-valve biologic replacement.

Acknowledgments. The authors are grateful to Anne M. Gale, ELS, for editorial assistance, Astrid Benhennour for bibliographic support, and Carla Weber for providing the graphics.

References

1. Yankah CA, Pasic M, Musci M, Stein J, Detschades C, Siniawski H, Hetzer R (2008) Aortic valve replacement with the Mitroflow pericardial bioprosthesis: durability results up to 21 years. J Thorac Cardiovasc Surg 136(3):688–696
2. Myken PSU, Bech-Hansen O (2009) A 20-year experience of 1712 patients with the Biocor porcine bioprosthesis. J Thorac Cardiovasc Surg 137(1):76–81
3. Jamieson WR, Burr LH, Miyagishima RT, Germann E, MacNab JS, Stanford E, Chan F, Janusz MT, Ling H (2005) Carpentier-Edwards supra-annular aortic porcine bioprosthesis: clinical performance over 20 years. J Thorac Cardiovasc Surg 130(4):994–1000
4. Borger MA, Ivanov J, Armstrong S, Christie-Hrybinsky D, Feindel CM, David TE (2006) Twenty-year results of the Hancock II bioprosthesis. J Heart Valve Dis 15(1):49–56
5. Khan SS, Trento A, DeRobertis M, Kass RM, Sandhu M, Czer LS, Blanche C, Raissi S, Fontana GP, Cheng W, Chaux A, Matloff JM (2001) Twenty-year comparison of tissue and mechanical valve replacement. J Thorac Cardiovasc Surg 122(2):257–69
6. Eichinger WB, Hettich I, Ruzicka D, Holper K, Schricker C, Bleiziffer S, Lange R (2008) Twenty-year experience with the St.-Jude medical biocor prosthesis in the aortic position. Ann Thorac Surg 86(4):1204–1211
7. Yankah CA, Schubel J, Buz S, Siniawski H, Hetzer R (2005) Seventeen-year clinical results of 1037 Mitroflow pericardial heart valve prostheses in the aortic position. J Heart Valve Dis 14(2):172–180
8. Aupart MR, Mirza A, Muerisse YA, Sirinelli AL, Neville PH, Marchand MA (2006) Perimount pericardial bioprosthesis for aortic calcified stenosis: 18-year experience with 1133 patients J Heart Valve Dis 15(6):768–776
9. David TE, Puschmann R, Ivanov J, Bos J, Armstrong S, Feindel CM, Scully HE (1998) Aortic valve replacement with stentless and stented porcine valves: a case-match study. J Thorac Cardiovasc Surg 116(2):236–241
10. McGiffin DC, Galbraith AJ, O'Brien MF, McLachlan GJ, Naftel DC, Adams P, Reddy S, Early L (1997) An analysis of valve re-replacement after aortic valve replacement with biologic devices. J Thorac Cardiovasc Surg 113(2):311–318
11. Smedira NG, Blackstone EH, Roselli EE, Laffey CC, Cosgrove DM (2006) Are allografts the biologic valve of choice for aortic valve replacement in nonelderly patients? Comparison of explantation for structural valve deterioration of allograft and pericardial prostheses. J Thorac Cardiovasc Surg 131(3):558–564

12. Lund O, Chandrasekaran V, Grocott-Mason R, Elwidaa H, Mazhar R, Khaghani A, Mitchell A, Ilsley C, Yacoub MH (1999) Primary aortic valve replacement with allografts over twenty-five years: valve-related and procedure-related determinants of outcome. J Thorac Cardiovasc Surg 117(1):77–91
13. O'Brien MF, Harrocks S, Stafford EG, Gardner MA, Pohlner PG, Tesar PJ, Stephens F (2001) The homograft aortic valve: a 29-year, 99.3% follow up of 1022 valve replacements. J Heart Valve Dis 10(3):334–344
14. Dittrich S, Alexi-Meskishvili V, Yankah CA, Dähnert I, Meyer R, Hetzer R, Lange PE (2000) Comparison of porcine xenografts and homografts for pulmonary valve replacement in children. Ann Thorac Surg 70(3):717–722
15. David TE (1997) Surgical management of aortic root abscess. J Card Surg 12 (2 Suppl):262–269
16. Haydock D, Barratt-Boyes B, Macedo T, Kirklin JW, Blackstone E (1992) Aortic valve replacement for active infectious endocarditis in 108 patients. A comparison of freehand allograft valves with mechanical prostheses and bioprostheses. J Thorac Cardiovasc Surg 103(1):130–139
17. Petrou M, Wong K, Albertucci M, Brecker SJ, Yacoub MH (1994) Evaluation of unstented aortic homografts for the treatment of prosthetic aortic valve endocarditis. Circulation 90(5 Pt 2):II198–204
18. Knosalla C et al (2000) Homograft versus prosthetic valve for surgical treatment of aortic valve endocarditis with periannular abscess Eur Heart J 21:490–497
19. Yacoub M, Rasmi NR, Sundt TM, Lund O, Boyland E, Radley-Smith R, Khaghani A, Mitchell A (1995) Fourteen-year experience with homovital homografts for aortic valve replacement. J Thorac Cardiovasc Surg 110(1):186–194
20. Yankah CA, Pasic M, Klose H, Siniawski H, Weng Y, Hetzer R (2005) Homograft reconstruction of the aortic root for endocarditis with periannular abscess: a 17-year study. Eur J Cardiothorac Surg 28(1):69–75
21. Ruel M, Kulik A, Lam BK, Rubens FD, Hendry PJ, Masters RG, Bédard P, Mesana TG (2005) Long-term outcomes of valve replacement with modern prostheses in young adults. Eur J Cardiothorac Surg 27(3):425–330
22. Emery RW, Erickson CA, Arom KV, Northrup WF 3rd, Kersten TE, Von Rueden TJ, Lillehei TJ, Nicoloff DM (2003) Replacement of the aortic valve in patients under 50 years of age: long-term follow-up of the St. Jude Medical prosthesis. Ann Thorac Surg 75(6):1815–1819
23. Gummert JF, Fumkat A, Beckmann A, Schiller W, Hekmat K, Ernst M, Haverich A (2008) Cardiac surgery in Germany during 2007: A report on behalf of the German Society for Thoracic and Cardiovascular Surgery. Thorac Cardiov Surg 56:328–336
24. Puvimanasinghe JP, Takkenberg JJ, Edwards MB, Eijkemans MJ, Steyerberg EW, Van Herwerden LA, Taylor KM, Grunkemeier GL, Habbema JD, Bogers AJ (2004) Comparison of outcomes after aortic valve replacement with a mechanical valve or a bioprosthesis using microsimulation. Heart 90(10):1172–1178
25. Jamieson WR, Burr LH, Miyagishima RT, Janusz MT, Fradet GJ, Ling H, Lichtenstein SV (2003) Re-operation for bioprosthetic aortic structural failure – risk assessment. Eur J Cardiothorac Surg 24(6):873–878
26. Lau L, Jamieson WR, Hughes C, Germann E, Chan F (2006) What prosthesis should be used at valve re-replacement after structural valve deterioration of a bioprosthesis? Ann Thorac Surg 82(6):2123–2132
27. Potter DD, Sundt TM 3rd, Zehr KJ, Dearani JA, Daly RC, Mullany CJ, McGregor CG, Puga FJ, Schaff HV, Orszulak TA (2005) Operative risk of reoperative aortic valve replacement. J Thorac Cardiovasc Surg 129(1):94–103

28. Awad WI, De Souza AC, Magee PG, Walesby RK, Wright JE, Uppal R (1997) Re-do cardiac surgery in patients over 70 years old. Eur J Cardiothorac Surg 12(1):40–46
29. Byrne JG, Aranki SF, Couper GS, Adams DH, Allred EN, Cohn LH (1999) Reoperative aortic valve replacement: partial upper hemisternotomy versus conventional full sternotomy. J Thorac Cardiovasc Surg 118(6):991–997
30. Sener E, Yamak B, Katirciolu SF, Ozerdem G, Karagöz H, Tademir O, Bayazit K (1995) Risk factors of reoperations for prosthetic heart valve dysfunction in the ten years 1984–1993. Thorac Cardiovasc Surg 43(3):148–152
31. McGrath LB, Fernandez J, Laub GW, Anderson WA, Bailey BM, Chen C (1995) Perioperative events in patients with failed mechanical and bioprosthetic valves. Ann Thorac Surg 60(2 Suppl):S475–478
32. O'Brien MF, Harrocks S, Clarke A, Garlick B, Barnett AG (2002) How to do safe sternal reentry and the risk factors of redo cardiac surgery: a 21-year review with zero major cardiac injury. J Card Surg 17(1):4–13
33. Ellman PI, Smith RL, Girotti ME, Thompson PW, Peeler BB, Kern JA, Kron IL (2008) Cardiac injury during resternotomy does not affect perioperative mortality. J Am Coll Surg 206(5):993–997
34. Cohn LH, Aranki SF, Rizzo RJ, Adams DH, Cogswell KA, Kinchla NM, Couper GS, Collins JJ Jr (1993) Decrease in operative risk of reoperative valve surgery. Ann Thorac Surg 56(1):15–21
35. Bortolotti U, Milano A, Mossuto E, Mazzaro E, Thiene G, Casarotto D (1994) Early and late outcome after reoperation for prosthetic valve dysfunction: analysis of 549 patients during a 26-year period. J Heart Valve Dis 3(1):81–87
36. Jamieson WR, Burr LH, Tyers GF, Miyagishima RT, Janusz MT, Ling H, Fradet GJ, MacNab J, Chan F, Henderson C (1995) Carpentier-Edwards supraannular porcine bioprosthesis: Clinical performance to twelve years. Ann Thorac Surg 60(2 Suppl):S235–S40
37. Magilligan DJ, Lewis JW, Stein P, Alan M (1989) The porcine bioprosthetic heart valve: Experience at 15 years. Ann Thorac Surg 48(3):324–330
38. Spampinato N, Gagliardi C, Pantaleo D, Fimiani L, Ascione R, De Robertis F, Musumeci A, Stassano P (1998) Bioprosthetic replacement after bioprosthesis failure: a hazardous choice? Ann Thorac Surg 66(6 Suppl):S68–S72
39. Körtke H, Körfer R (2001) International normalized ratio self-management after mechanical heart valve replacement: is an early start advantageous? Ann Thorac Surg 72(1):44–48
40. Walther T, Falk V, Kempfert J, Borger MA, Fassi J, Chu MWA, Schuler G, Mohr F (2008) Transapical minimally invasive aortic valve implantation; the initial 50 patients. Eur J Cardiothorac Surg 33(6):983–988
41. Walther T, Kempfert J, Borger MA, Fassl J, Falk V, Blumenstein J, Dehdashtian M, Schuler G, Mohr FW (2008) Human minimally invasive off-pump valve-in-valve implantation. Ann Thorac Surg 85:1072–1073

Predictors of patient's outcome

Predicted outcomes after aortic valve replacement in octogenarians with aortic stenosis

C. Piper, D. Hering, G. Kleikamp, R. Körfer, D. Horstkotte

Introduction

The epidemiology of valvar heart disease is changing with decreasing numbers of patients with "rheumatic" lesions and increasing numbers of patients with "degenerative" lesions (mainly calcific aortic valve stenosis (AS) and mitral regurgitation), which is accompanied by the constant increase in patient age at the time of surgical intervention [1, 2].

Valve replacement (AVR) is frequently not performed in due time in octogenarians with symptomatic AS, because the prognostic benefit is often underestimated and perioperative morbidity and mortality are overestimated [3–7]. The severely impaired prognosis and quality of life after myocardial decompensation then urges AVR with a significantly increased perioperative risk [8–10].

It was the aim of this prospective study to assess peri- and postoperative morbidity and mortality in octogenarians with severe AS and to compare the outcomes for patients with myocardial compensated versus chronically decompensated AS.

Methods

Study patients

We prospectively included 83 consecutive octogenarians (32 men, 51 women; age range 80–93 years, mean 83.5 ± 2.8 years) with isolated symptomatic AS (aortic valve opening area < 0.5 cm^2/m^2) in our survey during a 3-year period (2003–2006). All patients had echocardiography and right and left heart catheterization prior to surgery. According to hemodynamic parameters, the patients were divided into two groups: 38 patients (46%) with signs and symptoms of chronically myocardial decompensation had dilated left ventricle (left ventricular end-diastolic diameter (LVEDD) > 55 mm) and/or impaired left ventricular function (ejection fraction (EF)

Table 1. Clinical and hemodynamic characteristics of consecutive octogenarians presenting with symptomatic severe aortic stenosis before surgery. Group A: patients with chronic myocardial decompensation (ejection fraction (EF)<55% and/or left ventricular enddiastolic parameter (LVEDD)>55 mm); group B: myocardial compensated patients (EF≥55% and LVEDD≤55 mm). (Modified from [3])

	Group A	Group B	p
▪ Patients (n)	38 (45.8%)	45 (54.2%)	
▪ Gender: m/f (n)	12/26	20/25	
▪ Age (years)	83.7±2.3 [80–91]	83.3 ±3.2 [80–93]	n.s.
▪ NYHA	3.3±0.5	2.8±0.5	<0.01
▪ AVA (cm^2/m^2)	0.35±0.08	0.40±0.08	0.01
▪ EF (%)	43±8 [25–53]	59±4 [55–71]	<0.01
▪ LVEDD (mm)	57±8 [38–73]	47±5 [36–55]	<0.01
▪ Patients with syncope (n)	11 (29%)	0	<0.01

AVA aortic valve opening area

Table 2 Presents perioperative data of the two patient groups. (Modified from [3])

	Group A	Group B	p
▪ Ring enlargement (pericardial tissue) (n)	8 (21%)	12 (27%)	n.s.
▪ Prosthesis' size (mm)	23 [19–25]	23 [19–25]	n.s.
▪ Concomitant CABG (n)	11 (29%)	12 (27%)	n.s.

<55%) (group A). The remaining patients (group B) had normal left ventricular dimensions (LVEDD ≤55 mm), normal left ventricular ejection fraction (EF≥55%), and no clinical episodes of myocardial decompensation. The clinical and hemodynamic characteristics of both groups are given in Table 1. All patients underwent AVR, and 23 (27.7%) underwent simultaneous coronary revascularization (Table 2). Follow-up was 100% and ranged from 7 to 46 months.

▪ Statistics

Data are given as mean ±SD. For comparison of the two groups the Mann-Whitney U test was applied. Categorical variables were compared using the Chi square test. Kaplan-Meier survival curves were computed for patients with and without myocardial decompensation and differences compared using log-rank statistics. All analyses were performed using StatView 4.0. P values <0.05 were considered significant.

Results

Patients without myocardial decompensation (group B) had a 30-day mortality rate of 2.2% (1 out of 45). Two of the 38 octogenarians with symptomatic severe AS and chronically myocardial decompensation (group A) died perioperatively, resulting in a 30-day mortality rate of 5.3% (n.s.). The incidences of major postoperative complications, namely reversible acute renal failure (10.5% vs. 4.4%; n.s.), stroke (5.3% vs. 2.2%; n.s.), and myocardial failure requiring mechanical circulatory support (intraaortic balloon counterpulsation (n=5) and ventricular assist device (n=1)) (10.5% vs. 2.2%; n.s.), were higher in patients of group A. Due to the relatively low number of patients enrolled in the study, we also calculated the significance between the two groups for the composite endpoint renal failure, stroke plus indication for mechanical circulatory support, which was <0.05. Octogenarians not operated in due time demonstrated a higher postoperative morbidity (Fig. 1). More patients with chronic myocardial decompensation required mechanical circulatory support postoperatively (4 patients in group A vs. 1 in group B). During late follow-up (24.2±12.8 months), another 4 (11.1%) patients of group A and 5 (11.4%) of group B died. The cumulative survival rates after 24 months were 78% and after 36 months 68% for group A. Octogenarians of group B had a significantly (p<0.01) higher cumulative survival rate (87% after 24 months and 81% after 36 months) (Fig. 2). Six months after AVR, symptoms had improved in most patients. However, octogenarians with preoperative normal myocardial function (group B) according to NYHA classes performed better (Fig. 3). Figs. 4 and 5 demonstrate the negative influence of preoperative reduced ejection fraction and left ventricular dilation on the outcome.

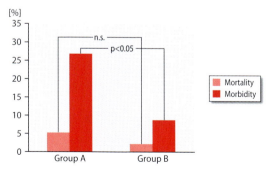

Fig. 1. Postoperative 30-day mortality and morbidity (major postoperative complications: reversible acute renal failure, stroke, and mechanical circulatory support) after AVR in octogenarians with symptomatic severe AS. (Modified from [3])

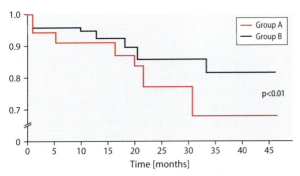

Fig. 2. Cumulative survival rates after AVR in octogenarians with chronically decompensated myocardial function (group A) are significantly poorer than in octogenarians with normal myocardial function (group B). (Modified from [3])

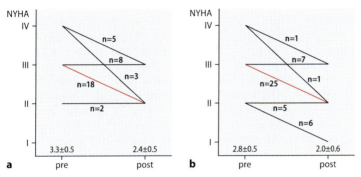

Fig. 3. Six months after AVR clinical outcome in octogenarians with severe AS: comparison of alterations in NYHA classes between patients with chronically myocardial decompensation (group A) and compensated myocardial function (group B) before AVR. (Modified from [3])

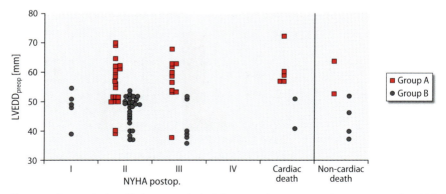

Fig. 4. Left ventricular dilation negatively influences the postoperative outcome after AVR in octogenarians. (Modified from [3])

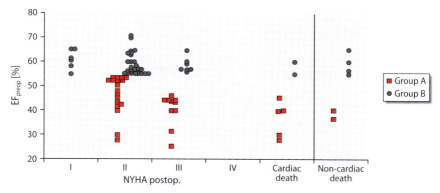

Fig. 5. The postoperative outcome after AVR in octogenarians is negatively influenced by preoperatively reduced left ventricular ejection fraction. (Modified from [3])

Discussion

Surgery in octogenarians should not be postponed until chronic myocardial decompensation finally convinces patients, relatives, and physicians that AVR is inevitable. In our survey, almost half of the consecutive patients (45.8%) with severe AS already suffered from chronic myocardial decompensation, which reflects that the benefits of AVR surgery in elderly patients are not really appreciated. With regard to patients' decision-making, Charlson et al. reported that 25% of their octogenarians with severe symptomatic AS had AVR surgery, 35% declined AVR surgery, while AVR surgery was not offered to 40% [9]. In the Euro Heart Survey on valvular heart disease, despite severe AS and significant symptoms, AVR surgery was refused in as many as 33% of elderly patients (≥75 years). Older age and left ventricular dysfunction (EF<50%) were the most striking characteristics of patients being refused, while comorbidities played a less important role [1].

There are also many reports documenting the safety of cardiac surgery in octogenarians [6–8, 10–14]. Presently, the largest series of 1100 octogenarians undergoing AVR reported a 30-day mortality of 6.6% with actuarial survival of 89% at 1 year, 79% at 3 years, 69% at 5 years, and 46% at 8 years [11]. Conservatively managed patients with severe AS and a mean age of 75±13 years had a grave prognosis. It was even worse in the presence of advanced age, left ventricular dysfunction, heart failure, and/or renal failure. The survival at 1, 5, and 10 years was 62%, 32%, and 18%, respectively [2]. In our survey, octogenarians with severe AS who were operated in due time had a low 30-day mortality rate (2.2%). The 30-day mortality rate, however, was more than twice as high (5.3%) in patients of the same age being operated in a stage of chronically myocardial maladaptation. Their long-term prognosis was significantly poorer. The cumulative survival rates at 46 months differed significantly between the two groups (68% vs. 81%). Similar results were obtained by Vaquette et al. who reported an operative mortality of 12% and a 5-year survival of 71% in elderly patients with severe AS and myocardial maladaptation [8]. In the survey of Langanay et al., the overall operative mortality rate of octogenarians with severe AS was 7.5%, though it increased dramatically from 5.6% to 42.9% if left ventricular EF was below 30%. This was partially due to the fact that mechanical circulatory support was refused in old age [7]. In our cohort, five patients required perioperative mechanical support, of whom only one died during the hospital stay. These data emphasize that AVR be performed in octogenarians with severe AS before the onset of myocardial maladaptation to chronic pressure overload.

AVR in this age group also results in significant clinical improvement [6, 7, 11–17]. Chiappini et al. reported that the mean NYHA functional class in their 84 long-term survivors improved from 2.9 ± 0.6 to 1.6 ± 0.6 after AVR [15]. In our cohort, the mean NYHA functional class improved during the first 6 months of AVR from 2.8 ± 0.5 to 2.0 ± 0.6, and from 3.3 ± 0.5 to 2.4 ± 0.5, if the patient already presented with chronic myocardial decompensation.

The incidence of stroke after AVR in octogenarians may be as low as 0.8% [15], while the average perioperative stroke rate was reported to be 6.5% [6, 16, 17]. The low incidence of nonfatal cerebral complications in our cohort is due to the meticulous removal of all debris and use of advanced perfusion techniques, including the use of arterial filters as well as short perfusion times [10].

Conclusion

In octogenarians, AVR can be performed with low mortality and morbidity, but it is important not to postpone the intervention until the onset of myocardial decompensation. Unfortunately, 46 of our consecutive series of patients with severe AS were referred only after manifestation of chronic myocardial decompensation. With respect to the poor natural history, the perioperative mortality even of these patients was acceptable but more than twice as high as in octogenarians being operated in due time. Patients not operated in due time also experienced a higher perioperative complication rate. Late survival was significantly lower in octogenarians, who suffered from myocardial decompensation before AVR. The indication for AVR may consider life-limiting comorbidities but should be made independent of patient's age.

As the average age of the western population continuous to increase, the frequency of degenerative AS requiring surgical or percutaneous interventions in the elderly will also increase. To further improve the prognosis of these patients, they should be referred early to a cardiologist for diagnostic and therapeutic decision making.

References

1. Iung B, Baron G, Butchart EG et al (2003) A prospective survey of patients with valvular heart disease in Europe: the Euro Heart Survey on valvular heart disease. Eur Heart J 24:1231–1243
2. Horstkotte D, Piper C (2008) Management of patients with heart valve disease 2008 – What has changed throughout the last three decades? Dtsch Med Wochenschr 133:S 280–284
3. Piper C, Hering D, Kleikamp G, Körfer R, Horstkotte D (2009) Valve replacement in octogenarians: argument for an earlier surgical intervention. J Heart Valve Dis 18:239–244
4. Iung B, Cachier A, Baron G et al (2005) Decision-making in elderly patients with severe aortic stenosis: why are so many denied surgery? Eur Heart J 26:2714–2720
5. Varadarajan P, Kapoor N, Bansal RC et al (2006) Clinical profile and natural history of 453 nonsurgically managed patients with severe aortic stenosis. Ann Thorac Surg 82:2111–2115
6. Horstkotte D, Hering D, Kleikamp G, Körfer R, Piper C (2005) Aortic valve stenosis in the senium: diagnostic and therapeutic strategies. Dtsch Med Wochenschr 130:741–746
7. Langanay Th, Verhoye J-PH, Ocampo G et al (2006) Current hospital mortality of aortic valve replacement in octogenarians. J Heart Valve Dis 15:630–637
8. Vaquette B, Corbineau H, Laurent M et al (2005) Valve replacement in patients with critical aortic stenosis and depressed left ventricular function: predicts of operative risk, left ventricular function recovery, and long term outcome. Heart 91:1324–1329
9. Charlson E, Legedza ATR, Hamel MB (2006) Decision-making and outcomes in severe symptomatic aortic stenosis. J Heart Valve Dis 15:312–321
10. Kleikamp G, Minami K, Breymann Th et al (1992) Aortic valve replacement in octogenarians. J Heart Valve Dis 1:196–200
11. Asimakopoulos G, Edwards MB, Taylor KM (1997) Aortic valve replacement in patients 80 years of age and older: survival and cause of death based on 1100 cases: collective results from the UK Heart Valve Registry. Circ 96:3403–3408
12. Vicchio M, Della Corte A, De Santo LS et al (2008) Tissue versus mechanical prostheses: quality of life in octogenarians. Ann Thorac Surg 85:1290–1295
13. De Vincentiis C, Kunkl AB, Trimarchi S et al (2008) Aortic valve replacement in octogenarians: is biologic valve the unique solution? Ann Thorac Surg 85:1296–1302
14. Urso St, Sabado R, Greco E et al (2007) One-hundred aortic valve replacements in octogenarians: outcome and risk factors for early mortality. J Heart Valve Dis 16:139–144
15. Chiappini B, Camurri N, Loforte A et al (2004) Outcome after aortic valve replacement in octogenarians. Ann Thorac Surg 78:85–89
16. Kolh P, Kerzmann A, Lahaye L et al (2001) Cardiac surgery in octogenarians. Eur Heart J 22:1235–1243
17. Sundt TM, Bailey MS, Moon MR et al (2000) Quality of life after aortic valve replacement at the age of >80 years. Circ 102(Suppl III):70–74

Predicted patient outcome after bioprosthetic AVR and the Ross operation

J. J. M. Takkenberg, M. W. A. van Geldorp

Determinants of survival after AVR

Multiple interrelated factors (patient-, physician-, and prosthesis-related) affect patient survival after aortic valve replacement. Every aortic valve replacement is associated with a risk of death due to the surgical procedure. This risk may vary with the type of prosthesis that is implanted, and obviously increases with patient age and with each reoperation. In addition, the etiology of the valve lesion, concomitant procedures, and other well-known risk factors may also affect operative mortality. Late survival of patients after aortic valve replacement differs considerably from survival of age-matched individuals in the general population. Fig. 1 shows that life expectancy of male patients after aortic valve replacement is significantly reduced compared to the age-matched population life expectancy. This difference in life expectancy is particularly evident in young adult patients. Operative mortality and the occurrence of valve-related events [1] *(valve-related mortality)* can only in part explain this difference, as is illustrated in Fig. 1 by the life expectancy of a patient who receives the – thus far hy-

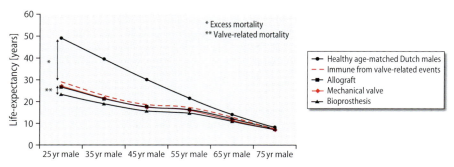

Fig. 1. Absolute life expectancy (years) after aortic valve replacement with stented bioprostheses, mechanical prostheses and allografts compared to the age-matched Dutch population. Hypothetical immunity from valve-related events is depicted by the uninterrupted solid line just above the life expectancy estimates of the different prosthetic valve types

pothetical – perfect valve substitute, i.e., a valve substitute that has no associated valve-related complications. The remaining loss in life expectancy compared to the general population is depicted by the term *excess mortality*.

For older patients after aortic valve replacement, survival is only slightly worse than observed survival in the general population. This is most likely due to the selection process that takes place prior to aortic valve replacement: recent studies have shown that a considerable proportion of older patients who require aortic valve replacement according to the current guidelines [4, 18] do not undergo surgery [3, 5, 7].

What are the causes of *excess mortality* after aortic valve replacement? Aortic valve disease is not limited to the aortic valve itself: it affects the entire heart. One can imagine that the strain posed on the myocardium by aortic valve disease will result in damage of the myocardium. Therefore, cardiac death is more common in patients with heart valve disease compared to the general population. Also, sudden unexplained unexpected death is probably more common in the former group. These may partly explain the observed differences in mortality. A landmark study by Kvidal et al. [12] investigated factors associated with *observed and relative survival* in a large patient cohort after aortic valve replacement. Risk factors associated with increased *observed* late mortality after aortic valve replacement included older patient age, pure aortic regurgitation, preoperative atrial fibrillation, advanced New York Heart Association class, and the presence of coronary artery disease. Interestingly, *relative* late survival (the ratio of observed late deaths in aortic valve replacement patients and expected deaths in the general age-matched population) was significantly greater in younger adult patients compared to older patients confirming the findings depicted in Fig. 1. In addition, pure aortic regurgitation, preoperative atrial fibrillation, and advanced New York Heart Association class were important factors associated with increased *relative* survival.

After AVR, life expectancy, total event-free life expectancy and reoperation-free life expectancy are highly dependent on the mortality in the general (reference/source) population. This 'background mortality' differs between countries and is different over time periods (life expectancy around the world has increased dramatically during in recent decades). Fig. 2 illustrates that even between developed countries, there are marked differences in population mortality that complicate the comparison of survival after aortic valve replacement between those countries. As can be seen in Fig. 2, the life expectancy of, for example, a 60-year-old individual in the Canadian population is approximately 21 years, about 4 years longer compared to a 60-year-old in the US population. This will result in a 2–3 year difference in life expectancy after aortic valve replacement between patients residing in Canada versus the US and may have implications for valve selection. The observed differences in general population mortality and their effect on survival after aortic valve replacement complicate the comparison of outcome after aortic valve replacement with different valve substitutes,

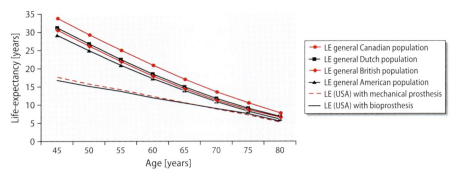

Fig. 2. Life expectancies for men in several general populations and life expectancy after implantation of a prosthetic aortic valve. Reprinted with permission from [20]; © American Association for Thoracic Surgery

and it therefore remains a challenge to study the possible survival advantage of certain biological valve substitutes (stentless bioprostheses and the Ross procedure). The following paragraphs provide an overview of reported patient outcome with different biological valve substitutes.

Predicted patient outcome after AVR

A microsimulation model was designed at Erasmus University Medical Center, Rotterdam, The Netherlands, to predict specific outcome of patients after AVR [17]. This computer model simulates a representative population at the individual patient level and offers a complementary tool to standard (e.g., Kaplan-Meier) methods of outcome analysis: it simulates the lives of virtual patients until death and takes into account all complications that may occur over time. The model can provide insight into age- and sex-specific life expectancy, event-free and reoperation-free life expectancy, and provides detailed information on the lifetime risk of valve-related events. Detailed descriptions on how to construct, test, and run this model have been published [14, 19]. The model including detailed instructions for use can be downloaded at *www.cardiothoracicresearch.nl*.

For conventional aortic valve surgery, one can choose between mechanical prostheses, biological stented or stentless prostheses, autografts and allo- (or homo-) grafts. The mechanical prosthesis has the major advantage of great durability and virtually zero technical valve failures. However, to prevent valve thrombosis and thromboembolism, lifelong coumadin anticoagulation is absolutely necessary. Unfortunately, this results in a higher bleeding risk, especially in the elderly. Limited availability of coumadin therapy and appropriate INR control in poorly developed countries result in a contraindication for the use of a mechanical prosthesis.

The main advantage of biological prostheses including allografts and autografts lies in the fact that there is no need for long-term anticoagulation, and the risk of bleeding approximates that of the normal population. The major downside of these biological valve types is structural deterioration of the valve apparatus which can lead to either regurgitation or stenosis of the valve leaflets, or root dilatation in case of autografts. This process of structural valve deterioration (SVD) increases with advancing time after implantation, decreases with age, and often – and in particular in younger adult patients and children – necessitates a reoperation.

In the following sections, microsimulation will be used to calculate patient outcome after aortic valve replacement with different biological valve substitutes.

Stented bioprostheses

Stented bioprostheses are the most commonly used biological valve substitutes. This prosthesis type is composed of a sewing ring and an artificial frame in which three porcine, bovine or equine pericardial leaflets are suspended. The prosthesis is relatively easy to implant and since it has been widely used large numbers of studies with long-term follow-up are available.

As mentioned before, the major downside of a (stented) bioprosthesis is the risk of SVD. This risk decreases as life-expectancy decreases (patients die before SVD develops). Therefore, current guidelines state that a bioprosthesis is generally preferable in patients over 65 years (without another indication for anticoagulation such as atrial fibrillation) [4]. However, from our microsimulation studies and the work of Jamieson and others [6], it seems this age-threshold could be lowered to around 60 years: compared with mechanical valves, around this age the risk reduction of bleeding that can be achieved with a bioprosthesis outweighs the increased risk associated with SVD. This results in a better event-free life expectancy, although total life expectancy after AVR remains comparable for mechanical and bioprosthesis patients. For a 60-year-old man, simulated life expectancy in years for biological versus mechanical prostheses was 11.9 versus 12.2, event-free life expectancy was 9.8 versus 9.3, and reoperation-free life expectancy was 10.5 versus 11.9. Lifetime risk of reoperation was 25% versus 3%. Lifetime risk of bleeding was 12% versus 41% [20].

Stentless bioprostheses

One of the downsides of the stented bioprosthesis is the relative obstruction that remains after the native valve has been replaced. This is caused by the valve opening, the sewing ring and its frame and could cause a 'patient-prosthesis mismatch' especially when the surgeon is forced to use a prosthesis of the smaller sizes (diameter 17–21 mm). Stentless bioprostheses have a larger effective orifice area (EOA) which provides lower transvalvular gradients, better hemodynamics and, therefore, more reduction of left ventricular hypertrophy. Furthermore, some consider stentless bioprostheses to be more durable than conventional stented bioprostheses, all contributing to a possible survival advantage. A disadvantage is they are more difficult and time-consuming to implant. A recent randomized trial comparing 96 patients who received a stented bioprosthesis versus 127 patients who received a stentless bioprosthesis showed that there was a late survival advantage for stentless valve recipients [13]. However, no cause-effect relationship between lower transvalvular pressure gradients and improved survival was found, and the need for additional trials studying this subject remains.

Microsimulation studies of the Medtronic stentless Freestyle valve predicted for a 65-year-old male a life expectancy of 13.1 years, which is close to that of the general population. The reoperation-free life expectancy was 11.2 years and the event-free life expectancy was 8.4 years [8].

Allografts

The human donor valve (allograft) has excellent hemodynamics, low occurrence of thromboembolic events and endocarditis, and does not require anticoagulation. It is most often used in aortic root disease or destructive endocarditis, because it has redundant tissue attached and provides more possibilities for reconstructive surgery than bio- or mechanical prostheses. On the other hand, the allograft is not an 'off the shelf' item and requires special preparation, storage, and considerable surgical skills. The number of studies on long-term allograft outcome is limited and affected by a considerable amount of bias/selection, since it is mostly used in a highly selected patient group. Microsimulation enabled multiple studies to be combined and predicted for a 65-year-old male a life expectancy of 12 years, a reoperation-free life expectancy of 10 years, and an event-free life expectancy of 9.7 years [15].

Finally, a microsimulation study that compared outcome after aortic valve replacement with either stented bioprostheses (Carpentier-Edwards supraannular and pericardial), stentless bioprostheses, or cryopreserved allografts showed that when assuming uniform patient characteristics and excess mortality, the difference in performance between the four biological valve types is small [9]. Patient selection and the timing of operation may explain most of the observed differences in prognosis after aortic valve replacement with biological prostheses.

Predicted patient outcome after the Ross operation in young adults

The Ross operation or autograft procedure is mainly performed in children and young adult patients. In this operation, the patient's pulmonary valve is used to replace the aortic valve either as a subcoronary implantation or as a full aortic root replacement, while the pulmonary valve is replaced with an alternative prosthesis, usually a pulmonary homograft. The potential advantages of the autograft or Ross procedure are the use of the patient's own living valve with favorable hemodynamic characteristics, low endocarditis risk, low thrombogenicity, avoidance of anticoagulant therapy, and autograft size increase in children. However, the Ross procedure is a technically demanding operation and both the autograft in aortic position and the valve substitute in the right ventricular outflow tract may develop structural failure over time. The Ross operation has been performed in small numbers, and long-term follow-up studies have been inconsistent, which makes analysis of long-term advantages and disadvantages difficult.

Although survival of young adult patients after this procedure is almost uniformly excellent and comparable with the general population, autograft durability is in some centers clearly superior to other biological valve conduits, while other centers report worrisome autograft reoperation rates. It remains unclear why these results diverge so much. A very recent systematic review and meta-analysis of reported outcome after the Ross procedure [16] shows that in young adult patients (mean age 39 years; range 11–71 years) the late survival pattern runs parallel to the general age-matched population (Fig. 3). Early pooled mortality was 3.24% (95% CI 1.47–6.58%), while the late mortality rate was 0.64%/patient year (95% CI 0.32–1.26%/patient year). Fig. 3 illustrates pooled estimated survival after the Ross operation in adults including 95% confidence intervals (best and worst case scenario). The review also illustrates that although the occur-

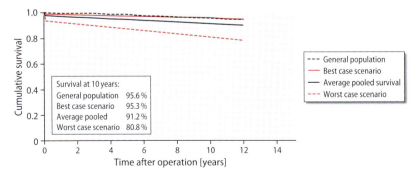

Fig. 3. Cumulative survival after the Ross procedure in young adult patients

rence rates of most valve-related complications are very low, the durability results of in particular the pulmonary autograft diverge considerably, especially 10 years postoperatively (95% CI for freedom from autograft failure at 10 years 86–96%). The question remains whether it is possible to optimize autograft durability through better patient selection, more optimal application of the root replacement technique, and perhaps postoperative antihypertensive treatment.

Remarkable is the excellent reported survival after the Ross operation in young adult patients, which appears to run parallel to the general population. This is in contradiction to the observed impaired *relative* survival in young adult patients after aortic valve replacement that was discussed in the first section of this chapter. It seems that *excess mortality* is virtually absent in patients after the Ross operation, and some authors suggest that this excellent survival advantage may be caused by the fact that the autograft provides a living and hemodynamically superior valve substitute [insert ref]. An update of the ongoing randomized trial in the United Kingdom (Harefield) between allograft and autograft aortic root replacement (personal communication) suggests indeed that autograft patients have superior survival compared to patients who receive an allograft [2]. On the other hand, the Ross operation is performed in a select group of patients, and their characteristics may also explain the observed survival pattern. For example, a single center observational study by Klieverik et al. [11] in young adult patients who underwent aortic valve replacement found that in a univariable Cox regression model for late survival the Ross procedure appeared to carry a survival advantage over allografts and mechanical prostheses. However, in a multivariable Cox regression model that also included preoperative renal impairment, preoperative impaired left ventricular function, concomitant mitral valve surgery, prior aortic valve surgery and patient age, the factor implanted valve substitute was no longer of influence on late survival. Another study by Klieverik et al. [10] that compared outcome after allograft or autograft aortic root replacement in young adult patients with congenital aortic valve disease showed no difference in survival between the two groups. These observations suggest that patient characteristics are important determinants of late survival and that the implanted valve type is of minor importance.

Summary and conclusions

Late patient survival after aortic valve replacement is impaired compared to the general population. This difference can only in part be explained by the occurrence of valve-related complications. In particular in younger adult patients there is a considerable amount of excess mortality that is due to patient-related factors. Regional differences in population mortality hamper studies on survival after aortic valve replacement and should be taken into account when assessing evidence on outcome after aortic valve replacement.

Microsimulation studies show that patient outcome after implantation of stented and stentless bioprostheses or cryopreserved allografts is acceptable and that differences in patient outcomes are most likely explained by patient selection and the timing of operation, rather than differences in the performance of these valve substitutes.

The pulmonary autograft appears to be the only biological valve substitute that carries a survival advantage. However, this survival advantage may very well be caused by patient selection. A randomized trial or a propensity score matching study of young adult patients who received either an autograft, allograft or mechanical prosthesis will elucidate whether there truly is a survival advantage. Durability of the autograft varies widely between reported series and may be optimized through through better patient selection, more optimal application of the root replacement technique, and perhaps postoperative antihypertensive treatment.

References

1. Akins CW, Miller DC, Turina MI, Kouchoukos NT, Blackstone EH, Grunkemeier GL, Takkenberg JJ, David TE, Butchart EG, Adams DH, Shahian DM, Hagl S, Mayer JE, Lytle BW (2008) Guidelines for reporting mortality and morbidity after cardiac valve interventions. Eur J Cardiothorac Surg 33:523–528
2. Aklog L, Carr-White GS, Birks EJ, Yacoub MH (2000) Pulmonary autograft versus aortic homograft for aortic valve replacement: interim results from a prospective randomized trial J Heart Valve Dis 9(2):176–188, discussion 188–189
3. Bach DS, Cimino N and Deeb GM (2007) Unoperated patients with severe aortic stenosis. J Am Coll Cardiol 50(20):2018–2019
4. Bonow RO, Carabello BA, Kanu C, de Leon AC, Jr., Faxon DP, Freed MD, Gaasch WH, Lytle BW, Nishimura RA, O'Gara PT, O'Rourke RA, Otto CM, Shah PM, Shanewise JS, Smith SC, Jr., Jacobs AK, Adams CD, Anderson JL, Antman EM, Faxon DP, Fuster V, Halperin JL, Hiratzka LF, Hunt SA, Lytle BW, Nishimura R, Page RL, Riegel B (2006) ACC/AHA 2006 guidelines for the management of patients with valvular heart disease: a report of the American College of Cardiology/American Heart Association Task Force on Practice Guidelines (writing committee to revise the 1998 Guidelines for the Management of Patients With Valvular Heart Disease): developed in collaboration with the Society of Cardiovascular Anesthesiologists: endorsed by the Society for Cardiovascular Angiography and Interventions and the Society of Thoracic Surgeons Circulation 114(5):e84–e231
5. Bouma BJ, van Den Brink RB, van Der Meulen JH, Verheul HA, Cheriex EC, Hamer HP, Dekker E, Lie KI, Tijssen JG (1999) To operate or not on elderly patients with aortic stenosis: the decision and its consequences. Heart 82(2):143–148
6. Chan V, Jamieson WR, Germann E, Chan F, Miyagishima RT, Burr LH, Janusz MT, Ling H, Fradet GJ (2006) Performance of bioprostheses and mechanical prostheses assessed by composites of valve-related complications to 15 years after aortic valve replacement. J Thorac Cardiovasc Surg 131(6):1267–1273

7. Iung B, Cachier A, Baron G, Messika-Zeitoun D, Delahaye F, Tornos P, Gohlke-Barwolf C, Boersma E, Ravaud P, Vahanian A (2005) Decision-making in elderly patients with severe aortic stenosis: why are so many denied surgery? Eur Heart J 26(24)2714–2720
8. Kappetein AP, Puvimanasinghe JP, Takkenberg JJ, Steyerberg EW, Bogers AJ (2007) Predicted patient outcome after aortic valve replacement with Medtronic Stentless Freestyle bioprostheses. J Heart Valve Dis 16(4)423–428, discussion 429
9. Kappetein AP, Takkenberg JJ, Puvimanasinghe JP, Jamieson WR, Eijkemans M, Bogers AJ (2006) Does the type of biological valve affect patient outcome? Interact Cardiovasc Thorac Surg 5(4)398–402
10. Klieverik LM, Bekkers JA, Roos JW, Eijkemans MJ, Raap GB, Bogers AJ, Takkenberg JJ (2008) Autograft or allograft aortic valve replacement in young adult patients with congenital aortic valve disease. Eur Heart J 29(11)1446–1453
11. Klieverik LM, Noorlander M, Takkenberg JJ, Kappetein AP, Bekkers JA, van Herwerden LA, Bogers AJ (2006) Outcome after aortic valve replacement in young adults: is patient profile more important than prosthesis type? J Heart Valve Dis 15(4)479–487, discussion 487
12. Kvidal P, Bergstrom R, Horte LG, Stahle E (2000) Observed and relative survival after aortic valve replacement. J Am Coll Cardiol 35(3)747–756
13. Lehmann S, Walther T, Kempfert J, Leontjev S, Rastan A, Falk V, Mohr FW (2007) Stentless versus conventional xenograft aortic valve replacement: midterm results of a prospectively randomized trial. Ann Thorac Surg 84(2)467–472
14. Puvimanasinghe JP, Steyerberg EW, Takkenberg JJ, Eijkemans MJ, van Herwerden LA, Bogers AJ, Habbema JD (2001) Prognosis after aortic valve replacement with a bioprosthesis: predictions based on meta-analysis and microsimulation. Circulation 103(11)1535–1541
15. Takkenberg JJ, Eijkemans MJ, van Herwerden LA, Steyerberg EW, Lane MM, Elkins RC, Habbema JD, Bogers AJ (2003) Prognosis after aortic root replacement with cryopreserved allografts in adults. Ann Thorac Surg 75(5)1482–1489
16. Takkenberg JJ, Klieverik LM, Schoof PH, van Suylen RJ, van Herwerden LA, Zondervan PE, Roos-Hesselink JW, Eijkemans MJC, Yacoub MH, Bogers AJ (2009) The Ross procedure: A systematic review and meta-analysis. Circulation 119:222–228
17. Takkenberg JJ, Puvimanasinghe JP, Grunkemeier GL (2003) Simulation models to predict outcome after aortic valve replacement. Ann Thorac Surg 75(5)1372–1376
18. Vahanian A, Baumgartner H, Bax J, Butchart E, Dion R, Filippatos G, Flachskampf F, Hall R, Iung B, Kasprzak J, Nataf P, Tornos P, Torracca L, Wenink A (2007) Guidelines on the management of valvular heart disease: The Task Force on the Management of Valvular Heart Disease of the European Society of Cardiology. Eur Heart J 28(2)230–268
19. van Geldorp MW, Jamieson WR, Kappetein AP, Puvimanasinghe JP, Eijkemans MJ, Grunkemeier GL, Takkenberg JJ, Bogers AJ (2007) Usefulness of microsimulation to translate valve performance into patient outcome: patient prognosis after aortic valve replacement with the Carpentier-Edwards supra-annular valve. J Thorac Cardiovasc Surg 134(3)702–709
20. van Geldorp MW, Jamieson WR, Kappetein AP, Ye J, Fradet GJ, Eijkemans MJ, Grunkemeier GL, Bogers AJ, Takkenberg JJ (2009) Patient outcome after aortic valve replacement with a mechanical or biological prosthesis: Weighing lifetime anticoagulant-related event risk against reoperation risk. J Thorac Cardiovasc Surg 137(4):881–886

Anticoagulation

Anticoagulation and self-management of INR: mid-term results

H. Körtke, J. Gummert

Following the implantation of a mechanical heart valve, permanent oral anticoagulation is a must. Despite progress in the development of artificial heart valves, thromboembolisms, and Marcumar-induced hemorrhages remain frequent complications after mechanical heart valve replacement. In the studies ESCAT I and II, we were able to show that INR self-management in conjunction with low-dose anticoagulation is able to reduce the rate of thromboembolism to 0.2% per patient/year and of hemorrhaging to 0.56% per patient/year [1]. The INR values measured by patients can now be monitored using telemedicine.

Of all the various cardiac diseases, chronic heart valve defects are particularly significant due to the severe hemodynamic changes they involve, leading in turn to reduced physical performance.

Since 1960, it has been possible to replace hemodynamically significant vitia using artificial heart valves, positively influencing prognoses in the process. Today, replacement of a diseased heart valve is the second most frequent cardiosurgical intervention, with approx. 18 000 patients per year receiving surgery for heart valve diseases in Germany alone. The perioperative mortality in experienced cardiosurgical centers for elective surgery on individual heart valves is currently 1–2% [2]. This means an expected 2–3 cases of valve-related complications per year [3].

Great efforts have been made in the field of heart valve development. After more than 30 years of continual improvements in hemodynamic function, numerous mechanical and biological valves are now available, and yet the question of biocompatibility regarding the materials used and the complications which can ensue still lacks an ultimate answer. Not all the demands made of an ideal replacement for defective human heart valves are currently being fulfilled.

Anticoagulation and general complications

Current biological heart valves display satisfactory hemodynamics; they are less thrombogenic and do not require permanent anticoagulation. They do have the disadvantage of degeneration, however, meaning that more than

50% of biological heart valve recipients are required to undergo reoperation after 12 years, in turn harboring a renewed perioperative risk. The vast majority of implanted heart valves are still so-called mechanical replacements and, despite progress in the development of these artificial valves, thromboembolism and hemorrhaging are still frequent complications following their implantation. Although this risk can be reduced through treatment with oral anticoagulants, the thromboembolism risk in conjunction with the new generation of valves is still approx. 1.5% per patient/year in the aortic position and 3% per patient/year in the mitral position. A hemorrhaging rate of varying severity has been recorded at 4.2 to 15.4% per patient/year, depending on the quality of the anticoagulation. The incidence of fatal hemorrhaging complications is recorded at approx. 0.2 per patient/year [4].

In 1991, Butchart et al. [5] were the first to introduce the concept of risk-adjusted anticoagulation intensity. They accepted that the thromboembolism risk is dependent on many factors. There are patient-related risk factors (the quality of postoperative anticoagulation required), cardiac-related and valve-specific risk factors. Butchart could show that postoperative oral anticoagulation following mechanical heart valve replacement was not usually adjusted to the levels required. He observed his patients for 88 months. The INR range, a measurement for anticoagulation control, was defined as between 3.0 and 4.5. Over the period in question, more than 60% of values were not within the predefined therapeutic range.

In addition, a high INR variation represents an increased risk factor for hemorrhaging or thromboembolic events. The number of hemorrhaging and thromboembolic complications in patients with anticoagulation – a permanent requirement in patients with mechanical heart valve replacement – is crucially bound to the stability of levels within the individually predefined therapeutic range. Following mechanical heart valve transplantation, permanent and stable anticoagulation is imperative and remains one of the chief causes of (thromboembolic or hemorrhagic) complications. Within the framework of secondary prophylaxis, anticoagulation with coumarin derivates has become established medical therapy.

Patient autonomy

Self-control and self-therapy in conjunction with chronic disease are not fundamentally new. Regular metabolism controls and autonomous adjustment of insulin dosage and diet are globally accepted measures for well-instructed diabetics and a crucial part of their diabetes therapy. Analogous to diabetics patients, anticoagulation patients are also capable of self-control or self-management for their long-term INR therapy. Thromboplastin time can currently be determined by more than 20 different thromboplastins. Due to the different thromboplastins various Quick values often describe the same coagulation state, making the many recordings still made using Quick values susceptible to a certain degree of error. For this reason, anticoagulation self-controls or self-management results should be given as INR (International Normalized Ratio) values. In Germany, approx. 120000 people with permanent oral anticoagulation currently perform INR self-management.

Self-management

In 1994, we began a new program at the Heart and Diabetes Center NRW (HDZ NRW) in Bad Oeynhausen for patients who have undergone mechanical heart valve replacement. For these patients the postoperative phase now begins with instruction about anticoagulation. About 7–10 days after surgery, INR management is taught to the patients. Instruction takes place in small groups of 3–5 patients and lasts for two 2-hour lessons, including an appropriate break. The patients are shown how to use the device, how to handle the test strips and how to transmit telemedical data. They are also told in simple terms how anticoagulation therapy (in this case phenprocoumon/Marcumar) works. Patients have to know that overdosing can lead to hemorrhaging, whereas underdosing can result in thromboembolic complications. They are encouraged to record their actions carefully and, should their lifestyle change or should they start to take any additional medication, to perform the tests not just once, but two or even three times per week. This will provide clear information about how the new medication is influencing anticoagulation. Patients are also

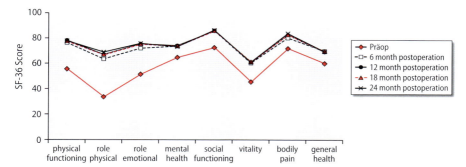

Fig. 1. The expected quality of life after mechanical valve replacement in the subject of INR self-management according to the questionnaire SF-36. Reprinted with permission from Koertke K, Koerfer R (2009) Postoperative Antikoagulation nach mechanischem Herzklappenersatz in Verbindung mit Telemedizin. In: Goss/Middeke/Mengden/Smetak (ed) Praktischen Telemedizin in Kardiologie und Hypertensiologie. Georg Thieme Verlag, Stuttgart, pp 113–117

told that they do not have to make any significant changes to their routines. On the contrary, anticoagulation treatment should be adjusted to suit their lifestyle. Finally, provided that their cardiac condition permits it, patients are encouraged to include exercise and sport (except competitive sport) in their leisure-time activities. We know that this strongly influences quality of life (Fig. 1), also in conjunction with anticoagulation therapy.

Handing over some of the necessary medical competence to patients is our attempt to answer the following question: "Does patient autonomy improve the quality of permanent oral anticoagulation and thus considerably reduce complications?" INR self-management is the first step towards improving postoperative anticoagulation. Nevertheless, there will always be at least some patients who require long-term medical help with their INR self-control. For this reason we began to experiment with telemedicine to assist this type of chronic disease therapy.

Telemedical monitoring

The term "telemedicine" covers all forms of medical information which can be exchanged long-distance using modern data transfer methods. In December 2003, we founded the Institute for Applied Telemedicine (IFAT) (Fig. 2).

Since then, IFAT has registered and medically monitors more than 900 Marcumar patients. They are instructed in INR self-control or self-management 7–10 d after surgery. They then receive a home monitor, in this case, a CoaguChek XS. Our own development team created a module which can read the INR self-control data as soon as the test has been performed and transmit it automatically to IFAT using SMS technology. There the data is matched to the corresponding electronic patient file. Physicians and trained staff monitor the incoming results and inform patients about further anticoagulation measures. The Institute works around the clock, 24 h/d and 7 d/week. The following safety requirements are fulfilled:

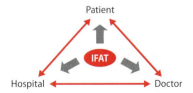

Fig. 2. The relationships of patients with medical institutions. Reprinted with permission from Koertke K, Koerfer R (2009) Postoperative Antikoagulation nach mechanischem Herzklappenersatz in Verbindung mit Telemedizin. In: Goss/Middeke/Mengden/Smetak (ed) Praktischen Telemedizin in Kardiologie und Hypertensiologie. Georg Thieme Verlag, Stuttgart, pp 113–117

- Availability: smooth functioning of technical equipment (regular maintenance and check-ups), as well as back-up systems for emergencies must be guaranteed.
- Addressed confidentiality: only addressed recipients can access and use information.
- Non-deniability: transmitter and recipient must be unequivocally identifiable.
- Pseudonyms: reestablishing the identity of a patient via a pseudonym must be possible (re-identification).
- Anonymity: patient master data must not be passed on.
- Originality: the source and time of creation must be discernible.
- Authenticity and authentication: medical staff must be able to be authenticated for (recognized by) the systems. Access rights must be allocated for particular roles.
- Data integrity: data must be transmitted without error or manipulation, or any error or manipulation must be detectable (routine check-ups and calibration).
- Auditability: establishing who has done what to which data and when must be possible.

Low-dose anticoagulation

Maintenance of the anticoagulation therapy required after mechanical heart valve replacement used to be very unsatisfactory, also in Germany. A study called ESCAT (Early Self-Controlled Anticoagulation Trial) was able to show that patients are capable of learning INR self-management and that

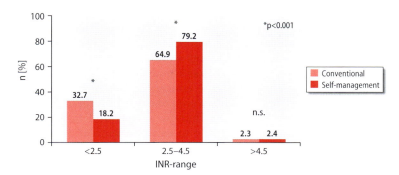

Fig. 3. INR self-management vs. conventional measurement with respect to reaching the target range (p < 0.001). Reprinted with permission from Koertke K, Koerfer R (2009) Postoperative Antikoagulation nach mechanischem Herzklappenersatz in Verbindung mit Telemedizin. In: Goss/Middeke/Mengden/Smetak (ed) Praktischen Telemedizin in Kardiologie und Hypertensiologie. Georg Thieme Verlag, Stuttgart, pp 113–117

Table 1. Proportion of thromboembolisms and hemorrhages (% per patient/year): ESCAT-I, n = 1155; ESCAT-II interim analysis, n = 1816

Adverse events (Level III)	ESCAT-I Conventional (1135.5 pat.-yr)	ESCAT-I Self-management (1116 pat.-yr)	ESCAT-II low-dose (1616 pat.-yr)
Overall	66 (5.8%)	58 (5.2%)	16 (0.76%)
Hemorrhages	34 (3.0%)	42 (3.7%)	13 (0.56%)
Thromboembolisms	32 (2.8%)	16 (1.5%)	3 (0.2%)

Table 2. INR target values according to valve position

Valve position	Risk factors and/or additional underlying cardiac diseases	INR range	Target value
Aortic	–	1.8–2.8	2.3
Mitral	–	2.5–3.5	2.8
Tricuspid/pulmonary	–	2.5–3.5	3.0
Aortic	±	2.0–3.0	2.5
Mitral	±	2.5–3.5	3.0
Tricuspid/pulmonary	±	2.5–3.5	3.0

they treat their autonomous handling of anticoagulation therapy carefully. Fig. 3 shows that the qualitative improvements achieved by INR self-management are highly significant.

It was important not only to achieve high-quality adjustments, but also to reduce the variability of INR values. In a follow-up study called ESCAT II, patients agreed to very low-dose anticoagulation. This enabled the stability of the anticoagulation therapy to be maintained, while at the same time reducing variability. Further reductions in thromboembolic and especially hemorrhaging complications were convincing (Table 1). These figures illustrate the superiority of INR self-management over conventionally managed patients, which is also true concerning low-dose anticoagulation with self-management. The patients were controlled by their family doctors.

Self-management led to the therapy ranges and target values shown in Table 2 – differentiated according to valve position and risk factors – which have become established as standards.

Patients with permanent anticoagulation sometimes encounter situations, even in their everyday routines, in which they feel unable to cope with this form of therapy. In such cases, it is of course imperative to renew medical supervision. Performing INR self-controls, possibly with the aid of family members or nurses, with added medical advice given telemedically could be a viable alternative. It makes INR self-control an option even to

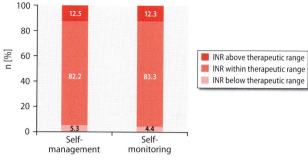

Fig. 4. INR self-management and INR self-monitoring patients having reached the therapeutic target range. Reprinted with permission from Koertke K, Koerfer R (2009) Postoperative Antikoagulation nach mechanischem Herzklappenersatz in Verbindung mit Telemedizin. In: Goss/Middeke/Mengden/Smetak (ed) Praktischen Telemedizin in Kardiologie und Hypertensiologie. Georg Thieme Verlag, Stuttgart, pp 113–117

patients who have become immobile or who cannot or will not practice autonomous anticoagulation management. Using the above plan, patients or their families can now record coagulation values using a home monitor. The values are then sent via an automatic connection to IFAT. Special staff, in particular trained physicians, can view the results by accessing the relevant electronic patient file. The results cannot be tampered with because automatic and immediate transmission prevents any intervention by patients or third parties. Regular weekly recommendations regarding adjustments to dosage are then sent to patients and their families, upholding the high quality described above.

Our evaluation of more than 900 patients (Fig. 4) shows that there are no significant differences between patients who are telemedically monitored and those practicing self-management.

INR self-control with telemedical transmission achieves comparable results to INR self-management, thus, making this an option for all patients. Even those patients who have become immobile can take advantage of this system, which is both high quality and readily available. Within the framework of a telemedical thrombosis service, INR self-control is already being practiced as an integrated care module in the German states of Saxony and Saxony-Anhalt.

Conclusion

The combination of medical autonomy coupled with telemedical service can achieve the highest qualitative improvements in oral anticoagulation following mechanical heart valve replacement. Therapy is now possible in close cooperation with local practitioners. Quality stabilization is guaranteed by data protection, as well as a transparency of data for treating physicians. Patients can discuss any problems they may have with this form of therapy with their local physicians. Documentation also gives physicians the opportunity to show patients their ongoing involvement in the treatment. The result is a minimum-risk anticoagulation therapy which can be practiced by and offered to nearly any patient with the relevant indication.

References

1. Koertke et al (2003) INR self-management permits lower anticoagulation levels after mechanical heart valve replacement. Circulation 108(Suppl 1)S:II75–II78
2. Turina J, Hess O, Selpulcri F et al (1987) Spontaneous course of aortic valve disease. Eur Heart J 8:S471–S483
3. Roiux C, Logeais Y, Leguerrier A et al (1988) Valvular replacement for aortic stenosis in patients over 70 years: immediate risk and long-term results (from a consecutive series of 355 patients). Eur Heart J 9(Suppl E):S121–S127
4. Forfar JC (1979) A 7-year analysis of hemorrhage in patients on long-term anticoagulant therapy. Brit Heart J 42:S128–S132
5. Butchart EG, Lewis PA, Bethel JA et al (1991) Adjusting anticoagulation to prosthesis thrombogenicity and patient risk factors – recommendations for the Medtronic Hall valve. Circulation 84(Suppl III):III61–III69

Tissue engineering

Biomatrix-polymer hybrid material for heart valve tissue engineering

C. Stamm, N. Grabow, G. Steinhoff

Heart valve tissue engineering

Fabrication of a viable heart valve with lifelong durability and growth potential during childhood is the common goal of all heart valve tissue engineering strategies. Despite significant improvements in valve design, patients carrying conventional prostheses remain burdened by the lifelong need for anticoagulation or the inevitable degeneration of nonvital biologic valve tissue. Research on tissue engineering of heart valves commenced in the 1990s, and several strategies have evolved ever since [29, 30]. Initially, biodegradable polymers were used as scaffolds to be seeded with the recipient's autologous cells. This approach is feasible with a wide variety of adult, neonatal, and prenatal cell types, but requires extensive in vitro conditioning to facilitate the adhesion of cells on the polymer surface and to induce the deposition of biologic extracellular matrix components prior to implantation [21, 22, 32, 33]. A similar strategy is the production of viable heart valves based on cells embedded in biological hydrogels, which also require elaborate technology for in vitro tissue growth [18]. Alternatively, the allogenic or xenogenic extracellularized heart valve matrix has been suggested as a conveniently preformed scaffold [24, 26, 36]. Here, the idea is to remove all cellular components by enzymatic digestion, physical destruction, or chemical detergents, and without using glutaraldehyde tanning and tissue fixation [2, 13–15]. The antigencity of cellular epitopes is thereby eliminated, while the biological integrity of extracellular matrix components is preserved. Originally, such decellularized matrix valves were designed to be reseeded with the recipient's cells in vitro. More recently, however, decellularized valves are nearly always being implanted as-is, without prior cell seeding, since it has become clear that spontaneous repopulation with circulating endothelial progenitor cells occurs rapidly and effectively in situ after implantation. However, there are at least two major problems: first, the mechanical tissue properties deteriorate when cells are removed and the tertiary structure of fibrous valve tissue constituents is altered during the decellularization process. Such valves do not withstand hemodynamic forces in the systemic circulation and have so far only been used for pulmonary valve replacement. Second, exposed collagen surfaces are highly thrombogenic, since collagen directly induces platelet activation as well as coagulation factor XII. To solve these problems, we developed biomaterial/polymer composite materials based on decellularized vascular matrix scaffolds that are coated with biodegradable polymers, and tested the hypothesis that such hybrid tissues exhibit improved the biocompatibility in vitro and in vivo [20, 34].

Hybrid tissue fabrication

Decellularization process

Enzymatic removal of cells without altering the biochemical characteristics of the extracellular matrix by exposure to chemical fixatives was performed as previously described by Steinhoff et al. [36]. Hearts were harvested from porcine cadavers; the aortic root was prepared, washed in phosphate buffered saline (PBS) and incubated in 0.05% trypsin solution for 48 h at 37 °C, followed by 3 washing steps for 1 h each. For longer storage, the specimens were lyophilized (at –40 °C and 0.05 mbar) and rehydrated prior to further use, but for implantation in sheep the valves were processed immediately. Biocompatibility tests in vitro and in rabbits were performed using human aortic wall tissue, which was obtained during routine CABG operations and was processed in identical fashion. The decellularization process removed all cellular components of the porcine aortic valve leaflets

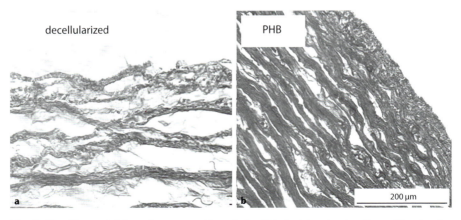

Fig. 1. Van Gieson staining of a cross-section of decellularized heart valve tissue. The decellularization process removes all cellular components of the valve tissue, while preserving its biologic integrity (**a**). By polymer coating or penetration of the matrix, the structure of the extracellular matrix is maintained, but the fiber architecture appears condensed (**b**)

and the aortic wall (Fig. 1). After enzymatic removal of the endothelial cell layer and cellular components of the media, the fibrous network of collagen, elastin and proteoglycans forms the luminal surface of the valve scaffold.

▌ Polymer coating

Polymers from the family of polyhydroxyalkanoates (PHA) were selected to investigate their structural performance in hybrid valve tissue: poly(3-hydroxybutyrate) (P3HB), poly(4-hydroxybutyrate) (P(4HB), also known as PHA4400), and the co-polymer poly(3-hydroxybutyrate-co-4-hydroxybutyrate) (P(3HB-co-4HB), also known as PHA3444) with a composition of 82% 3HB and 18% 4HB. Polymers in powder form were dissolved in chloroform at 50 °C according to the chosen concentration. Initially, a dip-coating process was used for fabrication of biomatrix/polymer hybrid tis-

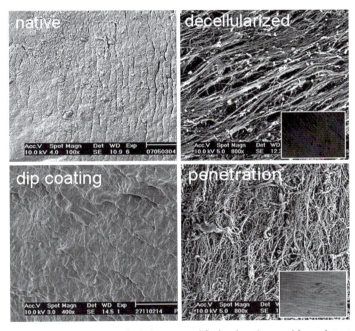

Fig. 2. Scanning electron microscopy images depicting unmodified valve tissue with an intact endothelial cell layer ("native"). The decellularization process exposes the subendothelial fiber network ("decellularized"). The insert shows a Nile red staining of PHB polymer, which is negative. The dip coating process ("dip coating") produces a smooth polymer surface but was shown to have negative effects on mechanic valve function. In contrast, the polymer penetration process ("penetration") preserves the porous structure of the subendothelial extracellular matrix. The insert shows a positive Nile Red stain, indicating that PHB is indeed present

sue: decellularized and lyophilized tissue was repeatedly immersed in 2–6% (w/v) polymer solution followed by solvent evaporation for two weeks until the chloroform content was <0.2%. Prior to further use, the tissue was rehydrated in cell culture medium (in vitro experiments) or in phosphate buffered saline (in vivo experiments). When it became evident that this coating may not withstand systemic hemodynamic forces (see section Valve testing), we developed a polymer impregnation process: freshly decellularized valve tissue was subjected to a wet dehydration process, replacing water with ethanol. Then, the specimens were immersed in 1% (w/v) polymer solution for 30 min, followed by rehydration and wet solvent elimination in PBS. As opposed to the initially used dip-coating procedure, the modified polymer penetration protocol did not alter the surface morphology of the decellularized matrix, preserving the tissue native texture and microporosity, hypothetically facilitating adhesion and migration of recipient cells (Fig. 2).

In vitro testing of hybrid valve tissue

Toxicity and cell proliferation

Whether biomatrix/polymer hybrid valve tissue can be repopulated with viable cells, without exhibiting cytotoxicity, was tested in series of in vitro experiments. Tissue samples were prepared as described above, seeded with L929 mouse fibroblasts and incubated under standard cell culture conditions for at least 72 h. Cell viability was then assessed using the CellTiter96® fluorescent cell proliferation assay (MTS test). Since cellular adhesion, proliferation, metabolic activity, and resistance to toxin are highly dependent on species and cell type, similar tests were performed using a mixed population of human vascular myofibroblasts and endothelial cells, which were prepared from saphenous vein samples of CABG patients. The MTS tests were performed in decellularized matrix treated with various polymer preparations, but also with pure polymer samples as well as with hydrid tissues following several sterilization and storage protocols such as lyophilization, plasma sterilization, FAD sterilization, ethylene oxide sterilization, and gamma sterilization. Initially, it appeared that P3HB almost completely inhibited murine cell growth on the matrix. These experiments were then repeated using human endothelial cells and myofibroblasts, and we now found that they proliferate very well on all matrix/polymer combinations. Hence, decellularized biomatrix/polymer hybrid tissue has the potential for repopulation even in the xenogenic setting.

Hemocompatibility

In addition to standard biocompatibility testing, hemocompatibility tests that specifically assess interference with the coagulation system need to be performed when implants are to be placed in the blood stream. Complement and coagulation system activation in response to different hybrid tissue preparations were studied in several in vitro assays. Activation of complement factor C3 was assessed by ELISA for C3a-des-Arg, the stable metabolite of activated C3, following incubation of human plasma with hybrid tissue samples. Representative for activation of the plasmatic clotting system, the concentration of the prothrombin fragments F1 and F2 was also measured by ELISA, again after incubation of human plasma with hybrid tissue. Finally, the response of the cellular clotting system to biomatrix/polymer hybrid tissue was studied by measuring the activation of platelet factor 4. Matrix impregnation with P3HB attenuated the activation of platelet factor 4 in human plasma, indicating less activation of the cellular clotting system. With P3/4HB co-polymer there was still some attenuation of PF4 release, while P4HB alone appeared not to change the matrix-induced PF4 activation. Activation of the plasmatic clotting cascade as assessed by the concentration of prothrombin fragments F1 and F2 was partially suppressed when the matrix was coated with biodegradable polymer, irrespective of the PHB-type used. Finally, activation of the complement system in response to hybrid tissue was estimated. Again, attenuation of C3a-des-Arg production in the presence of polymer-coated matrix compared to untreated decellularized matrix was observed.

Mechanical tissue properties

From the biomechanical point of view, the predominant problems of heart valve substitution arise from the enormous dynamic in vivo loads on the implant, even more so in the systemic circulation. Tissue engineered heart valves have to bear these loads during the time span of complete autologous tissue restoration in situ. As has been previously reported, the enzymatic digestion process inevitably weakens the mechanical characteristics of the valve, so that it may not be able to withstand hemodynamic forces in the systemic circulation [10, 20]. The mechanical properties of P(4HB), such as pliability and elasticity, compared to P(3HB) which is rather stiff and brittle, make it very suitable for applications in soft tissue engineering. We hypothesized that the polymer impregnation process would lead to improved physical properties, and investigated biomechanical tissue and valve performance in a series of mechanical in vitro tests. During the material selection process we analyzed selected mechanical and thermomechanical properties of P(4HB) and P(3HB-co-4HB) in comparison to P(3HB). In contrast to P(3HB), P(4HB) exhibits a tremendous ductility and appears far more pliable, and incorporation of relatively small amounts of 4HB into the copolymer (in our case 18% 4HB) results in major improvements of the material characteristics regarding the suitability for applications in soft tissue replacement.

▌ Suture retention strength

Specimens of the aortic conduits adjacent to the valves were placed in a tensile testing machine. The crosshead speed was set to 100 mm/min, and monofilament 4/0 suture material was used. The mean suture retention strength for native valve (aortic wall) specimens was 630 g, and this level was maintained or exceeded by all other specimen types tested. While decellularized and coated specimens showed values in the same range, suture retention strength was almost doubled in the impregnated specimens (1150–1190 g). Due to the cross-linking of collagen during glutaraldehyde fixation, the mechanical properties of glutaraldehyde-fixed control tissue were enhanced under multiaxial loading. This led to an intermediate suture retention in GA-fixed specimens of 1020 g.

▌ Leaflet testing

To assess the biomechanical behavior of the hybrid valves as compared to native and decellularized valves, leaflet specimens were subjected to tensile testing. Specimens, 1.5 mm wide, were cut out from the valve leaflets in the circumferential fiber direction. The tensile tests were performed at ambient temperature, and in controlled force mode with a force ramping of 1 N/min. Tensile strength, elongation to break, and the linear elastic modulus (tangent modulus) as the slope of the stress-strain curve in the linear elastic portion of the stress-strain curve were assessed. The latter parameter describes the biomechanical behavior of soft tissue, which is comprised of three distinct load corresponding stages. We found that decellularization led to a stiffening of the tissue (tangent modulus = 128 MPa) along with an increase of tensile strength (17 MPa) compared to the native state (74 MPa and 11 MPa, respectively). This effect may be attributed to the absence of cellular compartments and ground substance, which in native tissue act as water filled cushions and thereby decrease stiffness under uniaxial loading. It can further be assumed that in native tissue, cellular compartments add to the tension and crimp in the elastic network, leading to a preload of the fibers. This multiaxial preload is absent in the decellularized state leading to slack fibers in the unloaded state and an increase of tensile strength under load. Polymer impregnation further added to the stiffening effect and increased tensile strength. The coated specimens, however, exhibited a converse behavior with diminished stiffness and tensile strength. We conclude

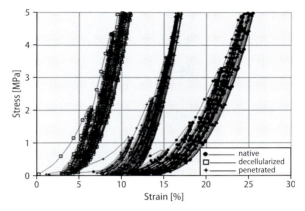

Fig. 3. Stress-strain relationship (SSR) in isolated heart valve leaflets. The tensile tests were performed on a Dynamic Mechanical Analyzer DMA 2980 (TA-Instruments, New Castle, Delaware, USA) in controlled force mode with a force ramping of 1 N/min until specimen fracture. Compared with a native valve leaflet ("native"), SSR is significantly altered in decellularized valves ("decellularized"), but partially restored by polymer impregnation ("penetrated")

that lyophilization and the associated shrinking processes lead to an impairment of the three-dimensional fiber architecture and thereby alter the structural properties of the decellularized matrix (Fig. 3).

Valve testing

Valve testing was conducted under physiological hemodynamic load conditions in a pulse duplicator system. The pulse rate was set to 60 bpm, systolic fraction was 32%, diastolic and systolic pressures were 80 mmHg and 130 mmHg, respectively. In addition to video morphometry recordings, transvalvular pressure gradient (TVP), closing volume fraction (Vclose), leakage volume fraction (Vleak) and total regurgitation volume fraction (Vreg%) were evaluated to characterize valve performance. A decrease of TVP was seen in both decellularized valve groups (before and after lyophilization). This effect, which was even more pronounced after lyophilization and the associated shrinking, was found to be caused by an easier opening of the leaflets due to a thickness reduction induced by the decellularization process. After polymer coating of the specimens, however, the TVP increased. The TVP increases with higher polymer solution concentration, since a thick polymer layer constricts valve opening. Due to leaflet stiffening, the effective orifice area (EOA) of coated valves also was reduced and the valves appeared stenosed. In the impregnated specimens, however, TVP was comparable to native valves. Regurgitation was found to be low in native and in decellularized specimens before lyophilization. Decellularized specimens after lyophilization showed increased regurgitation due to insufficiency caused by leaflet shrinkage. This effect was also apparent in the coated valves. Coating further affected the closing behavior as a result of the stiffness of the leaflets. Video morphometry of the working valves showed that in coated specimens the integrity of the polymer layer was disrupted, and the polymer coating of the leaflets partially peeled off the matrix when subjected to flexure under physiological loading. In contrast, the impregnated specimens functioned well and showed excellent structural integrity and low regurgitation.

In vivo biocompatibility testing

Intravascular biocompatibility of various hybrid tissue preparations was tested in a rabbit model. Adult New Zealand White rabbits were anesthetized, heparinized, intubated, and ventilated. The abdomen was opened, and then the abdominal aorta was dissected, clamped, and incised longitudinally. A patch of biomatrix/polymer hybrid tissue measuring approximately 5×3 mm was sutured in place using nonresorbable suture. After 1, 3, or 6 months, the animals were sacrificed and the aortic segment containing the patch was explanted and prepared for histology. Sections were stained with H & E and/or antibodies for immunohistology, and examined by light microscopy. A scoring system was designed to facilitate comparison of histologic findings. The following histologic characteristics were studied:
- endothelialization of the luminal patch surface,
- intima proliferation,
- inflammatory infiltration,
- calcification,
- cellular migration into the patch material,
- thrombus formation,
- formation of a neoelastica interna.

At follow-up, all rabbit aortas were patent, free from blood clot formation, except in one animal with a P4HB-treated patch. There were no patch aneurysms despite implantation in the high-pressure system. There was some early inflammatory cell infiltration (4 weeks) that later resolved in all patches (12 weeks). Recipient blood vessel cells had migrated into patch material in both the P3HB and P4HB coated matrices. Importantly, very little or no calcification occurred in the decellularized and P3HB-coated matrices, in contrast to autologous blood vessel control patches and some P4HB-coated matrices. Intimal thickening with formation of a neoelastica interna occurred in all hybrid tissue patches, but the vessel lumen was not narrowed in any of the P3HB-coated patches. As confirmed by immunohistology staining for CD31, there was complete endothelial cell lining of the luminal surface of matrix/polymer hybrid patches.

Large animal testing

The biocompatibility and mechanical screening tests of various hybrid material preparations indicated that P3HB-treated xenogenic matrix tends to exhibit better biocompatibility but is rather stiff and brittle, while the P4HB-coated matrix is soft and pliable, but probably at the cost of earlier calcification in vivo. Based on these results, we chose to prepare porcine hybrid tissue valves produced by decellularization followed by penetration with poly(3-hydroxybutyrate-co-4-hydroxybutyrate) consisting of 82% P3HB and 18% P4HB for further testing in a xenogenic large animal model. Two valves were implanted so as to replace the native pulmonary root in sheep, and three valves were implanted as freestanding aortic root replacement with coronary reimplantation. One animal died while undergoing aortic valve surgery and was excluded from the analysis. Three months after implantation, the animals underwent echocardiography and cardiac catheterization before they were sacrificed. Morphologic analysis of the hybrid valve was carried out before the valve tissue was divided in three parts and prepared for further analysis by light microscopy, immunohistology, and electron microscopy. The first valve implanted in pulmonary position was severely obliterated, with severe diffuse piogranulomatous valvular endocarditis, chronic lymphohistocytic and necrotizing bioprosthetic periarteritis, and intimal fibrous hyperplasia. Although microbiology at the time of sacrifice was negative, bacterial endocarditis was probably the cause. The second valve was in excellent condition, with near-normal gross morphology (Fig. 4). On histology, there was complete endothelial cell lining and moderate multifocal granulomatous inflammation limited to the leaflet hinge point. Particular attention was paid to the two valves im-

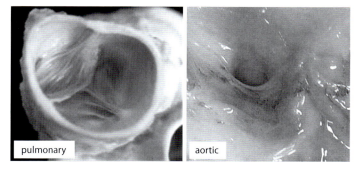

Fig. 4. Porcine biomatrix-polymer hybrid valves 3 months after implantation in a sheep model. In both the pulmonary and in aortic positions, the gross morphology of the valves is very satisfying. This was also mirrored by normal valve function on echocardiography. On histology, the valves were completely re-endothelialized, but cellular repopulation of the media was still scarce

planted in aortic position. At the time of sacrifice, both animals were in good condition without clinical signs of valve dysfunction. There were focal fibrinous deposits on the leaflets, and the leaflets contained homogeneous eosinophilic bundles of collagen, expanded by moderate multifocal granulomatous inflammation. There was some intimal thickening particularly of the luminal surface of the otherwise delicate leaflets. By immunohistology, complete endothelial cell lining of the leaflets and the conduit wall was found. Smooth muscle cells had migrated into the media of the leaflets, but there was very little cellular infiltration of the conduit wall.

Interpretation

It has recently been shown that mismatch of HLA-DR and ABO antigens on endothelial cells in unmodified valve allografts is associated with accelerated valve failure [3, 23]. Therefore, it appears preferable to reduce or eliminate donor cell immunogenicity by tanning or by decellularization [11]. In contrast to aldehyde-fixed tissue, enzymatically decellularized matrix without tanning-induced crosslinks possesses epitopes for cellular adhesion receptors, facilitating repopulation with tissue-specific cell types but also with inflammatory cells [2, 9]. Allogenic matrix constituents such as collagen, elastin, and proteoglycans have little immunogenicity, given that cellular components are entirely removed [37]. However, in the xenogenic setting or during immunologic stimulation (i.e., surgical stress, autoimmune disease, sepsis), exposed decellularized matrix can elicit a significant local immune response [8, 35]. Uncoated decellularized matrix valves are commercially available and have been implanted in the pulmonary position in hundreds of patients. Those include patients with congenital heart defects that require implantation of a valved conduit between the right ventricle and the pulmonary arteries [6, 31], as well as patients with aortic valve disease who undergo a Ross procedure [5, 7, 25]. However, their use with or without in vitro autologous preseeding for heart valve replacement remains controversial [28]. Preclinical large animal testing in the xenogenic and allogenic setting was very promising, with good hemodynamic function, morphologic reconstitution, and little calcification for almost one year [1, 12, 16, 19, 26, 27]. The initial enthusiasm has been muted, however, by reports of early failure decellularized xenogenic valves in humans [18, 19]. Decellularized homografts, i.e., allografts, appear to cause less problems in humans, but the actual long-term benefit remains to be determined [4, 17]. Moreover, aggressive decellularization weakens the valve tissue, so that the mechanical properties do not allow for implantation in the high pressure system [10]. Therefore, we sought to combine the advantageous properties of the native extracellular matrix scaffold with those of an artificial polymer, and we found that polymer-treated valve scaffolds indeed exhibit improved resistance to hemodynamic forces. Such impregnated hybrid valve structures are functional and readily implantable tissue engineering scaffolds with excellent biomechanical and structural characteristics [20]. Hybrid tissue heart valves can be produced and distributed as off-the-shelf items, and will are readily "revitalized", i.e., repopulated by recipient endothelial cells. The polymer coating is then degraded, while cells migrate into the extracellular matrix scaffold, restore the natural tissue structure of the native heart valve, and initiate the physiologic turnover of extracellular matrix components. Once these processes have been completed, the neovalve should have biological and mechanical characteristics identical to those of the native valve. The coating process also serves to attenuate the procoagulatory activity of bare matrix components. As long as re-endotheliazation is incomplete, platelets directly adhere by binding of platelet collagen receptor to integrins on exposed collagen, and the intrinsic clotting cascade is also initiated when prekallikrein, kininogen, factor XI, and factor XII are exposed to collagen. In the in vitro screening tests, we found that activation of both the cellular and the plasmatic coagulation system is indeed attenuated by polymer coating of decellularized matrix, reducing the risk of thrombembolic events after implantation.

In conclusion, we believe that decellularized heart valve matrix holds great potential for the creation of viable, long-lasting replacement valves, and that many of the problems in the xenogenic setting, including impaired biomechanics and residual antigenicity can be overcome by pretreatment with biodegradable polymers. However, more extensive long-term studies are clearly needed before clinical use can be considered.

References

1. Affonso da Costa FD, Dohmen PM, Lopes SV, Lacerda G, Pohl F, Vilani R, Affonso Da Costa MB, Vieira ED, Yoschi S, Konertz W, Affonso da Costa I (2004) Comparison of cryopreserved homografts and decellularized porcine heterografts implanted in sheep. Artificial organs 28:366–370
2. Bader A, Schilling T, Teebken OE, Brandes G, Herden T, Steinhoff G, Haverich A (1998) Tissue engineering of heart valves–human endothelial cell seeding of detergent acellularized porcine valves. Eur J Cardiothorac Surg 14:279–284
3. Baskett RJ, Nanton MA, Warren AE, Ross DB (2003) Human leukocyte antigen-DR and ABO mismatch are associated with accelerated homograft valve failure in children: implications for therapeutic interventions. J Thorac Cardiovasc Surg 126:232–239
4. Bechtel JF, Muller-Steinhardt M, Schmidtke C, Brunswik A, Stierle U, Sievers HH (2003) Evaluation of the decellularized pulmonary valve homograft (SynerGraft). J Heart Valve Dis 12:734-739; discussion 739–740
5. Bechtel JF, Stierle U, Sievers HH (2008) Fifty-two months' mean follow up of decellularized SynerGraft-treated pulmonary valve allografts. J Heart Valve Dis 17: 98–104, discussion 104

6. Cebotari S, Lichtenberg A, Tudorache I, Hilfiker A, Mertsching H, Leyh R, Breymann T, Kallenbach K, Maniuc L, Batrinac A, Repin O, Maliga O, Ciubotaru A, Haverich A (2006) Clinical application of tissue engineered human heart valves using autologous progenitor cells. Circulation 114:I132–137
7. Costa F, Dohmen P, Vieira E, Lopes SV, Colatusso C, Pereira EW, Matsuda CN, Cauduro S (2007) Ross Operation with decellularized pulmonary allografts: medium-term results. Rev Bras Cir Cardiovasc 22:454–462
8. Courtman DW, Errett BF, Wilson GJ (2001) The role of crosslinking in modification of the immune response elicited against xenogenic vascular acellular matrices. Journal of biomedical materials research 55:576–586
9. Courtman DW, Pereira CA, Kashef V, McComb D, Lee JM, Wilson GJ (1994) Development of a pericardial acellular matrix biomaterial: biochemical and mechanical effects of cell extraction. Journal of biomedical materials research 28:655–666
10. Courtman DW, Pereira CA, Omar S, Langdon SE, Lee JM, Wilson GJ (1995) Biomechanical and ultrastructural comparison of cryopreservation and a novel cellular extraction of porcine aortic valve leaflets. Journal of biomedical materials research 29:1507–1516
11. da Costa FD, Dohmen PM, Duarte D, von Glenn C, Lopes SV, Filho HH, da Costa MB, Konertz W (2005) Immunological and echocardiographic evaluation of decellularized versus cryopreserved allografts during the Ross operation. Eur J Cardiothorac Surg 27:572–578
12. Dohmen PM, Costa F, Lopes SV, Yoshi S, Souza FP, Vilani R, Costa MB, Konertz W (2005) Results of a decellularized porcine heart valve implanted into the juvenile sheep model. Heart Surg Forum 8:E100–E104, discussion E104
13. Dohmen PM, Ozaki S, Nitsch R, Yperman J, Flameng W, Konertz W (2003) A tissue engineered heart valve implanted in a juvenile sheep model. Med Sci Monit 9:BR97–BR104
14. Dohmen PM, Ozaki S, Verbeken E, Yperman J, Flameng W, Konertz WF (2002) Tissue engineering of an auto-xenograft pulmonary heart valve. Asian cardiovascular & thoracic annals 10:25–30
15. Dohmen PM, Ozaki S, Yperman J, Flameng W, Konertz W (2001) Lack of calcification of tissue engineered heart valves in juvenile sheep. Seminars in thoracic and cardiovascular surgery 13:93–98
16. Elkins RC, Dawson PE, Goldstein S, Walsh SP, Black KS (2001) Decellularized human valve allografts. The Annals of thoracic surgery 71:S428–432
17. Erdbrugger W, Konertz W, Dohmen PM, Posner S, Ellerbrok H, Brodde OE, Robenek H, Modersohn D, Pruss A, Holinski S, Stein-Konertz M, Pauli G (2006) Decellularized xenogenic heart valves reveal remodeling and growth potential in vivo. Tissue engineering 12:2059–2068
18. Flanagan TC, Cornelissen C, Koch S, Tschoeke B, Sachweh JS, Schmitz-Rode T, Jockenhoevel S (2007) The in vitro development of autologous fibrin-based tissue-engineered heart valves through optimised dynamic conditioning. Biomaterials 28:3388–3397
19. Goldstein S, Clarke DR, Walsh SP, Black KS, O'Brien MF (2000) Transpecies heart valve transplant: advanced studies of a bioengineered xeno-autograft. Ann Thorac Surg 70:1962–1969
20. Grabow N, Schmohl K, Khosravi A, Philipp M, Scharfschwerdt M, Graf B, Stamm C, Haubold A, Schmitz KP, Steinhoff G (2004) Mechanical and structural properties of a novel hybrid heart valve scaffold for tissue engineering. Artificial organs 28:971–979
21. Hoerstrup SP, Kadner A, Melnitchouk S, Trojan A, Eid K, Tracy J, Sodian R, Visjager JF, Kolb SA, Grunenfelder J, Zund G, Turina MI (2002) Tissue engineering of

functional trileaflet heart valves from human marrow stromal cells. Circulation 106:I143–150
22. Hoerstrup SP, Sodian R, Daebritz S, Wang J, Bacha EA, Martin DP, Moran AM, Guleserian KJ, Sperling JS, Kaushal S, Vacanti JP, Schoen FJ, Mayer JE Jr (2000) Functional living trileaflet heart valves grown in vitro. Circulation 102:III44–III49
23. Hogan PG, O'Brien MF (2003) Improving the allograft valve: does the immune response matter? The Journal of thoracic and cardiovascular surgery 126:1251–1253
24. Hopkins RA (2005) Tissue engineering of heart valves: decellularized valve scaffolds. Circulation 111:2712–2714
25. Konertz W, Dohmen PM, Liu J, Beholz S, Dushe S, Posner S, Lembcke A, Erdbrugger W (2005) Hemodynamic characteristics of the Matrix P decellularized xenograft for pulmonary valve replacement during the Ross operation. J Heart Valve Dis 14:78–81
26. Leyh RG, Wilhelmi M, Rebe P, Fischer S, Kofidis T, Haverich A, Mertsching H (2003) In vivo repopulation of xenogeneic and allogeneic acellular valve matrix conduits in the pulmonary circulation. Ann Thorac Surg 75:1457–1463, discussion 1463
27. O'Brien MF, Goldstein S, Walsh S, Black KS, Elkins R, Clarke D (1999) The SynerGraft valve: a new acellular (nonglutaraldehyde-fixed) tissue heart valve for autologous recellularization first experimental studies before clinical implantation. Seminars in thoracic and cardiovascular surgery 11:194–200
28. Sayk F, Bos I, Schubert U, Wedel T, Sievers HH (2005) Histopathologic findings in a novel decellularized pulmonary homograft: an autopsy study. The Annals of thoracic surgery 79:1755–1758
29. Shinoka T, Breuer CK, Tanel RE, Zund G, Miura T, Ma PX, Langer R, Vacanti JP, Mayer JE, Jr. (1995) Tissue engineering heart valves: valve leaflet replacement study in a lamb model. The Annals of thoracic surgery 60:S513–S516
30. Shinoka T, Ma PX, Shum-Tim D, Breuer CK, Cusick RA, Zund G, Langer R, Vacanti JP, Mayer JE, Jr. (1996) Tissue-engineered heart valves. Autologous valve leaflet replacement study in a lamb model. Circulation 94:II164–II168
31. Sievers HH, Stierle U, Schmidtke C, Bechtel M (2003) Decellularized pulmonary homograft (SynerGraft) for reconstruction of the right ventricular outflow tract: first clinical experience. Zeitschrift fur Kardiologie 92:53–59
32. Sodian R, Lueders C, Kraemer L, Kuebler W, Shakibaei M, Reichart B, Daebritz S, Hetzer R (2006) Tissue engineering of autologous human heart valves using cryopreserved vascular umbilical cord cells. Ann Thorac Surg 81:2207–2216
33. Sodian R, Sperling JS, Martin DP, Egozy A, Stock U, Mayer JE, Jr., Vacanti JP (2000) Fabrication of a trileaflet heart valve scaffold from a polyhydroxyalkanoate biopolyester for use in tissue engineering. Tissue engineering 6:183–188
34. Stamm C, Khosravi A, Grabow N, Schmohl K, Treckmann N, Drechsel A, Nan M, Schmitz KP, Haubold A, Steinhoff G (2004) Biomatrix/polymer composite material for heart valve tissue engineering. Ann Thorac Surg 78:2084–2092, discussion 2092–2083
35. Stamm C, Steinhoff G (2006) When less is more: go slowly when repopulating a decellularized valve in vivo! J Thorac Cardiovasc Surg 132:735–737, author reply 737
36. Steinhoff G, Stock U, Karim N, Mertsching H, Timke A, Meliss RR, Pethig K, Haverich A, Bader A (2000) Tissue engineering of pulmonary heart valves on allogenic acellular matrix conduits: in vivo restoration of valve tissue. Circulation 102:III50–III55
37. Wilson GJ, Courtman DW, Klement P, Lee JM, Yeger H (1995) Acellular matrix: a biomaterials approach for coronary artery bypass and heart valve replacement. Ann Thorac Surg 60:S353–358

Standards for the in vitro fabrication of heart valves using human umbilical cord cells

C. Lüders-Theuerkauf, R. Hetzer

Background

The most common therapy for end-stage valvular heart disease is valve replacement. Currently, 300 000 procedures are performed annually worldwide. Furthermore, 8 of 1000 children are born with congenital cardiac defects. Every fifth of these needs a heart valve replacement. Clinically available heart valve substitutes, including biological prostheses such as xenografts and homografts, and mechanical prostheses have satisfactory hemodynamic properties and function well but have several limitations in common, for example, an increased risk of infection and, particularly in pediatric patients, an increased potential for degeneration and calcification [1–3]. Furthermore, these substitutes consist of foreign, nonviable materials which entail the risk of thromboembolism and the lack of ability to remodel, repair, and grow. Pediatric patients are of particular interest in this context because they "outgrow" the prostheses so that multiple reoperations and considerable suffering for the patients and their families are the consequence [4]. Tissue engineering could be an alternative in overcoming these disadvantages. The interdisciplinary approach of tissue engineering combines principles of engineering and material science with biology and vascular surgery to fabricate viable and functional prostheses from autologous, living cells with the aim of long-lasting replacement or reconstruction of the dysfunctional native tissue. In the early 1990s tissue engineering emerged as a field of research with multiple clinical applications including reparative cartilage [5], trachea [6], skin [7], blood vessels [8], and heart valves [9, 10]. Research into producing a successful tissue engineered cardiovascular substitute has concentrated on three areas:
- a suitable 3-dimensional scaffold;
- the evaluation of suitable cell sources, if possible of autologous origin; and
- the cell seeding and in vitro conditioning process conducive of fabrication of the cell-matrix construct before implantation.

Scaffold materials

Several research experiments have demonstrated the possibility of fabricating a tissue-like structure in vitro, which remodels into functional tissue in vivo. The major problem is the composition of the scaffold. The scaffold serves as a physical and structural support and template for cell adhesion and tissue development. In recent years much effort has been expended on analyzing the optimal chemical and physical configuration of different biomaterials and their interaction with living cells to produce a functional tissue engineered construct. Therefore, the selection of an optimal scaffold is of particular interest. Several scaffold materials of different origin have been analyzed in vitro or are currently available for clinical application. All these biomaterials require a 3-dimensional structure and can be permanent or biodegradable. They can be of natural or biological origin, synthetic materials or hybrids. All these materials should be compatible with living cells in vitro and in vivo, should be without cytotoxic degradation products or immune response reactions, and should have adequate hemodynamic, biological, and mechanical functions and therefore life-long durability.

Natural scaffolds

For the tissue engineering of blood vessels, collagen-based matrices have been investigated in several approaches over the past 20 years [11–15]. The use of fibrin gel isolated from the patient's own blood as an autologous matrix has also been investigated [16]. One advantage is the homogenous distribution of cells within the gels from the beginning caused by the fast immobilization of the cells during polymerization of the gel.

Biological scaffolds

Biological scaffolds consist of decellularized material from animal donors (xenografts) or from human donors (homografts). Decellularization is achieved by enzymatic or detergent reactions [17]. The decellularized matrices offer the extracellular matrix (ECM), a mixture of functional proteins such as collagens, fibronectin, elastin and others, glycoproteins, and proteoglycans [18]. Theoretically, decellularized matrices are biodegradable but they will not work for all applications. They all have a heterologous origin, which makes immunosuppression therapy necessary. Several biological scaffolds are available for heart valve replacements, and the results so far have been satisfactory [19–24].

Synthetic scaffolds

Alternatively, synthetic biodegradable polymers such as polyglyclic acid (PGA), polylactide acid (PLA) or poly-4-hydroxy-butyrate (P4HB) have been demonstrated to be applicable in cardiovascular tissue engineering [25–28]. PGA was the first polymer used for the successful fabrication of a tissue engineered tissue. The original PGA is approved by the US Food and Drug Administration (FDA). It consists of a fibrous structure with several properties appropriate for cardiovascular tissue engineering. In our laboratory we use a 3-dimensional non-woven PGA structure fabricated exclusively for our applications. Due to its hydrophobic nature, it is absolutely necessary to precoat the scaffold with extracellular matrix proteins to improve the attachment of cells to the surface. PGA samples seeded with vascular human umbilical cord cells showed, after 5 weeks of incubation, a dense tissue-like structure. A large number of cells adhered to the surface and migrated into the polymeric structure (Fig. 1).

These data are reproducible but the PGA has to be modified and further optimized in working towards successful clinical application in the future. Recent studies have demonstrated the feasibility of combinations of different polymers resulting in copolymers which provide thermoplasticity and better mechanical properties [29, 30]. Major advantages of synthetic matrices are their controllable biodegradation properties and their high elasticity.

So far the fabrication of synthetic scaffolds for heart valve tissue engineering is reproducible but does not conform to good manufacturing practice (GMP) guidelines. For a prospective clinical application, it is important to set standards for the scaffold material itself and to establish a GMP protocol and quality control for a standardized fabrication technique. A basic requirement is the biocompatibility of the polymeric scaffold material. The

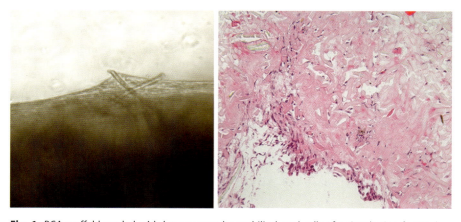

Fig. 1. PGA scaffold seeded with human vascular umbilical cord cells after incubation for 37 days

degradation process should not be attended by inflammation or immune response reactions. Furthermore, it is necessary to avoid cytotoxic degradation products when the seeded scaffold is implanted. The fabrication process needs to be reproducible and standardized with the aim of obtaining permission for fabrication according to the pharmaceutical laws.

Cell sources

Several potential cell sources for the tissue engineering of cardiovascular structures have been evaluated in recent years. The ideal cell source should be autologous and cells should be available in large quantities. Using autologous cells, the fabricated viable heart valve prostheses should have the potential to integrate, grow, remodel, and repair, thus, conceivably making reoperations unnecessary.

There are two major questions: which cell types and which cell source are feasible? With regard to heart valve substitutes, two cell types are required for the tissue engineered constructs:

- myofibroblast-like cells which have the potential to differentiate into fibroblasts and smooth muscle cells. These cells produce the extracellular matrix and are responsible for the development of tissue with the mechanical properties of native heart valves.
- Endothelial cells are necessary to cover the surface of the tissue engineered valves. These cells represent a blood compatible layer, thus, enabling thrombotic complications to be avoided.

There are a variety of approaches to harvest autologous cells, such as, biopsies from organs or segments from vascular vessels. During the past decade, venous and aortic human fibroblasts [31], human marrow stromal cells [32], and amniotic fluid-derived cells [33] have been investigated in intensive experiments. In recent years, interest in the use of stem cells has rapidly grown. Human stem cells and progenitor cells have been isolated from a variety of sources, e.g., human bone marrow, adipose tissue, umbilical cord blood and amniotic derived cells. Their autologous origin, high proliferation capacity, and potential for differentiation into vascular phenotypes make this cell type suitable for the tissue engineering of cardiovascular structures, such as heart valves. In comparison to embryonic stem cells, adult stem cells are less controversial and are associated with fewer ethical concerns. The human umbilical cord is of particular interest due to its possibility of originating different cell lines. The umbilical cord contains three vessels: two arteries and one vein (Fig. 2).

These vessels are a rich source of vascular cells and their progenitors for several potential clinical applications [34, 35]. The isolated cells could be used as a potential cell source of autologous origin, particularly for pedia-

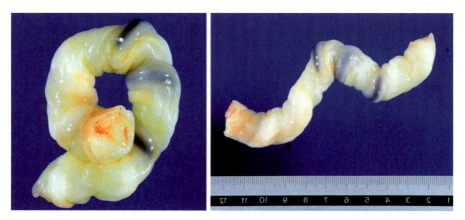

Fig. 2. The human umbilical cord contains three vessels: two arteries and one vein

tric patients and young adults with congenital heart defects. Naturally, harvesting autologous cells requires an invasive operation, to remove for example a small segment of an artery or vein. Using vascular cells from umbilical cords avoids the excision of pieces of vessels and, therefore, the risk of infectious complications. In view of all these advantages, our laboratory has focused on human vascular umbilical cord cells [34]. The ethics review board of the University Hospital Charité, Humboldt University of Berlin, Germany, approved the protocol and the human umbilical cords were collected after obtaining the written informed consent from each woman. Vascular cells were isolated, cryopreserved and afterwards thawed prior to use. These cells were cultured and expanded to achieve an appropriate cell number for seeding onto the scaffolds. After in vitro conditioning the cell-matrix construct should be implanted into the same patient from whom the cell material was isolated.

Cell seeding and in vitro conditioning

The cell seeding process is a critical procedure in fabricating tissue engineered constructs. First, it raises the question of whether a static or a dynamic cell seeding process is the better alternative. It is essential to obtain uniform distribution of the cells on the surface of a polymeric scaffold (Fig. 3).

After attachment to the surface, the cells start to migrate into the fibrous or porous structure of the polymer. It is absolutely necessary to supply the cells with nutrients to guarantee appropriate development of tissue-like structures. A prerequisite to achieve uniform distribution of the cells is

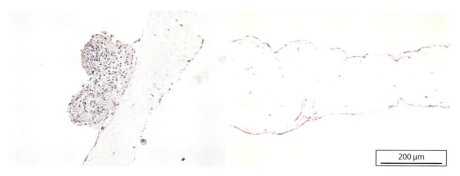

Fig. 3. Effect of a static cell seeding (left); effect of a dynamic cell seeding (right)

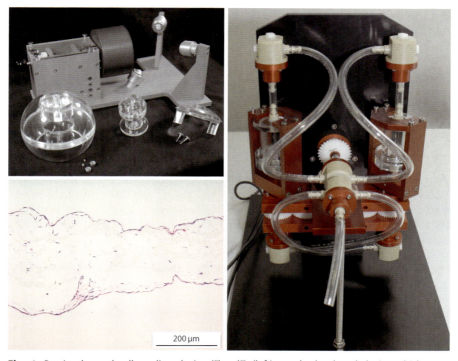

Fig. 4. Previously used cell seeding device ("bowl") (left); newly developed device which combines the cell seeding and the in vitro conditioning process (right)

that they be rotated together with the scaffold material. In our laboratory, we have developed various cell seeding devices. A few years ago, we started by developing a bowl which rotated with undirected movements [36]. The promising data in terms of cell distribution encouraged us to develop a new device that was to overcome some disadvantages of the bowl (Fig. 4).

In principle, the bowl was completely closed without any gas exchange. The new device consists of two individual cylindrical chambers rotating in one direction, the x-axis. These chambers are connected to a wheel that rotates in another direction, the y-axis. Gas permeable tubes are connected to seals which are able to rotate and this principle avoids twisting of the tubes. Previous studies have demonstrated that cells seeded onto biomaterials need specific cell culture conditions, so-called "in vitro conditioning" [37]. Before implantation the cells have to be "trained" for their intended function. The new device combines the cell seeding procedure and the in vitro conditioning process. It is not necessary to transfer the cell-matrix construct from one device to another, and therefore the risk of contamination is minimized. Thus, the cell culture conditions have to be optimized to guarantee a functional in vitro fabricated cardiovascular substitute. Taking supernatant samples helps to control and manage the in vitro conditioning process. Via a measuring unit, several parameters were monitored during the whole fabrication process to give an overview of the developing tissue inside the cylindrical chambers. This new principle set the first standards in fabricating tissue engineered heart valves independent of the cell source and the scaffold material.

Conclusion and perspectives

Progress has been made in engineering components of the cardiovascular system, i.e., blood vessels and heart valves. Tissue engineering could represent an alternative therapy to mechanical or biological heart valves prostheses. Recently, different human cell sources have been characterized and analyzed, and knowledge of biocompatible scaffolds and the in vitro conditioning process has rapidly increased. With the use of autologous cells, the tissue engineered constructs are very similar to native tissue and, thus, the risk of inflammation and rejection is minimized. The cell seeding and in vitro conditioning process function well but conditions need to be improved. There are still open questions: How many cells are needed? What is the optimal duration of incubation? Therefore, we need to further investigate manageable and controllable cell seeding processes. Each fabrication of tissue engineered heart valves using polymeric scaffolds is individual and does not yet conform to GMP. We need to set standards by establishing GMP protocols and quality control for the cell isolation, cryopreservation, cell seeding, and in vitro conditioning. Establishing standardized methods with controllable parameters is the basic requirement. It is necessary to monitor the whole process with concomitant in vivo studies and preclinical and clinical tests with the aim of obtaining the permission of regulatory boards for the fabrication of tissue engineered heart valves. Currently, the German guideline on human cell-based medicinal products from

September 1, 2008 is very strict. Furthermore, the characteristics of cell-based pharmaceuticals, such as tissue engineered heart valves, are regulated by EU edict 1394/2007. This means that for the first time, tissue engineered products have been defined in pharmaceutical legislation which stipulates GMP fabrication, quality control, and preclinical and clinical studies. A central element of EU 1394/2007 is EU-wide permission by the European Medicinal Agency (EMEA) from January 1, 2009. In summary, if it proves to be feasible to fabricate tissue engineered heart valves consisting of biodegradable polymers and human autologous cells according to the EU edict 1394/2007, tissue engineering will be on its way to becoming an alternative therapy to conventional therapies and is expected to play an important role in future human clinical applications.

References

1. Braunwald E (1997) Valvular heart disease. In: Braunwald E (ed) Heart disease 5th edition, Philadelphia: Saunders Company
2. Hammermeister KE, Sethi GK, Henderson WG et al (1993) A comparison of outcomes in men 11 years after heart-valve replacement with mechanical valve or bioprosthesis. N Engl J Med 328:1289–1296
3. Vongpatanasin W, Hillis D, Lange RA (1996) Prosthetic heart valves. N Engl J Med 335:407–416
4. Cannegieter SC, Rosendaal FR, Briet E (1994) Thromboembolic and bleeding complications in patients with mechanical heart valve prostheses. Circulation 89: 635–641
5. Moriya T, Wada Y, Watanabe A, Sasho T, Nakagawa K, Mainil-Varlet P, Moriya H (2007) Evaluation of reparative cartilage after autologous chondrocyte implantation for osteochondritis dissecans: histology, biochemistry, and MR imaging. J Orthop Sci 12(3):265–273
6. Macchiarini P, Jungebluth P, Go T, Asnaghi MA, Rees LE, Cogan TA, Dodson A, Martorell J, Bellini S, Parnigotto PP, Dickinson SC, Hollander AP, Mantero S, Conconi MT, Birchall MA (2008) Clinical transplantation of a tissue-engineered airway. The Lancet 372:2023–2030
7. Loss M, Wedler V, Künzi W, Meuli-Simmen C, Meyer VE (2000) Artificial skin, split-thickness autograft and cultured autologous keratinocytes combined to treat a severe burn injury of 93% of TBSA. Burns 26(7):644–562
8. Shinoka T, Imai Y, Ikada Y (2001) Transplantation of a tissue engineered pulmonary artery. N Engl J Med 344(7):532–533
9. Cebotari S, Lichtenberg A, Tudorache I, Hilfiker A, Mertsching H, Leyh R, Breymann T, Kallenbach K, Maniuc L, Batrinac A, Repin O, Maliga O, Ciubotaru A, Haverich A (2006) Clinical application of tissue engineered human heart valves using autologous progenitor cells. Circulation 114[suppl I]:I-132–I-137
10. Dohmen PM, Lembcke A, Hotz H, Kivelitz D, Konertz WF (2002) Ross operation with a tissue-engineered heart valve. Ann Thorac Surg 74(5):143814–42
11. Weinberg CB, Bell E (1986) A blood vessel constructed from collagen and cultured vascular cells. Science 231(4736):397–400

12. L'Heureux N, Germain L, Labbé R, Auger FA (1993) In vitro construction of a human blood vessel from cultures vascular cells: a morphologic study. J Vasc Surg 17(3):499–509
13. Hirai J, Kanda K, Oka T, Matsuda K (1994) Highly oriented tubular hybrid vascular tissue for a low pressure circulatory system. ASAIO J 40(3):M383–M388
14. Girton TS, Oegema TR, Tranquillo RT. (1999) Exploiting glycation to stiffen and strengthen tissue equivalents for tissue engineering. J Biomed Mater Res; 46(11): 87–92
15. Seliktar D, Black RA, Vito RP, Nerem RM (2000) Dynamic mechanical conditioning of collagen-based blood vessel constructs induces remodeling in vitro. Ann Biomed Engineering 28:351–362
16. Jockenhoevel S, Zünd G, Hoerstrup S, Chalabi K, Sachweh J, Demircan B, Turina M (2001) Fibrin gel – advantages of a new scaffold in cardiovascular tissue engineering. Europ J Cardio Thorac Surg 19:424–430
17. Dohmen PM, Konertz W (2008) Decellularization of xenogenic biologic tissue. Ann Thorac Surg 85(6):2163; author reply 2163–2164
18. Badylak SF (2002) The extracellular matrix as a scaffold for tissue reconstruction. Semin Cell Dev Biol 13 (5):377–383
19. Konertz W, Dohmen PM, Liu J, Beholz S, Dushe S, Posner S, Lembcke A, Erdbrügger W (2005) Hemodynamic characteristics of the Matrix P decellularized xenograft for pulmonary valve replacement during the Ross operation. J Heart Valve Dis 14(1):78–81
20. Dohmen PM, Lembcke A, Holinski S, Kivelitz D, Braun JP, Pruss A, Konertz W (2007) Mid-term clinical results using a tissue-engineered pulmonary valve to reconstruct the right ventricular outflow tract during the Ross procedure. Ann Thorac Surg 84(3):729–736
21. Erdbrügger W, Konertz W, Dohmen PM, Posner S, Ellerbrok H, Brodde OE, Robenek H, Modersohn D, Pruss A, Holinski S, Stein-Konertz M, Pauli G (2006) Decellularized xenogenic heart valves reveal remodeling and growth potential in vivo. Tissue Eng 12(8):2059–2068
22. Purohit M, Kitchiner D, Pozzi M (2004) Contegra bovine jugular vein right ventricle to pulmonary artery conduit in Ross procedure. Ann Thorac Surg 77(5):1707–1710
23. Bechtel JF, Stierle U, Sievers HH (2008) Fifty-two months' mean follow up of decellularized SynerGraft-treated pulmonary valve allografts. J Heart Valve Dis 17(1):98–104, discussion 104
24. Elkins RC, Dawson PE, Goldstein S, Walsh SP, Black KS (2001) Decellularized human valve allografts. Ann Thorac Surg 71:S428–S432
25. Shinoka T, Breuer CK, Tanel RE, Zund G, Miura T, Ma PX, Langer R, Vacanti JP, Mayer JE Jr (1995) Tissue engineering heart valves: valve leaflet replacement study in a lamb model. Ann Thorac Surg 60(6 Suppl):S513–S516
26. Ye Q, Zünd G, Jockenhoevel S, Schoeberlein A, Hoerstrup S, Grunenfelder J, Benedikt P, Turina M (2000) Scaffold precoating with human autologous extracellular matrix for improved cell attachment in cardiovascular tissue engineering. ASAIO J 46:730–733
27. Hoerstrup SP, Sodian R, Daebritz S, Wang J, Bacha EA, Martin DP, Moran AM, Guleserian KJ, Sperling JS, Kaushal S, Vacanti JP, Schoen FJ, Mayer JE Jr (2000) Functional living trileaflet heart valves grown in vitro. Circulation 102(19 Suppl 3): III44–III49
28. Sodian R, Lüders C, Krämer L, Kübler WM, Shakibaei M, Reichart B, Däbritz S, Hetzer R (2006) Tissue engineering of autologous human heart valves using cryopreserved vascular umbilical cord cells. Ann Thorac Surg 81(6):2207–2216

29. Brennan MP, Dardik A, Hibino N, Roh JD, Nelson GN, Papademitris X, Shinoka T, Breuer CK (2008) Tissue-engineered vascular grafts demonstrate evidence of growth and development when implanted in a juvenile animal model. Ann Surg 248(3):370–377
30. Wang W, Liu Y, Wang J, Jia X, Wang L, Yuan Z, Tang S, Liu M, Tang H, Yu Y (2008) A novel copolymer poly(lactide-co-beta-malic acid) with extended carboxyl arms offering better cell affinity and hemacompatibility for blood vessel engineering. Tissue Eng Part A
31. Schnell AM, Hoerstrup SP, Zund G, Kolb S, Sodian R, Visjager JF, Grunenfelder J, Suter A, Turina M (2001) Optimal cell source for cardiovascular tissue engineering: venous vs. aortic human myofibroblasts. Thorac Cardiovasc Surg 49(4):221–225
32. Hoerstrup SP, Kadner A, Melnitchouk S, Trojan A, Eid K, Tracy J, Sodian R, Visjager JF, Kolb SA, Grunenfelder J, Zund G Turina M (2002) Tissue engineering of functional trileaflet heart valves from human marrow stromal cells. Circulation 106(Suppl I):I143–I150
33. Schmidt D, Achermann J, Odermatt B, Genoni M, Zund G, Hoerstrup SP (2008) Cryopreserved amniotic fluid-derived cells: a lifelong autologous fetal stem cell source for heart valve tissue engineering. J Heart Valve Dis 17(4):446–455, discussion 455
34. Sodian R, Lüders C, Krämer L, Kübler WM, Shakibaei M, Reichart B, Däbritz S, Hetzer R (2006) Tissue engineering of autologous human heart valves using cryopreserved vascular umbilical cord cells. Ann Thorac Surg 81(6):2207–2216
35. Kadner A, Hoerstrup SP, Breymann C, Maurus CF, Melnitchouk S, Kadner G, Turina M (2002) Human umbilical cord cells: a new cell source for cardiovascular tissue engineering. Ann Thorac Surg 74(4):S1422–1428
36. Lueders C, Sodian R, Shakibaei M, Hetzer R (2006) Short-term culture of human neonatal myofibroblasts seeded using a novel three-dimensional rotary seeding device. ASAIO J 52(3):310–314
37. Hoerstrup SP, Sodian R, Daebritz S, Wang J, Bacha EA, Martin DP, Moran AM, Guleserian KJ, Sperling JS, Kaushal S, Vacanti JP, Schoen FJ, Mayer JE Jr (2000) Functional living trileaflet heart valves grown in vitro. Circulation 102(19 Suppl 3):III44–III49

Tissue engineering with a decellularized valve matrix

W. Konertz, S. Holinski, S. Dushe, A. Weymann,
W. Erdbrügger, S. Posner, M. Stein-Konertz, P. Dohmen

Tissue engineering requires scaffolds, which are of biologic or synthetic origin. Synthetic scaffolds have the advantage of sterility and no occurrence of immunologic barriers; however, the degradation process is unpredictable and thus the hemodynamic behavior is also unpredictable. Biologic scaffolds have the advantage that suitable animals, e.g., pigs, are abundant, the macroarchitecture is close to human anatomy which eases surgical handling and implantation, and their microarchitecture is adapted to load conditions. Disadvantages are the threats of rejection and infection, which also implies transmission of specific viruses. These drawbacks can be overcome only by complete decellularization.

In 1995, we started developing valve scaffolds. The first issue was to decellularize porcine tissue in order to:
- kill all cells
- preserve perfectly the extra decellular matrix and
- remove almost all cellular debris.

These goals can not be achieved with the implementation of enzymatic processes. A graft prepared in this manner came into clinical practice with the Synergraft® technology. This method showed suboptimal results with decellularized allografts [1] and catastrophic results with decellularized xenografts [2]. We used deoxycholate (DOA) for decellularization and were able to show a well-preserved collagen matrix and complete decellularization. The evaluation of the material was published previously [3]. In brief, the pulmonary valve was dissected free from hearts obtained from the slaughterhouse. Fine trimming was performed and the heart was exposed to an antibiotic solution for 24 h. Exposure to DOA for 14 h was followed by a validated physicochemical sterilization process including additional detergent and alcohol. In vitro evaluation of this tissue included quantitative real-time PCR to determine PERV-cDNA and PERV-DNA, radioligand binding for a_2-adrenoreceptors, electron microscopy, fluorescence microscopy, measurements of heart valve burst pressure, and other mechanical parameters. Preclinical in vivo evaluation was performed in a juvenile sheep model by Dohmen et al. [4]. These experiments showed that the decellularized xenografts were repopulated by host cells, where an overgrowth of endothelial cells on the inner surface of the implant and ingrowth of interstitial cells into the scaffold occurred over time, and the interstitial cells start producing procollagen and collagen. We were also able to demonstrate that additional blood supply to the implant is provided by vasa vasorum. Dohmen et al. were able to show that the valve grows in the animal experiment [5]. Thus, one can say that tissue, which was cell free at the time of implant, will be repopulated by the host over time and thus turns into living autologous tissue.

After extensive preclinical in vitro and in vivo experimentation in 2000, a trial with decellularized allografts was initiated, and the first operation was performed on May 20, 2000 [6]. During a Ross operation, a 43-year-old man received a decellularized pulmonary allograft, which was seeded in vitro with autologous endothelial cells. In 2001, we started to implant allografts without in vitro seeding. These allografts performed well and 5-year results have been published recently [7]. In 2002, xenograft trials were started with seeded and also with nonseeded implants. During this trial, complications occurred, which we had been unaware of previously and which were shown to be related to the porcine anatomy. In most pigs, the vessel wall of the posterior sinus portion of the pulmonary valve is extremely thin. In the presence of elevated pulmonary artery pressure, this led to the formation of aneurysms at the site of the sinus. In some patients, distal anastomotic narrowing also occurred. These complications were treated by repeat implantation of decellurized xenografts or in the case of anastomotic narrowing often simply by patch augmentation of the anastomosis. Complications observed in the early xenograft trials prompted the redesign of the valve with attached patches. This makes implantation easier. Most importantly, graft selection was scrutinized. In the end, only 2 or 3 out of 100 pulmonary valves were suitable for further processing.

The AutoTissue company is a spin-off from the Charité and was founded in 2000. The company worked intensively on the project and received the CE certification for Matrix P after ISO certification for valve producing facilities in 2004. The patch extended Matrix P plus was granted the CE certification in 2005 (Fig. 1).

With pulmonary valves readily available off the shelf, the number of Ross operations at our department increased tremendously (Fig. 2) Medi-

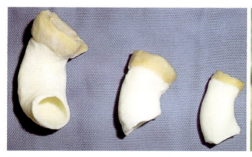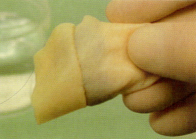

Fig. 1. Three sizes of Matrix P (left); patch extended Matrix P plus (right)

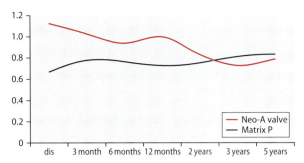

Fig. 2. Echocardiographically obtained flow (m/s) across the neoaortic valve and Matrix P during 5 years of follow-up

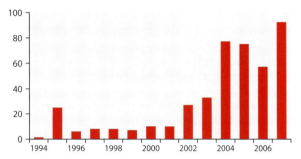

Fig. 3. Increase of Ross operations at the Department of Cardiovascular Surgery of the Charité from 1994 to 2007

um term performance of the valve is currently very satisfying (Fig. 3). In the year 2007, we performed the Ross operation in 91 patients. The patients' ages ranged from 9 days to 74 years and associated procedures were performed in 48% of the patients, most often CABG, mitral valve repair/replacement, or repair/replacement of the ascending aorta. Two hospital deaths occurred. One patient died early on the 5th postoperatively day from sepsis, and the other died on the 69th day as the result of abdominal surgery. Both deaths were not valve related. Mean gradient over the neoaortic valve was 5.1 ± 2.2 mmHg at discharge and 3.2 ± 1.0 mmHg one year postoperatively. Tissue engineered pulmonary valves showed a gradient of 2.8 ± 1.6 at discharge and 2.7 ± 1.2 one year postoperatively. No or trivial aortic regurgitation was shown in 88% of patients, while 12% showed mild I° aortic regurgitation. No patient had reoperation of the aortic valve. Two patients had reoperation of the pulmonary valve. In both cases, anastomotic narrowing had occurred 9 and 10 months postoperatively. In one case, it was obviously due to external compression from an organized hematoma that caused stenosis. In the other case, inappropriate selection of suture material may have been the cause.

The Matrix P plus heart valve was also used in pediatric implants at the Charité. From July 2006 to September 2008, 23 pediatric patients received the Matrix P plus. The mean age was 9.8 years (range 9 days to 22 years): 4 patients suffered from aortic stenosis, 10 tetralogy of Fallot, 1 neonatal truncus arteriosus, and 8 presented with degenerated right ventricular outflow allografts. In this cohort, 1 death occurred after redo operation. This patient died from nonvalve related bleeding from the ascending aorta. All except one are living and well. One is suffering from mitral stenosis which could be ameliorated only partially during initial neonatal surgery.

A 1-year follow-up echocardiography is available in 16 patients: 3 showed mild pulmonary regurgitation or stenosis and in 13 normal findings could be obtained.

Similar results were presented by Kroll at al. from Herzzentrum Duisburg [8]. They studied the Matrix P plus in 33 patients from April 2006 to April 2008. Patients had a mean age of 8.9 years (range from 11 days to 59 years): 8 patients suffered from aortic stenosis, 8 from TGA VSD PS, 14 patients had tetralogy of Fallot and 2 had hypoplastic left heart syndrome. In this complex patient population, 3 nonvalve-related deaths occurred, and a late follow-up showed that 11 patients had trivial pulmonary regurgitation or stenosis. The other 17 patients showed normal findings.

Since CE certification to the end of 2007, 711 valves have been implanted throughout Europe, including the countries of Germany, Italy, France, Great Britain, Spain, Poland, Estonia, and Croatia (Fig. 4). Surgery with tissue engineered heart valves is technically demanding. The valve has to be trimmed to absolutely proper length, every valve that is too long causes kinking and crimping with stenosis. A valve that is too short has too much tension and may cause suture hole bleeding. The correct implantation technique is that the valve is implanted in a manner that it comes under gentle tension once circulation is reestablished. Also the selection of the size (z-score ± 1) is absolutely important as oversizing may also result in distal anastomotic narrowing. Oversizing is a temptation especially for pediatric surgeons, who tend to oversize valves in order to prevent too early of a reoperation. As long as all technical demands of the implantation procedure

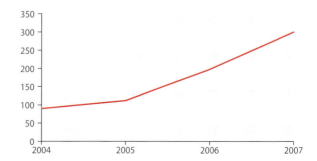

Fig. 4. Annual number of Matrix P/Matrix P plus manufactured from 2004 to 2007

are followed with Matrix P and Matrix P plus, we have perfect implants which have shown resistance to calcification and durability in a 7-year follow-up. Regeneration potential and potential for growth have been shown in animal experiments, and to assess this in human implants is the aim of ongoing international trials. In summary, this living tissue can be used for the Ross operation, for congenital RVOT reconstruction, and for exchange of calcified allografts or xenografts.

References

1. Sievers HH, Stierle U, Schmidtke C et al (2003) Decellularized pulmonary homograft (Synergraft) for reconstruction of the right ventricular outflow tract: first clinical experience. Z Kardiol 92:53–59
2. Simon P, Kasimir MT, Seebacher G et al (2003) Early failure of the tissue engineered porcine heart valves SYNERGRAFT™ in pediatric patients. Europ J Cardiothorac Surg 23:1002–1006
3. Erdbrügger W, Konertz W, Dohmen P et al (2006) Decellularized xenogenic heart valves reveal remodeling and growth potential in vivo. Tissue Engineering12:2059–2068
4. Dohmen PM, Ozaki S, Yperman J et al (2003) Results of tissue engineered autoxenograft implanted in the juvenile sheep model. Med Sci Monit 9:BR97–BR107
5. Dohmen PM, da Costa F, Holinski S et al (2006) Is there a possibility for a glutaraldehyde-free porcine heart valve to grow? Eur Surg Res 38:54–61
6. Dohmen PM, Lembcke A, Hotz H et al (2002) Ross operation with the tissue engineered heart valve. Ann Thorac Surg 74:1438–1442
7. Dohmen PM, Lembcke A, Holinski S et al (2007) Mid-term clinical results using a tissue engineered pulmonary valve to reconstruct the right ventricular outflow tract during the Ross procedure. Ann Thorac Surg 84:729–736
8. Kroll J, Buerbaum B, Beckmann A et al (2008) Kurzfristige Ergebnisse nach Pulmonalklappenersatz mit Matrix P plus Herzklappe. Clinical Research Cardiol 97:675

Regularatory issues on tissue valves

Human tissues for cardiovascular surgery: regulatory requirements

D. M. Fronk, J. D. Ferros

Introduction

The clinical use of cardiac allografts has been a mainstay in cardiovascular surgery for the past five decades for both the repair and reconstruction of congenital and acquired defects and anomalies. In order to meet these clinical needs, the tissue processors providing these tissues must comply with evolving governmental regulations established to ensure the safety and quality of the tissue. Generically considered as tissue for transplant, the history of these tissues from a regulatory perspective is both convoluted and complex. Though there are many general commonalities in the regulatory frameworks of two of the largest clinical markets for allograft cardiovascular tissue, the United States (US) and the European Union (EU), the pathway allowing for their distribution onto these markets is distinctly different. This chapter examines the governmental regulatory requirements for processed human cardiovascular tissue, with a specific focus on the regulations of the US and the EU.

United States

The US regulatory status of human heart valves has changed considerably in the past 20 years. Until 1991, there were no formal regulations for any type of processed human tissue. That changed in June 1991, when human heart valves became subject to regulation by the US Food and Drug Administration (FDA), and the FDA published a notice stating that human heart valves were to be de novo classified as a Class III medical device under the Food Drug and Cosmetic Act [15]. The notice required a formal regulatory application, i.e., investigational device exemption (IDE) or premarket approval (PMA) application, for continued distribution of human heart valves for transplantation. During this time, heart valve allografts were implanted under the control of a formal investigational clinical trial. In October 1994, the FDA rescinded their earlier decision [17] and announced that neither an approved application for PMA nor an IDE would be required for processors and distributors who had marketed heart valve allografts before June 1991. The revised notice further stated that allograft heart valves were to be "down-regulated" to Class II medical devices, subject to 510(k) premarket notification (and quality system regulations), and that any processor providing allograft heart valves prior to June 1991 would not be required to submit a premarket notification to continue their distribution of valves.

In 1997, the FDA began regulating other (non-heart valve) human tissue for transplantation under Section 361 of the Public Health Services Act to ensure the prevention of transmission of communicable diseases – 21 CFR 1270 [14]. The 1270 regulations focus on donor screening and testing procedures to help mitigate communicable disease transmission risk, e.g., human immunodeficiency virus and hepatitis virus. Though these regulations explicitly excluded human heart valves to be regulated as "human tissue for transplant," all donors, including heart valve donors, were required to comply with the screening and testing requirements of the 1270 regulations.

The FDA refined its rulemaking regarding human tissue intended for transplant with the proposed regulations for human cells, tissues, and cellular and tissue-based products (HCT/P) – 21 CFR 1271 [12]. These regulations included rules on establishment registration, donor eligibility, and good tissue practices (GTPs).

Through the 1271 regulations, the FDA further enhanced its efforts to ensure tissue safety to reduce the risk of relevant communicable diseases and disease agents. Human tissue donors are required to be screened and tested for human immunodeficiency virus types 1 and 2, hepatitis B virus, hepatitis C virus, and *Treponema pallidum*. Donors are further required to be screened for other infectious diseases such as bacteria and fungi, parasites, transmissible spongiform encephalopathy agents, sepsis, disease risks associated with xenotransplantation, vaccinia, and West Nile virus. The FDA issued a Guidance Document to assist in the compliance with the donor eligibility requirements associated with the 1271 regulations [18].

The development of the GTP regulations provided a regulatory goal to further prevent the introduction, transmission, or spread of communicable diseases by HCT/Ps by ensuring that the HCT/Ps do not become contaminated during manufacturing [9]. The GTP requirements provide a quality system-like framework to govern the methods used in, and the facilities and controls used for, the manufacture of HCT/Ps, including but not limited to all steps in recovery, donor screening, donor testing, processing, storage, labeling, packaging, and distribution. In addition, GTPs also include requirements for adequate personnel training, development of standard operating procedures, process validations, process change control procedures, record keeping and retention, tissue tracking, and complaint handling. (In general, the GTP regulations would be akin to Good Manufacturing Practice/Quality System Regulation used in the manufacture of pharmaceuticals and medical devices.)

On May 25, 2005, in conjunction with the promulgation of the GTP final rule, the FDA reclassified human heart valves, processed on or after that date, as human tissue subject to that rule. Any human heart valve processed prior to the implementation of the final rule, however, is still regulated as a medical device [16].

Even with the HCT/P regulations, there is still a tiered system for the regulation of human tissue. Tissue may be regulated as human tissue (i.e., an HCT/P), or, depending on the degree of its processing, its intended clinical use, and its overall composition, it may be regulated as a medical device or pharmaceutical product. In order for human tissue, to fall solely under the HCT/P regulations it must meet several criteria. Tissue that does not meet these criteria would be classified as a drug or device. These criteria [8] include:

- The tissue is minimally manipulated;
- the tissue is intended for homologous use only, as reflected by the labeling, advertising, or other indications of the manufacturer's objective intent; and
- the manufacture of the tissue does not involve the combination of the cells or tissues with another article, except for water, crystalloids, or a sterilizing, preserving, or storage agent, provided that the addition of water, crystalloids, or the sterilizing, preserving, or storage agent does not raise new clinical safety concerns with respect to the tissue.

As defined in the regulations, homologous use is the repair, reconstruction, replacement, or supplementation of a recipient's cells or tissues with an HCT/P that performs the same basic function or functions in the recipient as in the donor [10]. For structural tissues, such as heart valves, minimal manipulation is defined as processing that does not alter the original relevant characteristics of the tissue relating to the tissue's utility for reconstruction, repair, or replacement [11]. Examples of minimally manipulated processes are density gradient separation; selective removal of B-cells, T-cells, malignant cells, red blood cells, or platelets; centrifugation; cutting, grinding, or shaping; soaking in antibiotic solution; sterilization by ethylene oxide treatment or irradiation; cell separation; lyophilization; cryopreservation; or freezing [13]. Conventionally processed cardiac human tissue (i.e., antimicrobial decontamination with cryopreservation) meets the definition of minimal manipulation, and thus, falls under the HCT/P regulation.

European Union

Throughout the 1990s, Europe recognized a need to implement a scheme for placing EU-wide safety and approval requirements for medical products. The culmination of this activity was the implementation of two directives describing methods to ensure medical device safety and to set up a scheme for device approval, i.e., "placement on the market." The first of these two directives was the Active Implantable Medical Device Directive (AIMD) [4]. This directive focused only on those medical devices that were intended to be long-term implants and that used an internal power source to function. The AIMD was implemented first due to the recognition of these type of devices are more complex and are potentially a higher risk. Soon afterwards, the Medical Device Directive (MDD) was implemented [5]. This directive covered all other medical devices with a similar scheme for assuring product safety and describing a product approval process. As a result of the success with the Active Implantable and Medical Device Directive, European authorities identified a similar need for human tissue for transplantation.

The European Union Tissue and Cells Directives (EUTCD) were issued by the European Council to bring Europe under one set of requirements for control of tissue in order to provide comprehensive and umbrella coverage requirements. The first of these Directives [1] (also known as the "Parent Directive") lays down standards of quality and safety for the donation, procurement, and testing of all human tissue and cells intended for human applications. These standards in turn are further elaborated with two implementing measures that spell out specific technical requirements in each aspect of these activities in order to prevent the transmission of diseases by human tissue and cells.

The first measure [2] covers tissue donation, procurement, and testing, including factors such as staff training, facility design, and the creation of procedures for recovery and testing. This directive sets the requirements for screening and testing of donors for human immunodeficiency virus types 1 and 2, hepatitis B virus, hepatitis C virus, and syphilis. This directive also establishes criteria for donor selection to exclude donors with physical, medical, or behavioral evidence to include: death or disease of unknown etiologies, malignant disease, prion-based diseases (i.e., Creutzfeldt-Jakob disease, dementia), and systemic infection.

The second technical measure [3] establishes the provisions for processing, preservation, storage, and distribution of human tissue. This directive includes requirements for establishing a quality management system for all processing activities, validation of processing procedures, traceability of the tissues, and notification of serious adverse reactions and events.

Unlike the MDD, the EUTCDs do not describe a scheme for placement on the market; there is no mechanism described for review and conformity assessment by a single regulatory authority that is accepted by each of the Member States. As with other European Directives, the concepts and requirements found in the tissue directives must be transposed into local law. Each Member State is obligated to place the tissue directives requirements within its own legal system. Each European country has its own regulatory authority responsible for administering and ensuring compliance to the EUTCDs. Because there is no central scheme for "placement on the market," this has caused a patchwork system to be in place for meeting the requirements of the tissue directives within each individual country.

In the United Kingdom (UK), the governmental authority charged with administering the requirements of the tissue directives is the Human Tissue Authority (HTA). The HTA has been at the forefront of implementing the tissue directive requirements. The EUTCDs were fully implemented into UK law and set forth licensing requirements for establishments that procure, test, process, store, distribute, or import and export human tissue. In Germany, the EUTCD requirements are administered by the Paul Ehrlich Institute which is an agency under the Federal Ministry of Health with oversight of biologic medicinal products, which include human tissue (referred to as tissue preparations). The Paul Ehrlich Institute is responsible for processing of applications for marketing authorization for tissue preparations to ensure they meet the requirements as promulgated in the German Medicinal Products Act.

Decellularized cardiac tissues

The maintenance of donor cell viability has long been considered and argued as a potential immunologic source of both early and late tissue degeneration for cardiac allografts. In hopes of addressing these deleterious outcomes, numerous techniques have been developed to remove the donor cells and cellular debris from the tissue, while leaving an intact structural matrix. However, the development of these new decellularization technologies can result in changes to the regulatory status of these tissues.

In the US, human tissue falls only under the tissue regulations, if it is not more than minimally manipulated, that is, processed in a manner that does not alter the original relevant characteristics of the tissue relating to the tissue's utility for reconstruction, repair, or replacement. Should the processing be considered more than minimal manipulation, the tissue would be regulated as either a medical device or a drug and would require a formal regulatory submission to allow for its commercial distribution.

The FDA has deemed that removing cells from cardiovascular tissue is more than minimal manipulation in that the tissue's original characteristic of being populated with donor cells is relevant to the tissue's utility for reconstruction, repair, or replacement [19]. This decision was predicated on the opinion that the presence of donor cells in a graft relates to the tissue's antigenicity and to the fact that such donor cells may be foci for calcification, and is relevant even if the characteristic may not be critical or pivotal to the tissue's functionality for reconstruction, repair, or replacement. Therefore, decellularized cardiac allografts are regulated in the US as medical devices and require a premarket submission prior to commercialization.

To gain market clearance, these products would require extensive preclinical bench testing, animal testing, and possibly human clinical testing.

To date, two human cardiac tissue-based products have been introduced onto the US marketplace via the medical device regulatory pathway by receiving FDA 510(k) market clearance:

- The decellularized SynerGraft®-processed CryoValve® SG human pulmonary heart valve (CryoLife, Inc., Kennesaw, GA, USA) indicated for the replacement of diseased, damaged, malformed, or malfunctioning native or prosthetic pulmonary valves for both congenital and acquired valvular lesions, including use in the replacement of native pulmonary valves when the Ross procedure is performed [20].
- The MatrACELL™ decellularized pulmonary artery patch allograft (Lifenet Health, Virginia Beach, VA, USA) indicated for repair of the right ventricular outflow tract [21].

In the EU, the regulatory status of decellularized cardiac tissues is less clear due to the promulgation of the Advanced Therapy Medicinal Products (ATMP) regulation [7]. Similarly to the MDD, the ATMP sets up a scheme for an approval process for these products. In the case of ATMPs, the European Medicines Agency (EMEA), specifically the Committee for Medicinal Products for Human Use, reviews and approves products that are considered "advanced" such as gene therapy medicinal products, somatic cell therapy medicinal products, or tissue engineered products. Tissue engineered products may contain cells or tissues of human or animal origin, or both. Also, the cells or tissues may be viable or nonviable and may also contain additional substances, such as cellular products, biomolecules, biomaterials, chemical substances, scaffolds, or matrices [6]. Cardiac allograft tissues that have solely been decellularized should not fall into the definition of those products regulated by the ATMPs, since the definition of ATMP specifically excludes tissues "which do not act principally by pharmacological, immunological or metabolic action" [6]. However, currently no commercially available decellularized cardiac tissues have been fully vetted through the process to verify their regulatory status in the EU.

References

1. EU Commission Directive 2004/23/EC of 31 March 2004 on setting standards of quality and safety for the donation, procurement, testing, processing, preservation, storage and distribution of human tissues and cells
2. EU Commission Directive 2006/17/EC of 8 February 2006 implementing Directive 2004/23/EC of the European Parliament and of the Council as regards certain technical requirements for the donation, procurement and testing of human tissues and cells

3. EU Commission Directive 2006/86/EC of 24 October 2006 implementing Directive 2004/23/EC of the European Parliament and of the Council as regards traceability requirements, notification of serious adverse reactions and events and certain technical requirements for the coding, processing, preservation, storage and distribution of human tissues and cells
4. EU Council Directive 90/385/EEC of 20 June 1990 on the approximation of the laws of the Member States relating to active implantable medical devices
5. EU Council Directive 93/42/EEC of 14 June 1993 concerning medical devices
6. EU Regulation (EC) 1394/2007 Article 2, section 1(b)
7. EU Regulation (EC) 1394/2007 of the European Parliament and of the Council of 13 November 2007 on the advanced therapy of medicinal products and amending Directives 2001/83/EC and Regulation (EC) 726/2004
8. US Code of Federal Regulations, Chapter 21, Section 1271.10
9. US Code of Federal Regulations, Chapter 21, Section 1271.150
10. US Code of Federal Regulations, Chapter 21, Section 1271.3(c)
11. US Code of Federal Regulations, Chapter 21, Section 1271.3(f)
12. US Federal Register (January 19, 2001) 66 Fed Reg, p 5447
13. US Federal Register (January 19, 2001) 66 Fed Reg, p 5457
14. US Federal Register (July 29, 1997) 62 Fed Reg, p 40429
15. US Federal Register (June 26, 1991) 56 Fed Reg, p 29177
16. US Federal Register (November 24, 2004) 69 Fed Reg, p 68614
17. US Federal Register (October 14, 1994) 59 Fed Reg, p 52078
18. US Food and Drug Administration (2007) Guidance for industry: eligibility determination for donors of human cells, tissues, and cellular and tissue-based products. http://www.fda.gov/cber/gdlns/tissdonor.htm
19. US Food and Drug Administration, http://www.fda.gov/cber/tissue/trgfyrpts.htm
20. US Food and Drug Administration, http://www.fda.gov/cdrh/pdf3/K033484.pdf
21. US Food and Drug Administration, http://www.fda.gov/cdrh/pdf8/K081438.pdf

Concluding remarks

C. A. YANKAH

The excellent contributions in this volume have highlighted not only the continuing success, but also the progress and innovations made in aortic valve and root surgery during the past 50 years. Perioperative aortic root imaging techniques (echocardiography, computed tomography, and magnetic resonance imaging) have become important diagnostic tools in the planning and evaluation of surgical procedures in the aortic root. Aortic valve and root surgery is now routine with low perioperative morbidity and mortality as well as long-term improvement in survival and quality of life. Risk-adjusted operative mortality for aortic valve replacement is 3.9% and for aortic valve replacement with concomitant coronary artery bypass grafting, it is 6.3% according to the database of the German Society for Cardiothoracic and Vascular Surgery, whereas both operations carry a mortality rate of 5% according to the Society of Thoracic Surgeons. Reoperative mortality in many institutions did not differ statistically from that for primary aortic valve replacement and ranges from 1.5–6%. Reoperative risk for prosthetic valve endocarditis was 9–20%.

Despite more than 50 years of research and clinical application, the pursuit for the ideal valve substitute continues. This has led to the development of numerous aortic valve and root procedures such as the valve-sparing operations, the David and Yacoub operations, the relocation technique by Hetzer, and aortic valve repair by Schaefer and El Khoury. Aortic allograft and stentless bioprosthetic replacement, which were introduced in 1962 by Ross and Barratt-Boyes and in 1964 by Binet, Carpentier and O'Brien, has been relatively durable and free of thromboembolic problems. The allograft has an additional advantage over xenograft valves for aortic valve replacement in the setting of endocarditis, with a lower probability of recurrent endocarditis. Certainly, the mechanical valves with their requirement of anticoagulation and thromboembolic complications despite technology for home monitoring of the International Normalized Ratio (INR) are far from ideal, and the stented bioprostheses have inferior hemodynamics with a few exceptions, especially in the small valve sizes.

Bioprosthesis durability, expressed as freedom from structural valve deterioration or reoperation, is a great concern for any patient with a bioprosthesis especially in younger age groups. Many patients, particularly elderly patients, die before a biological valve requires replacement. Younger age at operation is a risk factor for the need for re-replacement of bioprostheses and cryopreserved allograft valves, and this effect is a result of the competing risks of death and replacement, as well as a biological predisposition to structural valve deterioration. Competing risk analysis provides the actual probability of requiring a re-replacement during the remainder of the patient's life after aortic valve replacement. This information is different from that provided by the Kaplan-Meier estimate, which reflects valve durability.

In patients older than 60 years at the time of aortic valve replacement, the probability of re-replacement for any reason before death was no different for bioprostheses and cryopreserved allografts. However, for patients younger than 60 years, in terms of the probability of re-replacement before death, the pulmonary autograft was superior to the cryopreserved allograft and bioprostheses. Therefore, the pulmonary autograft in the aortic position (the Ross operation) still comes close to meeting all the criteria for a perfect replacement valve; however, the operation does require an allograft or bioprosthetic replacement of the pulmonary valve and the right ventricular outflow tract.

The recent development of transcatheter valve-in-valve aortic valve implantation has contributed to the continued success of aortic valve surgery and offers an option for patients with a high operative risk of > 20%.

Research in tissue engineering has resulted in a potential valve tissue. The SynerGraft and AutoTissue, the decellularized allo- and xenograft valves may have some durability and biocompatibility, and therefore might represent close approximation to the perfect valve.

In the near future, it is expected that the emphasis will be on new technologies to perfect transcatheter aortic valve replacement and to improve the biocompatibility of bioprostheses for young patients.

Conclusion

Aortic valve replacement offers a wide range of choices for various age groups, each with advantages and disadvantages. The primary operative risk is similar to that of a second operation. Indications for aortic valve and root surgery have been refined to suit the available surgical options. Valve-sparing procedures have taken a significant role in the treatment of patients with aortic valve diseases.

The Ross procedure has earned an important place in the treatment of children and adolescents with aortic valve disease; however, it is associated with concomitant pulmonary valve replacement and reconstruction of the right ventricular outflow tract.

Transcatheter aortic valve implantation for dysfunctioned native and bioprosthetic valve offers an option for patients with a high operative risk of >20%, and there is potential for improvement of the delivery technology. Continuing research in the tissue engineering of biological valves to improve their biocompatibility and durability may offer better prognosis for young patients with valvular heart diseases. Improved technology for perioperative aortic root imaging has contributed significantly to the continued success of aortic valve and root surgery.

Acknowledgments

We are indebted to Dr. Sabine Hübler and her staff at the Department of Clinical Studies, German Heart Institute Berlin (GHIB), for their tireless efforts and excellent organization, preparation, and planning of the Berlin Heart Valve Symposium 2008. We are grateful to Ms. Ibkendanz, Dr. Gasser, Ms. Gossen, Mr. Schwind, and Ms. Denskus, of the publisher Springer-Verlag, for their excellent work and cooperation during the preparation of this multi-authored book. To all our contributors, and the heart valve manufacturers who provided photographs of biological valves for the atlas, we express our sincere appreciation. In particular, we would like to thank the Deutsches Herzzentrum Berlin (DHZB) for sponsoring the Symposium and the Gesellschaft der Freunde des Deutschen Herzzentrums Berlin (President: Prof. Fissenewert) for sponsoring the publication of the book. Similarly, we are indebted to Anne Gale for editorial assistance, Astrid Benhennour for bibliographic support, and for exceptional graphic design work Carla Weber and Holger Hasselbach.

Atlas of biological valves
C. A. Yankah

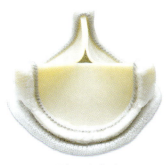
Carpentier-Edwards-Perimount Magna (Edwards Lifesciences) – 1984/2003

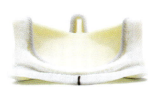
Carpentier-Edwards-Magna Ease (Edwards Lifesciences) – 2007

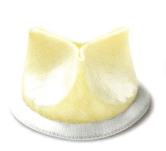
Mitroflow (Sorin) – 1982

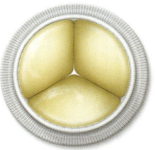
Soprano (Sorin) – 2003

Fig. 1. Stented bovine pericardial bioprostheses

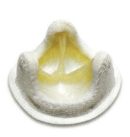
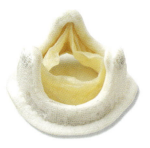
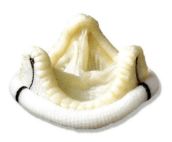

Hancock II (Medtronic) – 1982   Mosaic (Medtronic) – 1994   SJM Epic-Biocor (St. Jude Medical) – 1981

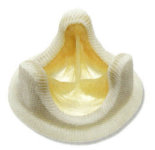
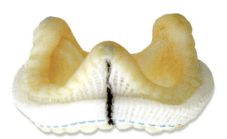

aspire ™ porcine valve (Vascutek) – 1979   Epci supra (St. Jude Medical) – 2003

Fig. 2. Stented porcine bioprostheses

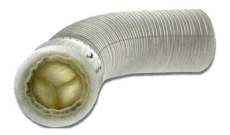

Fig. 3. BioValsalva™ – porcine stentless aortic valved conduit (Vascutek) – 2006

Fig. 4. Stentless bovine pericardial bioprostheses (Scalloped sinuses): Freedom Solo (Sorin) – 2004

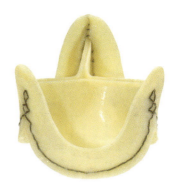

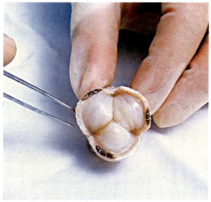

CryoLife O'Brien (CryoLife) – 1992

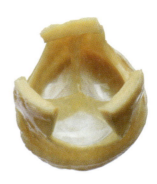

elan™ (Vascutek) – 1999

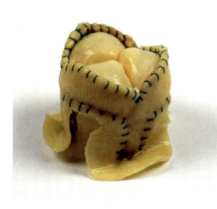

Shelhigh stentless – pericardial-covered (Shelhigh) – 1999

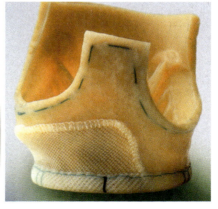

Prima Plus Baxter (Edwards Lifesciences) – 1991

Fig. 5. Stentless porcine bioprostheses (Scalloped sinuses)

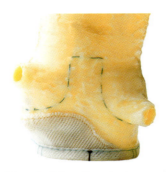 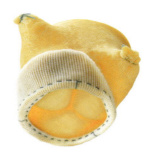 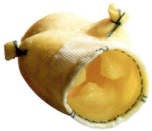

Edwards Prima Plus stentless (Edwards Lifesciences) – 1991

St. Jude Medical Toronto root (St. Jude Medical) – 1991

Freestyle stentless (Medtronic) – 1992

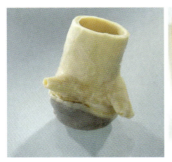 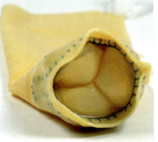 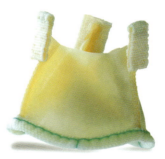

elan™ Root (Vascutek) – 1999

Shelhigh composite pericardial conduit – reinforced with pericardium (Shelhigh) – 1998

3F SAVR (Supraannular valve replacement) (ATS) – 2001

Fig. 6. Stentless porcine bioprostheses (Full root)

Atlas of biological valves | 595

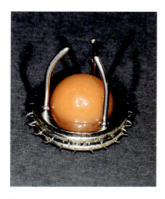 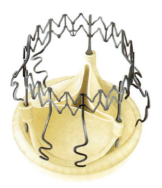 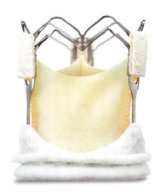

First sutureless prosthetic valve replacement: Magovern-Cromie – 1962. This prosthesis was explanted after 42 years (by courtesy of Prof. Zlotnick, Haifa, Israel)

Perceval bovine pericardial aortic valve replacement (Sorin) – 2007

3F Enable equine pericardial aortic valve replacement (ATS) – 2005

Fig. 7. Sutureless aortic bioprostheses for direct placement via ministernotomy in open heart surgery. History has repeated itself. From a rapid sutureless mechanical fixation of a mechanical prosthesis to a self-expandable sutureless fixation of a bioprosthesis

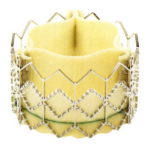 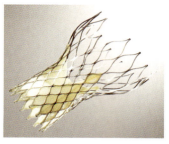 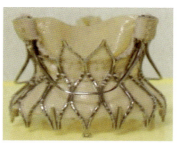

Edwards Sapien (Edwards Lifesciences): transfemoral aortic valve replacement – 2002 (Cribier), transapical aortic valve implantation – 2006 (Lichtenstein), and transapical aortic valve-in-valve replacement – 2007 (Walther)

CoreValve (Medtronic): transfemoral aortic valve replacement – 2005 (Grube), and transapical aortic valve replacement – 2007 (Walther)

Ventor Embracer (Medtronic): transapical aortic valve replacement – 2008 (Walther)

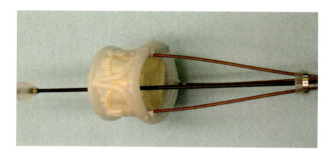

Direct Flow aortic valve replacement: transfemoral aortic valve replacement – 2007 (Direct Flow Medical), (Schofer/Reichenspurner)

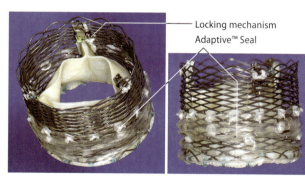

Sadra Lotus: transfemoral aortic valve replacement – 2007 (Sadra Lotus Medical), (Grube). The Sadra Lotus and Direct Flow Medical valves are undergoing safety and efficacy testing. They are repositionable, retrievable, and have smaller diameter sheath sizes

Fig. 8. Transcatheter percutaneous and transapical sutureless self-expandable pericardial aortic valve replacement

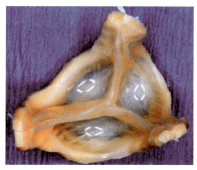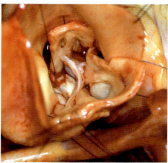

all three aortic sinuses scalloped – 1962 (Barratt-Boyes technique)

two aortic sinuses scalloped with retention of the noncoronary sinus – 1962 (Ross technique)

Fig. 9. Aortic allograft (scalloped 2-3 sinuses of Valsalva)

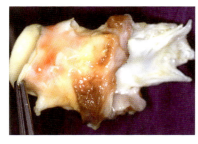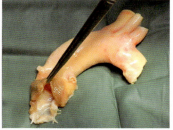

full root aortic allograft with a short segment of the ascending aorta (harvested from a heart transplant recipient)

full root aortic allograft with a long segment of the ascending aorta (harvested from a donor heart which was unsuitable for heart transplantation)

Fig. 10. Full root aortic allograft with ascending aorta

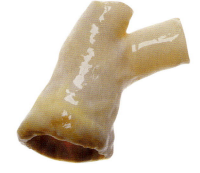

Fig. 11. Full root decellularized pulmonary allograft for the Ross operation: a decellularized pulmonary allograft – SynerGraft (CryoLife) – 2000

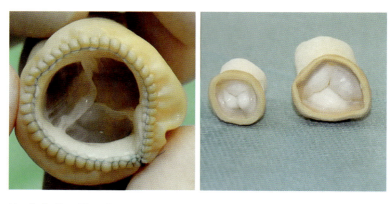

Matrix P (AutoTissue) – 2002   Matrix P Plus (AutoTissue) – 2005

Fig. 12. Full root decellularized bovine aortic xenograft for the Ross operation

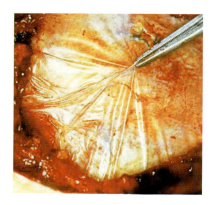

Fig. 13. GoreTex pericardial substitute for anticipated replacement of bioprostheses: Gore-Tex preclude pericardial membrane (WL Gore & Associates) – 1979

Subject index

A

ablation catheter   304, 307, 309
ablation line   309
– circumferential   304
ABO compatibility   264
abscess
– classification   229
– definition   227
– paravalvular   226
abscess cavity, incomplete resection   253
abscess development   227
abscess formation   212, 217, 402
acetylsalicyl acid   28, 411
acoronary sinus   374
acquired diseases   170
activated partial thromboplastin time   442
Active Implantable Medical Device Directive (AIMD)   584
active infective endocarditis (AIE)   23, 223, 243
actuarial analysis   443
acute endocarditis   67
acute myocardial infection   223
acute pericardial tamponade   481
adhesive embolization   187
adipose tissue   567
advanced age   460
Advanced Therapy Medicinal Products (ATMP)   586
afterload mismatch   47
age-dependent risk   460
age-matched Dutch population   530
age-matched population   530
aging population   46, 210
AIDS criteria   199

allograft   67, 263, 512, 532, 534
– undersized   254, 265
allograft anatomic insertion   277
allograft explanation   259, 515
allograft fixation   277
allograft heals in place   268
allograft implantation   155
allograft infection, recurrent   266
allograft patients, survival   267
allograft reoperation   68
allograft root distortion   275
allograft tissue decellularized   268
allograft valve indication   249
American College of Cardiology (ACC)   47
– guidelines   2006   291, 369
American Heart Association (AHA)   47
– guidelines   291
American Society of Echocardiography guidelines   291, 348
amino oleic acid (AOA)   470
amiodarone   309
amiodarone therapy   296
amniotic derived cells   567
analysis
– multivariate   255
– univariate   255
anatomic position   373
anesthetist   36
aneurismal wall, wrapping   180
aneurysms,
– ascending aortic   92
– supracoronary   120
angulation of LAO-10°   37
annular dilatation   5
annular abscess   352
annular base dilatation   115

annular implantation, subaortic 253
annular structures, destruction 234
annulectasia 71
annuloaortic ectasia 150, 183, 356
annuloplasty 95, 144
- subvalvular circular, techniques 159
- subcommisural 95
annulorrhaphy 265, 283
annulus
- crown-shaped 155
- sinotubular junction diameters 108
anomalous circumflex 364
antegrade route 35
antegrade transapical implantation 37
anterior axillary line 306
anterior incision 168
anterior mitral leaflet 157, 158, 164, 422
anterolateral sinus 18
anteromedial leaflet 18
antibiotic permeable 265
antibiotic prophylaxis 268
anticalcification 367
- treatment 33, 214
anticoagulant 424
anticoagulant therapy 503, 545
anticoagulant-related hemorrhage (ARH) 459
anticoagulation 357, 542, 544, 548
- contraindication 366
- long life, risk 107
- long-term 244
- low-dose 541, 546
- management 567
- therapy 347, 475, 484
antigenicity 470
antihypertensive treatment 537
antimineralization treatment 482
antiplatelet agents 347
antiplatelet drugs 444
antithromboembolic-related hemorrhage 470
aorta, disease 490
aorta pressure
- ascending 105
- left ventricular 105
aortic aneurysm 23, 178
aortic annuloplasty 144

- augmentation 144
- double sub- and supravalvular external 121
- reduction 144, 253, 282, 283
- subvalvular external 117, 161
aortic annulus 35
- crown-shaped 103
aortic arch 35, 182
aortic atherosclerosis 23
aortic bioprostheses 473
aortic clamp time (min) 297
aortic coarctation 151
aortic compliance 391
aortic cross-clamp time 61, 349
aortic dilatation 98
aortic dissection repair 186
aortic graft 284
aortic insufficiency, classification 123
aortic mitral fibrous septum 276
aortic mitral septum 245
aortic pericardial bioprostheses 468
aortic Perimount pericardial bioprostheses 441
aortic porcine bioprostheses 468
aortic prosthesis 164
aortic regurgitation 136, 137
aortic root 13, 182, 394, 552
- normal 106
- noninfected 68
aortic root abscess 67, 243, 244, 258
aortic root anatomy 103
aortic root aneurysm, surgical indication 107
aortic root annulus 16
aortic root disease 352
aortic root distance to left main coronary artery 16
aortic root dystrophy 106
aortic root enlargement 437
aortic root enlarging 281
aortic root expansion 104
aortic root geometry, normal 170
aortic root imaging 14
aortic root, porcine 346
aortic root procedure 588
aortic root repair 187
aortic root replacement (ARR) 250
-- allograft 244
-- technique 269
-- valve sparing 95

aortic root, tailoring 265
aortic root, valve dynamic 109
aortic root, valve sparing operation 133
aortic stenosis 341, 479
- operative risk 18
- symptomatic 18
aortic valve (AV) 216, 234, 471, 588
- close 13
- human, leaflets 149
- open 13
aortic valve disease 3, 490
aortic valve endocarditis 361
- intractable active infective 247
aortic valve implantation
- transapical 32
- transcatheter 7
aortic valve in systole 15
aortic valve incompetence 182
aortic valve leaflet
- shape 13
- topographic anatomy 13
aortic valve plane
- dislocation 178
- relocation 179
aortic valve prosthesis 22
aortic valve regurgitation 478
aortic valve reoperation 361
aortic valve repairing 107
aortic valve replacement (AVR) 308, 341, 397, 401, 454, 467, 474, 514, 537, 589
- conventional 18
- freehand subcoronary 252
- percutaneous transluminal 22
- predicted outcome 525
aortic valve sparing 107
- procedures 108
aortic valve stenosis 478
aortic valve surgery 590
- conservative 126
-- principles 126
- minimal invasive 48
aortic ventricular dehiscence 67
aortic wall, fibroelastic 145
aortic-mitral curtain 163, 165
aortography 27
aortoventricular dehiscence 228
aortoventricular junction 109
aorto-ventriculoplasty 166

apoptosis 89, 292
appendage obliteration 310
appendage occlude 303
applicator 187
Applied Telemedicine (IFAT) 544
argon 292
argon cryoenergy 304
artery injury, circumflex 296
artery stenosis, circumflex 299
ascending aorta 354, 380
- asymmetric growth 179
- dilatation 352
- enlargement 412
- replacement 246
ascending aortic aneurysms 92
associated procedures 349
asymptomatic patients 441
atrial fibrillation 291, 294, 302, 309, 370, 424, 448, 450, 453, 456, 479, 533
atrial fibrillation/flutter 475
atrial thrombus, left 305
ATS 3 f. Aortic Bioprosthesis 386, 391
ATS 3 f. Enable 57
ATS Medical 57
augmentation annuloplasty 170
autograft 532
autograft durability 537
autograft endocarditis 68
autograft failure 152
autograft regurgitation 79
autologous blood vessels 558
autologous cells 567, 568
autologous endothelial cells 575
autologous pericardial buttress 158
AutoTissue 575, 589

B

back to nature 154
bacterial infection, resistance 402
balloon valvuloplasty 26
balloon-expandable aortic valve prosthesis 22
Barratt-Boys, Sir Brian 67, 274
beating heart 302
Bentall, Hugh 107, 264, 274
Bentall-de Bono procedure 19
better science, better medicine 70

Subject index

better prognosis of survival with good quality of life 67
Biocor prosthesis 458
bicuspid aortic valve (BAV) 89, 92, 489, 410
- classification system 92
- fate 92
- prevalence 90
- repair 96
- syndrome 80, 89
- stenotic 94
bilateral lung ventilation 37
biocompatibility 552, 559, 590
- testing 555, 558
biocompatible heart valve 436
biocompatible scaffolds 570
biodegradable polymers 551, 561, 571
biofilm bacteria 250, 265
biofilm decolonization 250
biofilm microorganisms 264
BioGlue 185
biologic reconstruction 274
biological composite graft 381
biological scaffold 565
biological tissue, non-thrombogenic
biological valve 488, 503
biological valve conduit 496
biomatrix/polymer hybrid 553, 554
biomatrix/polymer hybrid tissue 558
Biomatrix-polymer 551
Biomatrix-polymer hybrid 559
bioprostheses 67, 211, 461, 498, 499, 501, 504, 512
- durability 513
- implantation 457
- replacement 505, 509, 511
- re-replacement 514
- second 509
bioprosthetic cardiac valve 470
BioValsalva 487, 496
BioValsalva conduit 489
BioValsalva graft 495
bipolar radiofrequency ablation 491
biventricular failure 247
bleeding events 445
blindness 226
blood test 305
body mass index (BMI) 297, 427
bovine pericardial 284
bovine pericardium 388, 414

Boyle's law 292
Brigham and Woman's Hospital 47
bundle of His 161

C

calcific degeneration 350
calcification 378
calcified aortic stenosis 441
calcified bicuspid aortic valve 363
cardiac allograft 581
cardiac complication 263
cardiac computed tomographic view 15
cardiac cycles 105
cardiac death 481
cardiac failure 443
cardiac injury 516
cardiac output 391
cardiac related death 404
cardiac surgery, previous 305
cardiogenic shock 234
cardiologist 36
cardiologist's discretion 442
cardioplegic arrest 33
cardiopulmonary bypass (CPB) 36, 61, 349, 442, 491
cardiorespiratory failure 255
cardiothoracic surgeon 27
cardiovascular event 94
cardiovascular tissue engineering 566
cardioversion 296, 309
care unit 381
carotid filtering devices 303
Carpentier, Alain 154
Carpentier's functional classification 5
Carpentier-Edwards Perimount 435
Carpentier-Edwards porcine valve 458
Catheter
- intracavitary 265
- intravascular 265
CAVIAAR trial 123
CD4 count 200
cell proliferation 554
cell seeding process 568
cell sources 567
cell-matrix construct 570
cerebral abscesses 248, 263
cerebral bleeding 215, 459

Subject index 603

cerebral complication   528
cerebral hematoma   479
cerebral hemorrhage   449
cerebrovascular events   78, 296
changes, cyclic   141
chest radiation, history   34
chest X-ray   305
Child B class   201
Child C class   201
cholecystitis   224
chordal elongation   5
chordal rupture   5
chordal shortening   5
chronic atrial brillation   442
chronic atrial fibrillation   473, 484
chronic myocardial decompensation   527
chronic obstructive pulmonary disease (COPD)   427
circular abscess   228
circular configuration   326
circulatory arrest   490
circumferential reduction   155
Cleveland Clinic   47
clinical outcome   224, 381
clinical performance   436
clinical safety   583
clopidrogrel   28
closing   334
clover-shaped aortic annular base and vortices   105
coagulation system   555
Cohn, Lawrence   47
collagenous condensation   145
color Doppler-flow studies   394
combined procedures   413
commissural area   104
commissural post   390, 394
commissure   19, 374
– fusion of thickening   5
– reattachment   96
Committee for Medicinal Products for Human   586
common cardiac malformation   98
common microorganisms   211
communicable disease transmission risk   582
comorbidity   511
comparable hemodynamic performance   343

competent system   555
competing risk analysis   589
complete endoscopic microwave ablation   304
composite valve   110
computed tomography   588
computer-aided design program   322
concomitant coronary artery bypass   418
concomitant procedures   472
conducting system   248
configuration of three adjacent hemispheric form   15
congenital aortic valve disease   536
congenital cardiac defects   564
congenital diseases   170
congenital heart repair   4
congestive heart failure   234, 454
conjoint cusps   91
contemporary bioprostheses   463
contraindications   83, 503
conventional AVR   18
copolymer   556
CoreValve   19
coronary angiography   305
coronary artery bypass   399
coronary artery bypass grafting (CABG)   246, 444, 493, 506
– concomitant   267
coronary artery bypass surgery   472
coronary artery disease   500
coronary artery reimplantation   278
coronary blood flow   495
coronary buttons, circumcised   283
coronary malpositioning and/or kinking   353
coronary perfusion   38
coronary reimplantation   491, 559
coronary revascularization   524
Cosgrove, Delos   47
Coumadin   424, 455
Cox classification, new   295
Cox MAZE procedure   291, 298
Cox's proportional hazards   255
Cribier   22
cross-clamp duration   78
cross-clamp times   349
cross-linking collagen   556
crown-shaped aortic annulus   102
croypresserved allograft   534

Subject index

cryoablation 292
– left atrial 295
cryoclamp 294
cryoenergy 293
CryoLife-O'Brien valve 410
– durability 364
– equates 364
– stentless porcine 356
CryoMaze surgical ablation system 293
cryopreserved allograft valves 537, 589
cryopreserved homograft 219
cumulative incidence 433
cusp closing displacement 106, 109
cusp free edge 104
cusp intervention 141
cusp nadir of insertion 118
cusp placation 95
cusp prolapse 120
cusp repair 114
cusp resuspension 121
cut-off diameter 34
cylinder inclusion technique 75
cystic medial necrosis 151
cytokine 150
cytotoxicity 554

D

database 506
David III 116
David IV 116
David V 116
David/Yacoub techniques 95
De Bono and Bentall 107
De Bono, Antony 264, 274
death valve related 359
decalcification 398, 421
– annulus 62
decellularization 436, 559
decellularization cardiac allograft 585
decellularization process 553
decellularization SynerGraft 586
decellularization technologies 585
decellularized cardiac tissue 585
decellularized heart valve matrix 561
decellularized homografts 560
decellularized matrix 554, 557

decellularized pulmonary allograft 575
decellularized valve matrix 551, 574
decellularized vascular matrix scaffolds 552
decellularized xenograft 574, 575
decision-making 434
deep hypothermia 179
defects, patch closure 95
degenerated right ventricular outflow allograft 577
degenerative aneurysm 489
delivery sheath 23
diagnostic
– clinical 201
– microbiological 201
diastolic dimension 397
different bioprosthetic 335
digital planimetry 318
dilated aortic sinuses 381
dilated ascending aorta 381
dimensional changes, dimensional 141
Direct Flow Medical 20, 51
Direct Flow Valve 51
diseases
– acquired 170
– complexity 202
– congenital 170
dissection 98
distance of coronary ostia to the annulus 373
distance of the left coronary ostia to the aortic annulus 35
DNA testing 203
donor age 70
Doppler 361
double patch variation 165
double valve endocarditis 223
double valve replacement 216
double-valve procedure 67
drug addicts 67
Duke diagnostic criteria 195
durability test 389, 391
– 20-year 463
– younger age group 268
dynamic anatomy 102
dynamic quantitative echocardiography 10
dystrophic AI 120
dystrophic calcification 459, 465

Subject index

E

early mortality   61
early referral of patients   268
early reoccurrence   309
early reoperation   514
Early Self-Controlled Anticoagulation Trial (ESCAT)   545
eccentric jet   122
echocardiographic assessment   350
echocardiographic follow-up   225, 516
echocardiographic investigations   224
echocardiographic studies   181, 268
echocardiography   361, 523, 588
– M-mode   3
– quantitative   10
– three-dimensional   233
– two-dimensional   233
Edmunds, criteria   452
Edwards Perimount valve   391, 392
Edwards Prima Plus stentless xenograft (EPP)   346
– contraindication   346
– overall survival   349
Edwards Sapien transcatheter valve   17
effective height, intraoperative   120
effective orifice area (EOA)   60, 314, 315, 318, 341, 366, 370, 478, 482, 557
– results   316
effective orifice area at discharge   61
effective orifice area index (EOAI)   316, 318
– chart   336
ejection fraction (EF)   524
Elan stentless valve   401, 403
Elan valve   488
elastin fragmentation   150
elective operation, mortality   114
elective replacement   516
electrical cardioversion   296
electron microscopy   559
ELISA   555
embolic complications   226, 360
embolism   297
end of systole   334
end-diastolic volumes   10
endocardial ablation   298
endocardial cryoablation   294
endocarditis   379, 445, 476, 480, 483, 503
– complication   225
– destructive form   226, 236
– left-sided   212
– native valve   224
– prosthetic   224
– right-sided   224
– treated   231
endoscopic ablation, totally   304
endoscopic method, single right unilateral   304
endothelial cells   567
endothelial surfaces, curetting   275
endothelial-mesenchymal transformation   89
end-stage liver failure   34
end-systolic volumes   10
energy loss, left ventricle   147
engineering concept   386
enzymatically decellularized matrix   560
epicardial ablation   304
equine pericardium   388
esophageal injury   296
esophageal perforation   304
Euro Heart Survery   527
European Clinical Trial   393
European Core-Valve registry   30
European Medicines Agency (EMEA)   586
European multicenter evaluation registry   29
European Union   583
EuroScore   23, 378, 399, 415
event-free life expectancy   531, 533
excellent hemodynamics   67
excessive leaflet motion   5
explantation   504
explants   480
extended infection   234
extended ischemic times   343
extra-anatomic position   373
extracardiac complication   263
extracardiac embolization   226
extracellular matrix   551
extracellular matrix protein   89
extracorporeal circulation   30

F

failure of the RVOT reconstruction   82
fatty acid alpha   470
femoral artery   26
fenestrations   134
fibrillin   150
fibrosis   150, 378
fibrotic retraction, secondary   141
fibrous structure, definite   145
first human implantation   22
fistulous communication   243
flow characteristic   394
flow dynamics   388
flow turbulence   394
fluoroscopic system   37
fluoroscopy   27, 36
focal trigger   302
Food and Drug Administration (FDA)   393, 581
Food Drug and Cosmetic Act   581
fractional shortening   397
Framingham Heart Study   291, 380
free of reoperation   69
Freedom Solo stentless   407
freehand subcoronary implantation   71
freehand subcoronary valve replacement (FAVR)   244
freestanding aortic root replacement   559
freestanding root with reimplantation   252
Freestyle bioprostheses   378
full root implantation   353
full root replacement   75
full root technique   376
function follows form   386, 387
functional tricuspid regurgitation   6

G

gastrointestinal bleeding   459, 479
gastrointestinal hemorrhage   483
gelatin-resorcine-formol (GRF)   136
gene therapy medicinal products   586
general population   531
genes mechanisms   89
geometric match   260
geometric mismatch   152, 161, 162, 265, 279
geometric orifice   13, 421
geometric orifice area (GOA)   313, 19, 323
German Federal Bureau of Population Statistics   513
German guidelines on human cell-based medicinal products   570
German Medicinal Products Act   585
German population   506
German Society of Cardiothoracic and Vascular Surgery database   506
glutaraldehyde fixed   362
governmental regulations   581
graft inclusion technique   180
graft replacement   110
granulomatous inflammation   559
greater effective orifice area   375
growth potential   74
Guidance Document   582
Guidelines for reporting mortality and morbidity   442

H

Hancock II prosthesis   470, 478
HCT/P, regulations   583
head perfusion, selective   179
heart block   298
heart failure
– congestive   219
– end-stage   403
– intractable   257
– progressive   212
heart transplantation   247, 257, 258
– orthotopic   202
heart valve   395
Hegar's dilators   116
helium   292
hemiarch   491
hemi-arch repair   188
hemiparesis   226
hemocompatibility   555
hemodialysis   498, 500
hemodialysis patients   210
hemodilution   442
hemodynamic advantages   366
hemodynamic data   402
hemodynamic deterioration   41
hemodynamic disturbance   4
hemodynamic evaluation   361
hemodynamic instability   218, 235
hemodynamic management   36

Subject index

hemodynamic performance   79, 389
hemodynamic superiority   390
hemolysis   445, 473
hemorrhage   433
hemorrhage-related death   433
hemorrhagic complications   360, 479
hemorrhagic shock   215, 460
hemostasis   185, 189, 265, 496
hepatitis virus   582
heritability   90
hi-frequency flutter   330
high risk patients   29
higher energy losses   336
higher mean pressure gradients   372
higher risk patients   516, 517
highest-risk candidates   203
highly challenging problem   204
high-risk patients   218
His bundle ablation   303
histologic characteristics   558
HIV infected patients   199
Holter monitor   296
home monitor   547
homograft   402, 532
– cryopreserved   274
horizontal aortotomy   398
hospital death, preoperative   267
hospital mortality   69, 255
hospital stay   400
hospital time   400
human aortic valve   389
human bone marrow   567
human immunodeficiency virus   582
Human Tissue Authority (HTH)   585
human tissue donors   582
human umbilical cord cells   564
human cells, tissues, and cellular and tissue based products (HCT/P)   582
hybrid procedure   505
hybrid tissue heart valves   561
hybrid valves   556
hybrid-OR   36
hypercalcemia   500
hypotension   235

I

immune response   70, 560, 565
immunosuppression   199
immune-histology   560
immunogenicity   560
immunohistology   558
impaired aortic growth   186
impaired left ventricular function   523
improper mismatch   313
Improved biocompatibility   415
improved durability   395
improving echocardiographic techniques (3D)   203
improving microbiological techniques   203
inclusion technique   347, 353
incomplete coaptation   335
increased cardiac output   326
infection
– recurrent, linearized rate   266
– resistance   268
infective endocarditis (IE)   195, 218, 484
– complex left sided   218
– contraindication   203
– diagnosis   197
– management   197
inferior vena cava   308
inflammation   567
inflammatory cell infiltration   558
inflammatory process   436
infraannular implantation   284
inheritance, autosomal dominant   90
inhospital stay   493
inotropes   41
intercommisural distances   373
intercostals space   306
interleaflet triangle   19, 104, 147, 156, 157, 368
– base   118
intermediate care   41
international Normalized Ratio (INR)   442, 453, 543
– target values   546
– self-management   541, 544, 545, 546, 547
interrupted sutures   155
interrupted Teflon pledgets   37
intertrigonal portion   158
intertrigonal running compression suture   158
inverting the valve into LVOT   410

Subject index

intraaortic balloon conterpulsation   525
intracellular signals   264
intracerebral hemorrhagic event   455
intraoperative assessment   10
intraoperative patient-prosthesis mismatch   433
intravenous drug abusers   210
irregular opening   333
ischemia   5
ischemic MVR   6
ischemic stroke   291, 460
ischemic time   400

J

jet lesion   230, 231
juvenile rheumatoid arthritis   83

K

Kaplan-Meier   425
– actuarial analysis   255
– method   474
kidney failures   234
kissing vegetation   230, 231
Konno technique   166

L

late death   397, 403, 427
late mortality   256, 447
leaflet
– high-frequency fluttering   322
leaflet cleft   5
leaflet disruption   435
leaflet flutter   330
leaflet perforation   5
leaflet prolapse   178, 351
leaflet shrinking   558
leaflet tears   435, 446, 465
leakage volume   334
learning curve   514
left anterior fibrous trigone   169
left anterolateral minithoracotomy   37
left atrial ablation   411
left atrial appendage   303
left coronary arteries   19
left coronary leaflet (LCL)   18
left coronary ostia   368
left fibrous trigones   145
left pulmonary veins   295
left scalloped sinus   280

left ventricular end diastolic pressure (LVEDP)   27
left ventricular hypertrophy   534
left ventricular mass   341, 397
left ventricular mass reduction   403, 414
left ventricular mass regression (LVMR)   307, 366, 342, 354, 428, 429
left ventricular myomectomy   169
left ventricular outflow tract (LVOT)   251, 275, 276
– obstruction   169
left ventricular reverse remodeling   406
left ventricular systolic   397
Leonardo da Vinci   104
life expectancy   506, 532
– in Germany   513
lifelong anticoagulation   449
life-long durability   565
limited life expectancy   447
linearized rate   78, 474, 483
– events   359
liver cirrhosis   200
liver failure, end stage   34
local disinfection   265
local metastases   230
local practitioners   548
localized abscess   228
loci minoris resistentiae   231
logistic EuroSCORE   23, 378, 399, 415
lone atrial fibrillation   303
long time survival, predictor   218
longest follow-up study   457
long-term anticoagulation   533
long-term durability   363, 434, 449
long-term prognosis   528
long-term results   460
long-term survival   426, 447
Lotus, Sandra   20
low cardiac output syndrome   235
low molecular heparin   42
low output syndrome   255
low reoperative rate   269
low transvalvular gradient   396
lower proximal line   276
lung function   305
lupus erythematosus   83
lyophilization   554, 557
lyophilized tissue   554

Subject index   609

M

magnet resonance imaging (MRI)   149
Magovern and Cromie Sutureless Valve   20
major bleeding events   379
Manouguian   164, 422
Manouguian procedures   166
Marcumar   543
Marfan syndrome   83
matched or oversized   153
matched valves   71
mathematic-based chart   317
matrix glycoprotein, extracellular   150
matrix metalloproteinases (MMPs)   150
Matrix P   575, 578
Matrix P plus heart valve   577, 578
matrix/polymer hybrid patches   558
mattress sutures   160, 277
– pledgeted   159
mechanical circulatory support   247, 257
mechanical heart valve replacement   548
mechanical prostheses   498, 499, 504, 532, 533, 537, 564
mechanical valves   461, 487
mechanical ventilation   30, 493
median survival time   381
mediastinistis   34
medical community awareness   203
Medical Device Directive (MDD)   584
medionecrosis   150
Medtronic Freestyle   367
meta-analysis   535
metalloproteinase release   436
metastatic abscess   248
microsimulation   533, 534, 537
minimal invasion MV surgery   297
minimal invasive aortic valve surgery   48
minimal invasive endoscopic ablation, beating heart   302
miniroot technique   348
mismatch   370
mitral leaflet, anterior   277
mitral prosthesis endocarditis   361
mitral regurgitation   5

mitral ring abscess   232
mitral valve   234, 471
mitral valve disease   3
– rheumatic   299
mitral valve endocarditis   232
mitral valve operation   291
mitral valve repair   248
mitral valve replacement (MVR)   216, 475
mitral valve surgery   225
– minimally invasive   293
Mitroflow   417
M-mode echocardiography   3
Model   11   422
Model   11   420
Model   12   422
moderate oversizing   34
molecular mechanisms   89
mortality
– by period   510
– 30-day mortality   32, 381, 443
– reoperative   514
Mosaic bioprostheses   472, 474
Mosaic porcine bioprostheses   463, 479, 480, 482
multiaxial loading   556
multiorgan failure   255
multivariate analysis   427, 443
muscular skirt, subvalvular   278
mutation   90
mycotic process   243
myocardial failure   215
– end-stage, without septicemia   267
myocardial infarction, ongoing   248
myocardial infection   358
myocardial maladaptation   528
myocardial support, aggressive   267
myofibroblast   554
myofibroblast-like cells   567

N

nadir   161
National Marfans Foundation   123
native aortic valve   393
native valve endocarditis, left-sided   219
natural leaflet structure   367
natural scaffolds   565
neopulmonary valve   79

neosinuses of Valsalva   108
neurological events   379
neurosurgeons   263
Nicks 281, 422
Nicks operation   164
Nicks procedure   254
nitrous oxide   292
no antigenicity   74
non structural valve deterioration   511
noncoronary leaflet (NCL)   18, 183
noncoronary sinus (NCS)   18
non-randomized trials   344, 470
nonstructural valve deterioration   400
nonstructural valve dysfunction   456
nonsurvivor   214
non-thrombogenic   74
nonvalve-related death   426, 456
normal leaflet motion   5
North American PARTNER Trial   52
nosocomial infections   210
NOTCH1 gene   90
NYHA class III/IV   29

O

octogenarians   32, 381, 523, 525, 527
– severe AS   526
open-button technique   494
opening configuration   324
operation, optimal time point   218
operative death   263
operative mortality   68, 358, 530
– increased risk   381
operative risk   18, 266
– profile   32
operative skin   377
operative steps   249
operative technique   409
Osler, Sir William   223, 243
osteomyelitis   224
outcomes, 30-day outcomes   29
outgrow the prostheses   564
outside-the-stent pericardial design   336
overall mortality   455
oversizing   393
– risk   371
– valve   358

P

pacemaker cables   233
pacemaker implantation   299, 303
pacemaker lead   26
papillary muscle elongation   5
paravalvular abscess   226
paravalvular leak   34, 262, 476, 480
paravalvular leakage   282, 411, 413, 456, 494
paravalvular regurgitation   8
partial sternotomy   32
partial upper sternotomy   58
patent bypass graft   34
patient characteristica   76, 398
patient selection   108
patient survival   69, 268, 400, 443, 510, 511
patient-at risk   466
patient-prosthesis mismatch   318, 435
patient-related factors   417, 536
patients under   65 years   437
patients' comorbidity   435
Paul Ehrlich Institute   585
percutaneous femoral-femoral cardiopulmonary bypass   36
percutaneous femoro-femoral by-pass   26
percutaneous transluminal aortic valve replacement   22
periannular abscesses   362
periannular structures, destruction   234
periarteritis   559
Pericarbon Freedom stentless valve   406
pericardial bioprostheses   464, 465, 466
pericardial effusion   78
pericardial patch closure   164
pericardial reconstruction   275
pericardial stay sutures   37
pericardial tissue   417
pericardial valve   329, 332, 364, 447, 484
– advantage   325
– self-expandable sutureless   17
– supraannular models   325
pericardium, drain   277
Peri-in valve   320, 323, 326, 333
Perimount pericardial valve   450

perioperative complication 528
perioperative conversion 116
perioperative imaging 3
perioperative morbidity 523
perioperative mortality 415
- overall 296
Peri-out Supra 333, 335
Peri-out valves 320, 323, 326
peripheral embolic events 351
peripheral embolization 226
perivalvular abscesses 201
perivalvular hematoma 369
permanent pacemaker 27
persistent sepsis 234
pharmaceutical legislation 571
physiologic root dynamic 109
physiological advantages 364
physiological loading 558
pigtail catheter 26
plasmatic clotting cascade 555
plasmatic coagulation system 561
plication 155
- subcommissural 156
polyhydroxyalkanoates (PHA) 553
polymer 553
polymer coating 557
polymer impregnation process 554
polymer layer 558
polymerase chain reaction 203
polymer-coated matrix 555
polymeric scaffold material 566, 568
polymerized glue emboli 186
polytetrafluoroethylene (PTFE) 487, 488
poor life expectancy 441
porcelain aorta 34, 364
porcine aortic bioprostheses 465, 466
porcine bioprostheses 452, 464
porcine stentless bioprostheses 488
porcine stentless heart valve 495
porcine valve 321, 330, 332, 336, 356
- advantage 325
- supraannular models 325
Porc-intact Supra 324
Porc-tricomp valve 335
- supra version 324
position, supine 306
postanesthetic care unit 41
posterior annuloplasty 422
posterior leaflet 18

postmortem pathological investigations 223
postoperative anticoagulation 453
postoperative atrial fibrillation 381
postoperative outcome 400
- early 298
potential for growth 578
potentially life threatening complications 299
predicted patient outcome 525, 531, 535
preoperative clinical characteristic 397
preoperative complication 247
preoperative imaging 507
preoperative NYHA status 444
preoperative risk assessment 203
pressure gradient 80
primary aortic valve replacement 426
primary cusp deterioration 459
primary tissue failure 436
primary valve failure 353
profound vasoconstriction 235
progressive annular dilatation 71
prolonged stay 381
proper match 313
prospective trial 470
3f-prosthesis 57
prosthesis mismatch 480
prosthesis of choice 503
prosthesis selection 506
prosthesis thrombosis 483
prosthesis-patient mismatch 162, 370
prosthetic endocarditis 480
prosthetic function 4
prosthetic valve 210, 245, 471
- bioprosthetic 245
- mechanical 245
prosthetic valve endocarditis (PVE) 202, 211, 455
protamine 41
proteoglycans 553
proximal isovelocity surface area (PISA) 6
proximal line sutures 278
proximal suture line 372
pseudoaneurysm 69, 263
pseudoaneurysmal formation 243
pseudosinuses 134
pulmonary allograft 264

Subject index

pulmonary autograft   67, 536, 589
pulmonary bleeding   215
pulmonary emboli   215
pulmonary homograft   535
pulmonary regurgitation   577
pulmonary stenosis   577
pulmonary valve replacement   589
purse-string suture   283
– method   160
push-and-pull technique   27

Q

quality assurance   203
quality control   571
quantification of MV regurgitation (MVR)   6

R

radial strain of anterior wall   9
radial stretch   149
radical debridement   265, 269
radiofrequency ablation (RF)   292, 294, 298, 304
radius
– inlet   148
– ridge   148
randomized clinical trials (RCTs)   342
randomized trials   344
rapid environmental changes, tolerating   264
rapid ventricular pacing   38
ratio St/aortic annular base   106
reattachment of the commissure   96
recipient   70, 583
reconstruction, biological   244
reconstructive surgery   236
recurrent bleeding   433
recurrent endocarditis   402
– hazard function   262
recurrent infection   262, 503
recurrent septic embolism   212
reduction annuloplasty   152, 157
re-endotheliazation   561
regional and global deformation   10
regional wall motion abnormalities   5
registry of birth and death   254
regulations of the EU   581
regulations of the US   581
regulatory requirements   581

regurgitant volume   335
reimplantation   108
reinfection   217, 235, 433
– low rate   268
relocation procedure   183, 588
remodeling procedure (Yacoub)   108, 135, 159
renal failure   255, 298, 358
– end-stage   498
renal transplantation   499
reoperation   68, 217, 359, 377, 401, 445, 456, 458, 459, 476
– autograft   82
– causes   258, 379
– predicting factors   260
– risk   448, 515
– technical causes   253
– valve-related   244
Replacement of Heart Valve, Guidance   453
rescue operation   71, 263
resistance to infection   67
resistant to biofilm bacterial infection   269
respiratory failure   358
respiratory infection   224
restrictive leaflet motion   5
results over
– 10 years   363
– 20 years   68
rethoracotomy   493
retrograde transfemoral implantation   37
retrospective studies   354
right atrial ablation   296
right chest cavity   307
right coronary arteries   19
right coronary leaflet (RCL)   18
right fibrous trigones   145
right Judkins catheter   38
right parasternal incision   47
right scalloped sinus   280
right sided endocarditis (RSE)   233
right ventricular outflow tract (RVOT)
risk of oversizing   371
risk stratification tools   53, 203
root abscesses   67
root distensibility   109, 141
root inclusion   375
root reconstruction   142

root repair   186
root replacement   368
- indication   249
root surgery   590
Ross operation   67, 74, 536, 575, 576, 578
- operative details   76
- technical artistry   71
Ross operation II   202
Ross procedure   156, 589
Ross registry
- German   75
- German-Dutch   75
Ross, Donald   67, 274
Ross-Konno procedure   168

S

safety net   36
scaffold materials   565
scientific basis   44
second generation   364
second suture line   371, 372
secondary prevention stroke   310
second-generation tissue valves   461
self-expandable sutureless pericardial valve   17
self-expanding nitinol external frame   57
self-management of International Normalized Ratio (INR)   541
septic emboli   234, 248
septic multiorgan failure   215
septic shock   218, 234
septicemia   481
serious disease   204
severe aortic stenosis   524
sewing ring diameter   329
Seybold-Epting   164
Sheath
- 14F   38
- 26 F transapical delivery   38
Shelhigh   211
short- and mid-term results   133
short/long axis view imaging   9
simple trigonometric function   318
sinotubular junction (STJ)   19, 181, 182, 279, 408, 409
- new   179
sinotubular junction/annulus ratio   149

sinus calcification   371
sinus configuration   140
sinus rhythm   296, 475
sinus of Valsalva   18, 390, 407
- aneurysm   243
sinus wall, noncoronary   281
sinus, noncoronary, enlarging   281
skin abscess   224
smooth muscle cells   560
society guidelines   198
Society of Thoracic Surgeons Board of Directors   54
somatic cell therapy medicinal products   586
sonographic appearance   227
sonomicrometry   105
Sorin Pericarbon Freedom stentless   414
space efficiency   313, 327, 332
spontaneous rupture   227
stable sinus rhythm   309
static cell seeding   569
statistical comparison   335
stent implantation   505
stent space efficiency   327, 328
stented bioprostheses   343, 377, 417, 533
stented bioprosthetic valve   313, 332
stented porcine   484
stentless aortic xenograft   352
stentless bioprostheses   371, 377, 532, 533, 534
stentless Freestyle valve   534
stentless porcine aortic valve   358
stentless prostheses   343, 532
stentless valve   202, 414
stentless valve bioprostheses   284
stentless valve prosthesis   211
stentless xenograft   263, 487
stentless xenograft roots   494
stent-mounted devices   364
stiffness   149
stress-strain curve   556
stroke   498, 528
- factors   380
stroke risk   35
structural valve deterioration (SVD)   348, 351, 360, 378, 400, 444, 446, 476, 500
- reoperation   382

Subject index

STS score   23
Study
- nonrandomized   220
- retrospective   220
subaortic obstructive septal hypertrophy   421
subclinical obstruction   97
subcoronary aortic valve, freehand replacement   280
subcoronary implantation (SC)   75, 82, 250, 367, 406, 535
subcoronary technique   158, 368, 376
subendothelial extracellular matrix   553
subpulmonary conal muscle skirt   168
subvalvular external aortic annuloplasty   117
subvalvular plane   118
sudden death   426
- unexplained   453
sufficient volume preload   38
supraannular implantation   421
supraannular pericardial valve   319
supraannular valve   467
- implantation   411, 471
supraanular positioning   421
supracoronary aorta   106
supracoronary replacement   183
supravalvular stenosis   284
supravalvular technique   412
surgeon's experience   36, 369
surgery   223
surgery for lone AF   310
surgery, indications   198, 398, 399, 411
surgical access   36
surgical bailout   36
surgical reexploration   78
surgical skills   534
surgical techniques   249
surpaannular stented porcine bioprostheses   470
survival advantage   363, 536, 537
survival after AVR, determinants   530
survival by age group   425
Survival rates   378
- cumulative   526
- 30 days   216
- 10-year   108, 516
- 20-year   69, 515
- 20-year cumulative   516
suture line
- distal   252
- lower (proximal)   251, 252
sutureless valve implantation   62
sutures
- continuous running   253
- lower line   276
syndrome, low output   255
SynerGraft   574, 589
synthetic biodegradable polymers   566
synthetic matrices   566
synthetic scaffolds   574
systemic embolization   186
systolic anterior motion   7
systolic ejection   315
systolic pressure above 120 mmHg   38

T

table of GOA   335
tale of the ring   102
technology, three-dimensional   233
telemedicine   544
telemetric surveillance   42
telephone interview   254
temporary blood   493
temporary dialysis   493
temporary pacemaker   27
tetralogy of Fallot   151
TGF-β signaling   150
therapy-resistant septic infection   212
thermomechanical properties   555
thoracic computer tomography (CT)   507
thoracotomy   30
thromboembolic complication   424, 588, 542
thromboembolic events   351
thromboembolism   434, 445, 456, 457, 476
thromboplastin time   542
thrombotic occlusion   478
tissue bonding   187
tissue engineered heart valves   570
tissue engineered pulmonary valves   576
tissue engineering   551, 555, 564, 590
tissue failure   68

Subject index | 615

tissue viability   70
tissue-engineered heart valve   436
tonsillitis   224
tooth extraction   224
topographic anatomy of the aortic valve leaflet   13
Toronto SPV valve   392
total regurgitant volume   334
total root technique   377
toxicity   186
tranesophageal echocardiography   305
transapical abortive valve implantation   32
transapical approach   7, 35
transapical valve-in-valve implantation   17
transcatheter aortic valve implantation   7, 33, 589
transcatheter valve-in-valve aortic valve implantation   589
transcatheter-based beating heart procedure   53
transcription factors   89
transesophageal echocardiography (TEE)   3
transfemoral access   33
transforming growth factor (TGF)β 150
transient ischemic   459
transmural lesion   294
transprosthetic gradients   369
transthoracic echocardiography   28, 494
trans-valvular flow dynamic   394
transvalvular gradients   60, 352, 361, 366, 374, 423, 482, 494
transvalvular pressure gradients at discharge   370
transvalvular regurgitation   477
transverse aortotomy   407
transverse sinus   308
treatment of AIE   218
triclopidine   347
tricuspid valve   234
tricuspid valve annulus   296
tricuspid valve reconstruction   246
trileaflet structure   104
Triplex Valsalva vascular graft   487
trivial pulmonary regurgitation   577
Trojan horse   74

truncated cone   148
tunnel-like subaortic stenosis   167
tunnel-type left ventricular outflow, reconstruction   264
turbulence   389
tutorial guidance   283
two apical purse-string sutures   37
two-dimensional area   314
type A dissection, acute   183

U

U stitches   118
ultrasonic micrometric transceiver-receiver crystal   141
umbilical cord   567
umbilical cord cells   568
undersized allograft   70
undersized valves   71
unexplained death   481, 482
Unimpeded laminar blood flow   420
United Kingdom (UK)   585
United States Food and Drug Administration (USFDA)
– approval   393, 581
univariate analysis   427

V

vale-sparing   142
Valsalva graft   109
valve, oversizing   358
valve coaptation   106
valve conduits, biological   284
valve deterioration
– nonstructural   261
– structural   259
– – age group   259
valve failure, mechanism   397
valve migration   29
valve related morbidity, linearized rated   379
valve related adverse event   477, 484
valve replacement   500
valve sparing, evolution   126
valve sparing procedures   112
valve specific risk factor   542
valve stenosis   446
valve testing   557
valve thrombosis   360

valve-in-valve implantation 8, 509, 517
– transapical of pump 510
valve-preserving technique 134
valve-related adverse events 348
valve-related complication 359, 444, 449, 452, 473, 500, 515, 531, 536, 541
valve-related death 404, 444, 454, 481
valve-related events 357, 530
valve-related morbidity 107, 382
valve-related mortality 349, 458
valve-related reoperations 136
valve-sparing operation 160, 588
valve-sparing procedure 157, 161
valvular endocarditis 360
valvular reconstruction 4
valvular regurgitation 8
valvuloplasty balloon, 20mm 38
vascular graft 140
vascular smooth muscle cells (VSMCs) 151
– apoptosis 151
vascular strictures 186
vasodilatory shock 235

Vasutek Elan aortic stentless bioprosthesis 396
velocity time curve 315
velocity-time integral (VTI) 314
ventricular aneurysme 5
ventricular assist device 525
ventricular hypertrophy 437
ventricular junction 162
ventricular outflow tract, left 160, 244
ventricular septum 170, 245
ventricular septum defect, closure 248
ventriculoaortic dehiscence 246
ventriculoarterial junction 146, 148
In vitro pulse duplication 322

W

warfarin 296, 309
warfarin therapy 421
wire handling 36
women of child-bearing age 417
wound healing 224